SCIENCE-BASED THERAPY

This is the first book to analyze empirically supported treatments by using the newest criteria from the *American Psychological Association*'s Society of Clinical Psychology, Division 12. Clinicians, scholars, and students all need to stay updated on the treatment research, and this book goes beyond providing updated treatment information by pointing readers to other useful treatment manuals and websites for continuing to stay up to date. The chapters, all written by prominent experts, highlight the best available evidence for specific disorders by breaking treatments down into credible components. With an emphasis on treatments for adults, chapters also share information about treatments for youth. Other variables that influence treatment are discussed, including assessment, comorbidity, demographics, and medication. Each chapter also corresponds with a chapter in the companion book, *Pseudoscience in Therapy*, presenting a full picture of the evidence base for common treatments.

STEPHEN HUPP is a professor, psychologist, author, and editor of the magazine *Skeptical Inquirer*. He has received the Great Teacher Award and the Champion for Diversity Award from Southern Illinois University Edwardsville, and holds a Guinness World Record for the "longest line of books."

DAVID F. TOLIN is the author of more than 200 scientific journal articles and several books, including *Doing CBT*. He has received the Award for Distinguished Contribution to the Science of Psychology, the Award for Distinguished Contribution to the Practice of Psychology, and the Award for Lifetime Contribution to Psychology from the Connecticut Psychological Association. He is the past-president of the Association for Behavioral and Cognitive Therapies, and past-president of the Clinical Psychology Division of the American Psychological Association.

T0372786

Other Books in this Series

- *Pseudoscience in Therapy: A Skeptical Field Guide*
- *Pseudoscience in Child and Adolescent Psychotherapy: A Skeptical Field Guide*
- *Child and Adolescent Psychotherapy: Components of Evidence-Based Treatments for Youth and Their Parents* (a second edition is forthcoming with the revised title, Science-Based Therapy for Children and Adolescents)

Other Books by Stephen Hupp

- *Investigating Clinical Psychology: Pseudoscience, Fringe Science, and Controversies*
- *Investigating School Psychology: Pseudoscience, Fringe Science, and Controversies*
- *Investigating Pop Psychology: Pseudoscience, Fringe Science, and Controversies*
- *Thinking Critically about Child Development: Examining Myths and Misunderstandings*
- *Great Myths of Child Development*
- *Great Myths of Adolescence*
- *Dr. Huckleberry's True or Malarkey? Superhuman Abilities*

Other Books by David F. Tolin

- *Doing CBT: A Comprehensive Guide to Working with Behaviors, Thoughts, and Emotions*
- *The Oxford Handbook of Obsessive-Compulsive and Related Disorders*
- *The Big Book of Exposures: Innovative, Creative, and Effective CBT-Based Exposures for Treating Anxiety-Related Disorders*
- *CBT for Hoarding Disorder: A Group Therapy Program Workbook*
- *Treating Trichotillomania: Cognitive-Behavioral Therapy for Hairpulling and Related Problems*
- *Face Your Fears: A Proven Plan to Beat Anxiety, Panic, Phobias, and Obsessions*
- *Buried in Treasures: Help for Compulsive Acquiring, Saving, and Hoarding*

SCIENCE-BASED THERAPY

Raising the Bar for Empirically Supported Treatments

Edited by

Stephen Hupp
Southern Illinois University Edwardsville

David F. Tolin
Institute of Living

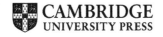

CAMBRIDGE
UNIVERSITY PRESS

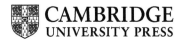

CAMBRIDGE
UNIVERSITY PRESS

Shaftesbury Road, Cambridge CB2 8EA, United Kingdom

One Liberty Plaza, 20th Floor, New York, NY 10006, USA

477 Williamstown Road, Port Melbourne, VIC 3207, Australia

314–321, 3rd Floor, Plot 3, Splendor Forum, Jasola District Centre,
New Delhi – 110025, India

103 Penang Road, #05–06/07, Visioncrest Commercial, Singapore 238467

Cambridge University Press is part of Cambridge University Press & Assessment,
a department of the University of Cambridge.

We share the University's mission to contribute to society through the pursuit of
education, learning and research at the highest international levels of excellence.

www.cambridge.org
Information on this title: www.cambridge.org/9781316514566

DOI: 10.1017/9781009086264

First published 2024

A catalogue record for this publication is available from the British Library.

Library of Congress Cataloging-in-Publication Data
Names: Tolin, David F., editor. | Hupp, Stephen, editor.
Title: Science-based therapy : raising the bar for empirically supported treatments / edited by David F.
Tolin, Southern Illinois University, Edwardsville, Stephen Hupp, Institute of Living.
Description: New York : Cambridge University Press, [2024] | Includes bibliographical references and
index.
Identifiers: LCCN 2024000815 | ISBN 9781316514566 (hardback) | ISBN 9781009087940 (paperback) |
ISBN 9781009086264 (ebook)
Subjects: LCSH: Evidence-based psychotherapy. | Mental illness – Treatment.
Classification: LCC RC455.2.E94 S35 2024 | DDC 616.89/14–dc23/eng/20240208
LC record available at https://lccn.loc.gov/2024000815

ISBN 978-1-316-51456-6 Hardback
ISBN 978-1-009-08794-0 Paperback

To my son, Henry Thomas Hupp – I'm proud of everything you do. (S. H.)
To Fiona, James, and Katie, with love and thanks. (D. T.)

Contents

Tables

Contributors

Damla E. Aksen is a clinical psychology doctoral student at SUNY Binghamton University (SUNY). Her research focuses on working memory, emotion dysregulation, dissociation, and impulsivity.

Erin F. Reto received her doctorate from Binghamton University, State University of New York. Her research on intimate partner violence led to a well-regarded review article in the journal *Trauma, Violence, & Abuse*.

Monica Ramirez Basco is a clinical psychologist and founding fellow of the Academy of Cognitive Therapy. She is author of the book *The Bipolar Workbook: Tools for Controlling Your Mood Swings, Second Edition*.

Jennifer A. Battles is a primary care clinical psychologist and a member of the Interdisciplinary Eating Disorder Team at the VA St. Louis Healthcare System.

Brooke L. Bennett is an assistant professor at Clemson University.

Cassandra L. Boness is a licensed clinical psychologist and a research assistant professor at the University of New Mexico Center on Alcohol, Substance use, And Addictions (CASAA). Dr. Boness' expertise is related to the etiology, assessment, and treatment of substance use disorder.

Kirsten Bootes is a doctoral student in clinical psychology at the University of Utah.

Emily Braley is a doctoral student in clinical psychology at the University of Utah.

Jennifer Brasch is the lead for addiction psychiatry at St. Joseph's Healthcare Hamilton and Associate Professor in the Department of Psychiatry and Behavioural Neurosciences at McMaster University. Dr. Brasch is the past president of the Canadian Society of Addiction Medicine.

Alfiee Breland-Noble is the founder of the mental health nonprofit The AAKOMA Project, which focuses on improving the mental health needs of intersectional Youth of Color via research, outreach, and media. Dr. Breland-Noble is the editor of the book *Community Mental Health Engagement with Racially Diverse Populations*.

Colleen Carney is a professor of psychology at Toronto Metropolitan University. Dr. Carney is author of the book *Goodnight Mind: Turn off Your Noisy Thoughts & Get a Good Night's Sleep*.

Frank R. Cicero is an associate professor and program director for the behavior analysis programs at Seton Hall University, New Jersey. He has published works in the fields of behavior analysis and autism over the past several decades.

Laura Nelson Darling is a doctoral student of clinical psychology at Boston University. Her research and clinical work centers on evidence-based treatments for anxiety and related disorders.

Claudia Drossel is an associate professor of psychology at Eastern Michigan University. She is coeditor of the book *Applications of Behavior Analysis in Healthcare and Beyond*.

Brandon A. Gaudiano is a professor in the Department of Psychiatry and Human Behavior at the Warren Alpert Medical School of Brown University and in the Department of Behavioral and Social Sciences at the School of Public Health. He is also director of the Transitional Outpatient Program at Butler Hospital, and a research psychologist at the Providence VA Medical Center.

Michael B. Himle is an associate professor of psychology at the University of Utah, where he teaches and conducts research on tic disorders.

Danae L. Hudson is a professor of psychology at Missouri State University. She is coauthor of the books *Revel Psychology 1st edition* and *Psychological Disorders: A Scientist-Practitioner Approach, 5th edition.*

Stephen Hupp is a professor of psychology at Southern Illinois University Edwardsville. He is editor of the book *Investigating Clinical Psychology* and editor of *Skeptical Inquirer: The Magazine for Science and Reason.*

Matthew D. Johnson is a professor of psychology and director of the clinical psychology PhD program at Binghamton University, State University of New York. He is the author of *Great Myths of Intimate Relationships: Dating, Sex, and Marriage.*

Christie P. Karpiak is Professor of Psychology and Department Chair at the University of Scranton. She is also a child clinical psychologist in part-time practice.

Parky Lau is a doctoral student in clinical psychology at Toronto Metropolitan University.

Kristine Lee is a doctoral student of clinical psychology at Boston University. Her research interests focus on increasing access to evidence-based treatments, specifically for marginalized youth of color.

Jamie M. Loor is a postdoctoral research fellow at the University of New Mexico Health Sciences Center with the Center for Healthcare Equity in Kidney Disease.

Andrew B. Lumb is a clinical and health psychologist in the Transitional Aged Youth Service, Substance Use and Concurrent Disorders Program at the Royal Ottawa Mental Health Centre and a faculty member in the School of Psychology of the University of Ottawa.

Amy D. Lykins is an associate professor of clinical psychology at the University of New England in New South Wales, Australia. She is a consulting editor for the *Journal of Sex Research* and coeditor of the book series Critical Topics in Sexuality Research.

Steven Jay Lynn is Distinguished Professor at Binghamton University (SUNY). He is coeditor of the book *Science and Pseudoscience in Clinical Psychology* and coauthor of *50 Great Myths of Popular Psychology: Shattering Widespread Misconceptions of Human Behavior.*

James MacKillop holds the Peter Boris Chair in Addictions Research and a Tier 1 Canada Research Chair in Translational Addiction Research, and is Professor of Psychiatry and Behavioural Neurosciences at McMaster University. Dr. MacKillop directs the Peter Boris Centre for Addictions Research and the Michael G. DeGroote Centre for Medicinal Cannabis Research at McMaster and St. Joseph's Healthcare Hamilton.

Onkar Marway is a doctoral student in clinical psychology at Toronto Metropolitan University.

Dean McKay is a professor of psychology at Fordham University. He is coeditor of the book *Complexities in Obsessive Compulsive and Related Disorders: Advances in Conceptualization and Treatment.*

Carmen P. McLean is a clinical psychologist at the National Center for PTSD, Dissemination and Training Division at the Palo Alto VA Health Care System and a clinical professor (affiliated) in the Department of Psychiatry and Behavioral Sciences, Stanford University.

John R. McQuaid is Chief of Psychology at the Palo Alto VA Health Care System and a vice chair in the Department of Psychiatry and Behavioral Sciences, Weill Center for Neuroscience, University of California, San Francisco. He served as cochampion for the VA/DoD Clinical Practice Guidelines for Major Depression.

Marta Meana is a professor of psychology at the University of Las Vegas. She is past president of the Society for Sex Therapy and Research, associate editor of the *Journal of Sex Research*, and was an advisor to the DSM-5 Sexual Dysfunctions Workgroup.

John C. Norcross is Distinguished Professor of Psychology at the University of Scranton and Clinical Professor of Psychiatry at SUNY Upstate Medical University. He is author of numerous books, including the third edition of *Psychotherapy Relationships That Work.*

John Otis is a research associate professor at Boston University. He is the author of the treatment manual *Managing Chronic Pain.*

Joel Paris is an emeritus professor of psychiatry at McGill University in Canada. He is author of the book *Treatment of Borderline Personality Disorder: A Guide to Evidence-Based Practice, Second Edition.*

Devon L. L. Polaschek is a professor of psychology at the University of Waikato. She is coeditor of *The Wiley International Handbook of Correctional Psychology.*

Eve A. Rosenfeld is an advanced postdoctoral fellow at the National Center for PTSD, Dissemination and Training Division at the VA Palo Alto Health Care System and at the Department of Psychiatry and Behavioral Sciences, Stanford University

Mary V. Solanto is Professor of Pediatrics and Psychiatry at Hofstra-Northwell School of Medicine, New York. She authored *Cognitive-Behavioral Treatment for Adult ADHD: Targeting Executive Dysfunction*, a treatment manual for clinicians.

Victoria E. Stead is a psychologist with the Young Adult Substance Use Program within the Concurrent Disorders Outpatient Service at St. Joseph's Healthcare Hamilton and an assistant professor (part-time) in the Department of Psychiatry and Behavioural Neurosciences at McMaster University.

Elizabeth Thompson is a clinical psychologist and an assistant professor of psychiatry and human behavior at the Warren Alpert Medical School of Brown University. She also is a research scientist and staff psychologist at Rhode Island and Bradley Hospitals.

David F. Tolin is the founder and director of the Anxiety Disorders Center at the Institute of Living and an adjunct professor of psychiatry at Yale University School of Medicine. He also maintains a private clinical and consulting practice.

Katherine Visser is a clinical psychologist and a clinical assistant professor of psychiatry and human behavior at the Warren Alpert Medical School of Brown University. She is also a staff psychologist with the Lifespan Physician Group in Providence, RI.

Madeline Ward is a clinical psychology doctoral student at Case Western Reserve University.

Brooke L. Whisenhunt is a professor of psychology at Missouri State University. She is coauthor of the books *Revel Psychology 1st edition* and *Psychological Disorders: A Scientist-Practitioner Approach, 5th edition.*

Preface

I attended graduate school in the 1990s when the movement to define and identify empirically supported treatments (ESTs) was really starting to take off. I fully embraced the model then, as I do today, because I was already concerned about some clinical practices that were commonly used despite research demonstrating they were ineffective and sometimes even harmful. In fact, my concern about pseudoscience in clinical psychology has grown stronger every year, leading me to publish books about great myths, fringe science, and critical thinking. Those books ultimately led to my recent role as the editor of *Skeptical Inquirer: The Magazine for Science and Reason*.

The use of pseudoscience in clinical psychology is especially perplexing when considered in the context of the large and growing number of available ESTs (see the Postscript to this book for a summary). When a task force from the American Psychological Association first defined well-established ESTs, they intentionally set the bar at a somewhat rigorous but also achievable level. Over the course of three decades, many treatments reached this bar and set a firm foundation for new developments and research endeavors.

It's now time to raise that bar. Even though it was set at a reasonable level, given the state of the literature three decades ago, the field has advanced tremendously. I sought out David Tolin – former president of the Association for Behavioral and Cognitive Therapies – as coeditor of this book because he's helped lead the movement toward setting a higher bar, colloquially referred to as the "Tolin criteria" – a term that I can't help but use even though he's modestly shared he doesn't love it. To be clear, the Tolin criteria were created by a team including scholars such as Dean McKay, Evan Forman, David Klonsky, and Brett Thombs, and greatly influenced by others such as Cassandra Boness, Scott Lilienfeld, Steven Jay Lynn, Daniel David, and Guy Montgomery. The biggest influencer of all was Dianne Chambless, who led the initial task force comprised of a similarly impressive group of clinicians and scholars in wisely (and bravely) setting the initial bar for ESTs. The development of the "Chambless criteria" was a giant leap forward for science-based therapies.

The Tolin criteria are meant to supplement, not supplant, the Chambless criteria, and both models are well represented in this book. The Society of Clinical Psychology (SCP), through their website (www.psychologicaltreatments.org), has been cataloging well-established ESTs based on the Chambless criteria for many years. To date, however, only a small number of treatments have been evaluated using the Tolin criteria, and I'm aware of only a small number of future planned reviews using the Tolin criteria. Thus, now is the time for more people to help us raise the bar by doing more reviews, and if you would like to review a particular treatment for a particular disorder, then please read the Postscript to this book for what to do next.

As you read through the chapters of this book, you'll get a better understanding for which treatments have the most research support. The chapters are written through the combined lenses of the Chambless criteria and the Tolin criteria, with an emphasis on high-quality research, systematic reviews, and credible components (or processes) of ESTs.

Focus and Structure

This book focuses on therapy with adults, while another book in this series (Child and Adolescent Psychotherapy [the forthcoming second edition will be titled Science-Based Therapy for Children and Adolescents]) focuses on therapy with youth. Chapter 1 defines ESTs, evidence-based practice, and science-based therapy. The chapters that follow focus on diagnoses and issues that are commonly the focus of clinical attention in an order that is generally consistent with how they appear in the *Diagnostic and Statistical Manual of Mental Disorders, Fifth Edition, Text Revision*. Almost all of the chapters include these sections:

- description of disorder(s) of focus
- etiology and theoretical underpinnings of treatment
- brief overview of treatments
- credible components of treatments
- approaches for youth
- other variables influencing treatment (i.e., assessment and diagnosis, comorbidity, demographics, and medication)
- conclusion

Expert Contributors

The chapters are written by both clinicians and researchers, the majority of whom are licensed psychologists who also engage in publishing university-based research. Several chapter authors have published books or edited journals related to the focus of their chapter. Some chapters are authored by just one scholar, while others represent collaborative efforts of multiple authors, sometimes including doctoral students – the next generation of clinicians and researchers. In sum, all of the authors are champions for the science of clinical psychology.

Target Audience

The goal of this book is to be a handy reference for all therapists, including psychologists, counselors, social workers, psychiatrists, and professionals in related disciplines. Relatedly, it may serve as a primary text for graduate courses in therapy and counseling. By covering the same broad topics, it works well in tandem with another book in this series: *Pseudoscience in Therapy*.

Stephen Hupp

Acknowledgments

We would like to thank everyone who contributed to the scholarship of ESTs, with special gratitude in particular to the late Dianne Chambless for leading the way. Sadly, Steven Jay Lynn died just a few months prior to publication. His contributions to critical thinking about therapy cannot be overstated, and we are so thankful that he generously co-authored a chapter in this book. We're also very thankful to the chapter authors, who worked diligently to summarize a large body of research in a small amount of time. Everyone at Cambridge University Press has been extremely helpful from beginning to end, and we're especially grateful to Stephen Acerra, who helped shape all of the books in this series. Also, Rowan Groat always had an answer when we needed one. As a project manager, Giridharan Gunasekaran expertly guided us through the final stages of production with considerable help from Helen B. Cooper (copy-editor), Laheba Alam (content manager), and Carol Bailey (indexer).

1

What Is Science-Based Therapy?

David F. Tolin and Stephen Hupp

For much of its history, psychotherapy was not particularly amenable to scientific inquiry. The psychoanalysis developed by Sigmund Freud (1933/1965), which set the stage for the development of more modern psychotherapeutic interventions, proposed several nonfalsifiable constructs, had rather nebulous aims, and was comprised largely of procedures that were difficult to operationalize (see Paniagua, 1987, for review; but see also Westen, 1998, for a counterargument). More contemporary psychodynamic therapies have resolved many (though not all) of these issues, and the past four decades have witnessed an increase in both the quantity and the quality of clinical trials of psychodynamic therapy (Thoma et al., 2012). In reaction to the untestable claims of Freud's psychoanalysis, science-based approaches began to emerge, and they focused on examining testable hypotheses.

For better or for worse, the origins of psychoanalysis were in the clinic, not in the laboratory. As such, psychoanalysis was based on clinical observations of patients, rather than on scientifically demonstrable processes of behavior, thought, and emotion. The first wave of one science-based approach to therapy development began with the early behaviorists, who developed their procedures based on laboratory science with animal and human subjects. Joseph Wolpe (1961) developed systematic desensitization based on earlier studies of classical fear conditioning (Watson & Watson, 1921). Soon thereafter, operant conditioning processes, which had been well established in animals and humans (Skinner, 1953), were used to create strategies such as token economies for patients with chronic mental illness (Ayllon & Azrin, 1968). These early practices served as proof of concept that laboratory science could be used to develop strategies to help patients suffering from psychological problems.

Shortly after the development of behavioral interventions, a second wave of this science-based approach, comprised of cognitive strategies (e.g., Beck, 1976; Meichenbaum, 1977), led to the development of what is now called cognitive-behavioral therapy (CBT). Of note, following Freud's tradition, cognitive interventions came largely from clinical observations, though some research at the time pointed toward the presence of dysfunctional, conscious cognitive processes in

1

patients that presumably could be addressed by this new form of therapy (Beck, 1963). Perhaps most importantly, CBT was based on procedures that could be operationalized and replicated, and targeted outcomes that could be measured, and it was predicated on purported mechanisms that could be examined scientifically. Thus, psychotherapy, like other aspects of health care, could readily be studied from a scientific perspective, as was done in early trials of CBT for depression (e.g., Blackburn et al., 1981; Rush et al., 1977). And studied it was, with a massive surge in research demonstrating the efficacy of CBT for depression, anxiety disorders, substance use disorders, and a slew of other problems. Under the broad umbrella of CBT, we are now seeing what has been called a "third wave," in which some of the cognitive elements are de-emphasized in favor of strategies such as acceptance and mindfulness. Dialectical behavioral therapy (Linehan, 1993), acceptance and commitment therapy (Hayes et al., 1999), and mindfulness-based stress reduction (Kabat-Zinn et al., 1985) are but a few examples of these interventions. Some have called the idea of a third wave into question, pointing out that in many respects these treatments resemble the first wave of behavioral therapies (e.g., Hofmann & Asmundson, 2008).

We do wish to be clear, however, that calling a treatment "science-based" does not necessarily mean that it must be CBT, nor can we safely assume that any new CBT is automatically based on scientific evidence (for example, see O'Donahue, Snipes, & Soto, 2016, for a critique of the scientific integrity of "third-wave" approaches). The developers of any psychological treatment, regardless of its theoretical origins, must demonstrate that their treatment works, for whom and how well it works, as well as why it works. This leads us to review several key terms: *empirically supported treatments*, *evidence-based practice*, and *science-based therapy* (the term we favor in this book).

Identifying Treatments that Work

Empirically Supported Treatment

The term "empirically supported treatment" (EST) became popular in clinical psychology when the Society of Clinical Psychology (SCP) (Division 12 of the American Psychological Association) first published criteria for what were initially termed "empirically validated psychological treatments" (Task Force on Promotion and Dissemination of Psychological Procedures, 1993) and later termed "empirically supported psychological treatments" (Chambless & Hollon, 1998; Chambless & Ollendick, 2001). In this framework, sometimes referred to as the "Chambless criteria," a treatment was characterized as being *well-established* (also called "strong research support") if it meets *both* of these basic criteria:

1. At least two well-done randomized control trials (RCTs) demonstrate the treatment group has greater symptom reduction than an active comparison group or a placebo group.

2. And at least two of these RCTs are conducted by at least two different research teams.

Alternatively, a treatment could be characterized as *probably efficacious* (also called "modest research support") if it meets *either* of these basic criteria:

1. At least one well-done RCT demonstrates the treatment group has greater symptom reduction than an active comparison group or a placebo group.
2. Or at least two well-done RCTs demonstrate the treatment group has greater symptom reduction than a control group. In this case the control group does not need to include an active comparison group or a placebo. Also, the two RCTs do not need to be from different research teams for this criterion.

Within this framework, a large number of treatment approaches have been identified as being well established, and many treatments are also probably efficacious. Most chapters in this book will identify the current level of support for the treatments being discussed. For adult patients, the best place to keep up-to-date on the status of ESTs is the website for the Society of Clinical Psychology (www.psychologicaltreatments.org). For youth, the website for the Society of Clinical Child and Adolescent Psychology (www.effectivechildtherapy.org) provides updated information (that resource uses the term "works well" for well-established treatments and "works" for probably efficacious treatments). However, it is important to note that changes in the way we identify ESTs are currently underway.

The initial criteria for ESTs were criticized for setting a low bar for efficacy and failing to account for mixed findings (Borkovec & Castonguay, 1998; Henry, 1998; Herbert, 2003), relying solely on symptom reduction over functional outcomes and quality of life (Cowen, 1991; Hayes, 2004; Seligman, 1995), and failing to account for variations in the internal validity and degree of research bias in clinical trials (Luborsky et al., 1999; Wachtel, 2010). In response to these concerns, the Society of Clinical Psychology updated their EST requirements (Tolin et al., 2015) to include broad and inclusive reviews of the scientific literature, taking methodological quality of the study into account and allowing for a multitude of outcomes.

The updated EST requirements suggested by Tolin et al. (2015), sometimes referred to as the "Tolin criteria," emphasize the role of high-quality evidence in the form of systematic reviews comprised of a wide range of well-done studies with consistent results. Based on this type of evidence, for a treatment to be provided a *very strong recommendation* it must meet *all* of the following criteria:

1. The treatment results in clinically meaningful symptom reduction.
2. The treatment results in clinically meaningful functional outcome improvement.
3. Symptom reduction and/or functional outcome improvement last at least three months once the treatment has ended.
4. At least one well-done study demonstrates a clinically meaningful effect in a nonresearch setting.

Alternatively, a treatment can be given a *strong recommendation* (as opposed to the aforementioned "very strong" recommendation) based on moderate- to high-quality evidence from systematic reviews and *at least one* of the following criteria:

1. The treatment results in clinically meaningful symptom reduction.
2. And/or the treatment results in clinically meaningful functional outcome improvement.

Overall, these updated criteria raise the bar for providing a recommendation about which treatments have adequate research support. Rather than relying on only two (possibly cherry-picked) studies, the revised criteria now require that *all* of the available evidence on a given treatment's effects be taken into account, not only those studies that are favorable to the treatment. Rather than relying on posttreatment symptom reduction alone, the revised criteria now highlight the importance of functional improvement and longer-term outcomes. And, finally, the effectiveness of a therapy in a "front-line" clinical setting is considered. To date, only a handful of treatments have been evaluated within this framework (see the Postscript for an overall summary).

Evidence-Based Practice

Work on ESTs was an important catalyst for an increased emphasis on *evidence-based practice* (EBP). EBP is a broad template of activities that include assessment, case formulation, relationship factors, and treatment decisions that are hoped to assist the clinician to achieve the best possible outcome. In 2006, a Presidential Task Force of the American Psychological Association (APA Presidential Task Force on Evidence-Based Practice, 2006) adapted the Institute of Medicine's (2001) definition of evidence-based medicine, defining EBP as practice that integrates three sources of information: patient characteristics, clinical expertise, and the best available research evidence. It is unclear as to whether EBP represents a step forward or a step backward from the EST movement. The emphasis not only on science but also on patient characteristics and clinical expertise seems intuitively logical, and it's hard to argue that these other factors *shouldn't* be taken into consideration. On the other hand, it is not clear, in this "three-legged stool" model, whether each leg of the stool should be weighted equally. What should a clinician do, for example, when the best scientific evidence points to exposure with response prevention for obsessive-compulsive disorder, yet the clinician's patient differs from the RCT participants in important ways and the clinician's expertise is in another aspect of therapy? Should the scientific findings be thrown out? One possible solution is to give priority to scientific research, with clinician expertise and patient characteristics serving as "filters" through which the research must pass (Tolin, 2012). However, that has not been codified into the EBP definition used by the American Psychological Association

(APA), and at present the term "evidence-based" has been used (and misused) so often that we fear its meaning has been degraded.

Science-Based Therapy

In this book, we're going to use the term "science-based therapy," which overlaps with the Chambless and Tolin criteria for ESTs and the more recent conceptualization of EBP. Although the Chambless criteria were silent on the ingredients of treatment (that is, the question at hand was simply whether or not a treatment worked), the Tolin criteria did note that the ingredients and mechanisms of therapy were also important:

> The Task Force may take into account the purported mechanism or active ingredient(s) of treatment, and may upgrade or downgrade the recommendation based on the quality of evidence supporting that mechanism or ingredient(s). It is conceptually difficult to standardize this consideration into the criteria, as admittedly the mechanisms of many efficacious treatments are unclear. However, to the extent that a given treatment is based on a specific purported mechanism, or relies strongly on a particular treatment ingredient, the [reviewers] can and should consider whether those assertions are supported.
>
> (Tolin et al., 2015, p. 331)

This added emphasis on not only *whether* a treatment works, but also *why* it works, represented a step forward in the EST movement, pointing toward what would later be termed "science-based practice." That term, proposed by Lilienfeld et al. (2018), denotes that "treatment outcome data are considered along with broader research evidence bearing on the *plausibility of the treatment's theoretical rationale* when evaluating an intervention's scientific status" (p. 44; italics added). Thus, science-based practice extends the idea of ESTs by focusing not just on outcomes but also on whether the treatment is based on mechanisms of change that are scientifically credible. Here, in addition to RCTs comparing a treatment to a control condition, dismantling studies become critical, in which elements of the treatment are systematically withdrawn to test whether those elements are indeed responsible for the clinical outcomes. Rosen and Davison (2003) illustrated the idea with a tongue-in-cheek description of "purple hat therapy," in which a practitioner uses well-established CBT principles while the patient also wears a purple hat, and then mistakenly attributes the patient's successful outcome to the purple hat, later packaging and selling this "new" therapy. In case you think this was just for laughs, consider for a moment the promulgation of what have been called "energy" therapies, in which noncredible (in our opinion) elements such as acupressure point tapping have been added to traditional elements of CBT, and are currently being marketed as "evidence-based" new treatments.

We had purple hat therapy firmly in mind as we compiled this book. We want you, the reader, to understand not only *what* treatments work for given psychological problems, but also *why* they work. Hence, we strove to eliminate therapeutic "filler."

> **Box 1.1 Pseudoscience-Based Therapy**
>
> Many of the components used in the so-called energy therapies can be characterized as *pseudoscience*. That is, saying that acupressure point tapping is evidence-based, when in fact no rigorous research supports this claim, represents the dissemination of false information under the cover of scientific-sounding language. Energy therapies are commonly used for anxiety- and trauma-based disorders, but pseudoscience abounds for just about every other type of disorder as well. Some of the more outrageous treatments include bee-sting therapy for depressive disorders, dolphin-assisted therapy for neurodevelopmental disorders, and homeopathy for just about every mental health affliction that ails you. In fact, there are so many dubious therapeutic approaches that two books in this series focus solely on the topic. The book *Pseudoscience in Therapy* (Hupp & Santa Maria, 2019) critiques dubious treatments for adults, and the clinical topics are covered in the same order they are covered in this book, making the two books great companions. Further, the book *Pseudoscience in Child and Adolescent Psychotherapy* (Hupp, 2019) critiques dubious treatments for youth.

We challenged our chapter authors to name the specific and credible ingredients of effective treatments, and to produce evidence showing why those ingredients are effective. Of course, we recognize that not every ingredient in therapy will have solid evidence from dismantling research. But, in the absence of such evidence, we should at least expect that there will be a scientific reason why these ingredients should be credible. That is, how well do these therapy ingredients match up with what is currently known about the brain and behavior? Elements such as acupressure tapping are disconnected from current scientific understanding of psychological processes, and as such lack credibility (let alone evidence). To be sure, we aren't saying that such things *can't* work, but we should remain skeptical until we see compelling evidence that they *do* work. And when an ingredient is credible yet unsupported, that should serve as a call for researchers to investigate.

Conclusion

Over the last few decades, the Society for Clinical Psychology has led the way in conceptualizing and identifying ESTs. Most, but not all, of these treatments tend to be from the behavioral and cognitive traditions, though it need not be so. The conceptualization of ESTs is continuing to evolve, and previously identified ESTs are just now starting to get reassessed using the newer science-based criteria that place a greater emphasis on systematic reviews, functional outcomes, lasting effects, and credible active ingredients.

We would argue that science-based therapy is not merely an academic issue, but also an ethical issue. That is, the ethical practice of psychological therapy is based on science. Patients receiving any form of health care have a right to expect that their provider will be aware of, understand, and apply the best available science to their condition. Behavioral health should be no different. The American Psychological Association's ethical guidelines state "Psychologists' work is based upon established scientific and professional knowledge of the discipline" (American Psychological Association, 2017, p. 5), though we note that the ethics code is silent on what constitutes "scientific and professional knowledge." We would take this a step further by suggesting that our patients have the right not only to receive treatments based on the best available science, but also to receive accurate information about their condition, why it has occurred, and what will help. Here, we suggest that an ethical practitioner appropriately applies knowledge from the science of psychology to explain the patient's condition and its resolution (see Sechrest & Smith, 1994). Accordingly, explanations based on empirically unsupported mechanisms such as energy meridians, chakras, eye movements, and similar features are not only scientifically unsound but also ethically unjustifiable.

In this book, you'll hear from leading clinician-scientists about their areas of expertise. One emphasis will be on what works, both for adult patients and, to a lesser extent, for their younger counterparts (other books in this series place a greater emphasis on children and adolescents). Each author will describe the psychological treatments known to be efficacious for a given condition, and will provide the scientific justification for how we know those treatments are efficacious. This aim will help you answer the basic question of "what treatment should be used with this patient?" But the chapters don't stop there. In keeping with the principle of science-based therapy, we have asked each author to also describe the credible mechanisms of change within and across ESTs. That is, rather than solely asking what treatment "package" works, we also wanted to clarify which mechanisms of change have empirical support or are at least scientifically plausible. In our opinion, a good therapist needs to be more like a chef than a cook – that is, able not only to follow a recipe (e.g., a manualized treatment approach), but also to use a case formulation approach to build a patient-focused treatment from the ground up, based on the best available science and the particular characteristics of the patient. You'll see in these chapters that even within a given therapeutic framework, there's a fair amount of wiggle room. So a good "chef" therapist will strive to maximize the elements of treatment that lead to the largest effects, rather than just sticking to a manual.

We also want you to see where the gaps are in our current knowledge. That is, what don't we know? Our hope is that clinicians, researchers, and clinician-researchers will find this book to be a useful guide toward further inquiry about what works and why. We recognize that the domain of science-based therapy is very much a work in progress, so nothing in this book should be taken as the last word on the topic. Science is constantly adding new information and new perspectives, and we hope to be able to update this book in the future with that new knowledge.

References

American Psychological Association. (2017). *Ethical principles of psychologists and code of conduct*. American Psychological Association.

APA Presidential Task Force on Evidence-Based Practice. (2006). Evidence-based practice in psychology. *American Psychologist*, 61(4), 271–285. https://doi.org/10.1037/0003-066X.61.4.271.

Ayllon, T., & Azrin, N. H. (1968). *The token economy: A motivational system for therapy and rehabilitation*. Appleton-Century-Crofts.

Beck, A. T. (1963). Thinking and depression. I. Idiosyncratic content and cognitive distortions. *Archives of General Psychiatry*, 9, 324–333. https://doi.org/10.1001/archpsyc.1963.01720160014002

Beck, A. T. (1976). *Cognitive therapy and the emotional disorders*. International Universities Press.

Blackburn, I. M., Bishop, S., Glen, A. I., Whalley, L. J., & Christie, J. E. (1981). The efficacy of cognitive therapy in depression: A treatment trial using cognitive therapy and pharmaco-therapy, each alone and in combination. *British Journal of Psychiatry*, 139(3), 181–189. https://doi.org/10.1192/bjp.139.3.181.

Borkovec, T. D., & Castonguay, L. G. (1998). What is the scientific meaning of empirically supported therapy? *Journal of Consulting and Clinical Psychology*, 66(1), 136–142. https://doi.org/10.1037/0022-006X.66.1.136.

Chambless, D. L., & Hollon, S. D. (1998). Defining empirically supported therapies. *Journal of Consulting and Clinical Psychology*, 66(1), 7–18. https://doi.org/10.1037/0022-006X.66.1.7.

Chambless, D. L., & Ollendick, T. H. (2001). Empirically supported psychological interventions: Controversies and evidence. *Annual Review of Psychology*, 52, 685–716. https://doi.org/10.1146/annurev.psych.52.1.685.

Cowen, E. L. (1991). In pursuit of wellness. *American Psychologist*, 46(4), 404–408. https://psycnet.apa.org/doi/10.1037/0003-066X.46.4.404.

Freud, S. (1933/1965). *New introductory lectures on psycho-analysis*. W. W. Norton & Company.

Hayes, S. C. (2004). Acceptance and commitment therapy, relational frame theory, and the third wave of behavioral and cognitive therapies. *Behavior Therapy*, 35(4), 639–665. https://doi.org/10.1016/S0005-7894(04)80013-3.

Hayes, S. C., Strosahl, K. D., & Wilson, K. G. (1999). *Acceptance and commitment therapy: An experiential approach to behavior change*. Guilford Press.

Henry, W. P. (1998). Science, politics, and the politics of science: The use and misuse of empirically validated treatment research. *Psychotherapy Research*, 8(2), 126–140. https://doi.org/10.1080/10503309812331332267.

Herbert, J. D. (2003). The science and practice of empirically supported treatments. *Behavior Modification*, 27(3), 412–430. https://doi.org/10.1177/0145445503027003008.

Hofmann, S. G., & Asmundson, G. J. (2008). Acceptance and mindfulness-based therapy: New wave or old hat? *Clinical Psychology Review*, 28(1), 1–16. www.ncbi.nlm.nih.gov/entrez/query.fcgi?cmd=Retrieve&db=PubMed&dopt=Citation&list_uids=17904260.

Hupp, S. (2019). *Pseudoscience in child and adolescent psychotherapy: A skeptical field guide*. Cambridge University Press.

Hupp, S. & Santa Maria, C. L. (2019) (Eds.), *Pseudoscience in therapy: A skeptical field guide*. Cambridge University Press.

Institute of Medicine. (2001). *Crossing the quality chasm: A new health system for the 21st century*. National Academy Press.

Kabat-Zinn, J., Lipworth, L., & Burney, R. (1985). The clinical use of mindfulness meditation for the self-regulation of chronic pain. *Journal of Behavioral Medicine*, 8(2), 163–190. www.ncbi.nlm.nih.gov/entrez/query.fcgi?cmd=Retrieve&db=PubMed&dopt=Citation&list_uids=3897551.

Lilienfeld, S. O., Lynn, S. J., & Bowden, S. C. (2018). Why evidence-based practice isn't enough: A call for science-based practice. *The Behavior Therapist*, 41(1), 42–47.

Linehan, M. M. (1993). *Cognitive-behavioral treatment of borderline personality disorder*. Guilford Press.

Luborsky, L., Diguer, L., Seligman, D. A., et al. (1999). The researcher's own therapy allegiances: A "wild card" in comparisons of treatment efficacy. *Clinical Psychology: Science and Practice*, 6, 95–106. https://doi.org/10.1093/clipsy.6.1.95.

Meichenbaum, D. (1977). *Cognitive-behavior modification: An integrative approach*. Plenum.

O'Donahue, W., Snipes, C., & Soto, C. (2016). The design, manufacture, and reporting of weak and pseudo-tests: The case of ACT. *Journal of Contemporary Psychotherapy*, 46(1), 37–40.

Paniagua, C. (1987). Can clinical psychoanalysis be scientific? *American Journal of Psychotherapy*, 41(1), 104–116.

Rosen, G. M., & Davison, G. C. (2003). Psychology should list empirically supported principles of change (ESPs) and not credential trademarked therapies or other treatment packages. *Behavior Modification*, 27(3), 300–312. https://doi.org/10.1177/0145445503027003003.

Rush, A. J., Beck, A. T., Kovacs, M., & Hollon, S. (1977). Comparative efficacy of cognitive therapy and pharmacotherapy in the treatment of depressed outpatients. *Cognitive Therapy and Research*, 1(1), 17–37.

Sechrest, L., & Smith, B. (1994). Psychotherapy is the practice of psychology. *Journal of Psychotherapy Integration*, 4, 1–29.

Seligman, M. E. (1995). The effectiveness of psychotherapy. The Consumer Reports study. *American Psychologist*, 50(12), 965–974. https://doi.org/10.1037/0003-066X.50.12.965.

Skinner, B. F. (1953). *Science and human behavior*. The Free Press.

Task Force on Promotion and Dissemination of Psychological Procedures. (1993). Training in and dissemination of empirically-validated psychological treatments: Report and recommendation. *The Clinical Psychologist*, 48, 3–23.

Thoma, N. C., McKay, D., Gerber, A. J., et al. (2012). A quality-based review of randomized controlled trials of cognitive-behavioral therapy for depression: An assessment and metaregression. *American Journal of Psychiatry*, 169(1), 22–30. https://doi.org/10.1176/appi.ajp.2011.11030433.

Tolin, D. F. (2012). Evidence-based practice: Three-legged stool or filter system? *The Clinical Psychologist*, 67(3), 1–3.

Tolin, D. F., McKay, D., Forman, E. M., Klonsky, E. D., & Thombs, B. D. (2015). Empirically supported treatment: Recommendations for a new model. *Clinical Psychology: Science & Practice*, 22, 317–338.

Wachtel, P. L. (2010). Beyond "ESTs": Problematic assumptions in the pursuit of evidence-based practice. *Psychoanalytic Psychology*, 27(3), 251–272. https://doi.org/10.1037/a0020532.

Watson, J. B., & Watson, R. R. (1921). Studies in infant psychology. *The Scientific Monthly*, 13(6), 493–515.

Westen, D. (1998). The scientific legacy of Sigmund Freud: Toward a psychodynamically informed psychological science. *Psychological Bulletin*, 124(3), 333–371.

Wolpe, J. (1961). The systematic desensitization treatment of neuroses. *Journal of Nervous and Mental Disease*, 132, 189–203. www.ncbi.nlm.nih.gov/entrez/query.fcgi?cmd=Retrieve&db=PubMed&dopt=Citation&list_uids=13786444.

2

Depressive Disorders

John R. McQuaid and Alfiee Breland-Noble

The *Diagnostic and Statistical Manual for Mental Disorders-5th Edition, Text Revision* (DSM-5-TR; American Psychiatric Association, 2022) defines major depressive disorder (MDD) as a period of at least two weeks in which the person experiences five or more symptoms of depression nearly every day, and at least one of the symptoms is either depressed mood or loss of interest/ pleasure. To meet the criteria for MDD, the symptoms must cause clinically significant distress or impairment of functioning; cannot be attributable to substance use, a medical condition, or better attributed to another disorder; and the patient must never have had a manic or hypomanic episode. Diagnostic specifiers include anxious distress, atypical features, mood congruent psychotic features, mood incongruent psychotic features, catatonia, peripartum onset, and seasonal pattern.

Persistent depressive disorder (PDD) is a chronic variation of a depressive disorder that can be less intense, with fewer symptoms, but of longer duration (at least two years in adults). The symptoms must cause clinically significant distress or impairment of functioning; must not be attributable to substance use, a medical condition, or better attributed to another disorder; and the patient has never had a manic or hypomanic episode. This chapter focuses primarily on MDD, for which there is a more extensive literature base.

Approximately 21% of the US population experiences a depressive episode in their lifetime, with an estimated 10% having an episode in any twelve-month period (Hasin et al., 2018). Due to the prevalence and severity of impairment, clinical depression generates the highest disease burden of any mental health disorder as measured in disability-adjusted life years (DALYs; a measure of years of life lost due to premature mortality, disability, or time lived in states of less than full health) and is the sixth highest contributor of DALYs of any cause for adults in 2019, up from eighth in 1990 (Global Burden of Disease Study, 2019). This impact highlights the importance of providing effective treatments for depression.

Etiology and Theoretical Underpinnings of Treatment

A recent literature review identified a broad range of factors associated with depression risk (Remes et al., 2021). Some of the factors have been long recognized, including genetic vulnerability, psychological and traumatic stress, cognitive factors, psychological vulnerability (e.g., both beliefs and thinking processes such as rumination that increase risk of depression), social determinants (including social support deficits, systematic biases based on individual characteristics such as race or gender, lack of access to resources), and gene–environment interactions. More recently identified risk factors include vulnerabilities involving the microbiome and inflammation. However, different treatment models focus on specific etiological mechanisms.

Behavioral theorists argue for a learning model of depression based on lack of reinforcement (e.g., engaging in behaviors that lead to positive affect and increase the likelihood of future behavior). Individuals with depression are thought to either have limited opportunity to engage in rewarding behaviors (e.g., being unable to find employment, losing a positive relationship) or to have experiences that are not reinforcing (e.g., being rejected in a relationship or fired from a job). These factors lead to withdrawal from or avoidance of possible reinforcing experiences. This reduction in reinforcement could lead to depressive symptoms, which in turn reduce the likelihood of engaging in reinforcing experiences, leading to a downward cycle of increased depression and decreased rewarding behavior and engagement in social networks which are protective factors against depression (Santini et al., 2015). They propose that treatments helping patients identify and engage in rewarding activities are key to countering the deprivation in reinforcement associated with depressive illness (Lewinsohn & Graf, 1973).

Cognitive theory posits that belief systems interact with life events to create risk for depression. They argue that certain cognitive schema (defined as "negatively toned representations of self-referent knowledge and information that guide appraisal and interact with information to influence selective attention, memory search, and cognitions"; Scher et al., 2005, p. 489) increase hopelessness and negative self-image, and reduce likelihood of engaging in healthy behavior. Examples of such schema include identifying one's value as arising from one's productivity (leading to vulnerability if out of work) or that one must be loved to have value (leading to depression in the face of rejection). The role of cognitive processes including schema as predictors of depression onset, as well as the efficacy of treatments designed to modify these processes, is well established (Scher et al., 2005). Therapies that incorporate cognitive theory teach patients to identify and change their thinking patterns, to engage in activities that help test and challenge unhelpful beliefs, and to focus on the present rather than delving deeply into past experiences (Beck et al., 1979).

"Third wave" approaches are derived from behavioral and cognitive theories and incorporate mindful observation, attentional control, distress tolerance, and acceptance of emotional experience. These models highlight that depressive episodes, and particularly recurrent or chronic depression, are associated with difficulty recognizing that thoughts may not be true or helpful and that individuals with depression often engage in ineffective coping strategies (e.g., attempts to avoid emotional experience; Hayes et al., 2001). In contrast to traditional cognitive and behavioral models, third-wave approaches focus on learning to observe and experience emotions and cognitions, particularly unpleasant or painful ones, rather than changing emotions. The intent of intervention is to be able to tolerate a broad range of experiences and continue to act on core beliefs and values to achieve goals rather than having depressive symptoms guide behavior.

Brief Overview of Treatments

Current clinical practice guidelines for the treatment of depressive disorders identify several psychotherapies as first-line treatments. The American Psychological Association clinical practice guidelines identified limited options with sufficient research support for either adolescents (only cognitive-behavioral therapy [CBT]) or older adults (CBT or interpersonal psychotherapy [IPT]). However, for adults, they identified a range of treatment options, including acceptance and commitment therapy (ACT), behavioral activation/behavior therapy (BA/BT), CBT, IPT, and short-term psychodynamic psychotherapy (STPP; American Psychological Association, 2019). Similarly, the Department of Veterans Affairs and Department of Defense CPG recommended a similar list of psychotherapies for adults, including ACT, BA/BT, CBT, IPT, mindfulness-based cognitive therapy (MBCT), problem-solving therapy (PST), and STPP (McQuaid et al., 2022). The United Kingdom's review process, NICE, recommends (depending on depression severity) BA/BT, CBT, counseling, IPT, mindfulness interventions such as MBCT, and STPP (NICE, 2022). Division 12 of the American Psychological Association (APA) has also characterized most of these variations of behavioral and cognitive therapies as being well-established based on the original criteria for empirically supported treatments (Chambless & Hollon, 1998). See the Postscript of this book for a more specific list. These conclusions (that there are multiple psychotherapeutic approaches that are efficacious and there is limited evidence of differences between them) are supported by multiple systematic reviews and meta-analyses. For example, a meta-analysis of 409 trials examining CBT found a moderate to large effect size ($g = 0.60$ to 0.79 depending on risk of bias of the studies included) when compared to control conditions. When compared to other psychotherapies, including BA/BT, IPT, PST, third-wave, and other models, CBT had a slight significant advantage ($g = 0.06$) that became nonsignificant in most sensitivity analyses, suggesting comparable effects across treatment models

(Cuijpers et al., 2023a). An earlier meta-analysis out of the same group with 228 studies, including 18 studies that included a comparison between two psychotherapies, found no difference in outcome between psychotherapies (Cuijpers et al., 2021).

Credible Components of Treatments

While there are a number of efficacious and effective treatment options available for depression, the evidence for the contribution of the specific treatment components that comprise these interventions is more limited. The most common tools for testing specific aspects of treatments are dismantling studies which compare key components of psychotherapies.

There are significant similarities undergirding current science-backed psychotherapeutic treatments including BA/BT, CT/CBT, and PST, and to a lesser extent IPT and SSPT. The common components of these theories include a biophysical and behavioral model of psychotherapy with demonstrated effectiveness in White populations. Less knowledge exists on the effectiveness of these treatments when considering sociocultural factors such as race, culture, and ethnicity. For example, each in some way focuses on more individual root causes for depression such as genetic precursors, interpersonal relationships, the development of negative behaviors, negative thought patterns, and negative conceptualizations of life events (Stark et al., 2000), rather than environmental or systemic factors that may disproportionately affect people of color or other marginalized populations.

Common components across treatment models that are held up as critical factors and levers of change in science-backed depression treatments are influenced in part by their testing in randomized controlled trials and grounding in manualized approaches. Components thought to underlie depression treatment effectiveness include "a) therapeutic relationship, b) activation of resources, c) actualization of the patient's problems, d) motivational clarification, and e) (active help for) problem solving" (Woike et al., 2019, p. 1), while established mediators include change in dysfunctional attitudes, negative "automatic" thoughts, mindfulness and worry skills, and rumination-mediated change in outcomes (e.g., depression symptoms).

Overall, theories undergirding the most established psychotherapeutic treatments for depression are grounded in a biopsychosocial model which suggests that strong rapport between provider and patient is crucial, along with a focus on individual behavior changes as the primary factors for improving depression outcomes. A consideration for future development of effective treatments is to incorporate strategies that address environmental/social/systemic factors (e.g., poverty, bias, disparities in access to resources) that exacerbate mental health concerns.

Behavioral Activation

In behavioral activation, patients are encouraged to hold a present orientation while engaging in collaborative efforts with providers. The label of "behavioral activation" was developed for a dismantling study that found no differences between three treatment conditions: behavioral activation alone; behavioral activation plus cognitive restructuring; and behavioral activation, cognitive restructuring, and schema change (Jacobson et al., 1996). Key targets of behavioral activation include increasing access to positive reinforcement of healthy behaviors, and working through barriers to utilizing the skills of activation (Uphoff et al., 2020). Behavioral activation also includes activity scheduling, the development of social skills to increase access to and success in social interactions, and mood monitoring linked to daily behaviors. Behavioral activation is used both as a component of depression treatment (mainly in CBT) and as a stand-alone treatment for depressive illness.

Multiple studies of behavioral activation have demonstrated its efficacy, though little of this data is based on racially/ethnically diverse samples (Mazzucchelli et al., 2009). As a result, while there is evidence that behavioral activation works for White populations, it remains unclear how generalizable behavioral activation approaches are for people of color across the life span. This is particularly concerning given the individual orientation of the approach with little consideration of systemic issues (e.g., environmental risks, systematic bias, disparities in access to resources) that disproportionately impact communities of color. This same point could be made for all of the components discussed in this chapter, so rather than repeating the point we'll discuss the value of cultural humility in Box 2.1.

Box 2.1 Cultural Humility

Even when providers make cultural adaptations to psychotherapeutic approaches, including cognitive-behavioral approaches, people of color demonstrate high attrition rates in treatment when compared to their White peers. Therefore, enhancements are necessary at the treatment engagement level to even allow diverse populations to receive adequate "doses" of the types of treatments described herein, to allow for the possibility of benefit from the critical components of cognitive-behavioral approaches (Breland-Noble & The AAKOMA Project, 2022; Breland-Noble et al., 2016).

When quantifying the various benefits of psychotherapies, researchers seek to better understand both how and why various approaches work. This research involves examining factors such as the utility of treatments for different types of illnesses, frequency and intensity of treatment needed to generate positive outcomes, changes in illness symptomatology over time, and role of patient–provider alliance. While data are available to help the field better understand these factors, two factors that continue to be absent from the literature are individual factors and social determinants of health. Historically, research on individual factors has focused heavily on certain patient characteristics (e.g., illness symptomatology and severity of symptoms), factors impacting attrition, and patient–provider alliance (Flückiger et al., 2012; Luborsky et al.,1971). Key factors studied regarding provider characteristics include provider level of training and fidelity to treatment approaches (Diebold et al., 2020; Mowbray et al., 2003). Research on patient–provider alliance suggests that a patient's positive regard for the therapist as someone who demonstrates support for them, level of agreement between patient and therapist on the goals of treatment, and agreement between therapist and patient on the effectiveness of approaches to achieving the goals set are all critical components necessary for positive outcomes (Miller & Moyers, 2021).

Missing from these factors related to outcomes are provider cultural competence, which has been described as "a constellation of the right personal characteristics (awareness, knowledge, and skills) that a counselor or therapist should have" (Sue et al., 2009, p. 4), individual patient demographic characteristics, and their impact on outcomes and social determinants of health.

An emerging body of literature has specified the ways in which cultural competence and attention to cultural differences in treatment enhance therapeutic alliance and clinical outcomes in psychotherapy, including depressive illness (Breland-Noble & Miranda, 2017; van Loon et al., 2013). Specifically, a combination of creating a welcoming space, allowing the patient to feel understood, recognizing cultural differences, and creating a sense of familiarity have profound positive impacts upon which patients can then build a repertoire of tools for their self-care between sessions. Regarding patient demographics, the field has historically failed to power treatment studies to allow for the examination of individual differences (e.g., race, LGBTQ identity, socioeconomic status) in depression treatment outcomes.

Most psychotherapeutic approaches widely promoted today do not have evidence of wide generalizability across diverse populations (e.g., race, gender, LGBTQ identity, and persons with disabilities). Therefore, we need to review the relationships among these key aspects of identity (including identity-based trauma exposure) and reflect on their relationship to depression treatment and its components (including help-seeking behaviors and treatment engagement).

Mental health disparities and equity scholars have examined key components important for improved outcomes in depression treatment. The majority of this literature points to possible efficacy and effectiveness, but too few treatments have been tested with samples adequately powered to establish scientific efficacy or effectiveness across diverse groups (American Psychological Association, 2019). Two meta-analyses of evidence-based mental health treatments (including those for depression) for youth of color found only modest support, reflecting possibly efficacious or probably efficacious outcomes (Huey & Polo, 2008). The same is true for adults of color across the lifespan, as recently examined by the American Psychological Association's depression guideline panel (American Psychological Association, 2019).

Cognitive Restructuring

An extensive body of literature has established that depression is associated with a number of cognitive variables, referred to as "cognitive vulnerabilities," that are associated with increased risk for depression onset, relapse, and recurrence (Scher et al., 2005). As noted, a cognitive schema is a style of thinking that when present in the context of a stressor is likely to lead to interpretations of the experience that increased the likelihood of a depressive episode. An example of a cognitive schema interacting with a stressor might be a person who believes "I need to be productive to be worthwhile" and who, after losing a job, determines they have no value and develops feelings of worthlessness and hopelessness.

The components of CBT are designed to address cognitive schemas and change the thoughts and behaviors that arise from them. Patients work with providers to recognize faulty thinking and behaviors, to better understand their learning history, and to develop skills to change beliefs and behaviors. Typical tools used to facilitate learning in CBT include learning to identify unhelpful thoughts and behaviors, conducting behavioral experiments to test beliefs and alternative behaviors, using role-play to practice new skills, and identification and modification of cognitive schema from which automatic thoughts and problematic behaviors arise. CBT has the largest body of supporting literature of any psychotherapy, with multiple studies across the age span (primarily in White western samples) finding it to be effective with these populations (American Psychological Association, 2019; Gould et al., 2012; Weersing et al., 2016).

Problem Solving

Problem solving therapy is a model rooted in cognitive and behavioral principles guided by the theory that psychopathology is best understood as an individual's use of maladaptive coping skills (Nezu, 1986; Nezu & Perri, 1989). The provider and patient collaborate to identify and illuminate a presenting problem (or set of problems) and then work on providing the patient with tools to develop and practice adaptive and positive coping to address the problem. In doing so, the patient develops a greater sense of self-efficacy, reduces the negative impacts of the presenting issue, and develops confidence in their ability to address similar problems in the future. The five core components of problem solving include a positive problem orientation (i.e., the ability to evaluate a problem with the belief that is it solvable and a normal part of life), problem definition and formulation, generation of alternatives, decision-making, and solution implementation and verification. Multiple meta-analyses show the largest effect sizes when all five components are incorporated within the course of treatment (Bell & D'Zurilla, 2009). Problem solving is considered effective and comparable to other psychotherapies for the treatment of depression (with modest effect sizes; Cuijpers et al., 2018).

Mindfulness

The development of MBCT reflects a model that epitomizes the use of an a priori evidence-based theory to identify an intervention based on hypothesized mechanisms of the disorder and evaluated in relation not only to outcomes but to the hypothesized mechanism. Originally developed as an intervention for the prevention of relapse in individuals with a history of depression, MBCT is predicated on evidence that individuals with a history of depression have cognitive vulnerabilities that can be activated by stress and increase the likelihood of depressive episodes. The developers of MBCT posited that the techniques of mindfulness, including nonjudgmental observation of internal experiences, would allow individuals to respond to experiences in a manner that was not driven by the underlying cognitive vulnerability and would in fact potentially modify the vulnerabilities to reduce the likelihood of future depressive episodes. In a series of key studies, the authors found that MBCT was associated with reduced risk of depression (Teasdale et al., 2000) and reduced distorted thinking indicative of a cognitive vulnerability (Teasdale et al., 2022). Further studies have demonstrated that MBCT is effective not only for preventing recurrence for those with a history of depression but also for treating individuals experiencing a current depressive episode (Strauss et al., 2014).

Acceptance and Commitment

The interventions in ACT derive from relational frame theory, which focuses on the nature of language (including thoughts) having emotional and representative meaning that is learned by association with the items to which the language is connected (Hayes et al., 2001). Because of the strength of these associations, thoughts can create emotional experiences that feel like the events with which they are associated (e.g., thinking of being criticized by a loved one) and these experiences can contribute to depression. The treatment therefore emphasizes developing the ability to observe one's internal experience, including thoughts and emotions, without letting it determine one's actions but learning instead to act based on values and goals even in the context of painful emotions. Components of ACT include a number of techniques designed to address six core processes: acceptance (particularly of negative experience); cognitive defusion (i.e., recognizing a thought as being just a statement in one's mind, like reading a sentence, rather than something that has inherent truth and power); being present; understanding the self as context (i.e., learning to connect with a stable sense of self from which to observe changing experiences such as emotions and thoughts); identifying values; and committing to act on values. While the specific components of ACT have not been evaluated for efficacy, the overall model led to significant improvement for treatment of depression and was not significantly different from CBT (Ost, 2014).

Addressing Interpersonal Targets

The IPT model draws upon attachment and interpersonal theories, which propose that early loss leads to increased vulnerability to depression and that negative life events, particularly in relational domains, can provoke depressive episodes. The developers designed an intervention that targets four domains: role transition (e.g., moving from employment to retirement); role conflict (e.g., disagreeing with a spouse regarding who has what responsibilities managing a household); loss (specifically loss of a loved one); and interpersonal skills deficits (Klerman et al., 1984). Each of these dimensions are associated with stressors that have been demonstrated to increase risk for depression (Brown & Harris, 1989). The IPT approach is a structured treatment that is administered over a set number of sessions. Interventions include an interpersonal inventory to identify the target domain for treatment and create an interpersonal formulation, conducting a communication analysis to identify targets for coaching and role-play, exploration of problems and facilitating the client in identifying their goals and the approach they would like to take to achieve them, facilitating grief and mourning when some goals cannot be achieved, and use of the termination/graduation process to facilitate a healthy role transition.

Comparing Components

While it is well established that psychotherapies in general are more effective than no treatment in reducing depressive symptoms, the efficacy of specific components has received only limited attention, and the studies, with a few exceptions, focus on CBT. An early example was a trial of CBT for depression that examined three separate conditions: cognitive restructuring, behavioral activation, and assertive skills training (Zeiss et al., 1979). The authors found that all three conditions led to decreases in depressive symptoms and improvements in target behaviors, including interpersonal skills, cognitive style, and pleasant activities. However, there was no evidence that effects were specific to the target in question and there were no differences among conditions on the improvements in any domain. The authors argued that the improvement in symptoms reflected an increase in self-efficacy in general, regardless of the domain in which it was occurring.

The study of behavioral activation compared to two cognitive therapy conditions cited earlier also found no differences in outcomes (Jacobson et al., 1996). The authors later developed behavioral activation as a separate intervention that is now considered evidence-based in its own right by the VA/DoD and APA guidelines.

Additional studies of specific components of effective treatments for depression are limited. A meta-analysis of dismantling or component studies found a total of fifteen trials that met the inclusion criteria (Cuijpers et al., 2017). Thirteen were trials of CBT (including MBCT and behavioral activation/behavior therapy) either adding or removing a component, one was a dismantling trial of IPT, and one was a dismantling trial of full self-control therapy, an intervention which currently is not included as an evidence-based practice.

The key conclusion was that all but one study did not have sufficient power to detect meaningful differences among different treatments. The one study exception that had adequate power found a significant benefit of the addition of emotion regulation skills to CBT on an inpatient unit (Berking et al., 2013). In addition, one other trial found a benefit from the addition of a component (hypnosis added to CBT; Alladin & Alibhai, 2007) and two found that the full intervention of PST was superior to partial or abbreviated PST (Nezu, 1986; Nezu & Perri, 1989).

In addition, there is evidence that a large portion of change in psychotherapy for depression is not associated with specific treatment components but rather with general factors shared across interventions. A meta-analysis found that only 17% of variance in treatment outcome for depression was attributable to treatment specific factors, while nearly half (49.6%) was attributable to nonspecific factors and 33% was attributable to natural recovery (Cuijpers et al., 2012). While there are several limitations to this conclusion due to constraints of meta-analytic designs (Cuijpers et al., 2018), it highlights the challenge of understanding the role of specific theoretically derived interventions in the treatment of depression.

Approaches for Youth

Depression in children and adolescents is a significant concern, with rates rising from 2% in childhood to as high as 20% by age eighteen (Bose & Pettit, 2018). Depression in youth may manifest with irritability rather than sadness. This can present as increased activity (i.e., engaging in nondirective behaviors with increasing frequency and consistency), aggressiveness, or antisocial behaviors. A clinical assessment is critical to accurately identify the diagnosis and appropriate treatment options.

There is a more limited literature regarding treatment of depression in youth, and particularly young children, when compared to adults. The APA depression guideline panel found insufficient evidence to make recommendations for treatment in children (American Psychological Association, 2019). For adolescents, two interventions had sufficient research to support a recommendation: CBT and IPT. Both interventions incorporate components of the adult versions of the interventions. Of note, one version of CBT, the Coping with Depression Course, was designed specifically for a group format and as a treatment to prevent depression in vulnerable adolescents (Clarke et al., 1995). In considering treatment of youth and young adults, there is less evidence about what treatments are effective for stigmatized youth, including youth of color or LGBTQ youth, and what data are available suggest they are less likely to receive treatment than their White counterparts (Price & Hollinsaid, 2022) and less likely to benefit from it when they do, particularly in high-stigma environments (e.g., states with more racist attitudes reported or more restrictive policies regarding LGBTQ people; Price & Hollinsaid, 2022). These findings highlight the need for increased outreach and engagement, particularly given recent increases in suicidal behavior among youth of diverse racial/ethnic backgrounds (Charpignon et al., 2022).

Other Variables Influencing Treatment

Assessment and Diagnosis

This chapter has focused on MDD in part because it is the most researched mood disorder. However, there is significant variability within MDD, as well as between MDD and other mood disorders, that influences treatment considerations. For patients with severe depression who are not responsive to initial treatment or with a history of multiple depressive episodes, most guidelines recommend combining psychotherapy with pharmacotherapy (American Psychological Association, 2019), and recent meta-analyses indicate that combined treatment is more effective for moderate depression as well (Cuijpers et al., 2023b). For recurrent depression, MBCT was specifically created to treat it, and there is evidence that it both is an effective intervention and reduces risk of relapse or recurrence (McCartney et al., 2021). However, in a comparison with CBT there was no difference in preventing relapse (Farb et al., 2018). Third-wave models have in general been advocated for persistent depressive disorder, and while there is some evidence that MBCT, cognitive-behavioral analysis system of psychotherapy (CBASP, a CBT model that includes a structured interpersonal focus), long-term psychoanalytic psycho-therapy, and IPT plus medication may be particularly effective for PDD (McPherson & Senra, 2022), the data are based on limited number of studies (generally 1 or 2 per model) and replication is required.

Once a diagnosis is established and treatment is initiated, a key effective treatment component is measurement-based care. The use of regular symptom assessment and incorporation of it into the planning and implementation of treatment has been demonstrated to improve outcomes across treatments, though additional research is indicated for underserved populations (Guo et al., 2015). While use of measurement-based care is an integral component of cognitive, behavioral, and third-wave models, it has been incorporated effectively across many approaches to treatment to increase the effectiveness of the approach.

Comorbidity

Depression is comorbid with a broad range of other disorders, including anxiety disorders, personality disorders, and substance use disorders (Richards & O'Hara, 2014). In addition, depression is associated with many medical disorders, including cancer, diabetes, heart disease, HIV/AIDS, multiple scler-osis, and pain associated with multiple causes. Depression can further exacerbate health problems such as diabetes and heart disease (Katon, 2003). Recently, researchers have begun to link exposure to racism and discrimination to depres-sive illness and disparate mental health outcomes (Williams, 2018). These comorbidities can complicate effective treatment and highlight the need to for providers to be thorough in assessing contributing factors. Currently, most research on effective treatments does not address comorbidities so clinicians need to draw on both the best information available as well as clinical judgment in developing treatment plans.

Demographics

There is limited data on the effectiveness of any approaches for the treatment of depression in people of color, people who identify as LGBTQ, those with disabilities, and people whose identities include intersections among these identities. Of the available evidence, the best assessments suggest CBT for depression as probably or possibly efficacious with people of color (e.g., Black and Latinx youth) (Pina et al., 2019). The American Psychological Association's clinical practice guidelines for depression note that

the limitations of the literature highlighted the need for funding agencies and investigators to explicitly address differences, in particular, culture, ethnicity, sex, sexual minority, gender identity, disability, nationality of origin, generation status, race, socioeconomic status, and others, as well as the intersection of these variables, which can further influence treatment. These are areas that could contribute to the experience and treatment of depression but for which the panel did not have an adequate literature to address.

(APA, 2019, pp. 22–23)

Little has changed in the years since the panel wrote that statement.

There are differences between patient populations both in frequency of depressive disorders, access to care, and response to treatment. Women consist-ently report twice the rate of depression that men do, and individuals under age sixty-five report higher rates than do those over sixty-five (Hasin et al., 2018). While White and Native American people are at higher risk than Black, Latinx, and Asian American populations, recent research has identified links between racism-based trauma and depressive illness (a heretofore understudied phenom-enon), suggesting a need to better explore depression and other mental health disorders in these populations (Breland-Noble et al., 2016; Torres & Ong, 2010). In addition, Black and Latinx populations with depressive disorders are less likely to receive treatment compared to White populations (McGregors et al., 2020), and data regarding treatment efficacy and effectiveness are very limited for these populations.

Medication

In addition to the psychotherapies that are efficacious and effective for treatment of depression, there is an extensive list of effective medications. While current guidelines recommend either an antidepressant medication or an evidence-based psychotherapy for uncomplicated major depression, they recommend combined treatment (medication and psychotherapy) for complicated, treatment nonresponsive, severe, or chronic depression (American Psychological Association, 2019; McQuaid et al., 2022). While evidence does demonstrate that combined treatment can improve treatment outcomes (Cuijpers et al., 2023b), it is not clear if the benefits of combined treatment are additive or interactive. It is possible that medication can reduce symptoms that interfere with engagement in psychotherapy, leading to additional benefit. Alternately, psychotherapy that incorporates strategies to improve adherence to medication may lead to better outcomes, in part due to increased effectiveness of the medication. Future research is needed to determine how to best combine psychotherapy and pharmacotherapy. One developing area where there is a great deal of interest is in psychedelic-assisted psychotherapy. Recent theories propose that psychedelic drugs can increase neural plasticity, which can allow greater modification of previously established neural connections and therefore increase the ability to encode changes being made in psychotherapy (e.g., Sarris et al., 2022). However, this area is early in development and further research is needed to establish the efficacy, effectiveness, and mechanisms of action.

Conclusion

While depression is treatable, the mechanisms of change in psychotherapy remain insufficiently tested to make strong conclusions about most specific components. While all the models of therapy currently identified as evidence-based are derived from testable theories, some have been much more strenuously tested than others. Even for an approach like CBT, the level of component evaluation has been limited, and specific hypothesis-driven predictions about the mechanism of change have frequently failed to be supported (Zeiss et al., 1979; Jacobson et al., 1996).

Nonetheless, we believe that a theory-driven rather than an atheoretical approach to treatment development and evaluation is critical to continued progress in psychotherapy development. There are several approaches currently not included as evidence-based with varying levels of scientific support for the underlying theory. What does it matter if there is a weak theoretical frame if the treatment is efficacious? We see three key concerns. First, while it is possible for a poorly elaborated model to have some benefit based on the strength of nonspecific factors, pursuit of hypotheses based on such outcomes to understand why such an intervention was efficacious can lead to elaborations on a model that are based on false assumptions and can draw effort and energy from interventions more likely to be of benefit both in terms of outcome and in terms of informing our understanding of mechanisms driving depression. Given the limited resources available, we believe in focusing efforts on treatments with a sound theoretical and evidentiary footing. Second, we believe that as providers we have a responsibility to tell clients why the model being offered may lead to change. Engaging with a model that is poorly understood or unsupported may lead patients to erroneous assumptions about the nature of their disorder and change, and contribute to difficulty in effective treatment engagement. Third, the reality is that none of the treatments currently available are as effective as we would wish. There is a critical need, as highlighted here, to determine the effective components of treatments, refine them, and deliver them more effectively.

There are also key deficits in both access of patient populations to any evidence-informed treatments and in what we know about the development and application of various psychotherapeutic techniques to underrepresented groups. In reviewing what is currently offered to patient populations, and particularly to intersectional people of color (including LGBTQ, persons with disabilities, and geographically and/or socio-economically diverse populations), little of the research upon which the guidelines rely offers assessments of efficacy or effectiveness with these populations. As a result, it remains unclear how these treatments work and whether they are equally effective for the widest range of persons possible.

Future research is needed that addresses whether treatments need to be modified/adapted for different groups and, if so, how. Focusing on addressing these research gaps requires directing resources in a targeted manner, and this is most likely to be successful when guided by scientifically sound theory and a desire to create generalizable outcomes for public health.

Useful Resources

Treatment Guidelines

- American Psychological Association clinical guideline for treatment of depression: www.apa.org/depression-guideline.
- VA/DoD clinical guideline for the treatment of depression: www.healthquality.va.gov/guidelines/MH/mdd/.

Guidance Regarding Cultural Competence and Psychotherapy

- Sue, S., Zane, N., Hall, G. C. N., & Berger, L. K. (2009). The case for cultural competency in psychotherapeutic interventions. *Annual Review of Psychology*, 60(1), 525–548.

- Breland-Noble, A. M. (2020). *Community mental health engagement with racially diverse populations*. Academic Press.
- Breland-Noble, A. M., Al-Mateen, C. S., & Singh, N. N. (2016). *Handbook of mental health in African American youth*. Springer.
- American Psychological Association guidance on culturally competent care: www.apa.org/monitor/2015/03/cultural-competence#:~:text=Cultural%20competence%20%E2%80%94%20loosely%20defined%20as,practice%20for%20some%2050%20years.

References

Alladin, A., & Alibhai, A. (2007). Cognitive hypnotherapy for depression: An empirical investigation. *International Journal of Clinical and Experimental Hypnosis*, 55(2), 147–166.

American Psychiatric Association. (2022). *Diagnostic and statistical manual of mental disorders: DSM-5-TR* (Fifth edition, text revision). American Psychiatric Association Publishing.

American Psychological Association. (2019). *Clinical practice guideline for the treatment of depression across three age cohorts*. US Department of Veterans Affairs.

Ardito, R. B., & Rabellino, D. (2011). Therapeutic alliance and outcome of psychotherapy: Historical excursus, measurements, and prospects for research. *Frontiers in Psychology*, 2, 270.

Arean, P., Hegel, M., Vannoy, S., Fan, M. Y., & Unuzter, J. (2008). Effectiveness of problem-solving therapy for older, primary care patients with depression: Results from the IMPACT project. *The Gerontologist*, 48(3), 311–323.

Beck, A. T., Rush, A. J., Shaw, B. F., & Emery, G. (1979) *Cognitive therapy of depression*. The Guilford Press.

Bell, A. C., & D'Zurilla, T. J. (2009). Problem-solving therapy for depression: A meta-analysis. *Clinical Psychology Review*, 29(4), 348–353.

Berking, M., Ebert, D., Cuijpers, P., & Hofmann, S. G. (2013). Emotion regulation skills training enhances the efficacy of inpatient cognitive behavioral therapy for major depressive disorder: A randomized controlled trial. *Psychotherapy and Psychosomatics*, 82(4), 234–245.

Bose, D., & Pettit, J. W. (2018). Depression. In S. Hupp (Ed), *Child and Adolescent Psychotherapy* (pp. 138–153). Cambridge University Press.

Breland-Noble, A. M., Al-Mateen, C., & Singh, N. (2016). *Handbook of mental health in African American youth*. Springer.

Breland-Noble, A., & The AAKOMA Project. (2022). *The AAKOMA Project Presents: The State of Youth of Color Mental Health 2022*.

Breland-Noble, A.M. & Miranda, J. (2017). Depression in racially diverse populations: Challenges and opportunities. In G. W. Cohen (Ed.) *Public Health Perspectives on Depressive Illness*. Johns Hopkins University Press.

Brown, G. W., & Harris, T. O. (1989). Depression. In G. W. Brown & T. O. Harris (Eds.), *Life events and illness*. New York: The Guilford Press, pp. 49–93.

Chambless, D. L., & Hollon, S. D. (1998). Defining empirically supported therapies. *Journal of Consulting and Clinical Psychology*, 66(1), 7–18. https://doi.org/10.1037/0022-006X.66.1.7.

Charpignon, M., Ontiveros, J., Sundaresan, S., et al. (2022). Evaluation of suicides among US adolescents during the COVID-19 pandemic. *JAMA Pediatrics*, 176(7), 724–726.

Chowdhary, N., Jotheeswaran, A. T., Nadkarni, A., et al. (2014). The methods and outcomes of cultural adaptations of psychological treatments for depressive disorders: A systematic review. *Psychological Medicine*, 44(6), 1131–1146.

Clarke, G. N., Hawkins, W., Murphy, M., et al. (1995). Targeted prevention of unipolar depressive disorder in an at-risk sample of high school adolescents: A randomized trial of a group cognitive intervention. *Journal of the American Academy of Child & Adolescent Psychiatry*, 34(3), 312–321.

Connolly Gibbons, M. B., Gallop, R., Thompson, D., et al. (2016). Comparative effectiveness of cognitive therapy and dynamic psychotherapy for major depressive disorder in a community mental health setting: A randomized clinical noninferiority trial. *JAMA Psychiatry*, 73(9), 904–911.

Constantino, M. J., Castonguay, L. G., Zack, S. E., & DeGeorge, J. (2010). Engagement in psychotherapy: Factors contributing to the facilitation, demise, and restoration of the therapeutic alliance. In D. Castro-Blanco & M. S. Karver (Eds.), *Elusive alliance: Treatment engagement strategies with high-risk adolescents* (pp. 21–57). American Psychological Association.

Cuijpers, P. (2017). Four decades of outcome research on psychotherapies for adult depression: An overview of a series of meta-analyses. *Canadian Psychology/psychologie canadienne*, 58(1), 7–19.

Cuijpers, P., Cristea, I. A., Karyotaki, E., Reijnders, M., & Hollon, S. D. (2019) Component studies of psychological treatments of adult depression: A systematic review and meta-analysis, *Psychotherapy Research*, 29(1), 15–29.

Cuijpers, P., de Wit, L., Kleiboer, A., Karyotaki, E., & Ebert, D. D. (2018). Problem-solving therapy for adult depression: An updated meta-analysis. *European Psychiatry*, 48, 27–37.

Cuijpers, P., Driessen, E., Hollon, S. D., et al. (2012). The efficacy of non-directive supportive therapy for adult depression: A meta-analysis. *Clinical Psychology Review*, 32(4), 280–291.

Cuijpers, P., Karyotaki, E., Ciharova, M., et al. (2021). The effects of psychotherapies for depression on response, remission, reliable change, and deterioration: A meta-analysis. *Acta Psychiatrica Scandinavica*, 144(3), 288–299.

Cuijpers, P., Miguel, C., Harrer, M., et al. (2023a). Cognitive behavior therapy vs. control conditions, other psychotherapies, pharmacotherapies and combined treatment for depression: A comprehensive meta-analysis including 409 trials with 52,702 patients. *World Psychiatry*, 22(1), 105–115.

Cuijpers, P., Miguel, C., Harrer, M., et al. (2023b). Psychological treatment of depression: A systematic overview of a "Meta-Analytic Research Domain." *Journal of Affective Disorders*, 335, 141–151. https://doi-org.ucsf.idm.oclc.org/10.1016/j.jad.2023.05.011.

Diebold, A., Ciolino, J. D., Johnson, J. K., et al. (2020). Comparing fidelity outcomes of paraprofessional and professional delivery of a perinatal depression preventive intervention. *Administration and Policy in Mental Health and Mental Health Services Research*, 47(4), 597–605.

Driessen, E., Hegelmaier, L. M., Abbass, A. A., et al. (2015). The efficacy of short-term psychodynamic psychotherapy for depression: A meta-analysis update. *Clinical Psychology Review*, 42, 1–15.

Ellis, A. (1962) *Reason and emotion in psychotherapy*. Lyle Stuart.

Farb, N., Anderson, A., Ravindran, A., et al. (2018). Prevention of relapse/recurrence in major depressive disorder with either mindfulness-based cognitive therapy or cognitive therapy. *Journal of Consulting and Clinical Psychology*, 86(2), 200–204.

Flückiger, C., Del Re, A. C., Wampold, B. E., et al. (2012). Valuing clients' perspective and the effects on the therapeutic alliance: A randomized controlled study of an adjunctive instruction. *Journal of Counseling Psychology*, 59(1), 18–26.

GBD 2019 Diseases and Injuries Collaborators (2020). Global burden of 369 diseases and injuries in 204 countries and territories, 1990–2019: A systematic analysis for the Global Burden of Disease Study 2019. *Lancet*, 396, 1204–1222.

Global Burden of Disease Study (2019). Data resources. https://ghdx.healthdata.org/gbd-2019.

Gould, R. L., Coulson, M. C., & Howard, R. J. (2012). Cognitive behavioral therapy for depression in older people: A meta-analysis and meta-regression of randomized controlled trials. *Journal of the American Geriatrics Society*, 60(10), 1817–1830.

Guo, T., Xiang, Y. T., Xiao, L., et al. (2015). Measurement-based care versus standard care for major depression: A randomized controlled trial with blind raters. *The American Journal of Psychiatry*, 172(10), 1004–1013.

Hasin D. S, Sarvet, A. L., Meyers, J. L., et al. (2018). Epidemiology of Adult DSM-5 Major Depressive Disorder and Its Specifiers in the United States. *JAMA Psychiatry*, 75(4), 336–46.

Hayes, S. C., Barnes-Holmes, D., & Roche, B. (Eds). (2001). *Relational frame theory: A post-Skinnerian account of human language and cognition*. Kluwer Academic/Plenum Publishers.

Huey, S. J., & Polo, A. J. (2008). Evidence-based psychosocial treatments for ethnic minority youth [Review]. *Journal of Clinical Child and Adolescent Psychology*, 37(1), 262–301.

Huey, S. J., Tilley, J. L., Jones, E. O., & Smith, C. A. (2014). The contribution of cultural competence to evidence-based care for ethnically diverse populations. *Annual Review of Clinical Psychology*, 10, 305–338.

Jacobson, N. S., Dobson, K. S., Truax, P. A., et al. (1996). A component analysis of cognitive-behavioral treatment for depression. *Journal of Consulting and Clinical Psychology*, 64(2):295-304. https://doi.org/10.1037//0022-006x.64.2.295. PMID: 8871414.

Katon, W. J. (2003). Clinical and health services relationships between major depression, depressive symptoms, and general medical illness. *Biological Psychiatry*, 54(3), 216–226.

Klerman, G. L., Weissman, M. M., Rounsaville, B. J., & Chevron, E. S. (1984). *Interpersonal psychotherapy of depression*. Basic Books Inc.

Lewinsohn, P. M., & Graf, M. (1973). Pleasant activities and depression. *Journal of Consulting and Clinical Psychology*, 41(2), 261–268.

Luborsky, L., Chandler, M., Auerbach, A. H., Cohen, J., & Bachrach, H. M. (1971). Factors influencing the outcome of psychotherapy: A review of quantitative research. *Psychological Bulletin*, 75(3), 145–185.

Management of Major Depressive Disorder Work Group (2022). *VA/DoD clinical practice guideline for the management of major depressive disorder*. Government Printing Office.

Martell, C. R., Dimidjian, S., & Lewinsohn, P. M. (2010). Behavioral activation therapy. In N. Kazantzis, M. A. Reinecke, & A. Freeman (Eds.), *Cognitive and behavioral theories in clinical practice* (pp. 193–217). Guilford Press.

Mazzucchelli, T., Kane, R., & Rees, C. (2009). Behavioral activation treatments for depression in adults: A meta-analysis and review. *Clinical Psychology: Science and Practice*, 16(4), 383–411.

McCartney, M., Nevitt, S., Lloyd, A., et al. (2021). Mindfulness-based cognitive therapy for prevention and time to depressive relapse: Systematic review and network meta-analysis. *Acta Psychiatrica Scandinavica*, 143(1), 6–21.

McGregor, B., Li, C., Baltrus, P., et al. (2020). Racial and ethnic disparities in treatment and treatment type for depression in a national sample of Medicaid recipients. *Psychiatric Services*, 71(7), 663–669.

McPherson, S., & Senra, H. (2022). Psychological treatments for persistent depression: A systematic review and meta-analysis of quality of life and functioning outcomes. *Psychotherapy (Chicago, Ill.)*, 59(3), 447–459.

McQuaid, J. R., Buelt, A., Capaldi, V., et al. (2022). The management of major depressive disorder: Synopsis of the 2022 US Department of Veterans Affairs and US Department of Defense clinical practice guideline. *Annals of Internal Medicine*, 175(10), 1440–1451.

Miller, R. W. & Moyers, T. B. (2021). *Effective psychotherapists: Clinical skills that improve client outcomes*. The Guilford Press.

Mowbray, C. T., Holter, M. C., Teague, G. B., & Bybee, D. (2003). Fidelity criteria: Development, measurement, and validation. *American Journal of Evaluation*, 24(3), 315–340.

Nezu, A. M. (1986). Efficacy of a social problemsolving therapy approach for unipolar depression. *Journal of Consulting and Clinical Psychology*, 54(2), 196–202.

Nezu, A. M., & Perri, M. G. (1989). Social problemsolving therapy for unipolar depression: An initial dismantling investigation. *Journal of Consulting and Clinical Psychology*, 57(3), 408–413.

NICE (2022). *Depression in adults: Treatment and management*. NICE.

Ost L. G. (2014). The efficacy of Acceptance and Commitment Therapy: An updated systematic review and meta-analysis. *Behaviour Research and Therapy*, *61*, 105–121.

Pina, A. A., Polo, A. J., & Huey, S. J. (2019). Evidence-based psychosocial interventions for ethnic minority youth: The 10-year update. *Journal of Clinical Child & Adolescent Psychology*, 48(2), 179–202.

Price, M. A., & Hollinsaid, N. L. (2022). Future directions in mental health treatment with stigmatized youth. *Journal of Clinical Child and Adolescent Psychology*, 51(5), 810–825.

Remes, O, Mendes, J. F., & Templeton, P. (2021). Biological, psychological, and social determinants of depression: A review of recent literature. *Brain Science*, 11(12), 1633.

Richards, C. S., & O'Hara, M. W. (Eds.) (2014). *The Oxford handbook of depression and comorbidity*. Oxford University Press.

Santini, Z. I., Koyanagi, A., Tyrovolas, S., Mason, C., & Haro, J. M. (2015). The association between social relationships and depression: A systematic review. *Journal of Affective Disorders*, 175, 53–65.

Sarris, J., Pinzon Rubiano, D., Day, K., Galvão-Coelho, N. L., & Perkins, D. (2022). Psychedelic medicines for mood disorders: Current evidence and clinical considerations. *Current Opinion in Psychiatry*, 35(1), 22–29.

Sher, C. D., Ingram, R. E., & Segal, Z. V. (2005). Cognitive reactivity and vulnerability: Empirical evaluation of construct activation and cognitive diatheses in unipolar depression. *Clinical Psychology Review*, 25, 487–510.

Soto, A., Smith, T. B., Griner, D., Domenech Rodríguez, M., & Bernal, G. (2018). Cultural adaptations and therapist multicultural competence: Two meta-analytic reviews. *Journal of Clinical Psychology*, 74(11), 1907–1923.

Stark, K. D., Sander, J. B., Yancy, M. G., Bronik, M. D., & Hoke, J. A. (2000). Treatment of depression in childhood and adolescence: Cognitive-behavioral procedures for the individual and family. In P. C. Kendall (Ed.), *Child & adolescent therapy: Cognitive-behavioral procedures* (2nd ed., pp. 173–234). Guilford Press.

Strauss, C., Cavanagh, K., Oliver, A., & Pettman, D. (2014). Mindfulness-based interventions for people diagnosed with a current episode of an anxiety or depressive disorder: A meta-analysis of randomised controlled trials. *PLoS One*, 9(4), e96110.

Sue, S., Zane, N., Hall, G. C. N., & Berger, L. K. (2009). The case for cultural competency in psychotherapeutic interventions. *Annual Review of Psychology*, 60(1), 525–548.

Teasdale, J. D., Moore, R. G., Hayhurst, H., et al. (2022). Metacognitive awareness and prevention of relapse in depression: Empirical evidence. *Journal of Consulting and Clinical Psychology*, 70(2), 275–687.

Teasdale, J. D., Segal, Z. V., Williams, J. M., et al. (2000). Prevention of relapse/recurrence in major depression by mindfulness-based cognitive therapy. *Journal of Consulting and Clinical Psychology*, 68(4), 615–623.

Torres, L., & Ong, A. D. (2010). A daily diary investigation of latino ethnic identity, discrimination, and depression. *Cultural Diversity and Ethnic Minority Psychology*, 16(4), 561–568.

Uphoff, E., Pires, M., Barbui, C., et al. (2020). Behavioural activation therapy for depression in adults with non-communicable diseases. *Cochrane Database of Systematic Reviews*, 8(8), Cd013461.

van Loon, A., van Schaik, A., Dekker, J., & Beekman, A. (2013). Bridging the gap for ethnic minority adult outpatients with depression and anxiety disorders by culturally adapted treatments. *Journal of Affective Disorders*, 147(1-3), 9–16.

Weersing, R., Jeffreys, M., Do, M., Schwartz, K., & Bolano, C. (2016). Evidence-based update: Treatment of depression in children and adolescents. *Journal of Clinical Child & Adolescent Psychology*, 46(1), 11–43.

Williams, D. R. (2018). Stress and the mental health of populations of color: Advancing our understanding of race-related stressors. *Journal of Health and Social Behavior*, 59(4), 466–485. https://doi.org/10.1177/0022146518814251.

Woike, K., Sim, E. J., Keller, F., et al. (2019). Common factors of psychotherapy in inpatients with major depressive disorder: A pilot study [original research]. *Frontiers in Psychiatry*, 10. https://doi.org/10.3389/fpsyt.2019.00463.

Zeiss, A. M., Lewinsohn, P. M., & Muñoz, R. F. (1979). Nonspecific improvement effects in depression using interpersonal skills training, pleasant activity schedules, or cognitive training. *Journal of Consulting and Clinical Psychology*, 47(3), 427–439.

3

Bipolar Disorder

Monica Ramirez Basco

Bipolar disorder is a severe mental illness characterized by significant mood swings that are accompanied by various cognitive (e.g., racing thoughts), behavioral (e.g., increased risk taking), and physical (e.g., decreased need for sleep) symptoms. It affects approximately 1% of the population, about equally in men and women, and generally has an age of onset in the early twenties (Merikangas et al., 2007).

People with bipolar disorder commonly suffer from episodes of mania and major depression across the course of their lives once the illness begins. The pattern of these episodes can vary greatly over time and across individuals. Between episodes, people can be asymptomatic, experience some residual symptoms, or may have milder episodes with limited functional impairment. If receiving pharmacotherapy, these milder symptoms are sometimes referred to as symptom breakthrough because the bipolar symptoms break through the protective effects of medication.

Depressive episodes that occur in the course of bipolar disorder are similar in symptom presentation to those experienced as part of unipolar major depressive disorder (MDD): significant and persistent sadness, loss of interest in usual activities, sleep disruption, appetite and/or weight loss, slowed cognitive functioning, reduced physical activity, and feelings of hopelessness (APA, 2022). When symptoms are severe and persistent, hopelessness and an inability to overcome them can lead some to consider suicide as an alternative. Across studies, Novick and colleagues (2010) found that approximately 30% of study participants (range 24–46%) with bipolar disorder reported at least one suicide attempt.

Episodes of mania can ramp up slowly before eventually reaching a peak that is identifiable by its severity. For some, manic symptoms can occur together but be less severe and not cause significant impairment. These are called hypomanic episodes. Those who have had episodes of MDD and hypomania, but never mania, would be diagnosed with bipolar II disorder (APA, 2022). That diagnosis changes to bipolar I disorder if and when the individual experiences a manic episode.

The symptoms, time course, severity, comorbidities, and amount of functional impairment experienced with bipolar disorder varies considerably across individuals.

30

Similarly, the subjective experiences and outward presentations of manic and major depressive episodes can vary within an individual over time. Some differences are due to age of onset of the disorder, ongoing treatment, season of the year, psychosocial stressors, comorbid problems such as substance abuse or dependence, or the presence of psychotic symptoms. These variations not only present diagnostic challenges for clinicians, but also make it difficult for people with bipolar disorder to understand what they are experiencing, anticipate future episodes, and take preventive actions.

However, even with considerable variability in symptom presentation, people with bipolar disorder can learn to become more attuned to the onset of hallmark symptoms such as difficulty sleeping, poor concentration, or irritability, and take some actions to control them. Such actions can include seeking or resuming medication treatment, reducing stimulation in their environment, improving sleep habits, and discontinuing use of substances that worsen depression or mania. These actions are often part of relapse prevention plans created as part of cognitive-behavioral therapy (e.g., Lam et al., 2003).

Etiology and Theoretical Underpinnings of Treatment

Science drives the psychotherapy treatment development process by informing the conceptualization of a problem based on evidence of its existence and characteristics and the choice of interventions that might ameliorate those documented symptoms. In the case of bipolar disorder, for example, there is ample scientific evidence that supports the characterization of bipolar disorder as consisting of manic and major depressive episodes (Merikangas et al., 2007). Similarly, we already know a great deal about the efficacy of cognitive therapy for the treatment of major depression based on numerous clinical trials (Cuijpers et al., 2013). Therefore, it stands to reason that depressive symptoms in the course of bipolar disorder could be similarly responsive to the same types of interventions.

Science also helps us understand the biological, psychological, and social aspects of mental illnesses. This knowledge helps the intervention developer identify possible targets for treatment. For example, one of the common challenges observed in the pharmacological treatment of bipolar disorder is the ability to consistently take medication (Sylvia et al., 2014), often due to unpleasant side effects, limited understanding of the role of medication treatment in bipolar disorder, and the complexity of treatment regimens (Loots et al., 2021). Targeting these challenges has become a common strategy in cognitive-behavioral therapy for bipolar disorder (CBT-BP).

In the case of psychotherapy development, evidence-supported therapeutic models for mental health disorders with similar symptom presentations can be adapted to address new problems. For CBT-BP, a cognitive-behavioral model developed for depression and other behavioral problems inspired the basic framework. For example, physical symptoms in bipolar disorder, such as sleep or energy changes, can lead to behavioral symptoms such as risk-taking, hypersexuality, or impulsivity in spending money. CBT largely focuses on slowing down poor decision-making to give a person time to use their reasoning skills before taking impulsive actions that might lead to negative consequences. The advantages of working through CBT exercises with a therapist is that the person in treatment learns about their illness, such as how to recognize mood episodes as they begin to emerge. This puts them in a stronger position to utilize interventions that can control the symptoms of bipolar disorder early in their development.

The stage of the illness is important when choosing a CBT intervention for bipolar disorder. For example, those newly diagnosed with bipolar disorder will need to gain a thorough understanding of their illness through patient education, especially its chronic and recurrent nature, as well as how treatment works. Those who take medication for bipolar disorder but continue to have symptoms might seek therapy to learn what they can do to make further improvements or how to better live with the illness. Symptoms can interfere with learning, especially manic symptoms that interfere with concentration, such as racing thoughts. CBT-BP methods may be easier to learn when symptoms are mild.

Brief Overview of Treatments

Historically, the focus of treatment for bipolar disorder has been on use of mood stabilizing medications solely or in combination with other drugs, which, when taken consistently, can help stave off symptoms (Bowden, 2004). The development of psychotherapy interventions for bipolar disorder began in the late 1970s as "add-ons" or adjunctive treatments that helped people understand their symptoms and the importance of consistent use of pharmacotherapy for the control of this chronic mental health condition. The psychotherapy interventions with the best research support will be discussed next.

Cognitive-Behavioral Therapy for Bipolar Disorder

Cognitive-behavioral therapy for bipolar disorder (CBT-BP, Basco & Rush, 1996, 2005) is a more comprehensive approach to psychotherapy for bipolar disorder and has shown promise in reducing the risk of relapse (Lam et al., 2005), improving adherence to medication treatment (Cochran, 1984), and enhancing day-to-day func-tioning (Ball et al., 2006). CBT-BP was designed to help people cope better with mood, cognitive, behavioral, and physical symptoms associated with this condition and to reduce the risk of relapse. It was not intended as a substitute for medication treatment, but instead is viewed as an adjunctive intervention to address the problems that medication alone is often insufficient to fully address. While the purpose of medication treatments is to resolve symptoms of depression and mania as well as to prevent future episodes, the goal of CBT-BP is to help people with bipolar disorder play an active role in treatment by doing what they can to manage those aspects of their illness over which they have control with the same end-points in mind. These include gaining a better understanding of bipolar disorder and how treatment works so that they are better prepared to take appropriate action as needed, learning how to be consistent with taking medication, as well as knowing the early warning signs that a new episode is emerging and working closely with their healthcare providers to forestall it. In addition, CBT-BP helps people understand how their thoughts and choices of actions may contribute to worsening of symptoms and what they can do about it.

Like other cognitive and behavioral therapies described in this book, CBT-BP is not a one-size-fits-all treatment. It is a group of interventions that are organized around a theoretical model that explains problems and how to address them. For example, the aspects of the treatment that are intended to help people recognize their symptoms and which are more educational in nature might be helpful for people who are new to the illness, had a recent onset, or are initiating treatment for the first time. It helps them make sense of what is happening to them, to distinguish between normal and symptomatic states, and to begin to draw a connection between treatment and changes in these symptoms. For example, Perry et al. (1999) conducted one of the first clinical trials with a psychoeducational focus using 7–12 individual therapy sessions with people who had experienced a manic episode in the prior year. They found that helping people understand their early symptoms of mania led to longer periods without manic episodes as well as a reduction in the number of relapses into mania. Similarly, Colom et al. (2003) found that in comparison to participation in support groups, a 21-session CBT-BP group treatment with a psychoeducational focus for people with bipolar disorder who were in remission helped to decrease hospitalizations and to increase time of wellness between episodes. The focus of the CBT-BP intervention was on increasing awareness of symptoms, improving consistency in use of medications, and promoting better understanding of the interplay between lifestyle choices and symptom relapse.

Those who have experienced several episodes of depression or mania, and are therefore more familiar with the symptoms of bipolar disorder, may benefit from learning new methods to control symptoms when medication is not enough. Evans et al. (2017), for example, focused on empowering people to take charge of their treatment by learning to recognize the onset of mania and do what they could do to help reduce their symptoms. Compared to treatment as usual (TAU), which consisted of medication management, those who received the CBT-BP intervention had fewer relapses and better psychosocial functioning over the 18 months following the intervention.

A third group of individuals who can benefit from CBT-BP are those who have had bipolar disorder for some time and have either had consistent difficulty managing their illness (refractory bipolar disorder), or who seek therapy to help them better adapt to or accept having the illness. Sometimes, people in this group describe being tired of having to deal with symptoms and medication; desire a break from pharmacotherapy; or need help managing their symptoms when starting a new job, new relationship, or having a child. For example, González-Isasi et al. (2010) found that participants receiving 20 sessions of CBT-BP in a group format as part of treatment for refractory bipolar disorder demonstrated better psychosocial functioning than did those receiving medication only. These examples illustrate the clinical flexibility of CBT-BP to address the pressing concerns of people with bipolar disorder with broadly different needs as well as to adapt the intervention to available treatment modalities and services.

The development of the first published treatment protocol of CBT-BP (Basco & Rush, 1996) was inspired by early efforts to provide psychotherapy to people with bipolar disorder (e.g., Benson, 1975; Powell et al., 1977) and the work of Susan Cochran (1984), who designed and tested a group-based intervention for improving medication adherence in people being treated for bipolar disorder, a key strategy to maximize the success of pharmacotherapy. Dr. John Rush, a protégé of the late Dr. Aaron Beck who developed cognitive therapy for depression (Beck et al. 1979), conducted some of the earliest clinical trials of cognitive therapy (Rush et al., 1977) that supported the efficacy of this intervention. Dr. Rush saw the potential for utilizing similar methods in the treatment of bipolar disorder as an adjunct to medication treatment. Dr. Basco, a psychologist and researcher (and the author of this chapter), had been developing cognitive-behavioral strategies for enhancing long-term treatment adherence in Type I diabetes (Basco, 1993) as part of a multicenter clinical trial. Together, Basco and Rush developed a protocol of cognitive-behavioral interventions that could address the common challenges to stabilizing bipolar disorder, the first of which was recognition and acknowledgment of the illness by the individual, their support network, and their healthcare provider. Symptoms that generally required treatment beyond pharmacotherapy included cognitive, behavioral, and affective changes during episodes of bipolar disorder that were exacerbated by psychosocial stress, inconsistent adherence to mood stabilizing medications, and actions that contributed to the onset of new episodes.

Chiang et al. (2017) conducted a meta-analysis of 19 randomized-controlled trials of CBT-BP with participants who had either bipolar I or bipolar II disorder. They found that CBT-BP demonstrated an ability to lower relapse rates especially among participants with bipolar I disorder, albeit with small to medium effect sizes. These studies also demonstrated CBT-BP's usefulness in helping participants to reduce symptoms of depression and mania and improve their overall psychosocial functioning.

Care should be taken in comparing studies and formats of CBT-BP as the differences in their delivery can make the intervention incomparable. For example, D'Souza et al. (2010) examined the effectiveness of 12 sessions of group psychoeducation for patients with bipolar disorder and their companions relative to TAU. The intervention was shown to decrease the likelihood of, and the time to, relapse in the CBT group relative to the TAU group. However, given that the CBT group differed in both the intervention provided and in types of participants (patients only versus patients and their companions), it is difficult to know to which aspects that success can be attributed.

Keep in mind that therapy may be more effective than a placebo intervention for many people, but it would be a mistake to assume it works for all people with bipolar disorder even for interventions with sufficiently large effect sizes in support of its efficacy. In fact, placebo interventions can sometimes be more effective than active treatments for those who need what the placebo provides, such as a friendly ear, some structure in their weekly schedule, or an activity that gets them out of the house. Friendly human contact with someone with whom you can share thoughts and feelings can be quite comforting. By the same token, the educational aspects of skills-oriented therapies like CBT-BP, though shown to be effective for reducing symptoms and preventing relapse, can feel rigid or unpleasantly academic for some patients. The same is true for the format of treatment. Although shown to be effective, group CBT-BP can be unpleasant for those who are socially uncomfortable, and individual therapy can be unhelpful if a trusting therapeutic alliance cannot be established.

Family-Focused Therapy for Bipolar Disorder

Family-focused therapy (FFT) for bipolar disorder (Miklowitz, 2010) is a manualized psychotherapy that capitalizes on the available support from family members, especially those who reside with the person who has bipolar disorder. Family therapy sessions include education for all about the nature and management of bipolar disorder, training to improve communication among family members, and strengthening of problem-solving skills to prevent or reduce stress. These skills, in turn, aim to lessen the risk of relapse, reduce symptoms, and improve outcomes. As a component of FFT, families create a relapse prevention plan that utilizes the skills developed during FFT (Miklowitz & Chung, 2016).

In an exploration of the efficacy of manualized psychotherapies including FFT, CBT, interpersonal therapy, and psychoeducation for bipolar disorder, Miklowitz et al. (2021) summarized the outcomes of 20 RCTs. Study designs included random assignment to either medication treatment in combination with either FFT, CBT, interpersonal therapy, or psychoeducation, or to medication treatment with a control condition such as supportive therapy or medication TAU. Results favored structured and manualized treatments over unstructured supports, including lower rates of mood episode recurrences.

Systemic Care for Bipolar Disorder

Unlike manualized psychotherapies such as CBT-BP or FFT, systemic care (Bauer, 2001), sometimes referred to as collaborative care, is a healthcare system-level model of care that provides education, support, and symptom monitoring by clinicians for people with bipolar disorder and assures that pharmacotherapy is consistent with accepted treatment guidelines. Mental health care teams who are part of managed care systems (Bauer et al., 2006a) are a central feature of systemic care and generally include a treatment coordinator or case manager that serves as the patient's point of contact for care. This individual (often a nurse) connects patients to resources, monitors symptoms and adherence to medication treatment, and facilitates crisis intervention or other care services as needed.

RCTs of systemic therapy for bipolar disorder have focused on both patient outcomes and costs of program implementation. Simon et al. (2006) recruited 441 patients from 4 behavioral health clinics that were part of a managed care organization. Monthly telephone calls were used to monitor symptoms and treatment adherence over the 2 years of the intervention, as well as to determine the needs for any additional mental health services. When compared to TAU, those who had clinically significant mood symptoms at baseline showed improvements in the severity and duration of manic symptoms, but not depressive symptoms. The added cost of the program over TAU was marginal. Similarly, Bauer et al. (2006b) randomly assigned 306 patients in 11 VA hospitals to systemic treatment or TAU and followed them for 3 years. They also found a reduction in duration of only manic symptoms with systemic care as compared to TAU, with the added program of care being cost neutral.

In contrast, Van der Voort et al. (2015) conducted an RCT of systemic care as compared to TAU for 138 patients with bipolar disorder in 16 outpatient mental health clinics. Compared to TAU, systemic care led to greater improvements in severity of depression at 12 months and duration of depressive symptoms at both 6 months and at 12 months. However, they did not observe differences in mania between the two groups.

Credible Components of Treatments

There are several treatment protocols that fall under the rubric of CBT-BP. They share similar theoretical foundations and treatment goals, but, depending on available therapy time, will vary in how many interventions are taught or problems addressed. There are also similar components across CBT-BP, FFT-BP, and systemic care such as psychoeducation, skills for tracking and preventing relapse, and emphasis on adherence to pharmacological treatment.

The research supporting the efficacy of CBT-BP is based on well-established research methods that aim to standardize as many aspects of the process as possible. That includes use of valid and reliable methods for verifying a diagnosis of bipolar disorder and measuring outcomes such as symptom level, appointment attendance, relapse, and consistency with which medication is taken. While these methods are critical to the ability to draw conclusions about the efficacy of CBT-BP, they can also make clinicians unwittingly vulnerable to making therapeutic errors that can affect clinical outcomes. The most common errors are those that send the wrong message to the person in treatment that they are not as important as the research, such as failing to sustain sufficient eye contact, seeming to lose track of what the person is saying while focusing on protocol materials, or pushing an intervention that does not match well to the what the person may need from the session.

For these reasons, the research therapists who provide CBT-BP in clinical trials are trained on all methods and observed and rated for their abilities to provide the care as it was intended while maintaining a strong therapeutic alliance. Not everyone is well-suited to being a research therapist. It requires an ability to listen on several channels at all times and to execute methods that, at times, might not feel like the right fit for the moment. It is particularly challenging for therapists who in their private practices would generally use a type of intervention that is different from the research protocol.

This being said, research therapists that contribute to clinical trials are usually exceptional clinicians who willingly submit to being evaluated on their performance and can tolerate corrective feedback. While it may not be necessary to perform CBT-BP at expert levels, to achieve the results found in clinical studies therapists should receive thorough training in psychopathology that includes bipolar disorder as well as good basic training in cognitive-behavioral treatment methods.

Psychoeducation

A commonly used method across CBT-BP protocols is psychoeducation regarding aspects of the illness and its treatment. Therapists can weave education around discussion of the patient's experiences with bipolar disorder, including symptoms, patterns of occurrence and course of episodes occurring over time, and how treatment works. Educational materials, pamphlets, workbooks, and worksheets can be used between sessions to reinforce information covered or to help reinforce concepts. Psychoeducation is easy to deliver within sessions, but therapists should be cautioned to use it judiciously so that they are engaging in conversation rather than talking at the patient for the full therapy hour. To facilitate rapport with a new therapy patient, effective therapists do the following: (a) begin by asking people what they already know about their bipolar disorder before providing additional information, (b) inquire about what they have been told by healthcare

Box 3.2 Overcoming Challenges

There are several challenges to learning and administering CBT-BP, especially early in one's career as a therapist. Mastering technical skills may seem fairly straightforward, especially when utilizing structured protocols, worksheets, and instructional manuals. The hard part is doing these things while learning how to be a therapist, trying to establish and maintain rapport with the person in treatment, learning about the myriad of presentations of bipolar disorder, and dealing with comorbidities (e.g., substance use, anxiety, significant life stress).

Another challenge is that mood swings and changes in thought processes and content (i.e., racing thoughts, poor attention and concentration) can make it difficult for the person with bipolar disorder to actively participate in therapy and to follow through with the homework that is a hallmark of most CBT treatments. When distractibility and a limited attention span make it difficult for the individual to focus during the session or retain information gained in therapy sessions, the therapist can encourage the patient to take notes and/or provide them with written materials. In some cases, it can be useful and appropriate for the therapist to provide the written notes or to schedule a brief phone call between sessions to follow-up on assigned homework, especially those tasks that are critical to preventing an imminent relapse.

The therapist less experienced in working with people who have bipolar disorder may also have trouble knowing when therapy progress is being stymied by the symptoms of bipolar disorder versus problems with the therapeutic alliance or the clinician's limited skills. Clinical supervision for trainees and clinical consultation for experienced therapists are useful tools when developing any new therapy skills, including CBT-BP. It is also helpful to elicit feedback from the patient during sessions about how the therapy is progressing, how they feel about homework assigned between sessions, or any change they think would make the therapy process more productive.

The fairly straightforward structure of most CBT-BP treatment protocols, especially the educational ones, can cause some clinicians to eagerly jump into an intervention before taking sufficient time to get to know the person they are treating and their unique symptom presentation and experiences with bipolar disorder, or to get a feel for what they already know about how to manage their illness. This mistake can diminish rapport if it inadvertently communicates disrespect for their knowledge and skills. Every person with bipolar disorder is different and has unique needs and abilities. In developing your treatment plan, take time to listen to the person's story before jumping too quickly into an intervention. On the flip side, some people may have had many years of experience with their bipolar disorder and its treatment, but still not be able to make the connection between what they have subjectively experienced and the symptoms and treatment effects. Helping people make that connection is a useful exercise that helps them prepare for the next episode and to know when treatment is helping and when it's not.

providers or family members and ask if they agree, (c) demonstrate respect for their experience with the illness by listening without correcting them, and (d) make notes about future educational needs (Basco & Rush, 2005). Psychoeducation is characterized by the Society of Clinical Psychology as having "*strong* research support for mania and *modest* research support for depression" (Society for Clinical Psychology, n.d., emphasis added).

Relapse Prevention

Patient education and improving adherence to medication treatment are two important aspects of preventing relapse, another goal common in CBT-BP protocols. Preventing episodes of depression and mania begins with education around common symptoms. The next step is to teach strategies for monitoring and detecting those symptoms, especially those that a person typically experiences early in the course of an episode. Examples of such methods include tracking mood swings, making note of changes in sleep patterns, or selecting a feeling or action that has previously preceded the onset of depression or mania (Basco, 2015).

Early detection of relapse provides an opportunity for early intervention. These might be self-help interventions taught during CBT-BP, strategies used by the therapist, or engaging a healthcare provider that manages medication treatment. Therapists should become knowledgeable of common things that trigger manic episodes, such as sleep loss or overstimulation, or that worsen feelings of depression, such as rumination or social isolation. Discussion of such triggers can become part of an action plan to avert a relapse.

Cognitive Restructuring

Traditional cognitive restructuring methods like those introduced by Beck et al. (1979) are also commonly used tools in CBT-BP. They can be used to educate people about common changes (distortions) in thinking that can occur during periods of depression and mania and how to reason through them. For example, discussions around the logical errors that discourage consistent use of pharmacotherapy can help people gain a better understanding of how medications work and can help them learn to distinguish between valid concerns and those driven by the symptoms of bipolar disorder. An example might be mistaking the onset of a manic episode for their new normal and seeing no need to continue taking medication. Cochran (1984), for example, taught cognitive restructuring skills to help medication group participants fight the urge to stop treatment. More consistent use of pharmacotherapy helped to increase the time to relapse and reduce the number of relapses as compared to a standard care comparison group focused on medication management.

Social Support

One of key advantages of FFT and systemic interventions is their engagement of other people to assist in treatment (Bauer, 2001; Miklowitz, 2010). FFT's engagement of family members and systemic care's use of care managers that communicate with treatment team members help with the monitoring, recognition, and response to emerging symptoms of depression and mania in the person with bipolar disorder. FFT has the added advantage of working directly with family members, strengthening their coping skills along with patients' skills.

Approaches for Youth

Research on the usefulness of psychotherapy for preventing or reducing the symptoms of bipolar disorder in youth is limited to date. In general, studies of psychotherapeutic interventions, such as FFT, Interpersonal/Social Rhythm Therapy, and CBT, have shown some evidence of their abilities to reduce symptoms and lengthen the time between mood episodes when compared to TAU such as medication clinic or supportive care (Miklowitz et al., 2021). Unfortunately, there have been no sufficiently powered studies to date that specifically compare CBT to other standardized psychotherapeutic interventions in youth with bipolar disorder.

Some information, however, might be gleaned from examining the treatment responses of people in psychotherapy clinical trials who are earlier in their course of illness of bipolar disorder, and therefore presumably younger. Ratheesh et al. (2023) found that when compared to those receiving TAU, study participants early in their course of bipolar disorder had improved symptoms and a reduced risk of relapse in studies of FFT (which included teens), and with CBT – with the youngest participants being primarily young adults. Similarly, Colom et al. (2010) found that psychoeducation focused on bipolar disorder was superior to supportive psychotherapy for participants with less than six episodes of illness compared to those with a longer course of bipolar disorder. Number of episodes can be a proxy for age in some cases.

CBT for major depressive episodes has not yet been tested in clinicals trials of youth with bipolar disorder. However, there have been studies of CBT for unipolar depression in adolescents, albeit with mixed findings (Kennard et al., 2006). See Chapter 2 for more information about unipolar depression with youth.

Other Variables Influencing Treatment

Assessment and Diagnosis

What distinguishes bipolar disorder from MDD is the occurrence of manic episodes. The mood changes in mania can be experienced as euphoric, excited, happy, up, or excessively irritable. These emotional shifts are intense and much more pronounced than reactions one might have to good or bad events. However, the experience of mood is very subjective. For people who are generally in good spirits, it's not unusual to be in an up mood that is not a symptom of mania. Likewise, in people that tend to be easily annoyed or are difficult to please, an irritable mood might not stand out as extreme. To be accurate in evaluating the presence of mania, clinicians must consider the full array of symptoms associated with bipolar disorder – those described in the *Diagnostic and Statistical Manual of Mental Disorders, Fifth Edition, Text Revision* (APA, 2022). These symptoms include a decreased need for sleep, uncharacteristic talkativeness, distractibility, racing thoughts, or restlessness. Because self-awareness can be limited when manic symptoms are present, it is useful to gather information from family members, friends, or other healthcare providers who have had more opportunities to observe the person when symptoms are present.

A definitive diagnosis of bipolar disorder is difficult to make during childhood and adolescence for many reasons. The behavior changes that occur during episodes of depression or mania can be misinterpreted as the primary problem rather than part of a symptom constellation consistent with depression or mania. Attention problems common to both phases of the illness might be viewed as attention-deficit/hyperactivity disorder (ADHD) if the additional mood symptoms are not carefully evaluated. Perhaps most challenging is to differentiate MDD from bipolar disorder in youth when depressive episodes present before the first manic episode. Occurrence of a manic episode is required before a diagnosis of bipolar disorder can be accurately determined. Given that CBT-BP is heavily weighted on patient education about the illness and its treatment, care should be taken to carefully assess the symptoms of bipolar disorder for initiating the intervention.

Comorbidity

Common comorbidities in youth with bipolar disorder include anxiety disorders, oppositional defiant disorder, and substance abuse (Post & Grunze, 2021), some of which may have predated the onset of the mood disorder. Duffy et al. (2019) studied Canadian youth who were offspring of adults with bipolar disorder, thereby making them at high risk for having the illness. They found that bipolar disorder was predated by a sequence of other mental health problems. Anxiety, ADHD, and sleep problems occurred before the onset of minor mood episodes and adjustment disorders. This sequence is supported by Merikangas et al.'s (2010) findings in the National Comorbidity Survey-Adolescent Supplement which showed a median age of onset for anxiety for adolescents of 6 years and a later median age of onset of 13 years for mood disorders such as bipolar disorder. Substance use disorders tended to occur later, with a median age of onset of 15 years.

The evolution of mental health problems in youth over time is a challenge for clinicians. They are in the position of treating current symptoms without the benefit of knowing what will happen next. For psychotherapists, any intervention that provides knowledge and coping skills can be helpful. If new symptoms emerge, psychothera-peutic methods such as CBT-BP can be added to address new problems. Healthcare providers that prescribe medication treatments for depression have the more daunting task of selecting drugs that could create new problems, such as triggering the onset of mania.

Demographics

The evaluation of the efficacy and effectiveness of CBT-BP is still in the early stages. Meta-analyses of studies to date (e.g., Miklowitz et al., 2021) show its promise, but more work must be done before conclusions can be drawn about for whom it is a preferred treatment option. Like with any other psychotherapy, clinicians should gather information about a person's demographic, cultural, social, and family back-ground to help inform their conceptualization of the presenting problem and the selection of treatment options.

Medication

A commonly used component of CBT-BP is establishing, improving, or maintaining adherence to medication regimens. This begins during the education phase of therapy by talking with the individual about current or past treatment, times when adherence has been challenging, and occasions when it has not been a problem. Studies that have compared medication clinic visits only to those with additional CBT-BP sessions have demonstrated the advantage of therapy as a complement to providing medication alone (Cochran, 1984; Evans et al., 2017; Perry et al., 1999). CBT-BP allows people to talk about their problems, address concerns about medications such as side effects, and correct negative and inaccurate thoughts about having a mental illness that requires pharmacotherapy. Once a person is ready to commit to medication treatment, therapists can help by establishing open communication about treatment adherence with the patient and the prescribing clinician, as well as assisting in the design of a personalized plan for taking medication consistently.

Conclusion

CBT-BP, FFT, and systemic care have been shown to be effective and useful psychotherapeutic tools for bipolar disorder, especially when part of a treatment package that includes pharmacotherapy. While there can be challenges to implemen-tation, the efficacy of empirically supported treatments is well worth the effort in helping to improve the quality of life of people with bipolar disorder. Because of the lifelong nature of the illness, the usefulness of therapy has the potential to be more helpful than can be measured in a clinical trial with limited treatment and follow-up periods. Each episode of depression, mania, and hypomania provides people with bipolar disorder, as well as their healthcare providers and family members, with opportunities to learn more about the illness, its triggers, and ways to prevent recurrences, thus improving quality of life.

For trainees who wish to gain skills in empirically supported treatments for bipolar disorder, there is much to be learned from formal training opportunities in the classroom and in clinical settings, especially those that provide supervision from clinicians with extensive experience in the treatment of bipolar disorder. In truth, savvy clinicians continue to learn from their successes and challenges in the course of providing care for people with bipolar disorder, particularly given the variety in symptom presentations of the illness and the many other things people bring with them to the therapy experience. Trainees are encouraged to view these experiences as not just clinical encounters, but as gifts of knowledge provided by people who will teach a great deal about how to be helpful and keep humble about therapeutic skills.

Useful Resources

- National Institute of Mental Health (NIMH), Bipolar Disorder, www.nimh.nih.gov/health/topics/bipolar-disorder.
- National Alliance on Mental Illness (NAMI), https://nami.org/About-Mental-Illness/Mental-Health-Conditions/Bipolar-Disorder.
- Depression and Bipolar Support Alliance (DBSA), www.dbsalliance.org/education/bipolar-disorder/.
- Substance Abuse, and Mental Health Services Administration (SAMHSA), www.samhsa.gov/serious-mental-illness/bi-polar.
- American Psychiatric Association. Bipolar Disorders, www.psychiatry.org/patients-families/bipolar-disorders.
- American Psychological Association. Bipolar Disorder, www.apa.org/topics/bipolar-disorder.
- US Department of Veteran Affairs. Bipolar Disorder. www.mentalhealth.va.gov/bipolar/index.asp.
- Basco, M. R. (2015). *The Bipolar Workbook: Tools for Controlling your Mood Swings*, 2nd ed. Guilford Press.

References

American Psychiatric Association [APA]. (2022). Bipolar and related disorders. In *Diagnostic and statistical manual of mental disorders* (5th ed., text revision) (pp. 139–175). American Psychiatric Association.

Ball, J. R., Mitchell, P. B., Corry, J. C., et al. (2006). A randomized controlled trial of cognitive therapy for bipolar disorder: Focus on long-term change. *Journal of Clinical Psychiatry*, 67(2), 277–286.

Basco, M. R. (1993). The cognitive behavioral therapist's role in diabetes management. *Behavior Therapist*, 16, 180–182.

Basco, M. R. (2015). *The bipolar workbook: Tools for controlling your mood swings.* Guilford Publications.

Basco, M. (2000). Cognitive-behavior therapy for bipolar I disorder. *Journal of Cognitive Psychotherapy*, 14, 287–304. https://doi.org/10.1891/0889-8391.14.3.287.

Basco, M. R., & Rush, A. J. (1995). Compliance with pharmacotherapy in mood disorders. *Psychiatric Annals*, 25(5), 269–270, 276, 278–279. https://doi.org/10.3928/0048-5713-19950501-03.

Basco, M. R., & Rush, A. J. (1996). *Cognitive-behavioral therapy for bipolar disorder.* Guilford Press.

Basco, M. R., & Rush, A. J. (2005). *Cognitive-behavioral therapy for bipolar disorder* (2nd ed.). Guilford Press.

Bauer M. S. (2001). The collaborative practice model for bipolar disorder: Design and implementation in a multi-site randomized controlled trial. *Bipolar Disorders*, 3(5), 233–244. https://doi.org/10.1034/j.1399-5618.2001.30502.x.

Bauer, M. S., McBride, L., Williford, W. O., et al. (2006a). Collaborative care for bipolar disorder: Part I. Intervention and implementation in a randomized effectiveness trial. *Psychiatric Services*, 57(7), 927–936.

Bauer, M. S., McBride, L., Williford, W. O., et al. (2006b). Collaborative care for bipolar disorder: Part II. Impact on clinical outcome, function, and costs. *Psychiatric Services*, 57(7), 937–945.

Beck, A. T., Rush, A. J., Shaw, B. F., & Emery, G. (1979). *Cognitive therapy of depression.* Guilford Press.

Benson, R. (1975). The forgotten treatment modality in bipolar illness: Psychotherapy. *Diseases of the Nervous System*, 36(11), 634–638. PMID: 1183307.

Bowden, C. L. (2004). Making optimal use of combination pharmacotherapy in bipolar disorder. *Journal of Clinical Psychiatry*, 65(Suppl 15), 21–24.

Chambless, D. L., & Hollon, S. D. (1998). Defining empirically supported therapies. *Journal of Consulting and Clinical Psychology*, 66(1), 7–18.

Chiang, K.-J., Tsai, J.-C., Liu, D., et al. (2017). Efficacy of cognitive-behavioral therapy in patients with bipolar disorder: A meta-analysis of randomized controlled trials. *PLoS One*, 12(5), e0176849. https://doi.org/10.1371/journal.pone.0176849.

Cochran, S. D. (1984). Preventing medical noncompliance in the outpatient treatment of bipolar affective disorders. *Journal of Consulting and Clinical Psychology*, 52(5), 873–878. https://doi.org/10.1037//0022-006x.52.5.873.

Colom, F., Reinares, M., Pacchiarotti, I., et al. (2010). Has number of previous episodes any effect on response to group psychoeducation in bipolar patients? A 5-year follow-up post hoc analysis. *Acta Neuropsychiatrica*, 22(2), 50–53. https://doi.org/10.1111/j.1601-5215.2010.00450.x.

Colom, F., Vita, E., Martinez-Aran, A., et al. (2003). A randomized trial on the efficacy of group psychoeducation in the prophylaxix of recurrences in bipolar patients whose disease is in remission. *Archives of General Psychiatry*, 60, 402–407. https://doi.org/10.1001/archpsyc.60.4.402. PMID: 12695318.

Cuijpers, P., Berking, M., Andersson, G., et al. (2013). A meta-analysis of cognitive-behavioural therapy for adult depression, alone and in comparison with other treatments. *The Canadian Journal of Psychiatry*, 58(7), 376–385. https://journals.sagepub.com/doi/epdf/10.1177/070674371305800702.

Curry, J., Rohde, P., Simons, A., et al. (2006). Predictors and moderators of acute outcome in the Treatment for Adolescents with Depression Study (TADS). *Journal of the American Academy of Child & Adolescent Psychiatry*, 45(12), 1427–1439. https://doi.org/10.1097/01.chi.0000240838.78984.e2.

D'Souza, R., Piskulic, D., & Sundrum, S. (2010) Brief dyadic group based psychoeducation program improves relapse rates in recently remitted bipolar disorder: A pilot randomized control trial. *Journal of Affective Disorders*, 120, 272–276. www.sciencedirect.com/science/article/abs/pii/S0165032709001311?via%3Dihub.

Duffy, A., Goodday, S., Keown-Stoneman, C., & Grof, P. (2019). The emergent course of bipolar disorder: Observations over two decades from the Canadian high-risk offspring cohort. *American Journal of Psychiatry*, 176(9), 720–729. https://doi.org/10.1176/appi.ajp.2018.18040461.

Evans, M., Kellett, S., Heyland, S., et al. (2017). Cognitive analytic therapy for bipolar disorder: A pilot randomised controlled trial. *Clinical Psychology and Psychotherapy*, 24, 22–35. https://doi.org/10.1002/cpp.2065.

González-Isasi, A., Echeburua, E., Liminana, J. M., & Gonzalez-Pinto, A. (2010). How effective is a psychological intervention program for patients with refractory bipolar disorder? A randomized controlled trial. *Journal of Affective Disorders*. 126, 80–87. https://doi.org/10.1016/j.jad.2010.03.026, PMID: 20444503.

Kennard, B., Silva, S., Vitiello, B., et al. (2006). Remission and residual symptoms after short-term treatment in the Treatment of Adolescents with Depression Study (TADS). *Journal of the American Academy of Child & Adolescent Psychiatry*, 45(12), 1404–1411. https://doi.org/10.1097/01.chi.0000242228.75516.21.

Lam, D. H., Bright, J., Jones, S., et al. (2000). Cognitive Therapy for Bipolar Illness: A Pilot Study of Relapse Prevention. *Cognitive Therapy and Research*, 24(5), 503–520. https://doi.org/10.1023/A:1005557911051.

Lam, D. H., Hayward, P., Watkins, E. R., Wright, K., & Sham, P. (2005). Relapse prevention in patients with bipolar disorder: Cognitive therapy outcome after 2 years. *American Journal of Psychiatry*, 162(2), 324–329.

Lam, D. H., Watkins, E. R., Hayward, P., et al. (2003). A randomized controlled trial of cognitive therapy for relapse prevention for bipolar affective disorder: Outcome of the first year. *Archives of General Psychiatry*, 60, 145–152. PMID: 12578431.

Loots, E., Goossens, E., Vanwesemael, T., et al. (2021). Interventions to improve medication adherence in patients with schizophrenia or bipolar disorders: A systematic review and meta-analysis. *International Journal of Environmental Research and Public Health*, 18, 10213. https://doi.org/10.3390/ijerph181910213.

Merikangas, K. R., Akiskal, H. S., Angst, J., et al. (2007). Lifetime and 12-month prevalence of bipolar spectrum disorder in the National Comorbidity Survey replication. *Archives of General Psychiatry*, 64(5), 543-552. https://doi.org/10.1001/archpsyc.64.5.543.

Merikangas, K. R., He, J. P., Burstein M., et al. (2010). Lifetime prevalence of mental disorders in US adolescents: Results from the National Comorbidity Survey Replication–Adolescent Supplement (NCS-A). *Journal of Clinical Child & Adolescent Psychology*, 49(10), 980–989. https://doi.org/10.1016/j.jaac.2010.05.017.

Miklowitz, D. J. (2010). *Bipolar disorder: A family focused treatment approach* (2nd ed.) Guilford Press.

Miklowitz, D. J., & Chung, B. (2016). Family-focused therapy for bipolar disorder: Reflections on 30 years of research. *Family Process*, 55(3), 483–499.

Miklowitz, D. J., Efthimiou, O., Furukawa, T. A., et al. (2021). Adjunctive psychotherapy for bipolar disorder: A systematic review and component network meta-analysis. *JAMA Psychiatry*, 78(2), 141–150. https://doi.org/10.1001/jamapsychiatry.2020.2993.

Novick, D. M., & Swartz, H. A. (2019). Evidence-based psychotherapies for bipolar disorder. *FOCUS, A Journal of the American Psychiatric Association*, 17(3), 238–248. https://doi.org/10.1176/appi.focus.20190004.

Novick, D. M., Swartz, H. A., & Frank, E. (2010). Suicide attempts in bipolar I and bipolar II disorder: A review and meta-analysis of the evidence. *Bipolar Disorder*, 12(1), 1–9. https://doi.org/10.1111/j.1399-5618.2009.00786.x. PMID: 20148862; PMCID: PMC4536929.

Perry, A., Tarrier, N., Morriss, R., McCarthy, E., & Limb, K. (1999). Randomised controlled trial of efficacy of teaching patients with bipolar disorder to identify early symptoms of relapse and obtain treatment. *British Medical Journal*, 318(7177), 149–153. https://doi.org/10.1136/bmj.318.7177.149.

Post, R. M. & Grunze, H. (2021). The challenges of children with bipolar disorder. *Medicina*, 57, e601. https://doi.org/10.3390/medicina57060601.

Powell, B. J., Othmer, E., & Sinkhorn, C. (1977). Pharmacological aftercare for homogeneous groups of patients. *Hospital & Community Psychiatry*, 28(2), 125–127. https://doi.org/10.1176/ps.28.2.125.

Ratheesh, A., Hett, D., Ramain, J., et al. (2023). A systematic review of interventions in the early course of bipolar disorder I or II: A report of the International Society for Bipolar Disorders Taskforce on early intervention. *International Journal of Bipolar Disorders*, 11(1), 1–24. https://doi.org/10.1186/s40345-022-00275-3.

Rush, A. J., Beck, A. T., Kovacs, M., & Hollon, S. (1977). Comparative efficacy of cognitive therapy and pharmacotherapy in the treatment of depressed outpatients. *Cognitive Therapy and Research*, 1(1), 17–37. https://doi.org/10.1007/BF01173502.

Simon, G. E., Ludman, E. J., Bauer, M. S., Unützer, J., & Operskalski, B. (2006). Long-term effectiveness and cost of a systematic care program for bipolar disorder. *Archives of General Psychiatry*, 63(5), 500–508. https://doi.org/10.1001/archpsyc.63.5.500.

Society for Clinical Psychology (n.d.). Psychoeducation for bipolar disorder. https://div12.org/treatment/psychoeducation-for-bipolar-disorder/.

Sylvia, L. G., Reilly-Harrington, N. A., Leon, A. C., et al. (2014). Medication adherence in a comparative effectiveness trial for bipolar disorder. *Acta Psychiatrica Scandinavica*, 129(5), 359–365. https://doi.org/10.1111/acps.12202.

Van der Voort, T., Van Meijel, B., Goossens, P., et al. (2015). Collaborative care for patients with bipolar disorder: Randomised controlled trial. *The British Journal of Psychiatry*, 206 (5), 393–400. https://doi.org/10.1192/bjp.bp.114.152520.

4

Anxiety Disorders

Dean McKay

Anxiety disorders are the most common category of psychiatric conditions, with base rates in the population actually increasing in the past several years. Recent population-based surveys suggest that as many as 33.7% of the population has been significantly affected by anxiety in their lifetime (Bandelow & Michaelis, 2022). As a category of diagnoses in the *Diagnostic and Statistical Manual of Mental Disorders* (DSM-5-TR; American Psychiatric Association, 2022), anxiety disorders are comprised of generalized anxiety disorder, panic disorder, specific phobia, social anxiety disorder, agoraphobia, separation anxiety disorder, and selective mutism.

Across the range of anxiety disorders, there are empirically supported treatment protocols and guidelines for developing evidence-based approaches in everyday clinical practice. As the scope of these protocols is extensive, this chapter focuses primarily on alleviating anxiety in general, and offers resources for readers to identify methods of interventions for specific anxiety disorders.

Anxiety disorders are marked by several core features. First, sufferers experience heightened sympathetic nervous system arousal, resulting in increased heart rate, muscle tension, respiration, and associated physiological arousal. This arousal is in response to specific feared stimuli or situations. Second, sufferers typically experience anticipatory anxiety, as they expect to encounter feared stimuli and situations. Third, anxiety disorder sufferers engage in avoidance of associated stimuli and situations, a process that may foster a wide range of cognitive distortions that perpetuate avoidance behavior. Collectively, these three domains contribute significantly to disability associated with anxiety disorders.

Etiology and Theoretical Underpinnings of Treatment

Contemporary models of anxiety disorder etiology emphasize its emergence from a personality predisposition connected with specific biological risks. Neuroticism, a broad personality trait that has been linked with sensitivity to aversive experiences and lower reward sensitivity, is associated with the full range of anxiety disorders, as well as depression (Barlow et al., 2014). This sensitivity to aversive experiences sets the occasion for a higher rate of acquired feared stimuli and situations. This higher rate of acquisition can come about through direct experience, or through information processing and cognitive biases toward feared stimuli (discussed in McKay, 2016).

Each of the distinct anxiety disorders listed in the DSM-5-TR have well-established cognitive-behavioral treatment protocols. The varied protocols all emphasize targeting behavioral avoidance and cognitive distortions associated with anxiety onset and maintenance. These strategies, collectively, can be viewed as targeting neuroticism (Barlow et al., 2014). In recognition of this common thread among the anxiety disorders, the Unified Protocol (UP; Farchione et al., 2012) was developed to alleviate anxiety disorders and depression. The remainder of this chapter emphasizes intervention with the UP, while also recognizing the contribution to understanding the mechanisms of specific anxiety disorders resulting from research on other specific treatment protocols.

Brief Overview of Treatments

As noted, the emphasis in this chapter is on the UP as a treatment for anxiety disorders. However, across all treatment protocols, there is an emphasis on several interventions to varying degrees: exposure, cognitive therapy, and general emotion-focused coping strategies. The UP specifically enumerates five broad intervention domains: increasing present-focused emotion awareness, increasing cognitive flexibility, identifying and preventing patterns of emotion avoidance/maladaptive emotion-based behaviors, increased tolerance of emotion-based physical reactions, and interoceptive and situational exposure. Each of these treatment components of the UP can be classified into exposure (interoceptive and situational exposure; increased tolerance of emotional-based physical reactions), cognitive therapy (increased cognitive flexibility), and general emotion-focused coping strategies (increasing present-focused emotion awareness, identifying and preventing patterns of emotion avoidance/maladaptive emotion-based behaviors). What has been valuable about the development of the UP has been the portability and ease of disseminating to a wide range of settings where clinicians might otherwise be overwhelmed by the choice of treatment packages for the various anxiety disorders (McHugh & Barlow, 2010).

Exposure-Based Interventions

A core behavioral intervention for all anxiety disorders, exposure is seductively simple in its description, but technically challenging to implement. The central feature of exposure therapy involves gradually and systematically presenting feared stimuli or situations to clients, so that these previously avoided stimuli and situations are better emotionally tolerated. When possible, in vivo exposure should be conducted. Research has demonstrated that live exposure is most effective in alleviating anxiety and reducing exposure. When practiced in vivo, the clinician's role is to facilitate the exposure experience with imagery that highlights the feared outcome from the exposure (discussed in Garner et al., 2021). This is in order to reduce any potential cognitive avoidance the client may engage in that would undermine the effectiveness of the live exposure.

Cognitive Therapy

Modern cognitive therapy is based on two broad components. The first is that individuals have biases of thinking that foster beliefs that have not been critically examined. Therefore, one component of cognitive therapy is to train clients to approach their beliefs scientifically, and test out the assumptions they hold regarding different situations. In the anxiety disorders, there are some broad themes into which these beliefs roughly fall, such as intolerance of uncertainty and overestimation of threat (see Clark & Beck, 2009). The second component is based on findings from cognitive science, in which individuals with anxiety disorders differentially attend to, and therefore differentially encode into memory and form judgments in response to, greater amounts of threat-related information from the environment (discussed in Williams et al., 1997). This line of experimental cognitive research has led to recent computer-based interventions aimed at retraining individuals to attend to nonthreatening stimuli (Hang et al., 2021). Regardless of the application of computer-based attention retraining methods, understanding cognitive biases is useful in informing clinicians about how anxious individuals may show differential attention and memory, and guide how to facilitate gathering of evidence for clients to use in challenging their assumptions about feared situations.

Emotion-Focused Coping Strategies

The range of interventions that fall in this category is diverse. It includes direct physical interventions such as relaxation training (Manzoni et al., 2010) up to more recent developments such as mindfulness meditation (Hofmann et al., 2010). These approaches are often integrated into existing treatment packages for anxiety disorders. Recent research suggests that mindfulness, and some related interventions (such as acceptance-based treatments; see Box 4.1), produce large effects on anxiety reduction (Vøllestad et al., 2012). Although these approaches have generated considerable enthusiasm among anxiety disorder specialists, their unique contribution to symptom reduction remains unclear.

Overall Level of Research Support

The aforementioned broad treatment approaches for anxiety disorders enjoy substantial research support when examined as full treatment packages. However, support for treatment packages does not provide information regarding which components are essential, whether the sequence of interventions is optimum, or whether any components may be benign or even detrimental to outcome. Discussion of dismantling research and investigations of individual components are presented in the following sections.

The standards for empirically supported treatments (ESTs) recently underwent revision (Tolin et al., 2015). In the revised EST standards, a well-established treatment had to have a sufficient body of research support, in high-quality investigations, that the protocol would fare well in systematic reviews and meta-analyses. When considered in this light, few research protocols for anxiety disorders yet reach that standard, including the UP that has served as the central protocol for this chapter. However, the accumu-lated research over the past four decades into exposure therapy and cognitive therapy suggests that together these serve clients with anxiety disorders well, and may be reasonably considered the basis for treatment. In particular, using the original EST criteria, the Society for Clinical Psychology (n.d.) indicates there is *strong research support* for: (a) exposure therapies for specific phobias, (b) cognitive and behavioral therapies for generalized anxiety disorder, (c) cognitive-behavioral therapy for panic disorder, and (d) cognitive-behavioral therapy for social anxiety disorder.

The addition of emotion-focused coping strategies, however, is less clear. As a stand-alone set of interventions, these would not be considered sufficient to alleviate anxiety. Indeed, research has demonstrated that relaxation training alone leads to moderate effect sizes (Manzoni et al., 2010), as does mindfulness meditation (Hofmann et al., 2010). Contrast that with the effect sizes for exposure, which are typically large (discussed in Garner et al., 2021).

The UP has accumulated sufficient research that a systematic review has been conducted, showing large effect sizes for the treatment protocol (Sakiris & Berle, 2019). However, this review included adaptations of the UP to other diagnostic groups (such as eating disorders), treatment-seeking adults with a range of emotional distress, and studies that were single-subject or nonrandomized in nature. So, while there is cause for optimism that the UP may reach a level of being considered an EST (based on the recent criteria, Tolin et al., 2015), there are not yet sufficient high-quality investigations for a systematic review to evaluate.

Credible Components of Treatments

The discussion to this point has emphasized multicomponent intervention programs to alleviate anxiety disorders. However, to be fair, there have been few dismantling studies to isolate the individual interventions that form the basis for the existing

Box 4.1 Acceptance and Commitment Therapy

Among psychosocial treatment packages, the vast majority emphasize cognitive-behavioral approaches. Some recent treatment programs have also included a role for acceptance and commitment therapy (ACT; Hayes et al., 2016). Briefly, ACT is based on a modern verbal-learning theoretical framework called relational frame theory (discussed in Hayes & Hayes, 1992; Zettle et al., 2015). In a review of meta-analyses (Gloster et al., 2020), eleven studies reported effect sizes for anxiety reduction applying this treatment approach, and these effect sizes were small to moderate. Although ACT may contribute significantly to anxiety reduction, at the present time it may be best viewed as a contribution to other comprehensive treatment programs rather than as a stand-alone intervention.

treatment protocols. The few investigations that have been conducted have compared exposure to cognitive therapy, with no significant difference between interventions (discussed in Kaczkurkin & Foa, 2015). It should be noted, however, that exposure and cognitive therapy each contain components of the other, thus complicating any "pure" comparison between the two.

Aspects of Exposure

The underlying science of exposure has evolved significantly in the past ten years. Foa and Kozak (1986) articulated the dominant conceptualization for the mechanisms underlying exposure, a perspective that has guided the treatment literature for decades. Specifically, the requirements for exposure to exert its effect on anxiety demanded that the intervention provoke adequate arousal to engage the neural circuitry associated with fear and its connection to memory structures that stored the fear information. However, this came with a risk that the therapist might evoke too much fear, leading to a breakdown in the ability to benefit from the intervention, and instead would further crystallize the memory for the fear. This model, where the minimum requirement in each session was the evocation of fear, led to some unfounded apprehensions among clinicians, including concerns that there would be higher rates of client drop-out and risk of litigation (Richard & Gloster, 2006).

More recently, exposure methods have shifted to the inhibitory learning model (ILM; Craske et al., 2014). In this approach to exposure, the emphasis is on new learning, irrespective of clients' emotional reaction during the session. This model details several major ways that exposure procedures may be adjusted to target facets of classically conditioned fear and/or the associated avoidance. The author of this chapter has described the ILM as an approach intuitively applied by clinicians who are successful in implementing exposure, given that there is a de-emphasis on provoking anxiety and an emphasis on new behavior (Frank & McKay, 2019). However, the empirical support for the ILM has not been systematically tested, and thus as of this writing may be best considered a potential format for administering exposure that deserves greater empirical scrutiny. Interested readers are directed to Craske et al. (2014), as well as Jacoby and Abramowitz (2016) for detailed descriptions of the approach.

Intersection of Exposure and Cognitions

The prescription of exposure to alleviate fear is not done in a vacuum. Indeed, if mere exposure were easily accomplished by direct instruction, there would be little use for the clinician. Instead, clients need to have the procedure explained to them, with suitable justification for the effects on their anxiety that it will produce. The process of demonstrating that exposure will, ultimately, have some benefit typically includes a direct confrontation with the feared consequences and some challenge to the veracity of these consequences: In short, cognitive therapy but without the actual disputation and direct targeting of cognitions (discussed in Kaczkurkin & Foa, 2015).

Exposure in general may also serve to facilitate cognitive therapy. The following are two major ways this can be accomplished.

Increase Relevance of Cognitions

As imagery is constructed in conjunction with exposure, the associated cognitions become more accessible. This increased accessibility makes exposure an important accompaniment to cognitive therapy in order that robust challenges to the automatic biases may be undertaken. Therapeutic situations that raise the relevance of cognitions increase their accessibility, and thus are more readily targeted as part of cognitive therapy (discussed in Abramowitz, Taylor, & McKay, 2006).

Hypothesis Test Additional Cognitions

Cognitive science models emphasize that automatic processing entails attentional biases, which in turn influence memory and judgment. Accordingly, imagery exercises that accompany exposure may also serve the purpose of testing hypotheses the clinician may have regarding the putative anxiety-related stimuli that the client may not readily identify (discussed in Mathews, 1997). Imagery exercises serve an important purpose by targeting biases in attention and memory that accumulate from a process of chronic avoidance. That is, the persistent avoidance allows anxiety disorder sufferers to maintain untested beliefs, and hypothesis testing allows for the systematic breakdown of these biases.

Addressing Cognitive Biases

Modern cognitive therapy for anxiety disorders builds on prior iterations of the approach by highlighting empirically validated cognitive biases commonly observed among individuals with this class of disorders. The original formulation of cognitions for anxiety disorders was most clearly described by Beck and Emery (1985), where future-oriented catastrophic cognitions were spontaneously accessible to anxiety sufferers. This general model has since been refined to emphasize the following cognitive biases. Each of the belief domains listed here warrant a range of cognitive therapy interventions, such as behavioral experiments (to directly test hypotheses), practice in disputation, and rehearsal in coping with circumstances where hypothetically the feared outcome might come true.

Intolerance of Uncertainty

This specific cognitive bias is highly prevalent in the anxiety disorders, with meta-analyses showing it correlates significantly with symptoms of generalized anxiety (Gentes & Ruscio, 2011). It has also been shown to be highly correlated with general symptoms of emotion dysregulation (Sahib et al., 2023).

Perfectionism

The tendency toward perfectionism has long been associated with anxiety (e.g., Antony et al., 1998), as well as representing a specific risk for depression and suicide (Blatt, 1995). Additional systematic data show that perfectionism is highly predictive of the full range of anxiety disorders (Egan et al., 2011), and that direct treatment of perfectionism has palliative effects on anxiety in general (Galloway et al., 2021).

Overestimation of Threat

When individuals with anxiety disorders describe the objects and situations that provoke fear, it is often through the perspective of the dangerousness of the stimuli. A reasonable question that clinicians ask, then, is what is the level of risk? This question demands the client provide an appraisal of the hazard associated with the stimuli. Thus, to use a basic example, when individuals suffer from spider phobia, the appraised dangerousness of spiders is high, even though the actual number of spiders that are deadly to humans is extremely low. This kind of danger appraisal breakdown could be done with any presenting anxiety concern. Further, findings from experimental cognition research show that as anxiety increases, attentional bias is increased for more subtle threats, which in turn biases memory for danger (Pergamin-Hight et al., 2015).

Approaches for Youth

As with adult anxiety disorders, there are numerous ESTs for childhood anxiety. These protocols generally emphasize exposure and cognitive therapy, scaled to address the unique developmental needs of youth. As with the UP for adults, there is a protocol that has gained wide adoption for the treatment of anxiety disorders in youth: the Coping Cat (Kendall, 1994). Key components of the Coping Cat program include exposure, cognitive reappraisal methods, and relaxation strategies. Reappraisal strategies in children involve presenting situations where the child has to describe hypothetical thoughts that might accompany it and then generate other reasonable options. For example, in Coping Cat, there is a cartoon image of a large, ostensibly aggressive dog on a leash, and a cat that is clearly out of reach of the dog. The child would be asked to generate potential thoughts the cat may have in this situation.

The Coping Cat treatment program has been modified for adolescents (Podell et al., 2010) and frameworks have been developed to flexibly adopt the program based on complex clinical presentations and comorbid conditions (Beidas et al., 2010). Meta-analytic findings suggest that, compared to waitlist or control treatment conditions, the effect of the Coping Cat program on reducing anxiety and associated psychopathology is large, and when compared to other credible treatments the effect is small (Lenz, 2015).

Treatment of child anxiety often engages the parents in the process. The majority of treatment programs, including the Coping Cat, specify a role for parents related to aiding the child in practicing the core components of the protocol. However, research has consistently shown that parental involvement based solely on assisting in exposure and cognitive interventions has a negligible effect on treatment (Reynolds et al., 2012). The current conceptual models of treatment emphasize anxiety reduction without examining the environmental context in which it develops or is maintained, despite the foundation of behavioral interventions being based on learning experiences. Thus, there have been calls for programmatic developments of interventions that integrate parent and family variables that might foster anxiety in children and target those in addition to the already established and effective components of existing protocols (Taboas et al., 2015).

Other Variables Influencing Treatment

Assessment and Diagnosis

The chapter thus far has described treatment approaches for the majority of cases, without necessarily considering potential complicating factors. Identifying these potential complicating factors can be critical in developing a case conceptualization that would increase the likelihood of a good outcome. Research has shown that variables such as comorbid psychopathology, personality disturbance, and medication may impact adherence to treatment and drop-out (Taylor et al., 2012). Several major areas of potential treatment complications are reviewed.

Comorbidity

Depression commonly co-occurs with anxiety disorders. The connection between anxiety and depression has been recognized for a long time (i.e., Dobson, 1985; Rapee & Barlow, 1991). While it is acknowledged that anxiety and depression are separate conditions, depression associated with anxiety disorders is generally understood to result from the loss of control over the emotional arousal and range of situations that are associated with feared stimuli and situations (Beuke et al., 2003).

Comorbid conditions are generally considered additional barriers to treatment outcome. Interestingly, the consequence of different comorbid conditions on treatment outcome has not been widely or systematically evaluated, despite the finding that the vast majority of participants in treatment trials have one or more additional diagnoses (Newman et al., 2010). In one meta-analysis that considered all treatments, and not solely evidence-based interventions, it was shown that any additional comorbid condition was associated with poorer outcome (Olatunji et al., 2010).

The one class of disorders that stands out for a potential adverse effect on anxiety disorder treatment outcome are substance use disorders. Interestingly, there is comparably limited research on this (McHugh, 2015). This gap in the research is surprising considering that survey data has shown that anxiety disorders are a risk factor for substance use (Marmorstein, 2012).

Demographics

Research into demographic factors that might impact anxiety disorders has been conducted, and generally does not reveal any substantive effects, with one exception. It has been noted that anxiety disorders tend to affect women more than men (Craske, 2003), with risk for anxiety disorders at about twice the rate as for men. There is limited research on the full range of gender identities as yet, and the majority of the body of research is on traditional binary gender definitions. It has been suggested that this increased liability for anxiety in women is multifaceted but centers on biological differences in hormonal regulation and, consequentially, brain area action. The explanation for these differences remain largely theoretical. Research has shown that there are no differences in treatment outcome based on gender (Grubbs et al., 2015).

Medication

There are a diverse range of practice guidelines for anxiety disorders that have originated from several professional organizations. Thus, these guidelines emphasize the treatments that are generally within the purview of that organization. For example, while the evidence for medication in the treatment of anxiety disorders is generally positive, it is less clear the extent to which psychopharmacology is additive to psychosocial interventions (Olatunji et al., 2010). Despite this, most psychiatric organizations make the blanket recommendation for a combination of CBT with psychopharmacology (i.e., Bandelow et al., 2012).

There is a large body of research that examines the conjoint role of medication (usually antidepressants) and CBT in the anxiety disorders. As noted, while the majority of psychiatric clinical practice guidelines suggest that the best outcome is a combination of both, the research actually suggests some medications (such as benzodiazepines) may interfere with long-term benefits of CBT (Otto et al., 2005; Tolin, 2017).

Benzodiazepines (or minor tranquilizers) are commonly prescribed for anxiety disorders. This class of medications alleviate acute anxiety, and many anxiety disorder sufferers may be prescribed one of these drugs to take daily, rather than as needed. The difficulty this poses is that benzodiazepines also lead to physical dependence, and withdrawal symptoms upon discontinuation (see Julien et al., 2010 for a detailed discussion). Frequently, when individuals with anxiety disorders initiate CBT, particularly exposure therapy, the clinician may suggest that the client refrain from taking benzodiazepine medications as the sedating effects interfere with the elicitation of arousal necessary for exposure to have its benefits. As a result, individuals who have developed benzodiazepine dependence may require additional treatment specifically directed at managing withdrawal. Cognitive-behavioral therapy procedures specifically aimed at facilitating benzodiazepine discontinuation have been developed, and are found to be efficacious (Takeshima et al., 2021).

Box 4.2 Personality and Anxiety Disorders

Anxiety disorders are most closely associated with the personality trait of neuroticism, and there has been a recent resurgence in interest in this attribute (Barlow et al., 2014). This is the specific target personality trait at the heart of the UP, and, given the broad recognition of its role in a wide range of internalizing disorders, it is reasonable that it would be the focus of attention in evidence-based treatment.

Other personality variables have also been examined in relation to treatment outcome for anxiety disorders. For convenience, relying on the personality factors that form the "Big 5" (Costa & McCrae, 2008), the additional four traits would be extraversion, conscientiousness, agreeableness, and openness to experience. Recent research has shown that extraversion is a protective factor against the development of anxiety disorders (Metts et al., 2021). Research on conscientiousness and openness to experience are fairly lacking, but one investigation showed no meaningful association between these two traits in predicting anxiety disorder onset or severity (Karsten et al., 2012). In one meta-analysis that examined the relation of all the personality factors in the Big Five to anxiety, depressive, and substance use disorders, it was shown that extraversion had the highest protective value, and conscientiousness also provided some protection, whereas conscientiousness and openness to experience were generally unrelated (Kotov et al., 2010).

Although personality assessment is a common procedure in clinical settings, and conceptual research frequently emphasizes the negative prognostic indicators for co-occurring personality disorders for virtually all psychopathology, there remains limited research on how personality traits or disorders impact treatment outcome for anxiety disorders. One recent review examined all the available research, dating from 1980 to 2019, and identified only 48 studies that evaluated personality traits or disorders in predicting anxiety disorder treatment outcome (Hovenkamp et al., 2021). They found that personality disorders did, in fact, tend to predict poorer treatment outcome. For personality traits, they found that low levels of extraversion were associated with poorer outcome, and higher levels of attributes often broadly associated with neuroticism were also associated with poor treatment outcome.

Conclusion

Anxiety disorders have been heavily investigated, and ESTs have been developed that emphasize cognitive-behavioral models of intervention. A recent protocol, the UP, served as a useful framework for discussing the critical components of evidence-based treatment as it emphasizes exposure, cognitive modification, and specific coping strategies. While the available research on these conditions shows that effective treatments are available, and that these alleviate symptoms as well as improve quality of life, there remain significant gaps in research knowledge.

Addressing stigma, a known impediment to treatment outcome in a wide range of psychiatric disorders (Hatzenbueler & Pachankis, 2021), has been underinvestigated in relation to anxiety disorder outcome. Considering that stigma also impacts quality of life (Marcussen et al., 2010), another under investigated area of anxiety disorder treatment, future research should prioritize targeting this important variable.

There remain significant gaps in the research on the benefits of existing evidence-based interventions on several demographic groups, particularly people of color and other underrepresented groups. While these are well-known limits, strategies for improving representation in research that would in turn permit greater generalization of treatment programs have not yet borne fruit. It is expected that in the coming years more robust evidence-based treatment recommendations may be made that address the needs of the widest swath of the population.

Useful Resources

Books for Professionals

- Abramowitz, J. S., Deacon, B. J., & Whiteside, S. P. H. (2019). *Exposure therapy for anxiety: Principles and practice* (2nd ed.). Guilford.
- Barlow, D. H. (2002). *Anxiety and its disorders: The nature and treatment of anxiety and panic* (2nd ed.). Guilford.
- Emmelkamp, P., & Ehring, T. (2014). *The Wiley handbook of anxiety disorders*. Wiley-Blackwell.
- Olatunji, B. O. (2018). *The Cambridge handbook of anxiety and related disorders*. Cambridge University Press.
- Sauer-Zavala, S., & Barlow, D.H. (2021). *Neuroticism: A new framework for emotional disorders and their treatment*. Guilford.

Books for Clients and Consumers

- Bourne, E. J. (2020). *The anxiety and phobia workbook*. New Harbinger.
- Shannon, J. (2017). *Don't feed the monkey mind: How to stop the cycle of anxiety, fear and worry*. New Harbinger.

Organizations and Websites

- Anxiety and Depression Association of America (ADAA): www.adaa.org
- Association for Behavioral and Cognitive Therapies (ABCT): www.abct.org

References

Abramowitz, J. S., Taylor, S., & McKay, D. (2006). Potentials and limitations of cognitive therapy for obsessive-compulsive disorder. *Cognitive Behavior Therapy*, 34, 140–147.

Alonso, J., Buron, A., Bruffaerts, R., et al. (2008). Association of perceived stigma and mood and anxiety disorders: Results from the World Mental Health Surveys. *Acta Psychiatrica Scandinavica*, 188, 305–314.

American Psychiatric Association. (2022). *Diagnostic and statistical manual of mental disorders* (5th ed., text revision). Arlington: American Psychiatric Association.

Antony, M. M., Purdon, C. L., Huta, V., & Swinson, R. P. (1998). Dimensions of perfectionism across the anxiety disorders. *Behaviour Research and Therapy*, 36, 1143–1154.

Bandelow, B., & Michaelis, S. (2022). Epidemiology of anxiety disorders in the 21st century. *Dialogues in Clinical Neuroscience*, 17, 327–335.

Bandelow, B., Sher, L., Bunevicius, R., et al. (2012). Guidelines for the pharmacological treatment of anxiety disorders, obsessive-compulsive disorder and posttraumatic stress disorder in primary care. *International Journal of Psychiatry in Clinical Practice*, 16, 77–84.

Barlow, D.H., Sauer-Zavala, S., Carl, J.R., Bullis, J.R., & Ellard, K.K. (2014). The nature, diagnosis, and treatment of neuroticism: Back to the future. *Clinical Psychological Science*, 2, 344–365.

Beck, A. T. & Emery, G. (1985). *Anxiety disorders and phobias: A cognitive perspective.* Basic Books.

Beidas, R. S., Benjamin, C. L., Puleo, C. M., Edmunds, J. M., & Kendall, P. C. (2010). Flexible application of the Coping Cat program for anxious youth. *Cognitive and Behavioral Practice*, 17, 142–153.

Beuke, C. J., Fischer, R., & McDowall, J. (2003). Anxiety and depression: Why and how to measure their separate effects. *Clinical Psychology Review*, 23, 831–848.

Blatt, S. J. (1995). The destructiveness of perfectionism: Implications for the treatment of depression. *American Psychologist*, 50, 1003–1020.

Bolles, R. C. (1972). Reinforcement, expectancy, and learning. *Psychological Review*, 79, 394–409.

Clark, D. A., & Beck, A. T. (2009). *Cognitive therapy of anxiety disorders: Science & Practice*. Guilford.

Corrigan, P. W., Druss, B. G., & Pertick, D. A. (2014). The impact of mental illness stigma on seeking and participating in mental health care. *Psychological Science in the Public Interest*, 15, 37–70.

Costa, P. T., & McCrae, R. R. (2008). The revised NEO Personality Inventory. In G. J. Boyles, G. Matthews, & D. H. Saklofske (Eds.), *The SAGE Handbook of Personality Theory and Assessment, Vol. 2. Personality Measurement and Testing* (pp. 179–198). Sage.

Craske, M. G. (2003). *Origins of phobias and anxiety disorders: Why more women than men?* Amsterdam: Elsevier.

Craske, M. G., Treanor, M., Conway, C. C., & Zbozinek, T. (2014). Maximizing exposure therapy: An inhibitory learning approach. *Behaviour Research and Therapy*, 58, 10–23.

Curcio, C., & Corboy, D. (2020). Stigma and anxiety disorders: A systematic review. *Stigma and Health*, 5, 125–137.

Dobson, K. S. (1985). The relationship between anxiety and depression. *Clinical Psychology Review*, 5, 307–324.

Egan, S. J., Wade, T. D., & Shafran, R. (2011). Perfectionism as a transdiagnostic process: A clinical review. *Clinical Psychology Review*, 31, 203–212.

Fang, A., Sawyer, A. T., Asnaani, A., & Hofmann, S. G. (2013). Social mishap exposures for social anxiety disorder: An important treatment ingredient. *Cognitive & Behavioral Practice*, 20, 213–220.

Farchione, T. J., Fairholme, C. P., Ellard, K. K., et al. (2012). Unified protocol for transdiagnostic treatment of emotional disorders: A randomized controlled trial. *Behavior Therapy*, 43, 666–678.

Foa, E. B., & Kozak, M. J. (1986). Emotional processing of fear: exposure to corrective information. *Psychological Bulletin*, 99(1), 20–35.

Frank, B., & McKay, D. (2019). The suitability of an inhibitory learning approach in exposure when habituation fails: A clinical application to misophonia. *Cognitive & Behavioral Practice*, 26, 130–142.

Gallagher, M. W., Sauer-Zavala, S. E., Boswell, J. F., et al. (2013). The impact of the Unified Protocol for Emotional Disorders on quality of life. *International Journal of Cognitive Therapy*, 6, 57–72.

Galloway, R., Watson, H., Greene, D., Shafran, R., & Egan, S. J. (2021). The efficacy of randomised controlled trials of cognitive behaviour therapy for perfectionism: A systematic review and meta-analysis. *Cognitive Behaviour Therapy*, 51, 170–184.

Garner, L., & Steinberg, E., McKay, D. (2021). Exposure therapy. In A. Wenzel (Ed.), *Handbook of cognitive behavioral therapy* (pp. 275–312). American Psychological Association Press.

Gentes, E.L., & Ruscio, A.M. (2011). A meta-analysis of the relation of intolerance of uncertainty to symptoms of generalized anxiety disorder, major depressive disorder, and obsessive-compulsive disorder. *Clinical Psychology Review*, 31, 923–933.

Gloster, A.T., Walder, N., Levin, M.E., Twohig, M.P., & Karekla, M. (2020). The empirical status of acceptance and commitment therapy: A review of meta-analyses. *Journal of Contextual Behavioral Science*, 18, 181–192.

Grubbs, K., Cheney, A., Fortney, J., et al. (2015). The role of gender in moderating treatment outcome in collaborative care for anxiety. *Psychiatric Services*, 66, 265–271.

Hang, Y., Xu, L., Wang, C., Zhang, G., & Zhang, N. (2021). Can attention bias modification augement the effect of CBT for anxiety disorders? A systematic review and meta-analysis. *Psychiatry Research*, 299, 113982.

Hatzenbueler, M. L., & Pachankis, J. E. (2021). Does stigma moderate the efficacy of mental- and behavioral-health interventions? Examining individual and contextual sources of treatment-effect heterogeneity. *Current Directions in Psychological Science*, 30, 476–484.

Hayes, S. C., & Hayes, L. J. (1992). Verbal relations and the evolution of behavior analysis. *American Psychologist*, 47, 1383–1395.

Hayes, S. C., Strosahl, K. D., & Wilson, K. G. (2016). *Acceptance and commitment therapy: The process and practice of mindful change* (2nd ed.). Guilford.

Helbig-Lang, S., & Peterman, F. (2010). Tolerate or eliminate? A systematic review on the effects of safety behavior across anxiety disorders. *Clinical Psychology: Science and Practice*, 17, 218–233.

Hofmann, S. G., Sawyer, A. T., Witt, A. A., & Oh, D. (2010). The effect of mindfulness-based therapy on anxiety and depression: A meta-analytic review. *Journal of Consulting and Clinical Psychology*, 78, 169–183.

Hofmann, S. G., Wu, J.Q., & Boettcher, H. (2014). Effect of cognitive-behavioral therapy for anxiety disorders on quality of life. *Journal of Consulting and Clinical Psychology*, 82, 375–391.

Hovenkamp, J. H. M., Jeronimus, B. F., Myroniuk, S., Riese, H., & Schoevers, R. A. (2021). Predictors of persistence of anxiety disorders across the lifespan: A systematic review. *Lancet Psychiatry*, 8, 428–443.

Jacoby, R. J., & Abramowitz, J. S. (2016). Inhibitory learning approaches to exposure therapy: A critical review. *Clinical Psychology Review*, 49, 28–40.

Jenkins, H. M. (1984). Time and contingency in classical conditioning. *Annals of the New York Academy of Sciences*, 423, 242–253.

Julien, R. M., Advokat, C. D., & Comaty, J. E. (2010). *A primer of drug action* (12th ed.). Worth Publishers.

Kaczkurkin, A. N., & Foa, E. B. (2015). Cognitive-behavioral therapy for anxiety disorders: An update on the empirical evidence. *Dialogues in Clinical Neuroscience*, 17, 337–346.

Karsten, J., Penninx, B. W. J. H., Riese, H., et al. (2012). The state effect of depressive and anxiety disorders on big five personality traits. *Journal of Psychiatric Research*, 46, 644–650.

Kendall, P. C. (1994). Treating anxiety disorders in children: Results of a randomized clinical trial. *Journal of Consulting and Clinical Psychology*, 62, 100–110.

Kotov, R., Gamez, W., Schmidt, F., & Watson, D. (2010). Linking "big" personality traits to anxiety, depressive, and substance use disorders: A meta-analysis. *Psychological Bulletin*, 136, 768–821.

Lenz, A. S. (2015). Meta-analysis of the Coping Cat program for decreasing severity of anxiety symptoms among children and adolescents. *Journal of Child and Adolescent Counseling*, 1, 51–65.

Manzoni, G.M., Pagnini, F., Castelnuovo, G., & Molinari, E. (2010). Relaxation training for anxiety: A ten-years systematic review with meta-analysis. *BMC Psychiatry*, 8, 41.

Marmorstein, N. R. (2012). Anxiety disorders and substance use disorders: Different associations by anxiety disorder. *Journal of Anxiety Disorders*, 26, 88–94.

Marcussen, K., Ritter, C., & Munetz, M. R. (2010). The effect of services and stigma on quality of life for persons with serious mental illness. *Psychiatric Services*, 61, 489–494.

Mathews, A. (1997). Information-processing biases in emotional disorders. In D. M. Clark & C. G. Fairburn (Eds.), *Science and practice of cognitive behaviour therapy* (pp. 47–66). Oxford University Press.

McHugh, R. K. (2015). Treatment of co-occurring anxiety disorders and substance use disorders. *Harvard Review of Psychiatry*, 23, 99–111.

McHugh, R. K., & Barlow, D. H. (2010). The dissemination and implementation of evidence-based psychological treatments: A review of current efforts. *American Psychologist*, 65, 73–84.

McKay, D. (2016). Anxiety disorders. In J. C. Norcross, G. R. Vandenbos, & D. K. Freedheim (Eds.), *APA handbook of clinical psychology* (Vol. IV: *Psychopathology & health*, Volume editor N. Pole) (pp. 61–96). American Psychological Association.

Metts, A., Zinbarg, R., Hammen, C., Mineka, S., & Craske, M.G. (2021). Extraversion and interpersonal support as risk, resource, and protective factors in the prediction of unipolar mood and anxiety disorders. *Journal of Abnormal Psychology*, 130, 47–59.

Newman, M., Przeworski, A., Fisher, A., & Borkovec, T. D. (2010). Diagnostic comorbidity in adults with generalized anxiety disorder: Impact of comorbidity on psychotherapy outcome and impact of psychotherapy on comorbid diagnoses. *Behavior Therapy*, 41, 59–72.

Ociskova, M., Prasko, J., Vrbova, K., et al. (2018). Self-stigma and treatment effectiveness in patients with anxiety disorders – A mediation analysis. *Neuropsychiatric Disease and Treatment*, 14, 383–392.

Olatunji, B. O., Cisler, J. M., & Deacon, B. J. (2010). Efficacy of cognitive behavioral therapy for anxiety disorders: A review of meta-analytic findings. *Psychiatric Clinics of North America*, 33, 557–577.

Otto, M. W., Smits, J. A. J., & Reese, H. E. (2005). Combined psychotherapy and pharmacotherapy for mood and anxiety disorders in adults: Review and meta-analysis. *Clinical Psychology: Science & Practice*, 12, 72–86.

Olatunji, B. O., Cisler, J. M., & Tolin, D. F. (2007). Quality of life in the anxiety disorders: A meta-analytic review. *Clinical Psychology Review*, 27, 572–581.

Pergamin-Hight, L., Naim, R., Bakermans-Kranenburg, M. J., van IJzendoorn, M. H., & Bar-Haim, Y. (2015). Content specificity of attention to threat in anxiety disorders: A meta-analysis. *Clinical Psychology Review*, 35, 10–18.

Podell, J. L., Mychailyszyn, M., Edmunds, J., Puleo, C. M., & Kendall, P. C. (2010). The Coping Cat program for anxious youth: The FEAR plan comes to life. *Cognitive and Behavioral Practice*, 17, 132–141.

Rachman, S., Radomsky, A. S., & Shafran, R. (2008). Safety behaviour: A reconsideration. *Behaviour Research and Therapy*, 46, 163–173.

Rapee, R. M., & Barlow, D. H. (1991). *Chronic anxiety: Generalized anxiety disorder and mixed anxiety-depression.* Guilford.

Rescorla, R. A. (1988). Pavlovian conditioning: It's not what you think it is. *American Psychologist*, 43, 151–160.

Rescorla, R. A. (2006). Deepened extinction from compound stimulus presentation. *Journal of Experimental Psychology: Animal Behavior Processes*, 32, 135–144.

Reynolds, S., Wilson, C., Austin, J., & Hooper, L. (2012). Effects of psychotherapy for anxiety in children and adolescents: A meta-analytic review. *Clinical Psychology Review*, 32, 251–262.

Richard, D. C. S., & Gloster, A. T. (2006). Exposure therapy has a public relations problem: A dearth of litigation amid a wealth of concern. In D. C. S. Richard & D. L. Lauterbach (Eds.), *Handbook of exposure therapies* (pp. 409–425). Academic Press.

Sahib, A., Chen, J., Cardenas, D., & Calear, A.L. (2023). Intolerance of uncertainty and emotion regulation: A meta-analysis and systematic review. *Clinical Psychology Review*, 101, 102270.

Sakiris, N., & Berle, D. (2019). A systematic review and meta-analysis of the Unified Protocol as a transdiagnostic emotion regulation based intervention. *Clinical Psychology Review*, 72, 101751.

Society for Clinical Psychology (n.d.). Diagnoses. https://div12.org/diagnoses/.

Stokes, T. F. & Baer, D. M. (1977). An implicit technology of generalization. *Journal of Applied Behavior Analysis*, 10, 349–367.

Taboas, W. R., McKay, D., Whiteside, S. P. H., & Storch, E. A. (2015). Parental involvement in youth anxiety treatments: Conceptual bases, controversies, and recommendations for intervention. *Journal of Anxiety Disorders*, 30, 16–18.

Takeshima, M., Otsubo, T., Funada, D., et al. (2021). Does cognitive behavioral therapy for anxiety disorders assist the discontinuation of benzodiazepines among patients with anxiety disorders? A systematic review and meta-analysis. *Psychiatry and Clinical Neurosciences*, 75, 119–127.

Taylor, S., Abramowitz, J. S., & McKay, D. (2012). Non-adherence and non-response in the treatment of anxiety disorders. *Journal of Anxiety Disorders*, 26, 583–589.

Tolin, D. F. (2017). Can cognitive behavioral therapy for anxiety and depression be improved with pharmacotherapy? A meta-analysis. *Psychiatric Clinics of North America*, 40, 715–738.

Tolin, D. F., McKay, D., Forman, E. M., Klonsky, E. D., & Thombs, B.D. (2015). Empirically supported treatment: Recommendations for a new model. *Clinical Psychology: Science & Practice*, 22, 317–338.

Vøllestad, J., Nielsen, M. B., & Nielsen, G. H. (2012). Mindfulness- and acceptance-based interventions for anxiety disorders: A systematic review and meta-analysis. *British Journal of Clinical Psychology*, 51, 239–260.

Williams, M. T., Beckmann-Mendez, D. A., & Turkheimer, E. (2013). Cultural barriers to African American participation in anxiety disorder research. *Journal of the National Medical Association*, 105, 33–41.

Williams, J. M. G., Watts, F. N., MacLeod, C., & Mathews, A. (1997). *Cognitive psychology and emotional disorders* (2nd ed.). Wiley.

Zettle, R. D., Hayes, S. C., Barnes-Holmes, D., & Biglan, A. (2015). *The Wiley handbook of contextual behavioral science*. Wiley.

Zvolensky, M. J., Garey, L., & Bakhshaie, J. (2017). Disparities in anxiety and its disorders. *Journal of Anxiety Disorders*, 48, 1–5.

5

Obsessive-Compulsive Disorder

Dean McKay

Obsessive-compulsive disorder (OCD) is a heterogeneous psychiatric condition, marked by intrusive and unwanted thoughts (obsessions) that provoke anxiety, and that may be accompanied by compulsive behaviors designed to alleviate the obsessions. Estimates of prevalence vary, but generally range from 0.7% (Adam et al., 2012) to 1.2% (Ruscio et al., 2010) over a one-year period. Early clinical descriptions date back to Freud's famous "Rat Man" (Freud, 1909).

The heterogeneity of OCD is illustrated by the wide variety of symptom presentations, and can be categorized roughly into the following dimensions: contamination fear and washing rituals, obsessions (aggressive, sexual, religious, and somatic) and checking compulsions, and symmetry obsessions and ordering/counting/repeating compulsions (McKay et al., 2004; Abramowitz et al., 2005).[1] Early descriptions of OCD by Janet (1908) emphasized a perceptual component to the condition, one marked by a sense of incompleteness for actions. Tests of incompleteness suggest that it, along with a drive for harm avoidance, were associated with each dimension of OCD (Taylor et al., 2014). The sense of incompleteness appears in the research as reward insensitivity (discussed in Gruner & Pittenger, 2017).

This chapter covers treatment for OCD. It should be noted that some overlap in treatment mechanisms apply to other diagnoses in the broader obsessive-compulsive related disorders, the category of which OCD is part in the *Diagnostic and Statistical Manual* (5th ed., text revision; 2022). These disorders share intrusive cognitions, repetitive behaviors, or both. Theoretically, these disorders are unified by a breakdown in behavioral inhibition (Fineberg et al., 2021). However, there have been critiques of the shared neural mechanisms and logical consistency with underlying cognitive domains among these disorders (i.e., Abramowitz, 2018; Abramowitz et al., 2009). Nonetheless, behavioral inhibition is relevant in the discussion of treatments that follows in this chapter.

---

[1] Hoarding was a symptom of OCD in earlier editions of the diagnostic manual, and was therefore an additional dimension of OCD in the research cited. It was not listed here, as the current diagnostic manual lists hoarding as a separate disorder.

Etiology and Theoretical Underpinnings of Treatment

Etiological models of OCD derive from two major sources: biogenetic and cognitive-behavioral. While the thrust of this chapter emphasizes psychosocial treatment – and thus cognitive-behavioral approaches – the biogenetic model looms large over much of the current evidence-based treatment models. This is because many treatment guidelines stress the conjoint benefit of medication with treatment (i.e., Koran et al., 2007; Anxiety and Depression Association of America, 2015). Further, recent research has evaluated the role of neural stimulation methods (i.e., transcranial direct stimulation; da Silva et al., 2019) in conjunction with cognitive-behavioral therapy (CBT).

Before directly addressing etiological models based on CBT approaches to treatment, OCD is compelling for its potential as a biologically based psychiatric condition. The aforementioned reward insensitivity is suggestive of a biological substrate, considering the expressly psychophysiological modeling for behavioral inhibition (Corr & Perkins, 2006), the apparent heritability (Mahjani et al., 2021), and seeming brain localization (discussed in Stein et al., 2019). Despite the theoretical assertions for a biological basis, definitive evidence has been elusive (Mahjani et al., 2021). To be fair to the biological modeling of OCD, it is reasonable to consider that due to the wide heterogeneity of the disorder, biological models cannot satisfactorily determine unique neural or genetic features. To cite one illustration of how the heterogeneity complicates determination of specific etiological factors, contamination obsessions and washing rituals have been found to be a result of disgust as well as anxiety (i.e., Mancusi & McKay, 2021), whereas other symptom dimensions have prominent anxiety without disgust (discussed in McKay et al., 2015). As a result of the compelling notion of a neurobiological basis for OCD, much of the treatment research literature includes a prominent role for medication or other neurobiological interventions in conjunction with CBT, and thus few studies have completely isolated the effects of CBT, either in total or for individual components. Interested readers are directed to Pittenger (2017) for detailed coverage of neurobiological conceptualizations of OCD.

Cognitive-behavioral accounts of the etiology of OCD have been evolving, beginning with purely behavioral descriptions that suggested compulsions arose as a negatively reinforced behavior to alleviate obsessions (for a review, see Clark, 2004). These early accounts were quickly confronted by the problem of obsessions themselves, which are unlike other stimuli that are usually the source of avoidance in negative reinforcement associated with fear learning. Specifically, obsessions are purely internal events and required a different explanatory framework. Based on these early observations, the first integrative cognitive-behavioral account comes from Rachman and Hodgson (1980), who suggested that OCD is essentially the result of the following cognitive vulnerabilities: dysphoric mood;

stress; intolerance of certain thoughts; increased sensitivity to threat; and personality variables, particularly neuroticism, introversion, and elevated emotionality. This conceptualization also broadly expanded the scope of obsessional and compulsive phenomena, and facilitated distinguishing the condition from obsessive-compulsive personality.

Since the time of Rachman and Hodgson (1980), the conceptualization of OCD has centered on how individuals with OCD differ from other people with respect to their reactions to specific thoughts. Unwanted, intrusive thoughts are a common experience in the general population (Freeston et al., 1991). Individuals with OCD differ in their obsessional experiences from everyday intrusive thoughts in the following ways: higher frequency, higher distress and lower acceptability, guilt provoked by the thought(s), resistance when the thought(s) occur, a sense of loss of control over the thought(s), intrusions appraised as meaningful, substantial time with the thought(s) as focus of consciousness, extensive concern over need to control the thought, and extensive interference with activities (Clark, 2004).

The research described has led to the development of a more comprehensive cognitive model of OCD. This conceptualization suggests that obsessions arise from a specific set of dysfunctional beliefs. These beliefs are activated in response to otherwise normal obsessions. One dysfunctional belief that has received considerable attention is an inflated sense of personal responsibility (Salkovskis, 1985). Recent research has shown that inflated responsibility is indeed associated with OCD, but is not a unique contributor to symptoms (McKay et al., 2014) and may be more relevant for mild symptoms (Kim et al., 2016). Several other major dysfunctional beliefs have been hypothesized to increase obsessional problems and associated compulsive behavior. Among these are beliefs such as the over-importance of thoughts (e.g., "My thoughts indicate something significant about me"), the need to control thoughts, overestimation of threat, perfectionism, and intolerance for uncertainty (see Taylor et al., 2007), and are relevant to the condition at all levels of severity (Kim et al., 2016).

Recent additional conceptualizations of obsessional phenomena have focused on the reasoning process that individuals with OCD undergo when appraising situations that are associated with obsessions, rather than the content of obsessions themselves. Termed the "inferential confusion" model, this has emerged to address the breakdown in how individuals with OCD distrust their own perceptual experiences (O'Connor & Robillard, 1995). Since this conceptual development, there have been several investigations comparing a specific form of cognitive therapy based on this model to control interventions (Julien et al., 2016). However, it has not yet undergone more rigorous comparisons, nor are the distinctions with cognitive therapy yet empirically evaluated. It is raised in this chapter to highlight an emerging potential direction in research on OCD.

Brief Overview of Treatments

The story of evidence-based treatment for OCD dates back to the mid-1960s. Aside from Freud's Rat Man, OCD was considered a chronic and untreatable condition (Kringlen, 1965). Soon after that demoralizing assessment Meyer (1966) showed that OCD could be treated by exposing clients to obsession-evoking stimuli followed by blocking the associated rituals. This has come to be known as exposure with response prevention (ERP), and is by far the most well-validated behavioral intervention for OCD (discussed in McKay et al., 2015). The conceptual model for the mechanisms underlying exposure therapy in general was described by Foa and Kozak (1986). According to that model, it is considered necessary to evoke anxiety in order that corrective processes take place. Since that time, the inhibitory learning model (ILM) has emerged, which emphasizes new learning rather than anxiety evocation in order to promote change. Interestingly, Meyer (1966) described ERP as altering expectancies in clients; expectancy violations (and thus expectancy change) is a major component of the ILM.

Since the emergence of ERP, cognitive interventions have emerged to either augment behavioral interventions or to supplant them entirely. These interventions build on the cognitive framework developed by Salkovskis (1985), and have been expanded based on the identification of a core set of cognitions associated with OCD (Obsessive Compulsive Cognitions Working Group, 2001). The extent that the unique mechanisms for cognitive therapy can be isolated is limited, however, as treatment often includes behavioral experiments, such as exercises that include exposure as a means to provoke core cognitions (discussed in Abramowitz et al., 2005). Research has demonstrated that cognitive change is an essential ingredient for substantial symptom change (Woody et al., 2011), and, as a result, contemporary treatment for OCD includes both cognitive and behavioral interventions, even if there is overlap in the mechanisms between them.

Description of Treatment Packages

There are several treatment protocols for OCD. As noted, these can be roughly broken down into either ERP or cognitive therapy. These will be considered separately, although most specialists in OCD combine the two in evidence-based treatment as part of routine care.

Numerous meta-analyses have been conducted that demonstrate ERP results in large effect sizes in change when compared to control interventions. These meta-analyses have considered ERP alone or in conjunction with cognitive therapy (reviewed in Spencer et al., 2023). Additionally, cognitive interventions have been shown to further moderate treatment efficacy (Ferrando & Selai, 2021), complicating the extent that ERP may be considered a sufficient stand-alone treatment.

Across all treatment packages that emphasize ERP, the common core includes: developing a hierarchy of feared/avoided stimuli; practice in approaching these stimuli, in vivo where possible; inclusion of imagery to enhance the exposure exercises when conducted in vivo; and relapse prevention strategies. This process is akin to that described for exposure treatment for anxiety disorders (see Chapter 4). The response prevention arm of ERP is intended to continue exposure, since the central function of rituals is to alleviate obsessional experiences and the associated emotional arousal.

The model of cognitive therapy specifically developed for OCD is the accepted and empirically supported approach, and is associated with large effect sizes when compared to control interventions (Rosa-Alcázar et al., 2008). This is in direct contrast to the original general cognitive therapy approach that includes direct disputation of erroneous beliefs about harm. Recent conceptualizations suggest that the more general cognitive therapy model is either benign or potentially harmful (McKay, 2021) as the average OCD sufferer already recognizes the senselessness of their symptoms.

The majority of research on core dimensions of beliefs in OCD has emerged from the Obsessive-Compulsive Cognitions Workgroup (OCCWG, 2001). This consortium of researchers developed a measure – the Obsessive-Beliefs Questionnaire (OBQ-44; OCCWG, 2005) – that taps into six major cognitive dimensions: inflated responsibility; overestimation of threat; perfectionism; intolerance of uncertainty; importance of thoughts; and control of thoughts. Treatment programs have been developed based solely on the cognitive model (i.e., Wilhelm & Steketee, 2006). Across all cognitive therapy programs of treatment, the central focus is on how individuals appraise situations, and then connect these appraisals to the core cognitive dimensions considered theoretically associated with OCD.

Box 5.1 Body Dysmorphic Disorder, Hoarding Disorder, Trichotillomania, and Excoriation

The publication of the fifth edition of the *Diagnostic and Statistical Manual of Mental Disorders* (DSM-5; American Psychiatric Association, 2013) included the development of a new category of diagnoses: the Obsessive Compulsive Related Disorders (OCRDs). This new category includes body dysmorphic disorder (BDD), which was formerly a somatoform disorder, and trichotillomania, which was formerly an impulse control disorder. The new category also includes a new disorder: hoarding disorder. Hoarding was formerly a symptom of OCD, but extensive research showed that individuals whose primary issue was hoarding behaviors exhibited significant differences in demographics, functionality of symptoms, and other psychopathological signs (Pertusa et al., 2010). The OCRDs also include a new diagnosis called excoriation (skin-picking) disorder, marked by repetitive skin-picking.

There are treatment protocols for each of the disorders in the OCRD category. Treatment protocols for BDD emphasize cognitive-behavioral approaches for managing body image and reducing compulsive behaviors typical for the disorder, such as mirror checking and reassurance seeking regarding appearance (Wilhelm et al., 2012). Among the OCRDs, treatment for BDD most closely resembles treatment for OCD, in that exposure plays a prominent role in alleviating symptoms.

Treatment programs for trichotillomania (TM) center on habit reversal, a specific behavioral procedure that involves training in competing responses that interfere with the problematic repetitive behavior (reviewed in Farhat et al., 2020). In light of research showing that TM is also associated with emotional regulation difficulties (Diefenbach et al., 2008), specific interventions to target this aspect of functioning have been added to programs of habit reversal (such as with dialectical behavior therapy; Keuthen et al., 2011).

Treatment programs for hoarding disorder emphasize organization strategies, attachment to objects, self-control methods to reduce acquisition of items, and skills for managing emotional distress (Tolin et al., 2013). Among the OCRDs, hoarding disorder is more likely to require intervention outside the office, given the extent to which sufferers have pervasive difficulty managing their home environment.

The newest diagnosis in the DSM-5 – excoriation (skin-picking; dermatillomania) disorder – has at this point limited specific treatment approaches. Treatment models for this condition emphasize functional analysis for environmental and emotional situations that result in urges to skin pick. As with TM, habit reversal programs have been developed and shown to reduce symptoms of excoriation disorder (reviewed in Lochner et al., 2017).

Overall Level of Research Support

Treatments involving ERP and CT together represent the standard of psychological care for OCD (discussed in McKay et al., 2015). Evidence-based care for OCD emphasizes the application of specialized CBT (i.e., ADAA, 2015), which collectively represents a combination of ERP and CT. However, the extent to which a clinician may rely more on ERP or more on CT hinges on several facets.

- General comfort with exposure-based therapy: There is an extensive body of work showing that some clinicians are hesitant to conduct exposure-based treatments due to a range of misconceptions about the approach (Deacon et al., 2013). To illustrate the extent to which this hesitancy is germane to clinicians, the treatment text by Wilhelm and Steketee (2006) emphasizes that with the program they describe, effective treatment can be delivered without conducting exposure.
- Symptom dimension: The availability of in vivo stimuli that can be safely encountered for exposure varies widely by symptom dimension. Individuals with washing rituals may more readily have accessible stimuli for exposure (i.e., contact with ostensibly contaminated surfaces), whereas individuals with intrusive thoughts of harm lack readily accessible directly relevant cues.

- <u>Lag between exposure and likely feared outcome</u>: When exposure is conducted, it is predicted by the client that the feared outcome may occur in some discrete period of time afterward. However, some obsessions have feared outcomes far in the future (i.e., contamination fears about hepatitis, where illness may be many months after exposure) or postmortem (i.e., concerns about intrusive thoughts of blasphemy). These can pose significant hurdles for clinicians in developing exposure procedures (discussed in McKay, Taylor, & Abramowitz, 2010).
- <u>Overvalued ideation</u>: This is discussed in greater depth later, under "Other Variables Influencing Treatment," but deserves brief mention here. Some individuals with OCD hold strong beliefs in the likelihood of aversive outcome when rituals are considered essential. In some cases, these beliefs can come close to delusional in nature (Kozak & Foa, 1994), and pose a significant barrier to implementing exposure.

In light of these considerations, the efficacy of CBT as a broader treatment program can be considered efficacious. Overall, using the Chambless and Hollon (1998) criteria for empirically supported treatments, the Society of Clinical Psychology characterizes both ERP and CBT as being *well-established* for OCD (Society of Clinical Psychology, n.d.). ERP is the only treatment to date that has been evaluated using the Tolin, McKay et al. (2015) criteria, receiving a *strong recommendation* but not yet a *very strong recommendation* (Tolin, Melnyk et al., 2015). Overall, considerable expertise is required to make proper treatment decisions about how to develop exposure methods and identify salient cognitive dimensions for individuals with OCD while accounting for the myriad symptom presentations.

Credible Components of Treatments

Empirically supported treatment for OCD emphasizes combined ERP and CT. As noted earlier, considering the overlap in methods for conducting exposure, whereby feared outcomes may include elements that resemble cognitions, and CT, which may include behavioral experiments that resemble exposure, it has been challenging to isolate the effects of either ERP or CT in alleviating symptoms. Further complicating the picture is the heterogeneity of symptoms, and hesitancy about conducting exposure among some clinicians. Nonetheless, procedurally ERP and CT are different, and training clinicians in the two methods requires clear delineation.

Aspects of Exposure

While discussed in the "Anxiety Disorders" chapter in this text (by the same author; see Chapter 4), it is worth briefly discussing the contemporary model for exposure-based treatment as it has undergone some changes in the past ten years. The original model for exposure therapies emphasized activation of fear through engagement specifically of neural structures that store memory for the emotional connection with the stimuli (Foa & Kozak, 1986). It is this model that many clinicians cited when expressing concerns over conducting exposure therapy (discussed in Richard & Gloster, 2006). While part of the expressed concerns by clinicians was that exposure therapy increased the risk of drop-out, in the case of OCD this has not been observed (Ong et al., 2016). While exposure therapy has always had behavior change as its intended goal, the more recent inhibitory learning model (ILM; Craske et al., 2014) explicitly focuses on change over emotional response. The methods for accomplishing behavior change are broken into different strategies in the service of exposure. The application of the ILM is, at this point, in the nascent stages of development when applied to OCD, but may have promise (i.e., expectancy violations; Elsner et al., 2022). Interested readers may consider formulations that translate the components of ILM to applications for OCD (Jacoby & Abramowitz, 2016), and detailed discussions of different components of the ILM are described in a series of articles (Frank & McKay, 2019).

Cognitive Therapy

Behavioral Experiments

As noted earlier, some clinical guides emphasize CT without the need for ERP (i.e., Wilhelm & Steketee, 2006). Most of these same guides include specific exercises aimed at providing clients with direct experiential tests of the cognitions that may contribute to their obsessional concerns. These are termed "behavioral experiments" (Bennett-Levy et al., 2004). While a small number of investigations have suggested that cognitive therapy addresses the central mechanisms of change in OCD (i.e., Woody et al., 2011), the overall evidence remains that CT without corresponding ERP is insufficient to produce lasting change in OCD treatment. It has been suggested that the behavioral experiments that are central in CT form a type of exposure that facilitates behavior change (Abramowitz et al., 2005). This view is consistent with the modern ILM approach to exposure.

This is not to suggest that CT is unnecessary or superfluous in the treatment of OCD. Research has suggested that the addition of CT to ERP produces the greatest change in symptoms (Rector et al., 2019). Again, it should be emphasized, however, that such additive investigations are limited by the extent to which CT expressly involves an exposure component via behavioral exercises.

Cognitive Reappraisal

In addition to behavioral experiments, treatment for OCD involves targeting cognitive distortions through systematic evidence-gathering in collaboration between therapist and client. The belief domains described earlier, such as intolerance of uncertainty or inflated responsibility, would be scrutinized for the extent that each may be valid in the daily life of the OCD sufferer, with between-session exercises aimed at finding disconfirming evidence (Salkovskis, 2007).

Approaches for Youth

As with adult treatment for OCD, the emphasis for treatment with children is on ERP and, where suitable, CT. Extensive multisite investigations of the efficacy of CBT, broadly defined, have demonstrated significant symptom reduction in children (i.e., the Pediatric OCD Treatment Study Team [POTS, 2004; Franklin et al., 2011]). Treatment programs for OCD in children emphasize developmental features in addition to highlighting exposure for feared situations in order to promote symptom reduction. As a result, in younger children there are added treatment components that address emotion regulation and significant family and caregiver components to alleviate disruptive behavior that children may exhibit when faced with otherwise fear-evoking stimuli (Freeman et al., 2014). Broad, multicomponent treatment models – including approaches for groups, school settings, and for complex symptom presentations – are available (Storch et al., 2018).

Other Variables Influencing Treatment

Assessment and Diagnosis

There is an extensive array of assessment tools for evaluating severity and symptom dimensions of OCD (Taylor et al., 2020). While there are numerous measures, two major instruments have been most frequently applied for assessing symptom dimensions and associated severity. The Yale–Brown Obsessive-Compulsive Scale (Goodman et al., 1989) has been extensively evaluated for its psychometric properties and, while there are limitations (such as the item assessing resistance to obsessions), it is widely considered the "gold standard" for clinician-administered severity assessment (Rapp et al., 2016).

The other major measure is a self-report scale: the Obsessive-Compulsive Inventory-Revised (OCI-R; Foa et al., 2002). This scale can be broken into subscales that evaluate dimensions of OCD based on washing, checking, ordering, obsessing, neutralizing, and hoarding. Severity benchmarks have been developed for this scale (Abramovitch et al., 2020), and a recent revision to the measure has been completed that provides benchmarks for severity based on a subset of items that eliminates hoarding (as that is a separate disorder in DSM-5-TR) and neutralizing (as that is a symptom management strategy rather than a symptom per se) (Abramovitch et al., 2021).

It should be noted that should other symptom dimensions appear relevant, or clinical assessment suggests that other mechanisms are involved (such as the sense of incompleteness), then additional assessment tools may be necessary to capture the full scope of symptom expression in OCD. These are described in detail in Taylor et al. (2020).

Although OCD is often described as a "fear," research over the past twenty years has suggested a prominent role for disgust as well. Disgust remains an understudied emotion (McKay, 2017). At its core, disgust protects from ingestion of harmful substances, but it is also more general in protecting from any illness or disease state. As a result, in the specific case of contamination fear and washing rituals, concerns over "spreading" of putative toxins forms the core aspect of avoidance behavior. Experimental research has shown that the perceived contaminating force can remain in place for up to 12 steps removed from the original source among individuals with this symptom dimension of OCD – a significantly greater degree than for individuals with other anxiety disorders or nonanxious controls (Tolin et al., 2004). Recent conceptualizations have expanded this model to consider the unique blend of disgust and fear, specifically over the prospect of contaminants penetrating the skin, with individuals with elevated contamination fear showing greater avoidance of stimuli perceived to have a high propensity for skin penetration (e.g., blood worms) compared to individuals with high levels of anxiety without contamination fear and nonanxious controls (Mancusi & McKay, 2021). This is salient as it is less clear that disgust responds to exposure in the same way that fear does, and may call for different conceptualizations for intervention (Mason & Richardson, 2012).

Kozak and Foa (1994) laid out a conceptual model for overvalued ideation (OVI) in OCD. This framework places obsessions on one end of a dimension that goes through to delusions, with OVI closer to the delusional end of the spectrum. When present, OVI is considered an impediment to treatment using ERP and other cognitive methods, given that the sufferer holds the conviction that their obsessions pose a genuine risk, or that the compulsive behavior is essential. At the present time, there are no clear treatment guidelines for addressing OVI in conjunction with OCD.

Comorbidity

In addition to being highly heterogeneous, OCD is also marked by commonly occurring comorbid conditions. There are two in particular that stand out for complicating symptom management.

While it is not uncommon for depressed mood to occur secondary to severe symptoms of OCD, when depression exists as a distinct comorbid condition it has long been recognized as a complicating aspect of treatment (Grabill et al., 2008). One aspect which explains this complication is that when conducting exposure treatment, depressed mood interferes with emotional activation and associated behavior change. On the other side of this challenge, implementation of interventions aimed expressly at depressed mood runs into difficulty due to the avoidance associated with OCD.

Recent research suggests that the inclusion of behavioral activation to target depression may overcome this clinical challenge (Wheaton & Gallina, 2019).

Some neurobiological models of OCD emphasize the involvement of the basal gaglia, with some recent reviews supporting this association (Pearlman et al., 2015). Similarly, tic disorders have been associated with dysfunction in the basal ganglia (discussed in Bronfeld & Bar-Gad, 2013). This putative neural overlap has resulted in observed cases of tics comorbid to OCD, or even subtypes of OCD termed "Tourettic OCD" (Mansueto & Keuler, 2005). This complex symptom presentation poses unique challenges in treatment as tics are often exacerbated by stress, which is induced as part of ERP. At the present time there are primarily case studies and conceptual models for how to address this complex symptom presentation, but little in the way of any systematic research.

Demographics

A significant limitation in the research into treatment for OCD is that the majority of studies undersample underrepresented groups. This problem has been known for some time (Williams et al., 2010), but has yet to be fully addressed. As a result, it is likely that many individuals from underrepresented groups are misdiagnosed. Indeed, OCD is frequently misdiagnosed (Stahnke, 2021), leading to inappropriate care. Misdiagnosis with more severe psychiatric conditions is common among underrepresented groups (i.e., African Americans; Williams et al., 2012).

Gender also plays a significant role in treatment efficacy for OCD. While OCD is slightly more common among females, males tend to report earlier age of onset and higher rates of intrusive blasphemous thoughts (Mathes et al., 2019). As noted earlier, blasphemous thoughts pose a unique challenge given the lag between exposure exercises and perceived aversive outcomes. However, there has been limited research into treatment outcome differences among genders.

Medication

The vast majority of individuals with OCD have likely been prescribed psychiatric medications, and thus treatment trials often include individuals who have been on one or more medication or have tried multiple courses of medications. The general "clinical wisdom" is that medication in conjunction with CBT is the best course of action (i.e., ADAA or American Psychiatric Association treatment guidelines). However, it has been observed that the incremental gain for medication is slight when added to CBT for OCD in adults (Skapinaki et al., 2016) and children (Tao et al., 2022). An overview of medication managements strategies for OCD is available in McKay (2019).

Conclusion

Research into treatment for OCD has expanded significantly in the past forty years, and there is now a well-developed set of interventions for the condition. The two major psychosocial interventions, ERP and CT, together form a comprehensive set of methods for addressing a large proportion of symptoms that are commonly experienced among OCD sufferers. The marked heterogeneity of the condition has been emphasized in this chapter, though, and thus treatment for OCD calls for a high degree of expertise to understand the nuances of the disorder. Aside from high variability in symptom dimensions, there are commonly occurring complications such as comorbid depression or OVI, and additional emotional dimensions (i.e., disgust) that may not respond to exposure-based interventions. Further, the majority of the treatment research is best generalized to majority white populations, and thus careful considerations need to be taken when developing treatment for members of underrepresented groups and people of color.

Useful Resources

- Anxiety & Depression Association of America Clinical Practice Guidelines: https://adaa .org/resources-professionals/practice-guidelines-ocd
- International Obsessive-Compulsive Disorder Foundation: www.iocdf.org
- Mental Health America: www.mentalhealthamerica.net/conditions/ocd
- National Institute of Mental Health Fact Sheets: www.nimh.nih.gov/health/topics/obses sive-compulsive-disorder-ocd/index.shtml
- Springer, K. S., & Tolin, D. F. (2020). *The big book of exposures: Innovative, creative, and effective CBT-based exposures for treating anxiety-related disorders*. New Harbinger.

References

Abramovitch, A., Abramowitz, J. S., & McKay, D. (2021). The OCI-12: A syndromally valid modification of the obsessive-compulsive inventory-revised. *Psychiatry Research*, 298, 113808.

Abramovitch, A., Abramowitz, J. S., Riemann, B.C., & McKay, D. (2020). Severity benchmarks and contemporary clinical norms for the Obsessive-Compulsive Inventory-Revised (OCI-R). *Journal of Obsessive-Compulsive and Related Disorders*, 27, 100557.

Abramowitz, J. S. (2018). Presidential address: Are the obsessive-compulsive related disorders related to obsessive compulsive disorder? A critical look at DSM-5's new category. *Behavior Therapy*, 49, 1–11.

Abramowitz, J. S., Storch, E. A., McKay, D., Taylor, S., & Asmundson, G. J. G. (2009). The obsessive-compulsive spectrum: A critical review. In D. McKay, J. S. Abramowitz, S. Taylor, & G. J. G. Asmundson (Eds.), *Current perspectives on anxiety disorders: Implications for DSM-V and beyond* (pp. 329–352). Springer.

Abramowitz, J. S., Taylor, S., & McKay, D. (2005). Potentials and limitations of cognitive treatments for obsessive-compulsive disorder. *Cognitive Behaviour Therapy*, 34, 140–147.

Abramowitz, J., McKay, D., & Taylor, S. (2005). Special series: Subtypes of obsessive-compulsive disorder. *Behavior Therapy*, 36, 367–369.

Adam, Y., Meinlschmidt, G., Gloster, A. T., & Lieb, R. (2012). Obsessive-compulsive disorder in the community: 12-month prevalence, comorbidity and impairment. *Social Psychiatry and Psychiatric Epidemiology*, 47, 339–349.

American Psychiatric Association (2013). *Diagnostic and statistical manual of mental disorders* (5th ed.). American Psychiatric Association.

American Psychiatric Association (2022). *Diagnostic and statistical manual of mental disorders* (5th ed., text revision). American Psychiatric Association.

Anxiety and Depression Association of America (2015). *OCD Clinical Practice Task Force – Clinical practice review for OCD*. Anxiety and Depression Association of America. https://adaa.org/resources-professionals/practice-guidelines-ocd.

Bennett-Levy, J., Butler, G., Fennell, M., et al. (Eds.) (2004). *Oxford guide to behavioural experiments in cognitive therapy*. Oxford University Press.

Bronfeld, M., & Bar-Gad, I. (2013). Tic disorders: What happens in the basal ganglia? *The Neuroscientist*, 19, 101–108.

Chambless, D. L., & Hollon, S. D. (1998). Defining empirically supported therapies. *Journal of Consulting and Clinical Psychology*, 66(1), 7–18. https://doi.org/10.1037/0022-006X.66.1.7.

Clark, D. A. (2004). *Cognitive-behavioral therapy for OCD*. Guilford.

Corr, P. J., & Perkins, A. M. (2006). The role of theory in the psychophysiology of personality: From Ivan Pavlov to Jeffrey Gray. *International Journal of Psychophysiology*, 62, 367–376.

Craske, M. G., Treanor, M., Conway, C. C., Zbozinek, T., & Vervliet, B. (2014). Maximizing exposure therapy: An inhibitory learning approach. *Behaviour Research and Therapy*, 58, 10–23.

Craske, M. G., Treanor, M., Zbozinek, T. D., & Vervliet, B. (2022). Optimizing exposure therapy and inhibitory retrieval approach and the OptEx Nexus. *Behaviour Research and Therapy*, 152, 104069.

da Silva, R.M.F., Batistuzzo, M.C., Shavitt, R.G., et al. (2019). Transcranial direct current stimulation in obsessive-compulsive disorder: An update in electric field modeling investigations for optimal electrode montage. *Expert Review in Neurotherapeutics*, 19, 1025–1035.

Deacon, B. J., Farrell, N. R., Kemp, J. J., et al. (2013). Assessing therapist reservations about exposure therapy for anxiety disorders: The Therapist Beliefs about Exposure Scale. *Journal of Anxiety Disorders*, 27, 772–780.

Diefenbach, G.J., Tolin, D.F., Meunier, S., & Worhunsky, P. (2008). Emotion regulation and trichotillomania: A comparison of clinical and nonclinical hair pulling. *Journal of Behavior Therapy and Experimental Psychiatry*, 39, 32–41.

Elsner, B., Jacobi, T., Kischkel, E., Schulze, D., & Reuter, B. (2022). Mechanisms of exposure and response prevention in obsessive-compulsive disorder: Effects of habituation and expectancy violation on short-term outcome in cognitive-behavioral therapy. *BMC Psychiatry*, 22, 66.

Farhat, L.C., Olfson, E., Nasir, M., et al. (2020). Pharmacological and behavioral treatment of trichotillomania: An updated systematic review and meta-analysis. *Depression & Anxiety*, 37, 715–727.

Ferrando, C., & Selai, C. (2021). A systematic review and meta-analysis on the effectiveness of exposure and response prevention therapy in the treatment of obsessive-compulsive disorder. *Journal of Obsessive-Compulsive and Related Disorders*, 31, 100684.

Fineberg, N. A., Apergis-Schoute, A. M., Vaghi, M. M., et al. (2021). Mapping compulsivity in the DSM-5 obsessive compulsive related disorders: Cognitive domains, neural circuitry, and treatment. *International Journal of Neuropsychopharmacology*, 21, 42–58.

Foa, E. B., & Kozak, M. J. (1986). Emotional processing of fear: Exposure to corrective information. *Psychological Bulletin*, 99, 20–25.

Foa, E. B., Huppert, J. D., Leiberg, S., et al. (2002). The obsessive-compulsive inventory: Development and validation of a short version. *Psychological Assessment*, 14(4), 485–496.

Frank, B., & McKay, D. (2019). Introduction to the special series: Clinical applications of the inhibitory learning model. *Cognitive & Behavioral Practice*, 26, 127–129.

Franklin, M. A., Sapyta, J., Freeman, J.B., et al. (2011). Cognitive behavior therapy augmentataion of pharmacotherapy in pediatric obsessive-compulsive disorder: The Pediatric OCD Treatment Study II (POTS II) Randomized Controlled trial. *JAMA*, 306, 1224–1232.

Freeman, J., Sapyta, J., Garcia, A., et al. (2014). Family-based treatment of early childhood obsessive-compulsive disorder: The Pediatric Obsessive-Compulsive Disorder Treatment Study for Young Children (POTS Jr) – A randomized clinical trial. *JAMA Psychiatry*, 71, 689–698.

Freeston, M. H., Ladouceur, R., Thibodeau, N., & Gagnon, F. (1991). Cognitive intrusions in a nonclinical population: I. Response style, subjective experience, and appraisal. *Behaviour Research and Therapy*, 29, 585–597

Freud, S. (1909). A case of obsessional neurosis. *Standard edn*, 10.

Goodman, W. K., Price, L. H., Rasmussen, S. A., et al. (1989). The Yale–Brown obsessive compulsive scale. II. Validity. *Archives of General Psychiatry*, 46, 1012–1016.

Grabill, K., Merlo, L., Duke, D., et al. (2008). Assessment of obsessive-compulsive disorder: A review. *Journal of Anxiety Disorders*, 22, 1–17.

Gratz, K. L., Weiss, N. H., & Tull, M. T. (2015). Examining emotion regulation as an outcome, mechanism, and target of psychological treatments. *Current Opinion in Psychology*, 3, 85–90.

Gruner, P., & Pittenger, C. (2017). Cognitive inflexibility in obsessive-compulsive disorder. *Neuroscience*, 345, 243–255.

Jacoby, R. J., & Abramowitz, J. S. (2016). Inhibitory learning approaches to exposure therapy: A critical review and translation to obsessive-compulsive disorder. *Clinical Psychology Review*, 49, 28–40.

Janet, P. (1908). *Les obsessions et la psychasthénie*. (2nd ed., M. W. Adamowicz, trans.). Alcan.

Julien, D., O'Connor, K., & Aardema, F. (2016). The inference-based approach to obsessive-compulsive disorder: A comprehensive review of its etiological model, treatment efficacy, and model of change. *Journal of Affective Disorders*, 202, 187–196.

Keuthen, N. J., Rothbaum, B. O., Falkenstein, M. J., et al. (2011). DBT-enhance habit reversal treatment for trichotillomania: 3- and 6-month follow-up results. *Depression & Anxiety*, 28, 310–313.

Kim, S.-K., McKay, D., Taylor, S., et al. (2016). The structure of obsessive-compulsive symptoms and beliefs: A correspondence and biplot analysis. *Journal of Anxiety Disorders*, 38, 79–87.

Koran, L. M., Hanna, G. L., Hollander, E., Nestadt, G., & Simpson, H. B. (2007). *Practice guideline for the treatment of patients with obsessive-compulsive disorder*. American

Psychiatric Association. https://psychiatryonline.org/pb/assets/raw/sitewide/practice_gui
delines/guidelines/ocd.pdf.

Kozak, M. J., & Foa, E. B. (1994). Obsessions, overvalued ideas, and delusions in obsessive-compulsive disorder. *Behaviour Research and Therapy*, 32, 343–353.

Kringlen, E. (1965). Obsessional neurotics: Long-term outcome. *British Journal of Psychiatry*, 111, 709–722.

Lochner, C., Roos, A., & Stein, D. J. (2017). Excoriation (skin-picking) disorder: A systematic review of treatment options. *Neuropsychiatric Disease and Treatment*, 13, 1867–1872.

Mahjani, B., Bey, K., Boberg, J., & Burton, C. (2021). Genetics of obsessive-compulsive disorder. *Psychological Medicine*, 51, 2247–2259.

Mancusi, L., & McKay, D. (2021). Behavioral avoidance tasks for eliciting disgust and anxiety in contamination fear: An examination of a test for a combined disgust and fear reaction. *Journal of Anxiety Disorders*, 78, 102366.

Mansueto, C. S., & Keuler, D. J. (2005). Tic or compulsion? It's Tourettic OCD. *Behavior Modification*. 29, 784–799.

Mason, E. C., & Richardson, R. (2012). Treating disgust in anxiety disorders. *Clinical Psychology: Science & Practice*, 19, 180–194.

Mathes, B. M., Morabito, D. M., & Schmidt, N.B. (2019). Epidemiology and clinical gender differences in OCD. *Current Psychiatry Reports*, 21, 36.

McKay, D. (2017). Presidential address: Embracing the repulsive: The case for disgust as a functionally central emotional state in the theory, practice, and dissemination of cognitive-behavior therapy. *Behavior Therapy*, 48, 731–738.

McKay, D. (2019). Pharmacological treatment of obsessive-compulsive disorder and related disorders. In S. Evans & K. Carpenter (Eds.), *APA handbook of psychopharmacology for psychologists* (pp. 245–265). Washington, DC: American Psychological Association.

McKay, D., Abramowitz, J., Calamari, J., et al. (2004). A critical evaluation of obsessive-compulsive disorder subtypes: Symptoms versus mechanisms. *Clinical Psychology Review*, 24, 283–313.

McKay, D., Abramowitz, J.S., & Storch, E.A. (2021). Mechanisms of harmful treatments for obsessive-compulsive disorders. *Clinical Psychology: Science & Practice*, 28, 52–59.

McKay, D., Kim, S.-K., Taylor, S., et al. (2014). An examination of obsessive-compulsive symptoms and dimensions using profile analysis via multidimensional scaling (PAMS). *Journal of Anxiety Disorders*, 28, 352–357.

McKay, D., Sookman, D., Neziroglu, F., et al. (2015). Efficacy of cognitive-behavior therapy for obsessive-compulsive disorder. *Psychiatry Research*, 227, 104–113.

McKay, D., Taylor, S., & Abramowitz, J.S. (2010). Obsessive-compulsive disorder. In D. McKay, J. S. Abramowitz, & S. Taylor (Eds.), *Cognitive-behavioral therapy for refractory cases: Turning failure into success* (pp. 89–109). Washington, DC: American Psychological Association Press.

Meyer, V. (1966). Modification of expectations in cases with obsessional rituals. *Behaviour Research and Therapy*, 4, 273–280.

O'Connor, K. P., & Robillard, S. (1995). Inference processes in obsessive-compulsive disorder: Some clinical observations. *Behaviour Research and Therapy*, 33, 887–896.

Obsessive Compulsive Cognitions Working Group (2001). Development and initial validation of the Obsessive Beliefs Questionnaire and the Interpretation of Intrusions Inventory. *Behaviour Research and Therapy*, 39, 987–1005.

Obsessive Compulsive Cognitions Working Group (2005). Psychometric validation of the obsessive belief questionnaire and interpretation of intrusions inventory – Part 2: Factor analysis and testing of a brief version. *Behaviour Research and Therapy*, 43, 1527–1542.

Ong, C. W., Clyde, J. W., Bluett, E. J., & Twohig, M. P. (2016). Dropout rates in exposure with response prevention for obsessive-compulsive disorder: What do the data really say? *Journal of Anxiety Disorders*, 40, 8–17.

Pearlman, D. M., Vora, H. S., Marquis, B. G., Najjar, S., & Dudley, L. A. (2015). Anti-basal ganglia antibodies in primary obsessive-compulsive disorder: Systematic review and meta-analysis. *British Journal of Psychiatry*, 205, 8–16.

Pediatric OCD Treatment Study (POTS) Team (2004). Cognitive-behavior therapy, sertraline, and the combination for children and adolescents with obsessive-compulsive disorder: The Pediatric Obsessive Compulsive Treatment Study (POTS) randomized controlled trial. *JAMA*, 292, 1969–1976.

Pertusa, A., Frost, R. O., Fullana, M. A., et al. (2010). Refining the diagnostic boundaries of compulsive hoarding: A critical review. *Clinical Psychology Review*, 30, 371–386.

Pittenger, C. (2017). *Obsessive-compulsive disorder: Phenomenology, pathophysiology, and treatment*. Oxford University Press.

Rachman, S., & Hodgson, R. J. (1980). *Obsessions and compulsions*. Prentice-Hall.

Rapp, A. M., Bergman, R. L., Piacentini, J., & McGuire, J. F. (2016). Evidence-based assessment of obsessive-compulsive disorder. *Journal of Central Nervous System Disease*, 8, 13–29

Rector, N. A., Richter, M. A., Katz, D., & Leybman, M. (2019). Does the addition of cognitive therapy to exposure and response preventions for obsessive compulsive disorder enhance clinical efficacy? A randomized controlled trial in a community setting. *British Journal of Clinical Psychology*, 58, 1–18.

Richard, D. C. S., & Gloster, A. T. (2006). Exposure therapy has a public relations problem: A dearth of litigation amid a wealth of concern. In D. C. S. Richard & D. L. Lauterbach (Eds.), *Handbook of exposure therapies* (pp. 409–425). Academic Press.

Rosa-Alcázar, A. I., Sánchez-Meca, J., Gómez-Conesa, A., & Marín-Martínez. F. (2008). Psychological treatment of obsessive-compulsive disorder: A meta-analysis. *Clinical Psychology Review*, 28, 1310–1325

Ruscio, A. M., Stein, D. J., Chiu, W. T., & Kessler, R. C. (2010). The epidemiology of obsessive-compulsive disorder in the National Comorbidity Survey Replication. *Molecular Psychiatry*, 15, 53–63.

Salkovskis, P. M. (1985). Obsessional-compulsive problems: A cognitive-behavioural analysis. *Behaviour Research and Therapy*, 25, 571–583.

Salkovskis, P. M. (2007). Psychological treatment of obsessive-compulsive disorder. *Psychiatry*, 6, 229–233.

Skapinakis, P., Caldwell, D. M., Hollingworth, W., et al. (2016). Pharmacological and psychotherapeutic interventions for management of obsessive-compulsive disorder in adults: A systematic review and network meta-analysis. *The Lancet Psychiatry*, 3, 730–739.

Society of Clinical Psychology (n.d.) Obsessive-compulsive disorder. https://div12.org/diagnosis/obsessive-compulsive-disorder/.

Spencer, S. D., Stiede, J. T., Wiese, A. D., et al. (2023). Cognitive-behavioral therapy for obsessive-compulsive disorders. *Psychiatric Clinics of North America*, 46, 167–180.

Stahnke, B. (2021). A systematic review of misdiagnosis in those with obsessive-compulsive disorder. *Journal of Affective Disorders Reports*, 6, 100231.

Stein, D. J., Costa, D. L. C., Lochner, C., et al. (2019). Obsessive-compulsive disorder. *Nature Reviews: Disease Primers*, 5, 52.

Storch, E. A., McGuire, J. F., & McKay, D. (2018). *The clinician's guide to cognitive-behavioral therapy for children with obsessive-compulsive disorder*. Academic Press.

Tao, Y., Li, H., Li, L., et al. (2022). Comparing the efficacy of pharmacological treatment, alone and in combination, in children and adolescents with obsessive-compulsive disorder: A network meta-analysis. *Journal of Psychiatric Research*, 148, 95–102.

Taylor, S., Abramowitz, J. S., & McKay, D. (2007). Cognitive-behavioral models of obsessive-compulsive disorder. In M. M. Antony, C. Purdon, & L. J. Summerfeldt (Eds.), *Psychological theories of obsessive-compulsive disorder: Fundamentals and beyond* (pp. 9–29). American Psychological Association.

Taylor, S., Abramowitz, J. S., McKay, D., & Garner, L. (2020). Obsessive compulsive and related disorders. In M. M. Antony & D. H. Barlow (Eds.), *Handbook of assessment and treatment planning for psychological disorders* (3rd ed.) (pp. 253–294). Guilford.

Taylor, S., McKay, D., Crowe, K. B., et al. (2014). The sense of incompleteness as a motivator of obsessive-compulsive symptoms: An empirical analysis of concepts and correlates. *Behavior Therapy*, 45, 254–262.

Tolin, D. F., Frost, R. O., & Steketee, G. (2013). *Buried in treasures: Help for compulsive acquisition and hoarding* (2nd ed.). Oxford University Press.

Tolin, D. F., McKay, D., Forman, E. M., Klonsky, E. D., & Thombs, B. D. (2015). Empirically supported treatment: Recommendations for a new model. *Clinical Psychology: Science and Practice*, 22(4), 317–338. https://doi.org/10.1111/cpsp.12122.

Tolin, D. F., Melnyk, T., & Marx, B. (2015). Exposure and response prevention for obsessive-compulsive disorder. www.div12.org/wp-content/uploads/2019/10/Treatment-Review-ERP-for-OCD.pdf.

Tolin, D.F., Worhunsky, P., & Maltby, N. (2004). Sympathetic magic in contamination-related OCD. *Journal of Behavior Therapy and Experimental Psychiatry*, 35, 193–205.

Wheaton, M. G., & Gallina, E. R. (2019). Using cognitive-behavioral therapy to treat obsessive-compulsive disorder with co-occurring depression. *Journal of Cognitive Psychotherapy*, 33, 228–241.

Wilhelm, S., & Steketee, G. (2006). *Cognitive therapy for obsessive-compulsive disorder: A guide for professionals*. New Harbinger.

Wilhelm, S., Phillips, K., & Steketee, G. (2012). *Cognitive-behavioral therapy for body dysmorphic disorder: A treatment manual*. Guilford Press.

Williams, M., Domanico, J., Marques, L., Leblanc, N. J., & Turkheimer, E. (2012). Barriers to treatment among African Americans with obsessive-compulsive disorder. *Journal of Anxiety Disorders*, 26, 555–563.

Williams, M., Powers, M., Yun, Y. G., & Foa, E. (2010). Minority participation in randomized controlled trials for obsessive-compulsive disorder. *Journal of Anxiety Disorders*, 24, 171–177.

Woody, S. R., Whittal, M. L., & McLean, P. D. (2011). Mechanisms of symptom reduction in treatment for obsessions. *Journal of Consulting and Clinical Psychology*, 79, 653–664.

6

Posttraumatic Stress Disorder

Carmen P. McLean and Eve A. Rosenfeld

Since acute stress disorder and posttraumatic stress disorder (PTSD) were first codified in the *Diagnostic and Statistical Manual for Mental Disorders* (DSM-III) in 1980, our understanding of how to treat these posttraumatic stress reactions has expanded considerably, and there are now a number of evidence-based psychotherapy (EBP) options available. The current (DSM-5-TR) criteria for PTSD requires exposure to a traumatic event, defined as actual or threatened death, serious injury, or sexual violence, as well as symptoms from each of four clusters: re-experiencing symptoms (e.g., intrusive distressing memories), avoidance symptoms (e.g., avoiding thoughts related to the trauma), alterations in cognitions and mood symptoms (e.g., feeling detached or estranged from others), and arousal symptoms (e.g., hypervigilance). Symptoms must be present for more than one month after trauma exposure; prior to one month, a diagnosis of acute stress disorder may be appropriate.

Exposure to traumatic events is relatively common. However, most individuals who experience trauma recover on their own, without any formal intervention, in the weeks and months following the traumatic event (e.g., Bonanno et al., 2015). Nevertheless, a substantial minority of those exposed to trauma develop acute stress disorder and go on to develop PTSD. Epidemiological research has found a lifetime prevalence for PTSD of 8.5% for women and 3.4% for men in the United States (McLean et al., 2011), although the rates of PTSD are higher among certain groups, such as military personnel (Institute of Medicine, 2014; Tanielian et al., 2008). In the absence of effective treatment, PTSD can be a chronic and disabling disorder associated with significant distress and overall functional impairment (e.g., Kachadourian et al., 2019). Most individuals with PTSD also meet criteria for at least one additional psychiatric diagnosis, most commonly depressive disorders, anxiety disorders, and substance use disorders (Kessler et al., 2005).

Etiology and Theoretical Underpinnings of Treatment

The most prominent theories of PTSD development can be defined broadly as cognitive-behavioral, with each having a slightly different focus. Behavioral theories are rooted in learning and conditioning models, including both classical and operant conditioning. Mowrer's (1960) influential two-factor theory purports that classical conditioning can explain the development of fear reactions to previously neutral stimuli that were paired with the traumatic event, which then elicit fear reactions at subsequent presentations. Traumatic reactions can spread to stimuli that are less clearly related to the traumatic event through the process of generalization. Operant conditioning explains how negative reinforcement of avoidance can maintain fear reactions by limiting opportunities for extinction – the process by which individuals learn that conditioned stimuli no longer signal threat.

Schema theories and cognitive theories focus on core assumptions or beliefs guiding the interpretation of new information. For example, Janoff-Bulman (1989) proposed that trauma disrupts core assumptions about the world as generally benevolent and meaningful and the self as intrinsically worthy. As a result of this disruption, trauma survivors either assimilate the experience into existing core assumption (e.g., blaming oneself for the trauma to protect the belief in a just world), which could increase risk for PTSD, or change their core assumption to accommodate the trauma (e.g., the world is not always benevolent). Early research among trauma survivors found that beliefs about safety, trust, power and control, esteem, and intimacy are particularly susceptible to disruptions after a trauma (Janoff-Bulman, 1985; McCann et al., 1988). Building on this work, as well as Beck et al.'s (1979) cognitive theory, Resick and Schnicke (1993) proposed that PTSD can develop when disruptions in beliefs keep trauma survivors "stuck" in distress, and that treatment should therefore involve identifying "stuck points" (i.e., inaccurate thoughts) and challenging them through Socratic questioning with the goal of developing accurate, balanced perspectives on the trauma. Ehlers and Clark's (2000) cognitive model proposed two key factors that interact to promote the development and maintenance of PTSD: (1) trauma-related beliefs or appraisals about threat (e.g., "the world is dangerous") and (2) the fragmented nature of the traumatic memory that does not incorporate other autobiographical memories. Consistent with this theory are findings that PTSD is associated with maladaptive appraisals of the trauma (e.g., Bryant & Guthrie, 2007) and fragmented trauma narratives (e.g., Amir et al., 1998). Recall of the fragmented memory elicits distress and promotes threat appraisals, which in turn biases recall of the trauma memory in ways that further reinforce threat appraisals. It follows that cognitive therapy focuses on correcting beliefs and assumptions thought to underlie PTSD and elaborating the trauma memory and integrating it into the context of the survivor's life narrative.

Emotional processing theory (Foa & Kozak, 1985) is based on Mowrer's (1960) theory and bioinformational models of fear (e.g., Lang, 1977). Emotional processing theory proposed that trauma-related emotions are represented in memory as cognitive structures that include information about stimuli, responses, and their meaning, which are interrelated such that inputs matching any part of the structure activate the entire structure. Pathological fear structures are characterized by over-generalization and excessive responding to safe stimuli. Consistent with this notion are findings of attentional biases to a wide range of threat cues among individuals with PTSD (e.g., Harvey et al., 1996). This theory proposes that activation of the fear structure (e.g., through approaching trauma memories) in the absence of anticipated harm promotes recovery via disconfirmation of the pathological elements of the fear structure. Inhibitory learning theory (Craske et al., 2008) is based on learning paradigms showing that return of fear is common following extinction (Bouton, 1993). After successful extinction or exposure therapy, associations between the trauma stimuli and threat remain and compete with the newly formed associations between the trauma-related stimuli and safety. When trauma-related stimuli are encountered, the time since extinction/exposure and contextual cues determine which of these two associations is activated.

Brief Overview of Treatments

A number of psychotherapies for PTSD have been found efficacious in randomized controlled trials (RCTs) relative to various control conditions. The most consistently supported treatments are referred to as "trauma-focused psychotherapies." These treatments directly target thoughts, feelings, and/or memories of the worst traumatic event. Trauma-focused psychotherapies include exposure therapies such as prolonged exposure therapy (Foa et al., 2019); cognitive approaches such as cognitive processing therapy (CPT; Resick et al., 2017) and cognitive therapy (Ehlers et al., 2003); and other types of cognitive-behavioral therapy (CBT; e.g., Blanchard et al., 2003). Trauma-focused psychotherapies for PTSD are CBTs: they are based on principles of learning theory and/or cognitive theory and focus on changing maladaptive patterns of behaving and/or thinking.

Results from several large meta-analyses and systematic reviews indicate that trauma-focused psychotherapies are associated with large treatment effects. For example, an analysis by Watts et al. (2013) of 112 RCTs found that cognitive therapy and exposure therapy were associated with the largest effects. Another meta-analysis (Cusack et al., 2016) included 64 RCTs and graded the overall strength of the evidence (SOE) for each treatment based on information about risk of bias among the relevant studies and the consistency, directness, and precision of the evidence supporting a given treatment. Based on this analysis, Cusack et al. concluded that prolonged exposure, cognitive therapy, and CPT had the highest SOE. Other CBT

Box 6.1 The Controversy Over Eye Movement Desensitization and Reprocessing

Eye movement desensitization and reprocessing (EMDR; Shapiro & Maxfield, 2002) is a controversial trauma-focused treatment. EMDR has been found efficacious, with effect sizes that are comparable to other trauma-focused treatments (Lewis et al., 2020; McLean et al., 2022; Watts et al., 2013), although there is some evidence of greater risk of bias among EMDR studies (Cusack et al., 2016; McLean et al., 2022). EMDR includes exposure to trauma-related images accompanied by a "bilateral stimulation" task, such as following the therapist's hand moving back and forth with the patient's eyes. The major points of contention are whether the revisiting of the trauma imagery (i.e., exposure) by itself is the primary driver of change in EMDR, and whether, as originally theorized (Shapiro, 1989), the concurrent bilateral stimulation component impacts outcomes (Rosen & Davison, 2003). Dismantling studies (Cahill et al., 1999; Pitman et al., 1996; Sanderson & Carpenter, 1992), reviews (Cahill et al., 1999), and meta-analyses (Davidson & Parker, 2001) found no evidence supporting the clinical value of eye movements. A meta-analysis by Lee and Cuijpers (2013) found that effect sizes were larger when eye movements were used. However, this study included mainly experimental studies with healthy participants and used subjective process measures as outcomes. A subsequent meta-analysis focused on PTSD clinical trials found no evidence supporting the eye movement component (Cuijpers et al., 2020). Interestingly, Sack et al. (2016) found that visual attention on the therapist produced superior treatment outcomes than no instruction on attentional focus, and the induction of eye movements by following the therapist's moving hand did not offer an advantage compared to visually fixating on a nonmoving hand. The necessity of the bilateral stimulation component of EMDR remains controversial (Jeffries & Davis, 2013; Schubert & Lee, 2009) and higher-quality studies are necessary in order to resolve this controversy (Cuijpers et al., 2020). For more about the EMDR controversy, see Rosen and colleagues (2023).

packages were associated with a moderate SOE. The most recent meta-analysis of PTSD psychotherapies (Lewis et al., 2020) included 114 RCTs and concluded that there was robust evidence to support the efficacy of trauma-focused CBTs, including CPT, prolonged exposure, and cognitive therapy.

Consistent with these findings, Clinical Practice Guidelines (CPGs) based on systematic reviews of the available research all recommend trauma-focused psychotherapy as first-line intervention for PTSD. Five major CPGs for PTSD (see Hamblen et al., 2019 for a summary) have been published by workgroups at the American Psychological Association (APA, 2017), the International Society for Traumatic Stress Studies (ISTSS, 2018), the National Institute for Health and Care Excellence (NICE, 2018), the Phoenix Australia Centre for Posttraumatic Mental Health (2013), and the Department of Veterans Affairs and Department of Defense (VA/DoD, 2017). Although some CPGs recommend trauma-focused psychotherapy in general while others name specific protocols (e.g., APA recommends CBT, prolonged exposure, CPT, and cognitive therapy), all five CPGs give their strongest recommendation to PE, CPT, and trauma-focused CBT.

Credible Components of Treatments

Psychoeducation

Psychoeducation is a common component of trauma-focused interventions in which a mental health provider delivers relevant, up-to-date information about trauma and posttraumatic stress (Brouzos et al., 2022). Psychoeducation may be delivered passively (e.g., leaflets, informational websites) or actively (e.g., therapist-guided activities; Donker et al., 2009). Psychoeducation has been used as a stand-alone intervention; however, a meta-analysis found that stand-alone psychoeducation interventions do not significantly affect PTSD symptoms, nor do they differ from treatment-as-usual (Brouzos et al., 2022). In contrast, psychoeducation is a fundamental component of PTSD treatment when used in combination with other components (Whitworth, 2016). Within trauma-focused treatment, psychoeducation focuses on increasing comprehension of common reactions to trauma, normalizing reactions to trauma, building rapport, highlighting the role of avoidance and/or unhelpful beliefs in perpetuating PTSD symptoms, and providing a rationale for therapeutic skills and tasks (Brouzos et al., 2022; Whitworth, 2016). Psychoeducation can be integrated throughout treatment for PTSD, but it may be particularly crucial in the early stages of treatment in order to stimulate motivation and buy-in (Phoenix, 2007). Indeed, psychoeducation is highly acceptable to (Brooks et al., 2021) and valued by patients, who report high satisfaction, improvements in awareness of treatment options, greater optimism, and increased motivation for treatment (Gray et al., 2004). This may be especially important in trauma-focused treatment, as patients are asked to confront trauma reminders and/or challenge beliefs that may serve a psychologically protective function. When patients considered dropping out of trauma-focused treatment, a major contributing factor in their decision to continue treatment was belief in the treatment rationale (Hundt et al., 2017), highlighting the importance of psychoeducation in facilitating buy-in and promoting treatment retention. Psychoeducation also reduces stigma surrounding PTSD and seeking help for it (Gould et al., 2007).

Homework

In PTSD treatment, "homework" refers to structured, therapeutic activities completed between sessions and reviewed in session (Kazantzis et al., 2010). The purpose of therapy homework is to facilitate the rehearsal of therapeutic skills and the generalization of learning to new settings (Cummings et al., 2014; Mausbach et al., 2010). While most practicing psychologists use homework with their clients (Kazantzis &

Deane, 1999), it is viewed as most integral to CBT (Cooper et al., 2017; Detweiler & Whisman, 1999). Indeed, the majority of trauma-focused interventions for PTSD involve homework as a core component. Additionally, the majority of patients view homework positively and find it beneficial (Fehm & Mrose, 2008). Meta-analyses have demonstrated that homework adherence (i.e., completion of agreed upon homework) is associated with positive outcomes in CBT (Kazantzis et al., 2000; Mausbach et al., 2010). This is also true for trauma-focused treatment specifically: homework adherence is associated with enhanced outcomes for both CPT (Stirman et al., 2018) and prolonged exposure (Cooper et al., 2017). Homework facilitates rehearsal of skills and generalization of learning to new settings. For instance, in prolonged exposure, listening to recordings of in-session imaginal exposures for homework facilitates between-session extinction (Brown et al., 2019), which is associated with positive treatment outcomes (Rupp et al., 2017). Quality of homework also appears to be important for outcomes (Kazantzis et al., 2016). As such, clinicians should reinforce not only homework completion but high-quality homework completion (e.g., "I can see you put a lot of effort into this worksheet"; "I'm impressed that you stuck with that exposure without using any safety behaviors"). While it is difficult to parse the effects of homework from those of other components (e.g., in prolonged exposure, in vivo exposures are conducted entirely as homework assignments), homework adherence is consistently linked with enhanced outcomes. Thus, homework is a crucial component of most trauma-focused treatments used to facilitate and reinforce therapeutic learning

Exposure Therapy

Exposure is one of the most commonly used components in effective PTSD treatments. Exposure therapy derives directly from learning theories and can be considered a clinical analogue for extinction learning paradigms. Because PTSD is characterized by behavioral and cognitive avoidance, exposure involves repeatedly approaching feared thoughts, images, objects, situations, or activities in the absence of the expected negative outcome, in order to reduce pathological fear, anxiety, and other symptoms. There are two types of exposure that are used in treatments for PTSD. The most common type is called "imaginal exposure," which involves revisiting the memory of the traumatic event in one's imagination and, typically, recounting the events that occurred. Early studies of exposure therapy for PTSD used a variation of imaginal exposure known as "implosive" (or flooding) therapy (Boudewyns & Hyer, 1990; Keane et al., 1989), in which clients were guided through graduated imaginal exposure to trauma-related scenes. Some exposure therapy protocols also include a second type of exposure called "in vivo exposure," which involves approaching trauma-related situations or stimuli in real life. Early studies of implosive therapy informed the development of prolonged exposure therapy (Foa et al., 2019), the most well-studied exposure protocol. Prolonged exposure includes both imaginal and in vivo exposures. Other exposure-based therapies for PTSD include narrative exposure therapy (NET; Schauer et al., 2011), written exposure therapy (WET; Sloan & Marx, 2019), and some trauma-focused CBT protocols (e.g., Blanchard et al., 2003). Exposure therapies also include psychoeducation and typically, but not always (notably, WET), also include homework.

Many PTSD treatments are comprised of multiple components that are also used as stand-alone therapies. This makes the distinction between dismantling research, augmentation research, and comparative efficacy research somewhat unclear. Regardless, all of these study designs aim to answer the question of which treatment components matter most for therapeutic change. For example, several studies have tested combinations of exposure therapy and cognitive therapy, which are both components of trauma-focused CBT protocols but are also stand-alone treatments for PTSD. Findings from these studies (Bryant et al., 2003; Foa et al., 2005; Marks et al., 1998; Paunovic & Öst, 2001) generally show that adding cognitive restructuring does not improve outcomes in the context of exposure therapy for PTSD. An exception to this are findings from Bryant et al., (2008) showing that cognitive restructuring and exposure led to superior outcomes than three exposure alone conditions: imaginal exposure, in vivo exposure, and both imaginal and in vivo exposure. It is worth noting that in prolonged exposure, imaginal exposure is followed by "processing," which involves discussing the experience of revisiting the trauma memory with a focus on new learning and changed beliefs or perspectives. Processing is not as structured or directive as cognitive restructuring, but the two techniques are conceptually similar and share similar therapeutic goals. Thus, it is possible that some sort of elaboration of the learning that occurs during exposure is beneficial, and that that this is couched as processing of the imaginal exposure in some protocols and as cognitive restructuring in others. It may be that combining exposure and cognitive approaches does not improve outcomes because they share the same underlying therapeutic mechanisms. Possibly, lower-order associative processes like extinction learning or inhibitory learning occur, in varying degrees, in both exposure and cognitive therapies, affecting higher-order cognitive processes such as changes in trauma-related beliefs, which in turn supports subsequent associative learning (see Cooper et al., 2017; LeDoux, 2014). At present, we know very little about the mechanisms underlying effective PTSD treatment.

Bryant et al. (2008) can also be considered a dismantling study of protocols that combine imaginal and in vivo exposure. Bryant et al. found that imaginal exposure, in vivo exposure, and their combination were all effective (and inferior to the condition combining imaginal and in vivo exposure with cognitive restructuring). Thus, although Devilly and Foa (2001) argued that it is important to integrate in vivo and imaginal exposure, Bryant et al.'s findings suggest that combining in vivo and imaginal exposure may not be necessary, as the in vivo and imaginal exposure conditions both did as well as the condition that combined them. To date, very little research has examined differential responses to imaginal exposure and in vivo exposure.

Exposure appears to be a robust and flexible treatment approach in that it has been found efficacious when delivered in a wide range of formats and delivery tempos. For example, imaginal exposure is effective when the trauma memory is recounted verbally (e.g., Foa et al., 2005) or through writing (e.g., Sloan et al., 2018), implemented for longer (~40 minutes) or shorter periods (~20 minutes; e.g., Foa et al., 2022), and when patients recount the trauma memory from their imagination or through virtual reality (e.g., Reger et al., 2019). Exposure therapy is effective when delivered once-weekly (e.g., Foa et al., 2013), twice-weekly (e.g., Foa et al., 1999), daily (e.g., Foa et al., 2018), or in intensive outpatient programs (e.g., Rauch et al., 2021), and delivered in-person or via video telehealth (e.g., Acierno et al., 2017). There is also preliminary evidence for web-based delivery (McLean et al., 2021).

Cognitive Therapy

Cognitive therapy is another commonly used component in effective PTSD treatments. Because disruptions in beliefs can keep trauma survivors "stuck" in distress, cognitive therapies aim to identify inaccurate or unhelpful cognitions about the trauma and the survivor's reaction to the trauma and challenge them through Socratic questioning. The two most well-supporting treatments for PTSD that focus on cognitive therapy are CPT (Resick et al., 2017) and the cognitive therapy protocol developed by Ehlers and Clark (2000). CPT derives from cognitive (e.g., Beck et al., 1979) and schema theories (e.g., Janoff-Bulman, 1989). Ehlers and Clark (2000) later developed a cognitive model of PTSD and a corresponding treatment protocol based on this model. Both involve identifying inaccurate or unhelpful beliefs and challenging them, using Socratic questioning with the goal of arriving at more accurate and balanced conclusions. Both treatments also include common CBT components of psychoeducation and homework. CPT also involves strategies to increase awareness and acceptance of natural trauma-related emotions (e.g., sadness, anger), identify cognitive distortions, and explore trauma-related themes (e.g., safety, trust) via cognitive restructuring. In addition, CPT originally included a written exposure component. Cognitive therapy typically includes some form of exposure (imaginal and/or in vivo), although these are conceptualized as techniques to promote elaboration and integration of the trauma memory and are integrated with cognitive restructuring techniques.

One of the first studies of CPT was a dismantling study to examine the relative efficacy of the theorized active elements of CPT. In this study, Resick and colleagues (2008) compared the full CPT protocol (which included written exposure) with a written exposure only condition and a cognitive therapy only condition. All three treatments were found to be effective in reducing PTSD symptoms; however, participants in the cognitive therapy only condition showed more improvement than did those in the written exposure only condition. These findings informed a revision to the CPT protocol to designate the written account of the trauma as optional versus standard. Sloan et al. (2018) later compared 5 sessions of written exposure therapy (WET) to 12 sessions of CPT (including written exposure) and found WET noninferior to CPT.

Approaches for Youth

Treatment guidelines for children and adolescents are less consistent than those for adults. However, all guidelines recommend trauma-focused CBT (TF-CBT; Cohen & Mannarino, 2017) as a first-line approach. TF-CBT typically incorporates a caregiver in treatment (e.g., a nonperpetrating parent) and includes psychoeducation, emotion regulation and coping skills training, cognitive processing/restructuring, imaginal exposure, and in vivo exposure. TF-CBT demonstrated effectiveness for children impacted by a wide range of traumatic events and in children as young as preschool age (e.g., Scheeringa et al., 2011). PTSD treatments designed for adults have also been modified for use with younger populations, including prolonged exposure (e.g., Foa et al., 2008), cognitive therapy (Perrin et al., 2017), and NET (e.g., Ruf et al., 2010). Consistent with the adult literature, research has found that exposure-based CBT leads to comparable PTSD change, as does trauma-focused cognitive therapy at posttreatment (Nixon et al., 2012) and up to one year posttreatment (Nixon et al., 2017).

Other Variables Influencing Treatment

Assessment and Diagnosis

The PTSD Checklist for DSM-5 (PCL-5; Weathers et al., 2013b) is a widely used self-report measure of PTSD symptoms that mirror the DSM-5 symptom criteria for PTSD. The PCL-5 has excellent psychometric properties (e.g., Bovin et al., 2016). A cut-off score of 31–33 is suggested for identifying probable PTSD (Bovin et al., 2016). Additional well-validated self-report measures include the Impact of Events Scale-Revised (IES-R; Weiss & Marmar, 1996) and Posttraumatic Stress Diagnostic Scale for DSM-5 (PDS-5; Foa et al., 2016). An important issue for assessing PTSD is the need to link the symptoms to a Criterion A traumatic event (i.e., "index" event). For this reason, self-report measures of PTSD symptoms that do not include an assessment of trauma exposure should be administered along with a measure of Criterion A trauma, such as the Life Events Checklist (LEC-5; Weathers et al., 2013a) whenever the client's index event (i.e., the worst/most bothersome traumatic event) is not known. Repeated administration of symptom rating scales (e.g., administering the PCL-5 at every other session) is recommended to inform shared clinical decision-making about the helpfulness of treatment and the need to terminate or consider alternate treatment (i.e., measurement-based care). Assessing key associated constructs, such as negative trauma-related cognitions (Foa et al., 1999; Wells et al., 2019), may also be useful to guide treatment planning.

Structured diagnostic interviews such as the Structured Clinical Interview for DSM-5 Axis I Disorders, PTSD Module (SCID-5; First et al., 2016) and the Clinician Administered PTSD Scale for DSM-5 (Weathers et al., 2018) are recommended and common in clinical research settings. The CAPS-5 is considered the gold-standard interview measure of PTSD and yields comprehensive information about diagnostic status and symptom severity. PTSD is a heterogenous disorder comprised of behavioral, emotional, and cognitive symptoms. Some of these symptoms overlap with other disorders, and PTSD is associated with a high rate of psychiatric comorbidity (Kessler et al., 2005). Thus, it is important to evaluate the presence of other commonly co-occurring disorders.

When the onset of PTSD symptoms is delayed by six months or longer from the traumatic event, PTSD is diagnosed with a delayed onset specifier. There is no evidence to suggest that a delay in symptom onset impacts treatment prognosis. When less than one month has passed since the traumatic event, a diagnosis of acute stress disorder may be appropriate. Implementing brief trauma-focused psychotherapy within the first few weeks or months following a traumatic event can promote recovery among those experiencing significant PTSD symptoms (e.g., Roberts et al., 2019).

Complex PTSD, which is now included in the International Classification of Diseases, version 11 (ICD-11; WHO, 2022), comprises the core symptoms of PTSD, as well as three symptom groups of affective, relationship, and self-concept changes (Maercker, 2021). Trauma-focused psychotherapies, including CBT and exposure therapy, have been found efficacious for complex PTSD (Karatzias et al., 2019). In the past, a "phase-based" approach was recommended for complex PTSD, wherein a stabilization phase precedes a trauma-focused phase (e.g., Benham, 1995; Fisher, 1999). Goals of the stabilization phase include ensuring the patient's safety by improving self-regulation and interpersonal skills. However, evidence does not support this recommendation and guidance has shifted away from it, given that it unnecessarily delays implementation of evidence-based components (Bicanic et al., 2015; De Jongh et al., 2016).

Comorbidity

As noted previously, PTSD is associated with very high rates of psychiatric comorbidity. Fortunately, trauma-focused PTSD treatments remain efficacious when comorbid disorders are present, even without major adaptations for some disorders. For example, prolonged exposure has been found effective among patients with comorbid major depressive disorder (e.g., Hagenaars et al., 2010) and mild to moderate traumatic brain injury (e.g., Ragsdale & Voss Horrell, 2016). Moreover, symptoms of comorbid disorders often improve alongside PTSD symptoms, such as for depression (e. g., Acierno et al., 2017; Foa et al., 2013) and associated problems including general anxiety (e.g., Foa et al., 2005), trauma-related guilt (e.g., McLean et al., 2019), state anger (e.g., Ford et al., 2018), and dissociation (e.g., Harned et al., 2012). For other comorbid disorders, trauma-focused PTSD treatment has been found efficacious when delivered concurrently or integrated with treatment targeting the comorbid condition. For example, a treatment that integrates prolonged exposure with CBT for substance use can effectively reduce symptoms of both PTSD and substance use (e.g., Back et al., 2019). Similarly, integrating prolonged exposure with dialectical behavior therapy (DBT; Linehan et al., 2006) is efficacious for individuals with PTSD and comorbid borderline personality disorder (e.g., Harned et al., 2014).

Demographics

Older age has been linked to lower effect sizes for PTSD treatment in general (Dewar et al., 2020), and for exposure therapies (McLean et al., 2022) but not CPT (Asmundson et al., 2019). Additional research is needed to clarify the impact of age on treatment response, and the interaction of age and treatment type (e.g., exposure-based vs. cognitive) on outcomes. In terms of gender, the scope of the literature is limited to binary categories of men and women. Results from meta-analyses indicate that women benefit more from trauma-focused treatment than men (Sloan et al., 2011; Wade et al., 2016; Watts et al., 2013). Specifically, it appears that women benefit more than men from CPT (Asmundson et al., 2019; Khan et al., 2020), but no gender effects have been observed in exposure-based treatments (McLean et al., 2022). In clinical trials of trauma-focused treatments, racial and ethnic disparities in treatment response are generally not observed (Galovski et al., 2016; Held et al., 2021; McLean et al., 2022; Rutt et al., 2018), though one study found that African Americans benefited more from prolonged exposure compared to other ethnicities (Jeffreys et al., 2014). In contrast, veterans who identify as racial or ethnic minorities tend to have worse clinical outcomes following routine outpatient PTSD care through the Veterans Affairs health care system (Maguen et al., 2014; Sripada et al., 2017). Because race and ethnicity are often conflated and the scope has been largely limited to examining differences among White, African American, and Latinx trauma survivors, our understanding of racial and ethnic difference in PTSD outcomes remains limited.

Box 6.2 Trauma Type

Different categories of traumatic events, or "trauma types" (e.g., combat, accidents, interpersonal trauma), have been linked to distinct clinical PTSD symptom profiles (e.g., Birkeland et al., 2021; Kelley et al., 2009; Smith et al., 2016), which may potentially impact differential response to various treatment approaches. Combat trauma and interpersonal traumas (e.g., sexual assault, domestic violence, armed robbery) appear to most reliably predict poorer response to trauma-focused treatment (e.g., Bradley et al., 2005; Karatzias et al., 2019; Straud et al., 2019). However, results are inconsistent (e.g., Khan et al., 2020; Tiet et al., 2015). It is difficult to disentangle trauma type from chronicity of trauma exposure, particularly given that combat and interpersonal traumas are more likely to involve repeated exposure to traumatic stressors compared to, for example, a natural disaster or accident. Importantly, individuals with more complex trauma histories may benefit less from group therapy formats (Sloan et al., 2011), so it may be helpful to prioritize individual therapy for these persons. Although it is unclear to what extent trauma type versus trauma chronicity contribute to differential outcomes, both impact clinicians' perceptions of appropriate treatment approaches. Specifically, providers perceive greater treatment barriers (e.g., concerns about worsening of symptoms and dropout) and attenuated suitability of imaginal exposure for patients with multiple childhood traumas (van Minnen et al., 2010). This may inadvertently limit access to evidence-based treatment for certain subgroups of trauma survivors.

Medication

Serotonin reuptake inhibitors (SRIs) such as paroxetine, venlafaxine, and fluoxetine are efficacious pharmacotherapies for PTSD in adults (e.g., Forman-Hoffman et al., 2018). To date, only a few trials have tested the effects of combining EBPs with SRIs, and these studies have generally found that adding medication to trauma-focused psychotherapy does not improve long-term outcomes over medication or psychotherapy alone (e.g., Popiel et al., 2015; Rauch et al., 2019). Benzodiazepines are not recommended for PTSD; although they can help with anxiety and sleep in the short-term, they are not efficacious for treating PTSD and are associated with adverse side effects over time (Guina & Merrill, 2018). There is also evidence that benzodiazepines interfere with the effects of exposure therapy (e.g., van Minnen et al., 2012), possibly by promoting avoidance (i.e., functioning as a safety behavior), attenuating fear activation, and/or interfering with fear extinction (see Guina et al., 2015).

Conclusion

The most well-supported treatments for PTSD are trauma-focused psychotherapies. All of these treatments include psychoeducation, which can be critical to building therapeutic rapport, treatment credibility, and expectancy for change during treatment.

Homework is used in most efficacious treatment for PTSD, primarily to extend learning through additional practice of skills learned in-session and generalization to new contexts. Exposure and cognitive therapy are the two most often used evidence-based components of PTSD treatments. These components have been found to be highly efficacious when used alone (with psychoeducation and often with homework) or when combined in various ways in different trauma-focused protocols. Most studies have not found benefit to combining exposure and cognitive therapy techniques relative to focusing on one approach only, possibly because these approaches share underlying mechanisms of therapeutic change. For example, a quantitative review of studies examining exposure therapy with and without additional treatment components (typically cognitive restructuring) found a small but not clinically meaningful advantage for treatments with additional components relative to exposure alone on interviewer-assessed PTSD, and no differences on self-reported PTSD, loss of a PTSD diagnosis, or rate of treatment dropout (Kehle-Forbes et al., 2013). While some research has begun to identify potential treatment moderators among demographic (e.g., gender) and clinical (e.g., trauma type) characteristics, additional research is needed to determine which treatment approach will be most effective for a given patient. Shared decision-making is recommended to promote patient-centered care and has been linked with improved clinical outcomes (Watts et al., 2015).

Useful Resources

- CPT Web https://cpt2.musc.edu
  Online training for CPT.
- International Society for Traumatic Stress Studies (ISTSS) https://istss.org/home
  ISTSS is a professional association that offers information and resources related to traumatic stress and its management. The website includes information about PTSD assessment and treatment in adults and children, as well as provider training, treatment guidelines, and provider self-care.
- National Center for PTSD (NCPTSD) www.ptsd.va.gov
  The NCPTSD is a research and educational center of excellence on PTSD. The website offers information about PTSD assessment and PTSD treatments, including guidance on shared decision-making, and the PTSD Consultation Program, which provides clinical didactics and free expert consultation to any provider working with veterans with PTSD.
- National Child Traumatic Stress Network (NCTSN) www.nctsnet.org
  The NCTSN provides clinical services, education, and training to address traumatic stress in children and their families. It includes information about treatment approaches, psychological first aid, and trauma-informed care.
- PE Web http://pe.musc.edu
  The Medical University of South Carolina is one of several institutions that offers training in evidence-based treatment for PTSD, including online training for prolonged exposure therapy.

References

Acierno, R., Knapp, R., Tuerk, P., et al. (2017). A non-inferiority trial of prolonged exposure for posttraumatic stress disorder: In person versus home-based telehealth. *Behaviour Research and Therapy*, 89, 57–65.

Amir, N., Stafford, J., Freshman, M. S., & Foa, E. B. (1998). Relationship between trauma narratives and trauma pathology. *Journal of Traumatic Stress*, 11, 385–392. https://doi.org/ 10.1023/A:1024415523495.

Asmundson, G. J. G., Thorisdottir, A. S., Roden-Foreman, J. W., et al. (2019). A meta-analytic review of cognitive processing therapy for adults with posttraumatic stress disorder. *Cognitive Behaviour Therapy*, 48(1), 1–14. https://doi.org/10.1080/16506073.2018.1522371.

Back, S. E., Killeen, T., Badour, C. L., et al. (2019). Concurrent treatment of substance use disorders and PTSD using prolonged exposure: A randomized clinical trial in military veterans. *Addictive Behaviors*, 90, 369–377.

Beck, A. T, Rush, A. J., Shaw, B. F., & Emery, G. (1979). *Cognitive therapy of depression.* New Guilford Press.

Benham, E. (1995). Coping strategies: A psychoeducational approach to post-traumatic symptomatology. *Journal of Psychosocial Nursing and Mental Health Services*, 33(6), 30–35. https://doi.org/10.3928/0279-3695-19950601-07.

Bicanic, I., de Jongh, A., & Ten Broeke, E. (2015). Stabilisatie in traumabehandeling bij complexe PTSS: Noodzaak of mythe? [Stabilisation in trauma treatment: Necessity or myth?]. *Tijdschrift Voor Psychiatrie*, 57(5), 332–339.

Birkeland, M. S., Skar, A. M. S., & Jensen, T. K. (2021). Do different traumatic events invoke different kinds of post-traumatic stress symptoms? *European Journal of Psychotraumatology*, 12(sup1), 1866399. https://doi.org/10.1080/20008198.2020.1866399.

Blanchard, E. B., Hickling, E. J., Devineni, T., et al. (2003). A controlled evaluation of cognitive behaviorial therapy for posttraumatic stress in motor vehicle accident survivors. *Behaviour Research and Therapy*, 41(1), 79–96. https://doi.org/10.1016/S0005-7967(01)00131-0.

Bonanno, G. A., Romero, S. A., & Klein, S. I. (2015). The temporal elements of psychological resilience: An integrative framework for the study of individuals, families, and communities. *Psychological Inquiry*, 26(2), 139–169. https://doi.org/10.1080/ 1047840X.2015.992677.

Bosch, J., Mackintosh, M.-A., Wells, S. Y., et al. (2020). PTSD treatment response and quality of life in women with childhood trauma histories. *Psychological Trauma: Theory, Research, Practice and Policy*, 12(1), 55–63. https://doi.org/10.1037/tra0000468.

Boudewyns, P. A., & Hyer, L. (1990). Physiological response to combat memories and preliminary treatment outcome in Vietnam veteran PTSD patients treated with direct therapeutic exposure. *Behavior Therapy*, 21(1), 63–87.

Bouton, M. E. (1993). Context, time, and memory retrieval in the interference paradigms of Pavlovian learning. *Psychological Bulletin*, 114(1), 80–99. https://doi.org/10.1037/0033-2909.114.1.80.

Bovin, M. J., Marx, B. P., Weathers, F. W., et al. (2016). Psychometric properties of the PTSD checklist for diagnostic and statistical manual of mental disorders – fifth edition (PCL-5) in veterans. *Psychological assessment*, 28(11), 1379.

Bradley, R., Greene, J., Russ, E., Dutra, L., & Westen, D. (2005). A multidimensional meta-analysis of psychotherapy for PTSD. *American Journal of Psychiatry*, 162(2), 214–227. https://doi.org/10.1176/appi.ajp.162.2.214.

Brooks, S. K., Weston, D., Wessely, S., & Greenberg, N. (2021). Effectiveness and accept-ability of brief psychoeducational interventions after potentially traumatic events: A systematic review. *European Journal of Psychotraumatology*, 12(1), 1923110. https://doi.org/10.1080/20008198.2021.1923110.

Brouzos, A., Vatkali, E., Mavridis, D., Vassilopoulos, S. P., & Baourda, V. C. (2022). Psychoeducation for adults with post-traumatic stress symptomatology: A systematic review and meta-analysis. *Journal of Contemporary Psychotherapy*, 52(2), 155–164. https://doi.org/10.1007/s10879-021-09526-3.

Brown, L. A., Zandberg, L. J., & Foa, E. B. (2019). Mechanisms of change in prolonged exposure therapy for PTSD: Implications for clinical practice. *Journal of Psychotherapy Integration*, 29(1), 6–14. https://doi.org/10.1037/int0000109.

Bryant, R. A. (2003). Early predictors of posttraumatic stress disorder. *Biological Psychiatry*, 53(9), 789–95.

Bryant, R. A., & Guthrie, R. M. (2007). Maladaptive self-appraisals before trauma exposure predict posttraumatic stress disorder. *Journal of Consulting and Clinical Psychology*, 75(5), 812. https://doi.org/10.1037/0022-006X.75.5.812.

Bryant, R. A., Moulds, M. L., Guthrie, R. M., Dang, S. T., & Nixon, R. D. (2003). Imaginal exposure alone and imaginal exposure with cognitive restructuring in treatment of post-traumatic stress disorder. *Journal of Consulting and Clinical Psychology*, 71(4), 706-712. https://doi.org/10.1037/0022-006X.71.4.706

Bryant, R. A., Moulds, M. L., Guthrie, R. M., et al. (2008). A randomized controlled trial of exposure therapy and cognitive restructuring for posttraumatic stress disorder. *Journal of Consulting and Clinical Psychology*, 76, 695.

Cahill, S. P., Carrigan, M. H., & Frueh, B. C. (1999). Does EMDR work? And if so, why? A critical review of controlled outcome and dismantling research. *Journal of Anxiety Disorders*, 13(1), 5–33. https://doi.org/10.1016/S0887-6185(98)00039-5.

Cohen, J. A., & Mannarino, A. P. (2017). Evidence based intervention: Trauma-focused cognitive behavioral therapy for children and families. In D. M. Teti (Ed.), *Parenting and family processes in child maltreatment and intervention* (pp. 91–105). Springer International Publishing. https://doi.org/10.1007/978-3-319-40920-7_6.

Cooper, A. A., Kline, A. C., Graham, B., et al. (2017). Homework "dose," type, and helpful-ness as predictors of clinical outcomes in prolonged exposure for PTSD. *Behavior Therapy*, 48(2), 182–194. https://doi.org/10.1016/j.beth.2016.02.013.

Craske, M. G., Kircanski, K., Zelikowsky, M., et al. (2008). Optimizing inhibitory learning during exposure therapy. *Behaviour Research and Therapy*, 46(1), 5–27. https://doi.org/10.1016/j.brat.2007.10.003.

Cuijpers, P., Veen, S. C. Van, Sijbrandij, M., Yoder, W., & Cristea, I. A. (2020). Eye movement desensitization and reprocessing for mental health problems: A systematic review and meta-analysis. *Cognitive Behaviour Therapy*, 49(3), 165–180. https://doi.org/10.1080/16506073.2019.1703801.

Cummings, C. M., Kazantzis, N., & Kendall, P. C. (2014). Facilitating homework and generaliza-tion of skills to the real world. In E. S. Sburlati, H. J. Lyneham, C. A. Schniering, & R. M. Rappe (Eds.), *Evidence-based CBT for anxiety and depression in children and adolescents* (pp. 141–155). John Wiley & Sons, Ltd. https://doi.org/10.1002/9781118500576.ch11.

Cusack, K., Jonas, D. E., Forneris, C. A., et al. (2016). Psychological treatments for adults with posttraumatic stress disorder: A systematic review and meta-analysis. *Clinical Psychology Review*, 43, 128–141. https://doi.org/10.1016/j.cpr.2015.10.003.

Davidson, P. R., & Parker, K. C. H. (2001). Eye movement desensitization and reprocessing (EMDR): A meta-analysis. *Journal of Consulting and Clinical Psychology*, 69(2), 305–316. https://doi.org/10.1037/0022-006X.69.2.305.

De Jongh, A., Resick, P. A., Zoellner, L. A., et al. (2016). Critical analysis of the current treatment guidelines for complex PTSD in adults. *Depression and Anxiety*, 33(5), 359–369. https://doi.org/10.1002/da.2246.

Department of Veterans Affairs and Department of Defense (2017). *VA/DoD clinical practice guideline for the management of posttraumatic stress disorder and acute stress disorder.* Department of Veterans Affairs and Department of Defense.

Detweiler, J. B., & Whisman, M. A. (1999). The role of homework assignments in cognitive therapy for depression: Potential methods for enhancing adherence. *Clinical Psychology: Science and Practice*, 6(3), 267–282. https://doi.org/10.1093/clipsy.6.3.267.

Devilly, G. J., & Foa, E. B. (2001). The investigation of exposure and cognitive therapy: Comment on Tarrier et al. (1999). *Journal of Consulting and Clinical Psychology*, 69, 114–116.

Dewar, M., Paradis, A., & Fortin, C. A. (2020). Identifying trajectories and predictors of response to psychotherapy for post-traumatic stress disorder in adults: A systematic review of literature. *The Canadian Journal of Psychiatry*, 65(2), 71–86. https://doi.org/10.1177/0706743719875602.

Donker, T., Griffiths, K. M., Cuijpers, P., & Christensen, H. (2009). Psychoeducation for depression, anxiety and psychological distress: A meta-analysis. *BMC Medicine*, 7(1), 79. https://doi.org/10.1186/1741-7015-7-79.

Ehlers, A., & Clark, D. M. (2000). A cognitive model of posttraumatic stress disorder. *Behaviour Research and Therapy*, 38(4), 319–345.

Ehlers, A., Clark, D. M., Hackmann, A., et al. (2003). A randomized controlled trial of cognitive therapy, a self-help booklet, and repeated assessments as early interventions for posttraumatic stress disorder. *Archives of General Psychiatry*, 60, 1024–1032.

Fehm, L., & Mrose, J. (2008). Patients' perspective on homework assignments in cognitive-behavioural therapy. *Clinical Psychology & Psychotherapy*, 15(5), 320–328. https://doi.org/10.1002/cpp.592.

First, M. B., Williams, J. B., Karg, R. S., & Spitzer, R. L. (2016). *User's guide for the SCID-5-CV structured clinical interview for DSM-5® disorders: Clinical version.* American Psychiatric Publishing, Inc.

Fisher, J. (1999). The work of stabilization in trauma treatment. *Trauma Center Lecture Series*, 1–13.

Foa, E. B., & Kozak, M. J. (1985). Treatment of Anxiety Disorders: Implications for Psychopathology. In H. Tuma & J. Maser (Eds.), *Anxiety and the anxiety disorders*. Routledge.

Foa, E. B., Bredemeier, K., Acierno, R., et al. (2022). The efficacy of 90-min versus 60-min sessions of prolonged exposure for PTSD: A randomized controlled trial in active-duty military personnel. *Journal of Consulting and Clinical Psychology*, 90(6), 503–512. https://doi.org/10.1037/ccp0000739.

Foa, E. B., Chrestman, K. R., & Gilboa-Schechtman, E. (2008). *Prolonged exposure therapy for adolescents with PTSD emotional processing of traumatic experiences, therapist guide.* Oxford University Press.

Foa, E. B., Dancu, C. V., Hembree, E. A., et al. (1999). A comparison of exposure therapy, stress inoculation training, and their combination for reducing posttraumatic stress disorder in female assault victims. *Journal of Consulting and Clinical Psychology*, 67, 194–200.

Foa, E. B., Ehlers, A., Clark, D. M., Tolin, D. F., & Orsillo, S. M. (1999). The posttraumatic cognitions inventory (PTCI): Development and validation. *Psychological Assessment*, 11, 303–314. https://doi.org/10.1037/1040-3590.11.3.303.

Foa, E. B., Hembree, E. A., Cahill, S. P., et al. (2005). Randomized trial of prolonged exposure for posttraumatic stress disorder with and without cognitive restructuring: Outcome at academic and community clinics. *Journal of Consulting and Clinical Psychology*, 73, 953–964.

Foa, E. B., Hembree, E. A., Rothbaum, B. O., & Rauch, S. A. M. (2019). *Prolonged exposure therapy for PTSD: Emotional processing of traumatic experiences: Therapist guide*, 2nd ed. Oxford University Press. https://doi.org/10.1093/med-psych/9780190926939.001.0001.

Foa, E. B., McLean, C. P., Zang, Y., et al. (2016). Psychometric properties of the Posttraumatic Diagnostic Scale for DSM–5 (PDS–5). *Psychological assessment*, 28(10), 1166–1171. https://doi.org/10.1037/pas0000258.

Foa, E. B., McLean, C. P., Zang, Y., et al. (2018). Effect of prolonged exposure therapy delivered over 2 weeks vs 8 weeks vs present-centered therapy on PTSD symptom severity in military personnel: A randomized clinical trial. *Journal of the American Medical Association*, 319, 354–364.

Foa, E. B., Yusko, D. A., Mclean, C. P., et al. (2013). Concurrent naltrexone and prolonged exposure therapy for patients with comorbid alcohol dependence and PTSD. *Journal of the American Medical Association*, 310, 488–495.

Ford, J. D., Grasso, D. J., Greene, C. A., Slivinsky, M., & DeViva, J. C. (2018). Randomized clinical trial pilot study of prolonged exposure versus present centered affect regulation therapy for PTSD and anger problems with male military combat veterans. *Clinical Psychology & Psychotherapy*, 25, 641–649.

Forman-Hoffman, V., Middleton, J. C., Feltner, C., et al. (2018). *Psychological and pharmacological treatments for adults with posttraumatic stress disorder: A systematic review update*. Agency for Healthcare Research and Quality (US), Rockville (MD).

Galovski, T. E., Harik, J. M., Blain, L. M., et al. (2016). Identifying patterns and predictors of PTSD and depressive symptom change during cognitive processing therapy. *Cognitive Therapy and Research*, 40(5), 617–626. https://doi.org/10.1007/s10608-016-9770-4.

Goetter, E. M., Blackburn, A. M., Stasko, C., et al. (2020). Comparative effectiveness of prolonged exposure and cognitive processing therapy for military service members in an intensive treatment program. *Psychological Trauma: Theory, Research, Practice, and Policy*, 13(6), 632. https://doi.org/10.1037/tra0000956.

Gould, M., Greenberg, N., & Hetherton, J. (2007). Stigma and the military: Evaluation of a PTSD psychoeducational program. *Journal of Traumatic Stress*, 20(4), 505–515. https://doi.org/10.1002/jts.20233.

Gray, M. J., Elhai, J. D., & Frueh, B. C. (2004). Enhancing patient satisfaction and increasing treatment compliance: Patient education as a fundamental component of PTSD treatment. *Psychiatric Quarterly*, 75(4), 321–332. https://doi.org/10.1023/B:PSAQ.0000043508.52428.6e.

Guina, J., & Merrill, B. (2018). Benzodiazepines I: Upping the care on downers: the evidence of risks, benefits and alternatives. *Journal of Clinical Medicine*, 7(2), 17. https://doi.org/10.3390/jcm7020017.

Guina, J., Rossetter, S. R., DeRhodes, B. J., Nahhas, R. W., & Welton, R. S. (2015). Benzodiazepines for PTSD: A systematic review and meta-analysis. *Journal of Psychiatric Practice®*, 21(4), 281–303.

Hagenaars, M. A., van Minnen, A., & Hoogduin, K. A. (2010). The impact of dissociation and depression on the efficacy of prolonged exposure treatment for PTSD. *Behaviour Research and Therapy*, 48(1), 19–27.

Hamblen, J. L., Norman, S. B., Sonis, J. H., et al. (2019). A guide to guidelines for the treatment of posttraumatic stress disorder in adults: An update. *Psychotherapy*, 56(3), 359–373. https://doi.org/10.1037/pst0000231.

Harned, M. S., Korslund, K. E., & Linehan, M. M. (2014). A pilot randomized controlled trial of dialectical behavior therapy with and without the dialectical behavior therapy prolonged exposure protocol for suicidal and self-injuring women with borderline personality disorder and PTSD. *Behaviour Research and Therapy*, 55, 7–17.

Harned, M. S., Korslund, K. E., Foa, E. B., & Linehan, M. M. (2012). Treating PTSD in suicidal and self-injuring women with borderline personality disorder: Development and preliminary evaluation of a dialectical behavior therapy prolonged exposure protocol. *Behaviour Research and Therapy*, 50(6), 381–386.

Harvey, A. G., Bryant, R. A., & Rapee, R. M. (1996). Preconscious processing of threat in posttraumatic stress disorder. *Cognitive Therapy and Research*, 20, 613–623. https://doi.org/10.1007/BF02227964.

Held, P., Smith, D. L., Bagley, J. M., et al. (2021). Treatment response trajectories in a three-week CPT-Based intensive treatment for veterans with PTSD. *Journal of Psychiatric Research*, 141, 226–232. https://doi.org/10.1016/j.jpsychires.2021.07.004.

Hundt, N. E., Barrera, T. L., Arney, J., & Stanley, M. A. (2017). "It's worth it in the end": Veterans' experiences in prolonged exposure and cognitive processing therapy. *Cognitive and Behavioral Practice*, 24(1), 50–57. https://doi.org/10.1016/j.cbpra.2016.02.003.

International Society for Traumatic Stress Studies (2018). ISTSS PTSD prevention and treatment guidelines: Methodology and recommendations. www.istss.org/getattachment/Treating-Trauma/New-ISTSS-Prevention-and-TreatmentGuidelines/ISTSS_Prevention TreatmentGuidelines_FNL.pdf.aspx.

Janoff-Bulman, R. (1985). The aftermath of victimization: Rebuilding shattered assumptions. In C. R. Figley (Ed.), *Trauma and its wake: The study and treatment of post-traumatic Stress Disorder* (pp. 15–35). Brunner/Mazel.

Janoff-Bulman, R. (1989). Assumptive worlds and the stress of traumatic events: Applications of the schema construct. *Social Cognition*, 7(2), 113–136.

Jeffreys, M. D., Reinfeld, C., Nair, P. V., et al. (2014). Evaluating treatment of posttraumatic stress disorder with cognitive processing therapy and prolonged exposure therapy in a VHA specialty clinic. *Journal of Anxiety Disorders*, 28(1), 108–114. https://doi.org/10.1016/j.janxdis.2013.04.010.

Jeffries, F. W., & Davis, P. (2013). What is the role of eye movements in eye movement desensitization and reprocessing (EMDR) for post-traumatic stress disorder (PTSD)? A review. *Behavioural and Cognitive Psychotherapy*, 41(3), 290–300.

Kachadourian, L. K., Harpaz-Rotem, I., Tsai, J., Southwick, S. M., & Pietrzak, R. H. (2019). Posttraumatic stress disorder symptoms, functioning, and suicidal ideation in US military veterans: A symptomics approach. *The Primary Care Companion for CNS Disorders*, 21(2), 22914. https://doi.org/10.4088/PCC.18m02402.

Karatzias, T., Murphy, P., Cloitre, M., et al. (2019). Psychological interventions for ICD-11 complex PTSD symptoms: Systematic review and meta-analysis. *Psychological Medicine*, 49(11), 1761–1775. https://doi.org/10.1017/S0033291719000436.

Kazantzis, N., & Deane, F. P. (1999). Psychologists' use of homework assignments in clinical practice. *Professional Psychology: Research and Practice*, 30(6), 581–585. https://doi.org/10.1037/0735-7028.30.6.581.

Kazantzis, N., Arntz, A. R., Borkovec, T., Holmes, E. A., & Wade, T. (2010). Unresolved issues regarding homework assignments in cognitive and behavioural therapies: An expert panel discussion at AACBT. *Behaviour Change*, 27(3), 119–129. https://doi.org/10.1375/bech.27.3.119.

Kazantzis, N., Deane, F. P., & Ronan, K. R. (2000). Homework assignments in cognitive and behavioral therapy: A meta-analysis. *Clinical Psychology: Science and Practice*, 7(2), 189–202. https://doi.org/10.1093/clipsy.7.2.189.

Kazantzis, N., Whittington, C., Zelencich, L., et al. (2016). Quantity and quality of homework compliance: A meta-analysis of relations with outcome in cognitive behavior therapy. *Behavior Therapy*, 47(5), 755–772. https://doi.org/10.1016/j.beth.2016.05.002.

Keane, T. M., Fairbank, J. A., Caddell, J. M., & Zimering, R. T. (1989). Implosive (flooding) therapy reduces symptoms of PTSD in Vietnam combat veterans. *Behavior Therapy*, 20(2), 245–260. https://doi.org/10.1016/S0005-7894(89)80072-3.

Keefe, J. R., Wiltsey Stirman, S., Cohen, Z. D., et al. (2018). In rape trauma PTSD, patient characteristics indicate which trauma-focused treatment they are most likely to complete. *Depression and Anxiety*, 35(4), 330–338. https://doi.org/10.1002/da.22731.

Kehle-Forbes, S. M., Polusny, M. A., MacDonald, R., et al. (2013). A systematic review of the efficacy of adding nonexposure components to exposure therapy for posttraumatic stress disorder. *Psychological Trauma: Theory, Research, Practice, and Policy*, 5(4), 317.

Kelley, L. P., Weathers, F. W., McDevitt-Murphy, M. E., Eakin, D. E., & Flood, A. M. (2009). A comparison of PTSD symptom patterns in three types of civilian trauma. *Journal of Traumatic Stress*, 22(3), 227–235. https://doi.org/10.1002/jts.20406.

Kessler, R. C., Berglund, P., Demler, O., et al. (2005). Lifetime prevalence and age-of-onset distributions of DSM-IV disorders in the National Comorbidity Survey Replication. *Archives of General Psychiatry*, 62(6), 593–602.

Khan, A. J., Holder, N., Li, Y., et al. (2020). How do gender and military sexual trauma impact PTSD symptoms in cognitive processing therapy and prolonged exposure? *Journal of Psychiatric Research*, 130, 89–96. https://doi.org/10.1016/j.jpsychires.2020.06.025.

Lang, P. J. (1977). Imagery in therapy: An information processing analysis of fear. *Behavior Therapy*, 8(5), 862–886. https://doi.org/10.1016/S0005-7894(77)80157-3.

LeDoux, J. E. (2014). Coming to terms with fear. *Proceedings of the National Academy of Sciences*, 111(8), 2871–2878.

Lee, C. W., & Cuijpers, P. (2013). A meta-analysis of the contribution of eye movements in processing emotional memories. *Journal of Behavior Therapy and Experimental Psychiatry*, 44(2), 231–239.

Lewis, C., Roberts, N. P., Andrew, M., Starling, E., & Bisson, J. I. (2020). Psychological therapies for post-traumatic stress disorder in adults: Systematic review and meta-analysis. *European Journal of Psychotraumatology*, 11(1), 1729633. https://doi.org/10.1080/20008198.2020.1729633.

Linehan, M. M., Comtois, K. A., Murray, A. M., et al. (2006). Two-year randomized controlled trial and follow-up of dialectical behavior therapy vs therapy by experts for suicidal behaviors and borderline personality disorder. *Archives of General Psychiatry*, 63(7), 757–766.

Maercker, A. (2021). Development of the new CPTSD diagnosis for ICD-11. *Borderline Personality Disorder and Emotion Dysregulation*, 8(1), 1–4.

Maguen, S., Madden, E., Neylan, T. C., et al. (2014). Timing of mental health treatment and PTSD symptom improvement among Iraq and Afghanistan veterans. *Psychiatric Services*, 65(12), 1414–1419. https://doi.org/10.1176/appi.ps.201300453.

Markowitz, J. C., Neria, Y., Lovell, K., Van Meter, P. E., & Petkova, E. (2017). History of sexual trauma moderates psychotherapy outcome for posttraumatic stress disorder. *Depression and Anxiety*, 34(8), 692–700. https://doi.org/10.1002/da.22619.

Mausbach, B. T., Moore, R., Roesch, S., Cardenas, V., & Patterson, T. L. (2010). The relationship between homework compliance and therapy outcomes: An updated meta-analysis. *Cognitive Therapy and Research*, 34(5), 429–438. https://doi.org/10.1007/s10608-010-9297-z.

McCann, I. L., Sakheim, D. K., & Abrahamson, D. J. (1988). Trauma and victimization: A model of psychological adaptation. *The Counseling Psychologist*, 16(4), 531–594.

McLean, C. P., Asnaani, A., Litz, B. T., & Hofmann, S. G. (2011). Gender differences in anxiety disorders: Prevalence, course of illness, comorbidity and burden of illness. *Journal of Psychiatric Research*, 45(8), 1027–1035. https://doi.org/10.1016/j.jpsychires.2011.03.006.

McLean, C. P., Foa, E. B., Dondanville, K. A., et al. (2021). The effects of web-prolonged exposure among military personnel and veterans with posttraumatic stress disorder. *Psychological Trauma: Theory, Research, Practice, and Policy*, 13(6), 621–361. https://doi.org/10.1037/tra0000978.

McLean, C. P., Levy, H. C., Miller, M. L., & Tolin, D. F. (2022). Exposure therapy for PTSD: A meta-analysis. *Clinical Psychology Review*, 91, 102115. https://doi.org/10.1016/j.cpr.2021.102115.

McLean, C. P., Zang, Y., Gallagher, T., et al. (2019). Trauma-related cognitions and cognitive emotion regulation as mediators of PTSD change among treatment-seeking active-duty military personnel with PTSD. *Behavior Therapy*, 50(6), 1053–1062.

Mowrer, O. H. (1960). Two-factor learning theory: Versions one and two. In *Learning theory and behavior* (pp. 63–91). John Wiley & Sons Inc. https://doi.org/10.1037/10802-003.

National Institute for Health and Clinical Practice (2018). *Guideline for post-traumatic stress disorder*. National Institute for Health and Clinical Practice.

Nixon, R. D. V., Sterk, J., & Pearce, A. (2012). A randomized trial of cognitive behaviour therapy and cognitive therapy for children with posttraumatic stress disorder following single-incident trauma. *Journal of Abnormal Child Psychology*, 40(3), 327–337.

Nixon, R. D. V., Sterk, J., Pearce, A., & Weber, N. (2017). A randomized trial of cognitive behavior therapy and cognitive therapy for children with posttraumatic stress disorder following single-incident trauma: Predictors and outcome at 1-year follow-up. *Psychological Trauma: Theory, Research, Practice, and Policy*, 9(4), 471–478. https://doi.org/10.1037/tra0000190.

Perrin, S., Leigh, E., Smith, P., et al. (2017). Cognitive therapy for PTSD in children and adolescents. In M. A. Landolt, M. Cloitre, & U. Schnyder (Eds.), *Evidence-based treatments for trauma related disorders in children and adolescents* (pp. 187–207). Springer.

Phoenix Australia Centre for Posttraumatic Mental Health (2013). *Australian guidelines for the treatment of acute stress disorder and posttraumatic stress disorder*. Phoenix Australia Centre for Posttraumatic Mental Health.

Phoenix, B. J. (2007). Psychoeducation for survivors of trauma. *Perspectives in Psychiatric Care*, 43(3), 123–131. https://doi.org/10.1111/j.1744-6163.2007.00121.x.

Pitman, R. K., Orr, S. P., Altman, B., et al. (1996). Emotional processing during eye movement desensitization and reprocessing therapy of Vietnam veterans with chronic posttraumatic stress disorder. *Comprehensive Psychiatry*, 37(6), 419–429. https://doi.org/10.1016/S0010-440X(96)90025-5.

Popiel, A., Zawadzki, B., Pragłowska, E., & Teichman, Y. (2015). Prolonged exposure, paroxetine and the combination in the treatment of PTSD following a motor vehicle accident: A randomized clinical trial – The "TRAKT" study. *Journal of Behavior Therapy and Experimental Psychiatry*, 48, 17–26.

Ragsdale, K. A., & Voss Horrell, S. C. (2016). Effectiveness of prolonged exposure and cognitive processing therapy for US veterans with a history of traumatic brain injury. *Journal of Traumatic Stress*, 29(5), 474–477.

Rauch, S. A., Kim, H. M., Powell, C., et al. (2019). Efficacy of prolonged exposure therapy, sertraline hydrochloride, and their combination among combat veterans with posttraumatic stress disorder. *JAMA Psychiatry*, 76, 117–126. https://doi.org/10.1001/jamapsychiatry.2018.3412.

Rauch, S. A., King, A. P., Abelson, J., et al. (2015). Biological and symptom changes in posttraumatic stress disorder treatment: A randomized clinical trial. *Depression and Anxiety*, 32, 204–212.

Rauch, S. A., Yasinski, C. W., Post, L. M., et al. (2021). An intensive outpatient program with prolonged exposure for veterans with posttraumatic stress disorder: Retention, predictors, and patterns of change. *Psychological Services*, 18(4), 606–618. https://doi.org/10.1037/ser0000422.

Reger, G. M., McClure, M. L., Ruskin, D., Carter, S. P., & Reger, M. A. (2019). Integrating predictive modeling into mental health care: An example in suicide prevention. *Psychiatric Services*, 70(1), 71–74.

Resick, P. A., & Schnicke, M. (1993). *Cognitive processing therapy for rape victims: A treatment manual*. Sage.

Resick, P. A., Galovski, T. E., Uhlmansiek, M. O., et al. (2008). A randomized clinical trial to dismantle components of cognitive processing therapy for posttraumatic stress disorder in female victims of interpersonal violence. *Journal of Consulting and Clinical Psychology*, 76(2), 243–258. https://doi.org/10.1037/0022-006X.76.2.243.

Resick, P. A., Monson, C. M., & Chard, K. M. (2017). *Cognitive processing therapy for PTSD: A comprehensive manual*. Guilford Press.

Roberts, N. P., Kitchiner, N. J., Kenardy, J., et al. (2019). Multiple session early psychological interventions for the prevention of post-traumatic stress disorder. *Cochrane Database of Systematic Reviews*, (8). https://doi.org/10.1002/14651858.CD006869.pub3.

Rosen, C. S., Greenbaum, M. A., Schnurr, P. P., et al. (2013). Do benzodiazepines reduce the effectiveness of exposure therapy for posttraumatic stress disorder? *The Journal of Clinical Psychiatry*, 74(12), 1855.

Rosen, G. M., & Davison, G. C. (2003). Psychology should list empirically supported principles of change (ESPs) and not credential trademarked therapies or other treatment packages. *Behavior Modification*, 27(3), 300–312. https://doi.org/10.1177/0145445503027003003.

Rosen, G. M., Otgaar, H., & Merckelbach, H. (2023). Trauma. In S. Hupp & C. L. Santa Maria (Eds.), *Pseudoscience in therapy: A skeptical field guide* (pp. 69–93). Cambridge University Press.

Ruf, M., Schauer, M., Neuner, F., et al. (2010). Narrative exposure therapy for 7- to 16-year-olds: A randomized controlled trial with traumatized refugee children. *Journal of Traumatic Stress*, 23(4), 437–445.

Rupp, C., Doebler, P., Ehring, T., & Vossbeck-Elsebusch, A. N. (2017). Emotional processing theory put to test: A meta-analysis on the association between process and outcome measures in exposure therapy. *Clinical Psychology & Psychotherapy*, 24(3), 697–711. https://doi.org/10.1002/cpp.2039.

Rutt, B. T., Oehlert, M. E., Krieshok, T. S., & Lichtenberg, J. W. (2018). Effectiveness of cognitive processing therapy and prolonged exposure in the Department of Veterans Affairs. *Psychological Reports*, 121(2), 282–302. https://doi.org/10.1177/003329411 7727746.

Sack, M., Zehl, S., Otti, A., et al. (2016). A comparison of dual attention, eye movements, and exposure only during eye movement desensitization and reprocessing for posttraumatic stress disorder: Results from a randomized clinical trial. *Psychotherapy and Psychosomatics*, 85(6), 357–365.

Sanderson, A., & Carpenter, R. (1992). Eye movement desensitization versus image confrontation: A single-session crossover study of 58 phobic subjects. *Journal of Behavior Therapy and Experimental Psychiatry*, 23(4), 269–275. https://doi.org/10.1016/0005-7916(92) 90049-O.

Schauer, M., Neuner, F., & Elbert, T. (2011). *Narrative exposure therapy: A short-term treatment for traumatic stress disorders*. Hogrefe Publishing GmbH.

Scheeringa, M. S., Weems, C. F., Cohen, J. A., Amaya-Jackson, L., & Guthrie, D. (2011). Trauma-focused cognitive-behavioral therapy for posttraumatic stress disorder in three-through six year-old children: A randomized clinical trial. *Journal of Child Psychology and Psychiatry*, 52(8), 853–860. https://doi.org/10.1111/j.1469-7610.2010.02354.x.

Schubert, S., & Lee, C. W. (2009). Adult PTSD and its treatment with EMDR: A review of controversies, evidence, and theoretical knowledge. *Journal of EMDR Practice and Research*, 3(3), 117–132.

Shapiro, F., & Maxfield, L. (2002). Eye movement desensitization and reprocessing (EMDR): Information processing in the treatment of trauma. *Journal of Clinical Psychology*, 58(8), 933–946.

Sloan, D. M., & Marx, B. P. (2019). *Written exposure therapy for PTSD: A brief treatment approach for mental health professionals*. American Psychological Association.

Sloan, D. M., Feinstein, B. A., Gallagher, M. W., Beck, J. G., & Keane, T. M. (2011). Efficacy of group treatment for posttraumatic stress disorder symptoms: A meta-analysis. *Psychological Trauma: Theory, Research, Practice, and Policy*, 5(2), 176–183. https://doi.org/10.1037/a0026291.

Sloan, D. M., Marx, B. P., Lee, D. J., & Resick, P. A. (2018). A brief exposure-based treatment vs cognitive processing therapy for posttraumatic stress disorder: A randomized noninferiority clinical trial. *JAMA Psychiatry*, 75, 233–239.

Smith, H. L., Summers, B. J., Dillon, K. H., & Cougle, J. R. (2016). Is worst-event trauma type related to PTSD symptom presentation and associated features? *Journal of Anxiety Disorders*, 38, 55–61. https://doi.org/10.1016/j.janxdis.2016.01.007.

Sripada, R. K., Pfeiffer, P. N., Rampton, J., et al. (2017). Predictors of PTSD symptom change among outpatients in the US Department of Veterans Affairs Health Care System. *Journal of Traumatic Stress*, 30(1), 45–53. https://doi.org/10.1002/jts.22156.

Stirman, S. W., Gutner, C. A., Suvak, M. K., et al. (2018). Homework completion, patient characteristics, and symptom change in cognitive processing therapy for PTSD. *Behavior Therapy*, 49(5), 741–755. https://doi.org/10.1016/j.beth.2017.12.001.

Straud, C. L., Siev, J., Messer, S., & Zalta, A. K. (2019). Examining military population and trauma type as moderators of treatment outcome for first-line psychotherapies for PTSD: A meta-analysis. *Journal of Anxiety Disorders*, 67, 102133. https://doi.org/10.1016/j.janxdis.2019.102133.

Tanielian, T. L., & Jaycox, L. (2008). *Invisible wounds of war: Psychological and cognitive injuries, their consequences, and services to assist recovery*. RAND.

Tanielian, T. L., Jaycox, L. H., Schell, T. L., et al. (2008). *Invisible wounds of war: Summary and recommendations for addressing psychological and cognitive injuries*. RAND.

Tiet, Q. Q., Leyva, Y. E., Blau, K., Turchik, J. A., & Rosen, C. S. (2015). Military sexual assault, gender, and PTSD treatment outcomes of US veterans. *Journal of Traumatic Stress*, 28(2), 92–101. https://doi.org/10.1002/jts.21992.

van Minnen, A., Harned, M. S., Zoellner, L., & Mills, K. (2012). Examining potential contraindications for prolonged exposure therapy for PTSD. *European Journal of Psychotraumatology*, 3(1), 18805.

van Minnen, A., Hendriks, L., & Olff, M. (2010). When do trauma experts choose exposure therapy for PTSD patients? A controlled study of therapist and patient factors. *Behaviour Research and Therapy*, 48(4), 312–320. https://doi.org/10.1016/j.brat.2009.12.003.

Wade, D., Varker, T., Kartal, D., et al. (2016). Gender difference in outcomes following trauma-focused interventions for posttraumatic stress disorder: Systematic review and meta-analysis. *Psychological Trauma: Theory, Research, Practice, and Policy*, 8(3), 356–364. https://doi.org/10.1037/tra0000110.

Watts, B. V., Schnurr, P. P., Mayo, L., et al. (2013). Meta-analysis of the efficacy of treatments for posttraumatic stress disorder. *The Journal of Clinical Psychiatry*, 74(6), 11710. https://doi.org/10.4088/JCP.12r08225.

Watts, B. V., Schnurr, P. P., Zayed, M., et al. (2015). A randomized controlled clinical trial of a patient decision aid for posttraumatic stress disorder. *Psychiatric Services*, 66(2), 149–154. https://doi.org/10.1176/appi.ps.201400062.

Weathers, F. W., Blake, D. D., Schnurr, P. P., et al. (2013a). *The Life events checklist for DSM-5 (LEC-5)*. Instrument available from the National Center for PTSD: www.ptsd.va.gov.

Weathers, F. W., Bovin, M. J., Lee, D. J., et al. (2018). The clinician-administered PTSD scale for DSM–5 (CAPS-5): Development and initial psychometric evaluation in military veterans. *Psychological Assessment*, 30(3), 383.

Weathers, F. W., Litz, B. T., Keane, T. M., et al. (2013b). The PTSD checklist for DSM-5 (PCL-5). Scale available from the National Center for PTSD: www.ptsd.va.gov.

Weiss, D. S., & Marmar, C. R. (1996). The Impact of Event Scale - Revised. In J. Wilson & T. M. Keane (Eds.), *Assessing Psychological Trauma and PTSD* (pp. 399–411). Guilford.

Weiss, D. S., & Marmar, C. R. (2004). Impact of event scale-revised (IES-R). *Cross-Cultural Assessment of Psychological Trauma and PTSD*, 219–238.

Wells, S. Y., Morland, L. A., Torres, E. M., et al. (2019). The development of a brief version of the Posttraumatic Cognitions Inventory (PTCI-9). *Assessment*, 26(2), 193–208.

Whitworth, J. D. (2016). The role of psychoeducation in trauma recovery: Recommendations for content and delivery. *Journal of Evidence-Informed Social Work*, 13(5), 442–451. https://doi.org/10.1080/23761407.2016.1166852.

World Health Organization. (2022). *ICD-11: International classification of diseases* (11th revision). https://icd.who.int/.

Zalta, A. K., Held, P., Smith, D. L., et al. (2018). Evaluating patterns and predictors of symptom change during a three-week intensive outpatient treatment for veterans with PTSD. *BMC Psychiatry*, 18, 1–15. https://doi.org/10.1186/s12888-018-1816-6.

Zalta, A. K., Tirone, V., Orlowska, D., et al. (2021). Examining moderators of the relationship between social support and self-reported PTSD symptoms: A meta-analysis. *Psychological Bulletin*, 147(1), 33–54. https://doi.org/10.1037/bul0000316.

7

Dissociative Disorders

Damla E. Aksen and Steven Jay Lynn

The *Diagnostic and Statistical Manual of Mental Disorders* (DSM-5-TR) defines dissociative disorders as "disruption[s] of and/or discontinuity in the normal integration of consciousness, memory, identity, emotion, perception, body representation, motor control, and behavior" (American Psychiatric Association, 2022, p. 329). Dissociative experiences range from mild (e.g., absorption in everyday experiences) to serious and debilitating, as in the case of dissociative identity disorder (DID). Dissociative disorders encompass depersonalization (detachment from self, body), derealization (e.g., detachment from surroundings feelings of unreality), dissociative amnesia (e.g., gaps in autobiographical memory not accounted for by ordinary forgetting), and DID, formerly called multiple personality disorder (i.e., presence of distinct personality states, recurrent dissociative amnesia). Other mental health disorders (e.g., posttraumatic stress disorder, borderline personality disorder [BPD]) consider dissociative symptoms in formulating a diagnosis. Finally, "other specified dissociative disorder" and "unspecified dissociative disorder" are characterized by dissociative symptoms (e.g., dissociative seizures) that do not meet the threshold for any other disorder and were previously called "dissociative disorder not otherwise specified" (DDNOS).

Dissociative disorders (DD) are not uncommon, generally falling in the prevalence range of 1–3% (see Lynn et al., 2019), roughly equivalent to that of schizophrenia or bipolar disorder. Prevalence rates are higher in clinical populations and vary with diagnostic methods (e.g., structured versus unstructured interviews), interviewer reliability, examiner biases, local base-rates, and cultural factors discussed later in the chapter (see Lilienfeld & Lynn, 2003).

Because clinicians and researchers may be unaware of the prevalence of dissociative conditions, they may fail to assess and treat symptoms and to systematically develop and evaluate evidence-based interventions. Concerningly, Langeland et al. (2020) reviewed four studies regarding the economic burden of DD and tentatively concluded that DD are "costly to society and that there is a reduction in service utilization and associated costs over time with diagnosing of and specialized treatments for DDs" (p. 730).

Apart from societal costs, patients with DD often suffer from severe psychiatric symptoms; complex emotional, social, and physical health difficulties; and diverse functional impairments (Myrick, Webermann, Langeland, et al., 2017). Dissociative experiences are related to ratings of poor quality of life (Polizzi et al., 2022) and are associated with recurrent hospitalizations, suicide, and high rates of disability (Langeland et al., 2020). Clearly, effective treatments must be a high priority.

Etiology and Theoretical Underpinnings of Treatment

To underscore this point, the evaluation of treatments for DD has received sparse attention compared with other DSM-5-TR disorders. Evidence-based treatments arguably lag far behind the treatment of most other DSM conditions. One reason is that the theoretical underpinnings of the treatment of DD are highly controversial. Some experts have asserted that DD are byproducts of trauma and advocated for a posttraumatic model (PTM) of dissociation (Dalenberg et al., 2012; Gleaves, 1996). According to the PTM, processing of past traumatic events should be accorded the highest priority.

In contrast, proponents of the sociocognitive model (SCM; Lilienfeld et al., 1999; Lynn et al., 2014; Spanos, 1994) have claimed that while DD may be associated with severe psychopathology, their genesis often resides in cognitive, social, and cultural influences (e.g., media, suggestibility, fantasy, symptom overreporting, suggestive psychotherapies). This model is compatible with cognitive-behavioral interventions (CBT) and with research from a transdiagnostic/transtheoretical perspective that considers multiple determinants of dissociation as treatment targets. Research supports a role for an array of such determinants, including sleep disturbances, cognitive-affective dysregulation and avoidance, alexithymia, and meta-cognitive processes (Aksen et al., 2021; Lynn et al., 2019; Serrano-Sevillano et al., 2017; Van der Kloet et al., 2012).

PTM advocates have maintained that skepticism regarding DD and a lack of clinician training might account for why DD are not routinely assessed and treated (Brand et al., 2014, 2016; Leonard et al., 2015; Şar & Ross, 2006). However, SCM proponents have contended that iatrogenic influences (e.g., suggestive methods, hypnosis) in psychotherapy, and/or patients' attribution of puzzling symptoms to a fragmented self, may produce false positive diagnoses (Lynn et al., 2014). We will consider diagnostic issues in greater depth before we conclude. Nevertheless, regardless of one's theoretical perspective, we recommend that clinicians routinely screen for and carefully evaluate dissociative symptoms. Furthermore, (a) reliable diagnoses can be achieved in psychotherapy studies using structured interviews, regardless of the origin of the symptoms (Leonard et al., 2015), and (b) participants can be reliably "categorized" and diagnosed in treatment studies.

Brief Overview of Treatments

Research on the treatment of dissociation is deficient in rigorous controlled studies, although abundant case studies exist (but will not be the focus of our review; see Maxwell et al., 2018). This state of affairs is arguably attributable largely to the controversial nature of dissociative conditions spurred, in part, by (a) dramatized depictions of DD in the media (e.g., movies such as *The Three Faces of Eve*, *Sybil*, *Split*) and (b) by early and influential depictions of the treatment of DD based on the PTM. Such portrayals are exemplified in Putnam's 1989 influential work that presented suggestive interventions and memory recovery techniques, which some clinicians rejected based on concerns about false memories and iatrogenic DID. Such interventions veered sharply from behavioral, cognitive, and cognitive-behavioral methods, which came into vogue among psychotherapists and researchers who practiced and researched evidence-based psychotherapies. The negative reputation of suggestive interventions likely persists among some contemporary clinicians and researchers who do not identify DID treatment with well-researched empirically grounded methods.

Additionally, treatment research has likely been deterred by the intensive, costly, and long-term nature of DID treatment necessitated by the combination of serious dissociative conditions alongside comorbid psychopathology. Accordingly, we speculate that many researchers have been dissuaded from conducting treatment studies and pursuing grant funding. Still, researchers have developed and begun to evaluate promising treatments for dissociative conditions that span a diversity of approaches.

In this chapter, we will review treatments for dissociation and spotlight DID, given that most concerted research efforts have centered on DID. Nevertheless, we will allude to other dissociative conditions, such as depersonalization/derealization and dissociative seizures (e.g., "psychogenic nonepileptic" or "functional" seizures), and provide recommendations for future research. Given the limited research on DD, we will depart from other chapters and focus on emerging and promising treatments rather than on credible components of science-based treatments.

Emerging and Promising Treatments

Phase-Oriented Treatment

We would be remiss in not discussing a commonly used phase-oriented approach to treating DID and DDNOS, even though it is not yet grounded in systematic controlled research. This intervention is recommended in guidelines promulgated by the

International Society for the Study of Trauma and Dissociation (ISSTD). Although the phases are presented in a sequential order, they are usually implemented recursively, whereby each phase is evaluated and implemented based on the patient's unique needs (Courtois, 1999).

Phase 1 focuses on establishing the therapist alliance (Cronin et al., 2014) and symptom control. The goal is to build skills necessary to achieve symptom stabilization (e.g., reduce self-harm, suicide attempts) and emotion regulation (Nester et al., 2022; Şar et al., 2007). Symptom control can be facilitated by targeting emotional dysregulation via providing structure, behavioral change, emotion regulation strategies (e.g., grounding, breathing techniques), and medications, as well as devising safety management strategies (Nester et al., 2022).

Phase 2 focuses on confronting, integrating, and working through memories. This phase aims to recall, fully experience, process, and incorporate memories of past events to develop control over them and transform traumatic memories to narrative memories (Subramanyam et al., 2020). We suggest that clinicians exert due caution in avoiding aggressive and suggestive memory recovery techniques (e.g., hypnosis, reifying/mapping alters) throughout treatment.

Finally, phase 3 focuses on integration and rehabilitation with the goal of stabilizing identity (Pollock et al., 2017) and enhancing mindfulness skills (Sharma et al., 2016). The guidelines encourage other modalities such as CBT, schema therapy, family or expressive therapy, and dialectical behavior therapy (DBT) (Lilienfeld et al., 2013), although group therapy is not recommended as the primary treatment modality because traditional process-oriented groups tend to encourage discussion of traumatic experiences and identities that may exacerbate dissociation symptoms.

In Bækkelund et al.'s (2022) study, based on these guidelines, individuals diagnosed with complex DD did not report immediate improvement after group and individual therapy. However, they did report significant reductions in symptoms during the 6-month follow-up.

The ISSTD guidelines certainly merit study. However, as of this writing, it is not known (a) which intervention in any phase is necessary or sufficient, (b) which intervention takes precedence over others, and (c) how one or all components fare when compared with any other (non-phase) treatment.

Treatment of Patients with the Dissociative Disorders Network Program

The prospective longitudinal Treatment of Patients with Dissociative Disorders (TOP DD) study is the most comprehensive outcome study to date. In this web-based psychosocial intervention based on 111 international patients, Myrick, Webermann, Langeland, et al. (2017) reported that individuals diagnosed with DID benefit from specialized treatment. The research evaluated whether participants evidenced reduced symptoms over two years following the utilization of highly diverse interventions across therapists including educational videos, written and behavioral exercises, prolonged exposure, eye movement desensitization and reprocessing, grief management, CBT, and behavior chain analysis of dissociative episodes. Therapists were trained to treat DD, and educational materials were developed based on the ISSTD guidelines (Brand et al., 2012). During the program, participants reported only small improvements in dissociation; however, at the two-year mark, patients with high levels of dissociation initially experienced the greatest improvements in emotion regulation, PTSD, and dissociation. However, regression to the mean is a plausible explanation for these findings, as a no-treatment control or other comparison condition (e.g., placebo) was not evaluated.

Cognitive-Behavioral Therapy

Emerging evidence supports CBT in treating dissociation symptoms (Goldstein et al., 2020; Hoeboer et al., 2020). The use of CBT is based on the rationale that it can be utilized to reduce avoidance behaviors, linked with persistent posttraumatic stress, via challenging (inaccurate) meta-cognitive beliefs regarding the existence of separate indwelling "identities" (see Lynn et al., 2022). These dysfunctional beliefs promote cognitive-affect-behavioral avoidance of negative emotions and negative reinforcement of symptoms of depersonalization and derealization that represent maladaptive safety behaviors present in DD (Chiu et al., 2017; Şar et al., 2017). Derealization and depersonalization, in turn, can be treated with CBT using psychoeducation, diary entries to highlight symptom variability, grounding in present-moment experience, symptom avoidance-reduction, reducing safety behaviors and self-focused attention, and challenging catastrophic and motivation-degrading assumptions (Hunter et al., 2003; Hunter et al., 2005; Hunter, 2013). However, these potential symptom mediators and moderators have not been systematically isolated or evaluated to date in conjunction with treatment. Van Minnen and Tibben (2001) relied on CBT principles in a case study of a woman with PTSD and DID diagnoses. The intervention involved eight days of trauma-focused treatment, psychoeducation, and participation in physical activities. After two weeks, the participant no longer met the full criteria for PTSD or DID and maintained gains at three and six months. Research with larger samples and appropriate comparison conditions is warranted.

Goldstein et al. (2020) evaluated dissociative seizures in a multicenter randomized controlled trial in England, Scotland, and Wales based on 313 patients who received CBT plus standardized medical care or medical care alone. Although no differences were reported for primary outcome measures, secondary measures (e.g., better quality of life, less overall psychological distress, seizures rated as less bothersome) provided evidence for predicted differences favoring CBT.

The Unified Protocol

Lynn et al. (2019, 2022) have called for research investigating transtheoretical and transdiagnostic variables, noted earlier, in and apart from psychotherapy. The relevance of a transdiagnostic and transtheoretical approach is exemplified in the Unified Protocol (UP) for the Treatment of Emotional Disorders (Barlow et al., 2017), with demonstrated effectiveness in treating BPD, mood, anxiety, and somatoform disorders. The UP enhances emotion regulation by providing psychoeducation, cognitive reappraisal strategies, emotional and interoceptive awareness training, modifying metacognitions, exposure to stress/trauma-related triggers, and affect tolerance interventions.

Mohajerin et al. (2020) used the UP to treat five participants diagnosed with DID in individual 60–90-minute sessions for six months. At treatment termination, none of the participants met full criteria for DID diagnosis, and results were maintained at six-month follow-up. Interventions such as the UP, which target variables theoretically germane to DID, hold promise in treating severe dissociative conditions. Efforts to promote sleep hygiene would be a valuable addition to the UP and other DID interventions, given that sleep disturbances (e.g., narcolepsy, sleep paralysis, nightmares), inadequate sleep, and daytime napping, for example, increase dissociative symptoms (Arora et al., 2020), whereas improvements in sleep hygiene and sleep quality decrease dissociative symptoms (Van Heugten et al., 2015).

Dialectical Behavioral Therapy

Comorbidity of BPD and DID, in the range of 31–83% (Foote & Van Orden, 2016; Korzekwa et al., 2009), may be a function of overlap in transdiagnostic symptoms such as emotion dysregulation, fluctuations in identity, and poor affect tolerance (Brand & Lanius, 2014). Foote and Van Orden (2016) adapted DBT, commonly used to treat BPD, to treat DID in an 18-month case study of a single participant that included weekly individual DBT, medication management, and participation in a weekly DBT group.

The researchers relied on three principles (Foote & Van Orden, 2016). The first involved stabilizing symptoms of behavioral dysregulation or dissociative behaviors that engender self-harm and interfere with treatment. The second principle utilized behavioral and solution analysis to target "identities" that are adjudged to harm or threaten the patient's life or interfere with treatment. The third principle was to not consider "switching" between "identities" as maladaptive unless it interferes with treatment or proves harmful. At six-year follow-up, no notable self-harm behaviors or suicide attempts were reported, and the patient was able to establish a "life-worth-living," defined as a life that includes love, meaning, and compassion for imperfections (Linehan, 2014) Clearly, more research is required to establish DBT as a worthwhile treatment for DD.

Schema Therapy

Unlike the ISSTD guidelines, which incorporate the idea of dissociated "identities," schema therapy normalizes and reframes these "identities" by labeling them as modes that are present in all humans to varying degrees (Young et al., 2003). Huntjens et al. (2019) educated 10 participants with DID on the functions of the modes as well as allied behaviors and states linked with these modes. Treatment consisted of 2 individual weekly sessions, followed by 40 individual weekly sessions. This study is ongoing and findings are not yet available; however, the laudable aim of the research is to establish a standardized, evidence-based treatment for DID.

Approaches for Youth

Research on science-based treatments for children and adolescents with DD is lacking (Nilsson et al., 2019). Assessment of dissociation in children is not done consistently, and dissociative symptoms may be mistaken for other psychopathology (e.g., schizophrenia, bipolar disorder, ADHD; Diseth & Christie, 2005). Accordingly, treatment of dissociation may be overlooked or require more time than is optimal due to misdiagnosis.

Early detection of dissociative symptoms and intervention are important in achieving a favorable response. Macfie et al. (2001) argue that maltreatment is a risk factor in developing dissociation, primarily during preschool. Accordingly, effective treatment should prioritize ending maltreatment and processing traumatic experiences (Macfie et al., 2001). Emotion dysregulation is also associated with severity of dissociation symptoms in preschool children (Hébert et al., 2020). Combining individual psychotherapy, pharmacotherapy, and family therapy is thought to be necessary to alleviate dissociation in children (Diseth & Christie, 2005). Diseth and Christie (2005) recommend that therapists create a strong alliance and demonstrate empathy and continuity toward the child's experiences with possible imaginary friends or self-states. Creating science-based therapies is imperative to fill a glaring gap in meeting the needs of children with dissociative conditions.

Other Variables Influencing Treatment

Assessment and Diagnosis

Some experts have claimed that DD are overdiagnosed and have gone so far as to argue that they are a "fad" (Paris, 2012). In contrast, other experts have, with equal ardor, contended that DD are underdiagnosed or misdiagnosed (Şar & Ross, 2006). Unfortunately, few clinicians report adequate training in diagnosing and treating DD, and some clinicians question the validity of DD (Brand et al., 2014, 2016; Leonard et al., 2005). On average, misdiagnosed DID patients spend 5 to 12.4 years receiving

Box 7.1 Recommendations for Research on Dissociative Conditions

We proffer six recommendations for research regarding dissociative conditions.

1. We recommend clinical trials include waitlist, placebo, and alternate treatment comparison conditions. We further recommend (a) assessment by trained experimenters and exploration of alternative explanations including regression to the mean, demand characteristics, and nonspecific factors (see Lilienfeld et al., 2014) and (b) the development of standardized/manualized treatment protocols, which can be valuable resources, yet not adhered to slavishly or mindlessly.

2. It can be particularly challenging to not reify "separate selves" while engaging with patients who steadfastly believe in their existence. When objective measures are employed, researchers have found no support for the actual separation of identities within a single person (see Lynn et al., 2022). DID appears to be a disorder of belief in which a person is convinced in the reality of separate indwelling selves. We recommend that therapists skillfully negotiate these beliefs while working with the patient to develop a narrative of a single integrated "self." Research on the UP (Mohajerin et al., 2020) and schema-based therapy (Huntjens et al., 2019) provide useful suggestions for how to accomplish this.

3. We recommend that therapists avoid the use of hypnosis or other suggestive techniques to recover memories, as such procedures risk ratifying the patient's belief in a fractured self. Hypnosis is contraindicated because (a) it is based on the mistaken idea that memory can be stored forever and later accessed in pristine form, and (b) hypnosis poses risks of false memory creation (Lynn et al., 2020). Fetkewicz et al. (2000) surveyed 20 individuals diagnosed with DID who reported suicidal ideation and a history of suicide attempts. Unfortunately, after memory recovery treatment, 60% of the patients reported suicide attempts, a number higher post-treatment than pretreatment. The researchers concluded that memory recovery treatment could be hazardous and detrimental, and we concur.

4. We recommend that researchers develop treatments (e.g., UP, DBT schema-based interventions) that target transdiagnostic variables and assess mechanisms (e.g., emotion regulation, metacognition, sleep disturbances) in studies with follow-ups at three months, preferably extending to a year or more.

5. We recommend that research be conducted on pharmacological interventions and whether they can be used effectively with different treatments versus on a stand-alone basis.

6. We recommend that researchers evaluate not only positive outcomes but also negative or harmful effects of psychotherapies among individuals with diverse socioeconomic backgrounds.

mental health treatment before being accurately diagnosed with DID (Spiegel et al., 2011). Assessing, isolating, and targeting dissociative symptoms is imperative, as dissociative symptoms persist and worsen absent effective assessment and treatment (Brand et al., 2014).

Comorbidity

Dissociative symptoms have received sparse attention and pose problems for psychotherapy researchers due to high rates of comorbidity, with many conditions including BPD, psychotic spectrum disorders, depression, anxiety, avoidant personality, substance abuse, and eating disorders. These disorders might overshadow or mask diagnosis of dissociative symptoms, eventuate in misdiagnosis and false-negatives (Şar & Ross, 2006), and relegate treatment and research to a low priority (Ellickson-Larew et al., 2020; Foote & Van Orden, 2016; Korzekwa et al., 2009). Jepsen et al. (2014) concluded that patients need dissociation-specific treatment to achieve positive results, although this assertion awaits systematic evaluation. Belli (2014) found that, among patients with OCD, dissociation correlated with severity of OCD symptoms, and patients who did not improve after treatment experienced high levels of dissociative symptoms. However, Hoeboer et al. (2020), in their meta-analytic review of 1,714 patients, found no evidence that dissociation mediated effectiveness of psychotherapy for PTSD.

Demographics

Ghosh et al. (2021) identified racial, socioeconomic, ethnic, and age group backgrounds as impacting DD, with women more affected than men. DSM-5-TR criteria do not adequately address unusual yet culturally relevant dissociative experiences such as possession. Dorahy et al. (2014) posit that cultural identity with a deity and other sociocultural factors impact and complicate research and treatment of DD. For example, religious practices impact mental disorders, including the expression of dissociation, possession experiences, and out-of-body phenomena (Dorahy et al., 2014). Anglin et al.'s (2015) research, which accounted for cultural variation among ethnic minority groups, revealed that dissociation mediates the association between traumatic life events and attenuated positive psychotic symptoms, particularly among Black participants. Similarly, Brand et al. (2006) reported that a high prevalence of DD was associated with unique cultural manifestations. In some cultures, recurrent recall gaps may be considered ordinary forgetting, and experiences of two or more distinct personality states may be regarded as possession. Brand et al. (2016) studied 48 institutions in 16 countries and reported that possession experiences and DD occurred at different rates, possibly depending on whether clinicians endorse common myths about dissociation (e.g., "DID is a fad"). For example, prevalence

Box 7.2 Access to Treatment

Even when patients are diagnosed correctly, they might encounter barriers to accessing treatment, such as high cost. Myrick, Webermann, Langeland, et al. (2017) compared the changes in inpatient and outpatient costs for individuals diagnosed with DID. The researchers found that (a) estimated costs are lower for patients who receive treatment, (b) treatments for dissociation typically take years to complete, and (c) treatments are often costly. In contrast, patients with DD in Norway can seek free care at a three-month inpatient treatment program; similar programs are nonexistent in the United States (Jepsen et al., 2014).

rates for DID were two to three times higher in the United States compared to Canada and European countries such as the Netherlands and Germany.

Medication

Psychopharmacology interventions are not very effective and therefore have been utilized as a second-line treatment for dissociation, particularly when psychotherapy alone does not produce relief (Bridley et al., 2022). Commonly prescribed medications include serotonin reuptake inhibitors and monoamine oxidase and tricyclic antidepressant inhibitors (Kolla et al., 2016). Monoamine oxidase inhibitors are somewhat effective and are primarily utilized to treat DD with co-occurring major depressive disorder symptoms (Kolla et al., 2016). Sutar and Sahu (2019) systematically reviewed 214 participants with DD who received psychopharmacological treatment and concluded that paroxetine and naloxone are the only agents that improve dissociation (e.g., depersonalization) symptoms in individuals with comorbid PTSD and BPD. However, the role of placebo effects has not been adequately evaluated in the treatment of dissociation. Additionally, Gentile et al. (2013) caution practitioners against using benzodiazepines in patients with DD to prevent exacerbating symptoms of dissociation. To our knowledge, no research exists regarding the efficacy of combining medication and psychotherapy for dissociation.

Conclusion

Individuals who suffer from dissociative conditions are in great need of science-based treatments that are currently minimally studied or nonexistent. Commendably, researchers are beginning to accord the treatment of dissociation the attention that it deserves. Still, science-based treatments are in their infancy: No intervention has been investigated systematically, and promising initial findings must be replicated in order to be regarded as robust and convincing. For example, no extant treatment meets the Tolin et al. (2015) criteria or David and Montgomery's (2011) criteria for well-supported and evidence-based psychosocial interventions, which include rigorous evaluation of hypothesized change mechanisms. Unfortunately, RCTs are virtually absent, controlled case studies are scant, and mechanistic studies are nonexistent. We hope that our chapter spurs researchers to undertake the necessary research to meet the needs of people with DD, and that they do so in a timely manner.

Useful Resources

- Bridley, A., Daffin, L. W., & Washington State University. (2022). *Fundamentals of psychological disorders (formerly abnormal psychology) 3rd edition (5-TR)* (3rd ed.). Press Books.
- Chien, W. T., & Fung, H. W. (2022). The challenges in diagnosis and treatment of dissociative disorders. *Alpha Psychiatry*, 23(2), 45–46. https://doi.org/10.5152/alphapsychiatry.2022.0001.
- Diseth, T. H., & Christie, H. J. (2005). Trauma-related dissociative (conversion) disorders in children and adolescents – An overview of assessment tools and treatment principles. *Nordic Journal of Psychiatry*, 59(4), 278–292.
- Kring, A. M., & Johnson, S. M. (2018). *Abnormal psychology: The science and treatment of psychological disorders* (14th ed.). John Wiley & Sons, Inc.
- Maxwell, R., Merckelbach, H., Lilienfeld, S. O., & Lynn, S. J. (2018). The treatment of dissociation: An evaluation of effectiveness and potential mechanisms In D. David, S. J. Lynn, & G. H. Montgomery (Eds.), *Evidence-based psychotherapy: The state of the science and practice* (pp. 329–361). Wiley Blackwell.
- Mohajerin, Lynn, S. J., Bakhtiyari, M., & Dolatshah, B. (2020). Evaluating the Unified Protocol in the treatment of dissociative identify disorder. *Cognitive and Behavioral Practice*, 27(3), 270–289.
- Pieper, S., Out, D., Bakermans-Kranenburg, M. J., & van Ijzendoorn, M. H. (2011). Behavioral and molecular genetics of dissociation: The role of the serotonin transporter gene promoter polymorphism (5-HTTLPR). *Journal of Traumatic Stress*, 24(4), 373–380.
- Şar, V., Dorahy, M., & Krüger, C. (2017). Revisiting the etiological aspects of dissociative identity disorder: A biopsychosocial perspective. *Psychology Research and Behavior Management, Volume* 10(10), 137–146. https://doi.org/10.2147/prbm.s113743
- Young, J. E., Klosko, J. S., & Weishaar, M. E. (2003). *Schema therapy: A practitioner's guide*. The Guilford Press.

References

Aksen, D. E., Polizzi, C., & Lynn, S. J. (2021). Correlates and mediators of dissociation: Towards a transtheoretical perspective. *Imagination, Cognition and Personality*, 40: 372–392. https://doi.org/10.1177/0276236620956284,

American Psychiatric Association. (2022). *Diagnostic and statistical manual of mental disorders: DSM-5-TR*. Washington, DC: American Psychiatric Association.

Anglin, D. M., Polanco-Roman, L., & Lui, F. (2015). Ethnic variation in whether dissociation mediates the relation between traumatic life events and attenuated positive psychotic symptoms. *Journal of Trauma & Dissociation*, 16(1), 68–85.

Arora, T., Alhelali, E., & Grey, I. (2020). Poor sleep efficiency and daytime napping are risk factors of depersonalization disorder in female university students. *Neurobiology of Sleep and Circadian Rhythms* 9:100059. https://doi.org/10.1016/j.nbscr.2020.100059.

Bækkelund, H., Ulvenes, P., Boon-Langelaan, S., & Arnevik, E. A. (2022). Group treatment for complex dissociative disorders: a randomized clinical trial. *BMC Psychiatry*, 22(1), 338–338. https://doi.org/10.1186/s12888-022-03970-8.

Belli, H. (2014). Dissociative symptoms and dissociative disorders comorbidity in obsessive compulsive disorder: Symptom screening, diagnostic tools and reflections on treatment. *World Journal of Clinical Cases: WJCC*, 2(8), 327–331.

Brand, B. L., & Lanius, R. A. (2014). Chronic complex dissociative disorders and borderline personality disorder: disorders of emotion dysregulation? *Borderline Personality Disorder and Emotion Dysregulation*, 1(1), 1–12. https://doi.org/10.1186/2051-6673-1-13.

Brand, B. L., Classen, C. C., McNary, S. W. & Zaveri, P. (2009). A review of dissociative disorders treatment studies. *The Journal of Nervous and Mental Disease*, 197 (9), 646–654. https://doi.org/10.1097/NMD.0b013e3181b3afaa.

Brand, B. L., Loewenstein, R. J., & Spiegel, D. (2014). Dispelling myths about dissociative identity disorder treatment: An empirically based approach. *Psychiatry*, 77(2), 169-89. https://doi.org/10.1521/psyc.2014.77.2.169

Brand, B. L., Myrick, A. C., Loewenstein, R. J., et al. (2012). A survey of practices and recommended treatment interventions among expert therapists treating patients with dissociative identity disorder and dissociative disorder not otherwise specified. *Psychological Trauma: Theory, Research, Practice, and Policy*, 4(5), 490–500. https://doi.org/10.1037/a0026487.

Brand, B. L., Sar, V., Stavropoulos, P., et al. (2016). Separating fact from fiction: An empirical examination of six myths about dissociative identity disorder. *Harvard Review of Psychiatry*, 24(4), 257–270. https://doi.org/10.1097/hrp.0000000000000100.

Brand, B. L., Schielke, H. J., Putnam, K. T., et al. (2019). An online educational program for individuals with dissociative disorders and their clinicians: 1-year and 2-year follow-up. *Journal of Traumatic Stress*, 32(1), 156–166. https://doi.org/10.1002/jts.22370.

Brand, B. L., Webermann, A. R., & Frankel, A. S. (2016). Assessment of complex dissociative disorder patients and simulated dissociation in forensic contexts. *International Journal of Law and Psychiatry*, 49, 197–204.

Bridley, A., Daffin, L. W., & Washington State University. (2022). *Fundamentals of psychological disorders (formerly abnormal psychology) 3rd edition (5-TR)* (3rd ed.). Washington State University.

Chalavi, S., Vissia, E. M., Giesen, M. E., et al. (2015). Abnormal hippocampal morphology in dissociative identity disorder and post-traumatic stress disorder correlates with childhood trauma and dissociative symptoms. *Human Brain Mapping*, 36(5), 1692–1704. https://doi.org/10.1002/hbm.22730.

Chien, W. T., & Fung, H. W. (2022). The challenges in diagnosis and treatment of dissociative disorders. *Alpha Psychiatry*, 23(2), 45–46. https://doi.org/10.5152/alphapsychiatry.2022.0001.

Chiu, C.-D., Chang, J.-H., & Hui, C. M. (2017). Self-concept integration and differentiation in subclinical individuals with dissociation proneness. *Self & Identity*, *16*: 664–683. https://doi.org/10.1080/15298868.2017.1296491.

Courtois, C. (1999). *Recollections of sexual abuse: Treatment principles and guidelines*. W. W. Norton & Co.

Cronin, E., Brand, B. L., & Mattanah, J. F. (2014). The impact of the therapeutic alliance on treatment outcome in patients with dissociative disorders. *European Journal of Psychotraumatology*, 5. https://doi.org/10.3402/ejpt.v5.22676.

Dalenberg, C. J., Brand, B. L., Gleaves, D. H., et al. (2012). Evaluation of the evidence for the trauma and fantasy models of dissociation. *Psychological Bulletin*, 138(3), 550–588. https://doi.org/10.1037/a0027447.

David, D., & Montgomery, G. H. (2011). The scientific status of psychotherapies: A new evaluative framework for evidence-based psychosocial interventions. *Clinical Psychology: Science and Practice*, 18(2), 89–99.

Delmonte, Lucchetti, G., Moreira-Almeida, A., & Farias, M. (2016). Can the DSM-5 differentiate between nonpathological possession and dissociative identity disorder? A case study from an Afro-Brazilian religion. *Journal of Trauma & Dissociation*, 17(3), 322–337. https://doi.org/10.1080/15299732.2015.1103351.

Diseth, T. H., & Christie, H. J. (2005). Trauma-related dissociative (conversion) disorders in children and adolescents–an overview of assessment tools and treatment principles. *Nordic Journal of Psychiatry*, 59(4), 278–292. https://doi.org/10.1080/08039480500213683.

Dorahy, M. J., Brand, B. L., Şar, V., et al. (2014). Dissociative identity disorder: An empirical overview. *Australian & New Zealand Journal of Psychiatry*, 48(5), 402–417. https://doi.org/10.1177/0004867414527523.

Ellickson-Larew, S., Stasik-O'Brien, S. M., Stanton, K., & Watson, D. (2020). Dissociation as a multidimensional transdiagnostic symptom. *Psychology of Consciousness.: Theory., Research, and Practice*, 7, 126–150. https://doi.org/10.1037/cns0000218.

Foote, B., & Van Orden, K. (2016). Adapting dialectical behavior therapy for the treatment of dissociative identity disorder. *American Journal of Psychotherapy*, 70(4), 343–364.

Gentile, J. P., Dillon, K. S., & Gillig, P. M. (2013). Psychotherapy and pharmacotherapy for patients with dissociative identity disorder. *Innovations in Clinical Neuroscience*, 10(2), 22.

Ghosh, D., Mukhopadhyay, P., Chatterjee, I., & Roy, P. K. (2021). Arousability, personality, and decision-making ability in dissociative disorder. *Indian Journal of Psychological Medicine*. https://doi.org/10.1177/0253717620981555.

Giesbrecht, T., Smeets, T., Leppink, J., Jelicic, M., & Merckelbach, H. (2013). Acute dissociation after 1 night of sleep loss. *Psychology of Consciousness: Theory, Research, and Practice*, 1(S), 150–159. https://doi.org/10.1037/2326-5523.1.S.150.

Gleaves, D. H. (1996). The sociocognitive model of dissociative identity disorder: A reexamination of the evidence. *Psychological Bulletin*, 120, 42–59 https://doi.org/10.1037/0033-2909.120.1.42.

Goldstein, L. H., Robinson, E. J., Mellers, J. D. C., et al. (2020). Cognitive behavioural therapy for adults with dissociative seizures (CODES): A pragmatic, multicentre, randomised controlled trial. *The Lancet Psychiatry*, 7(6), 491–505. https://doi.org/10.1016/s2215-0366(20)30128-0.

Hébert, Langevin, R., & Charest, F. (2020). Disorganized attachment and emotion dysregulation as mediators of the association between sexual abuse and dissociation in preschoolers. *Journal of Affective Disorders*, 267, 220–228. https://doi.org/10.1016/j.jad.2020.02.032.

Hoeboer, C. M., De Kleine, R. A., Molendijk, M. L., et al. (2020). Impact of dissociation on the effectiveness of psychotherapy for post-traumatic stress disorder: Meta-analysis. *BJPsych Open*, 6(3). https://doi.org/10.1192/bjo.2020.30.

Hunter, E. C. M. (2013). Understanding and treating depersonalization disorder. In F. Kennedy, H. Kennerley, & D. Pearson (Eds.), *Cognitive behavioural approaches to the understanding and treatment of dissociation*. Routledge.

Hunter, E. C. M., Baker, D., Phillips, M. L., Sierra, M., & David, A. S. (2005). Cognitive-behaviour therapy for depersonalization disorder: An open study. *Behaviour Research and Therapy*, 43, 1121–1130. https://doi.org/10.1016/j.brat.2004.08.003

Hunter, E. C. M., Phillips, M. L., Chalder, T., Sierra, M., & David, A. S. (2003). Depersonalisation disorder: A cognitive-behavioural conceptualisation. *Behaviour Research and Therapy*, 41, 1451–1467. https://doi.org/10.1016/S0005-7967(03)00066-4.

Huntjens, R. J. C., Rijkeboer, M. M., & Arntz, A. (2019). Schema therapy for Dissociative Identity Disorder (DID): Rationale and study protocol, *European Journal of Psychotraumatology*, 10(1), 1571377. https://doi.org/10.1080/20008198.2019.1571377.

Jepsen, E. K., Langeland, W., Sexton, H., & Heir, T. (2014). Inpatient treatment for early sexually abused adults: A naturalistic 12-month follow-up study. *Psychological Trauma: Theory, Research, Practice, and Policy*, 6(2), 142. https://doi.org/10.1037/a0031646.

Karadag F., Şar V., Tamar-Gurol D., et al. (2005) Dissociative disorders among inpatients with drug or alcohol dependency. *Journal of Clinical Psychiatry*, 66, 1247–1253.

Kikuchi, H., Fujii, T., Abe, N., et al. (2010). Memory repression: Brain mechanisms underlying dissociative amnesia. *Journal of Cognitive Neuroscience*, 22(3), 602–613. https://doi.org/10.1162/jocn.2009.21212.

Kolla, N. J., Chiuccariello, L., Wilson, A. A., et al. (2016). Elevated monoamine oxidase: A distribution volume in borderline personality disorder is associated with severity across mood symptoms, suicidality, and cognition. *Biological Psychiatry*, 79(2), 117–126. https://doi.org/10.1016/j.biopsych.2014.11.024.

Korzekwa, M. I. Dell, P. F., Links, P. S., Thabane, L., & Fougere, P. (2009). Dissociation in borderline personality disorder: A detailed look. *Journal of Trauma & Dissociation*, 10(3), 346–367. https://doi.org/10.1080/15299730902956838.

Kring, A. M., & Johnson, S. L. (2018). *Abnormal psychology: The science and treatment of psychological disorders*. John Wiley & Sons.

Krüger, C. (2019). Culture, trauma, and dissociation: A broadening perspective for our field. *Journal of Trauma & Dissociation*, 21(1), 1–13. https://doi.org/10.1080/15299732.2020.1675134.

Langeland, W., Jepsen, E. K., Brand, B. L., et al. (2020). The economic burden of dissociative disorders: A qualitative systematic review of empirical studies. *Psychological Trauma: Theory, Research, Practice, and Policy*, 12(7), 730. https://doi.org/10.1037/tra0000556.

Leonard, D., Brann, S., & Tiller, J. (2005). Dissociative disorders: Pathways to diagnosis, clinician attitudes and their impact. *Australian & New Zealand Journal of Psychiatry*, 39(10), 940–946. https://doi.org/10.1080/j.1440-1614.2005.01700.x.

Lilienfeld, S. O., & Lynn, S. J. (2003). Dissociative identity disorder: Multiple personalities, multiple controversies. In S. O. Lilienfeld, S. J. Lynn, & J. M. Lohr (Eds.), *Science and pseudoscience in clinical psychology* (pp. 109–142). Guilford Press

Lilienfeld, S. O., Ritschel, L. A., Lynn, S. J., Cautin, R. L., & Latzman, R. D. (2014). Why ineffective therapies work: A taxonomy of causes of spurious therapeutic effectiveness. *Perspectives on Psychological Science*, 9, 355–387. https://doi.org/10.1177/1745691614 535216.

Lilienfeld, S. O., Lynn, S. J., Kirsch, I., et al. (1999). Dissociative identity disorder and the sociocognitive model: Recalling the lessons of the past. *Psychological Bulletin*, 125(5), 507–523.

Lilienfeld, S. O., Ritschel, L. A., Lynn, S. J., Cautin, R. L., & Latzman, R. D. (2013). Why many clinical psychologists are resistant to evidence-based practice: Root causes and constructive remedies. *Clinical Psychology Review*, 33, 883–900. https://doi.org/10.1016/j.cpr.2012.09.008.

Linehan, M. (2014). *DBT skills training manual*. Guilford Publications.

Luckenbaugh, D. A., Niciu, M. J., Ionesc, D. F., et al. (2014). Do the dissociative side effects of ketamine mediate its antidepressant effects. *Journal of Affective Disorders* 159: 56–61 https://doi.org/10.1016/j.jad.2014.02.017.

Lynn, S. J., Kirsch, I., Terhune, D. B., & Green, J. P. (2020). Myths and misconceptions about hypnosis and suggestion: Separating fact and fiction. *Applied Cognitive Psychology*, 34(6), 1253–1264. https://doi.org/10.1002/acp.3730.

Lynn, S. J., Lilienfeld, S. O., Merckelbach, H., et al. (2014). The trauma model of dissociation: Inconvenient truths and stubborn fictions: Comment on Dalenberg et al. (2012). *Psychological Bulletin*, 140, 896–910. https://doi.org/10.1037/a0035570.

Lynn, S. J., Maxwell, R., Merckelbach, H., et al. (2019). Dissociation and its disorders: Competing models, future directions, and a way forward. *Clinical Psychology Review*, 73, 101755. https://doi.org/10.1016/j.cpr.2019.101755.

Lynn, S. J., Polizzi, C., Merckelbach, H., et al. (2022). Dissociation and dissociative disorders reconsidered: Beyond sociocognitive and trauma models toward a transtheoretical framework. *Annual Review of Clinical Psychology*, 18. https://doi.org/10.1146/annurev-clinpsy-081219-102424.

Lynn, S. J., Sleight, F., Polizzi, C., et al. (2023). Dissociation. In S. Hupp, & C. Santa Maria (Eds.). *Pseudoscience in psychotherapy: A skeptical field guide* (pp. 94–110). Cambridge University Press.

Macfie, J., Cicchetti, D., & Toth, S. L. (2001). The development of dissociation in maltreated preschool-aged children. *Development and Psychopathology*, 13(2), 233–254. https://doi .org/10.1017/S0954579401002036.

Macfie, J., Cicchetti, D., & Toth, S. L. (2001). The development of dissociation in maltreated preschool-aged children. *Development and Psychopathology*, 13(2), 233–254. https://doi.org/10.1017/s0954579401002036.

Martinez-Taboas, A., & Rodriguez-Cay, J. R. (1997). Case study of a Puerto Rican woman with dissociative identity disorder. *Dissociation*, 10, 141–147.

Maxwell, R., Merckelbach, H., Lilienfeld, S. O., & Lynn, S. J. (2018). The treatment of dissociation: An evaluation of effectiveness and potential mechanisms. *Evidence-Based Psychotherapy: The State of the Science and Practice*, 329–361.

Mohajerin, B., Lynn, S. J, Bakhtiyari, M., & Dolatshah, B. (2020). Evaluating the unified protocol in the treatment of dissociative identity disorder. *Cognitive and Behavioral Practice*, 27(3), 270–289. https://doi.org/10.1016/j.cbpra.2019.07.012.

Myrick, A. C., Webermann, A. R., Langeland, W., Putnam, F. W., & Brand, B. L. (2017). Treatment of dissociative disorders and reported changes in inpatient and outpatient cost estimates. *European Journal of Psychotraumatology*, 8(1), 1375829. https://doi.org/ 10.1080/20008198.2017.1375829.

Myrick, A. C., Webermann, A. R., Loewenstein, R. J., et al. (2017). Six-year follow-up of the treatment of patients with dissociative disorders study. *European Journal of Psychotraumatology*, 8(1), 1344080. https://doi.org/10.1080/20008198.2017.1344080.

Myrick, A. C., Webermann, A. R., Loewenstein, R. J., et al. (2017). Six-year follow-up of the treatment of patients with dissociative disorders study. *European Journal of Psychotraumatology*, 8(1), 1344080.

Nester, M. S. Brand, B. L., Schielke, H. J., & Kumar, S. (2022) An examination of the relations between emotion dysregulation, dissociation, and self-injury among dissociative disorder patients, *European Journal of Psychotraumatology*, 13(1). https://doi.org/10.1080/ 20008198.2022.2031592.

Nester, M. S., Boi, C., Brand, B. L., & Schielke, H. J. (2022). The reasons dissociative disorder patients self-injure. *European Journal of Psychotraumatology*, 13(1), 2026738 https://doi.org/ 10.1080/20008198.2022.2026738.

Nilsson, D., Green, S., Svedin, C. G., & Dahlström, Ö. (2019). Psychoform and somatoform dissociation among children and adolescents: An evaluation of a new short screening instrument for dissociation, DSQ-12. *European Journal of Trauma & Dissociation = Revue Europâeenne Du Trauma et de La Dissociation*, 3(4), 213–220. https://doi.org/ 10.1016/j.ejtd.2019.07.001.

Norton, P. J., & Paulus, D. J. (2016). Toward a unified treatment for emotional disorders: Update on the science and practice. *Behavior Therapy*, 47(6), 854–868. https://doi.org/ 10.1016/j.beth.2015.07.002.

Paris, J. (2012). The rise and fall of dissociative identity disorder. *The Journal of Nervous and Mental Disease*, 200(12), 1076–1079. https://10.1097/NMD.0b013e318275d285.

Polizzi, C. P., Aksen, D. E., & Lynn, S. J. (2022). Quality of life, emotion regulation, and dissociation: Evaluating unique relations in an undergraduate sample and probable PTSD subsample. *Psychological Trauma: Theory, Research, Practice, and Policy*, 14(1), 107–15.

Putnam, F. W. (1989). *Diagnosis and treatment of multiple personality disorder*. Guilford.

Reinders, A., Marquand, A., Schlumpf, Y., et al. (2019). Aiding the diagnosis of dissociative identity disorder: Pattern recognition study of brain biomarkers. *British Journal of Psychiatry*, 215(3), 536–544. https://doi.org/10.1192/bjp.2018.255.

Ross, C. A. (2007) Borderline personality disorder and dissociation, *Journal of Trauma & Dissociation*, 8(1), 71–80. https://doi.org/10.1300/J229v08n01_05.

Roydeva, M. I., & Reinders, A. A. T. (2021). Biomarkers of pathological dissociation: A systematic review. *Neuroscience and Biobehavioral Reviews*, 123, 120–202. https:// doi.org/10.1016/j.neubiorev.2020.11.019.

Sar, V., & Ross, C. (2006). Dissociative disorders as a confounding factor in psychiatric research. *Psychiatric Clinics*, 29(1), 129–144.

Şar, V., Akyuz, G., & Dogan O. (2007) Prevalence of dissociative disorders among women in the general population. *Psychiatry Research*, 149, 169–176 https://doi.org/ 10.1016/j.psychres.2006.01.005.

Sar, V., Dorahy, M., & Krüger, C. (2017). Revisiting the etiological aspects of dissociative identity disorder: A biopsychosocial perspective. *Psychology Research and Behavior Management*, 10(10), 137–146. https://doi.org/10.2147/prbm.s113743.

Selvi, Y., Kiliç, S., Aydin, A., & Güzel Özdemir, P. (2015). The effects of sleep deprivation on dissociation and profiles of mood, and its association with biochemical changes. *Noro psikiyatri arsivi*, 52(1), 83–88. https://doi.org/10.5152/npa.2015.7116.

Serrano-Sevillano, Á., González-Ordi, H., Corbí-Gran, B., & Vallejo-Pareja, M. Á. (2017). Psychological characteristics of dissociation in general population. *Clínica y Salud* 28(3): 101–106. https://doi.org/10.1016/j.clysa.2017.09.003.

Sharma, T., Sinha, V. K., & Sayeed, N. (2016). Role of mindfulness in dissociative disorders among adolescents. *Indian Journal of Psychiatry*, 58(3), 326–328. https://doi.org/10.4103/0019-5545.192013.

Sharma, T., Sinha, V. K., & Sayeed, N. (2016). Role of mindfulness in dissociative disorders among adolescents. *Indian Journal of Psychiatry*, 58(3), 326–328.

Spanos, N. P. (1994). Multiple identity enactments and multiple personality disorder: a sociocognitive perspective. *Psychological Bulletin*, 116(1), 143–165.

Spanos, N. P. (1996). Multiple identities & false memories: A sociocognitive perspective. *American Psychological Association*. https://doi.org/10.1037/10216-000.

Spiegel, D., Loewenstein, R. J., Lewis-Fernández, R., et al. (2011). Dissociative disorders in DSM-5. *Depression and Anxiety*, 28(9), 824–852. https://doi.org/10.1002/da.20874.

Spitzer, C., Klauer, T., Grabe, H.-J., et al. (2003). Gender differences in dissociation. *Psychopathology*, 36(2), 65–70. https://doi.org/10.1159/000070360.

Subramanyam, A. A., Somaiya, M., Shankar, S., et al. (2020). Psychological interventions for dissociative disorders. *Indian Journal of Psychiatry*, 62(Suppl 2), S280–S289. https://doi.org/10.4103/psychiatry.IndianJPsychiatry_777_19.

Sutar, R. & Sahu, S. (2019). Pharmacotherapy for dissociative disorders: A systematic review. *Psychiatry Research*, 281, 112529–112529. https://doi.org/10.1016/j.psychres.2019.112529.

Tolin, D. F., McKay, D., Forman, E. M., Klonsky, E. D., & Thombs, B. D. (2015). Empirically supported treatment: Recommendations for a new model. *Clinical Psychology: Science and Practice*, 22(4), 317–338.

van der Kloet, D., Merckelbach, H., Giesbrecht, T., Lynn, S. J. (2012). Fragmented sleep, fragmented mind: The role of sleep in dissociative symptoms. *Perspectives on Psychological Science*, 7, 159–175. https://doi.org/10.1177/1745691612437597.

van Heugten–van der Kloet, D., Giesbrecht, T., & Merckelbach, H. (2015). Sleep loss increases dissociation and affects memory for emotional stimuli. *Journal of Behavior Therapy and Experimental Psychiatry*, 47, 9–17. https://doi.org/10.1016/j.jbtep.2014.11.002.

van Minnen, A., & Tibben, M. (2021). A brief cognitive-behavioural treatment approach for PTSD and Dissociative Identity Disorder, a case report. *Journal of Behavior Therapy and Experimental Psychiatry*, 72, 101655. https://doi.org/10.1016/j.jbtep.2021.101655.

Vermetten, E., Schmahl, C., Lindner, S., Loewenstein, R. J., & Bremner, J. D. (2006). Hippocampal and amygdalar volumes in dissociative identity disorder. *American Journal of Psychiatry*, 163(4), 630–636. https://doi.org/10.1176/ajp.2006.163.4.630.

Young, J. E., Klosko, J. S., & Weishaar, M. E. (2003). *Schema therapy: A practitioner's guide*. The Guilford Press.

8

Pain

Laura Nelson Darling, Kristine Lee, and John Otis

Pain is defined as an unpleasant sensory and emotional experience associated with actual or potential tissue damage or described in terms of such damage (Classification of Chronic Pain; Merskey & Bogduk, 1994). The experience of pain is typically an adaptive reaction to injury and serves to limit movement and allow healing to occur. Often referred to as "acute" pain, this type of pain is associated with injuries such as a burn, sprained ankle, or broken bone, and resolves on its own following conservative treatment. Chronic pain differs due to persistence, sometimes lasting years, without a continued underlying physical cause. When pain persists for more than three months in duration it is considered "chronic" (Merskey & Bogduk, 1994).

Chronic pain is one of the most common reasons people seek health care in the United States. In fact, a survey by the Centers for Disease Control and Prevention indicated that about 21% of adults reported having "pain most days or every day" for the past six months (Rikard et al., 2023). Chronic pain can have a devastating impact on all aspects of a person's life; thus, there are high rates of comorbidity with emotional disorders (Kroenke et al., 2013; Staerkle et al., 2004).

Given the high prevalence, costs, and distress associated with the experience of chronic pain, efforts to develop evidence-based psychological approaches to help patients learn more effective pain coping strategies have expanded in the last decade. This chapter will provide a review of the theoretical models that have contributed to our understanding of psychological approaches to chronic pain management. The chapter describes two evidence-based treatments for pain – cognitive-behavioral therapy (CBT) and Acceptance and Commitment Therapy (ACT) – and presents data supporting their use. The chapter then turns to describing individual components in each treatment approach that have been found to be essential. Since pain can occur across the lifespan, the chapter also addresses pain in children.

Box 8.1 Somatic Symptom Disorder

Individuals with chronic pain may present in ways that are consistent with the diagnostic criteria associated with Somatic Symptom and Related Disorders, with predominant pain. For example, consider the case of a person who experiences pain secondary to an injury that requires rest and rehabilitation or medical intervention for healing to occur. Once the injury has been medically addressed, the person may still experience painful sensations. In these situations, the person may intensely focus on the sensations of pain, and may even be hypervigilant to noticing sensations that would have previously been ignored. These sensations may trigger worry that pain is indication of underlying pathology or that some type of damage is being done. As a result, the person may seek medical interventions or pharmaceuticals to reduce pain, alter their gait, or limit their involvement in work or other activities that they believe have the potential to increase pain. In this example, given the excessive thoughts, feelings, and behaviors related to pain, and the disruption to daily life, clinicians might consider a diagnosis of Somatic Symptom Disorder, with predominant pain from the *Diagnostic and Statistical Manual of Mental Disorders, 5th Edition-Text Revision* (DSM-5-TR; American Psychological Association, 2022).

Etiology and Theoretical Underpinnings of Treatment

The onset of chronic pain may be associated with a number of different health issues, including medical illness or injury, changes in the body associated with aging, or neurological conditions. Chronic pain can be experienced in many different ways: from neuropathic pain that may be described as "burning" or "shooting" sensations; to somatic, meaning activation of pain receptors on the surface of the body or musculo-skeletal tissues; or visceral, referring to the activation of pain receptors located in internal organ systems. Individuals who experience chronic pain may seek medical consultation with the goal of determining the underlying cause of the pain sensation and advice on treatment. While early theoretical conceptualizations of pain centered exclusively on biological or pathophysiological processes, we now understand that pain is a complex experience that is influenced not only by the presence of underlying pathology, but also by an individual's thoughts, emotions, and behaviors. In the past, psychology was only involved in patient care when medical interventions failed to obtain a desired patient outcome; however, given our evolving understanding of pain, providers are increasingly involving psychology early in the treatment process.

Vlaeyen and Linton (2000) proposed a Cognitive-Behavioral Fear–Avoidance Model of chronic pain to explain the role of fear and avoidance in the transition from acute to chronic pain. In this model, a person might interpret the experience of pain as overly threatening (a process called "catastrophizing"), leading them to fear the experience of pain and avoid activities that they believe might potentially cause pain. "Guarding" behaviors may follow, such as tensing or bracing muscles to prepare for movement, using caution while walking, or otherwise altering posture in preparation for pain. Heightened alert to the mistaken belief that any pain is a sign of damage or yet-to-be-identified pathology may cause the individual to become hypervigilant to sensations, and may cause the amplification of low-intensity painful sensations. As the fear and avoidance of physical activity grows, the world in which the individual functions becomes more restricted. Avoidance of physical activity also limits opportunities to test and correct pain expectations. Decreased engagement in pleasurable and reinforcing activities may lead to depression. On the other hand, in the absence of serious somatic pathology, an individual who interprets pain as nonthreatening, and who engages in adaptive problem-solving instead of catastrophizing, is more likely to have a speedier recovery. Since the introduction of this model, studies have shown that fear and avoidance of movement is an even better predictor of disability than underlying biomedical pathology (Crombez et al., 1999). This model has served as the basis of research and clinical practice for decades and has helped in our formulation of treatments designed to help patients adaptively cope with the experience of chronic pain. As our understanding of the factors that may contribute to the etiology and maintenance of pain disorders has advanced, so has our repertoire of empirically supported strategies that are available to help patients cope more effectively.

Brief Overview of Treatments

Empirically supported psychological approaches to chronic pain management primarily target improvements in physical, emotional, social, and occupational functioning, rather than eliminating the pain itself. A number of studies have demonstrated that both CBT and ACT may result in improvements in various pain-relevant outcomes for patients with a variety of pain disorders; however, when evaluating the evidence supporting the use of a treatment it is important to consider the quality of the evidence (i.e., presence of high-quality meta-analytic reviews) and contextual factors (i.e., treatment effects are observed across several patient populations) when determining an overall treatment recommendation (Tolin et al., 2015).

CBT interventions for chronic pain utilize psychological principles to help introduce flexibility in ways of thinking, modify negative thoughts and behaviors that serve to maintain and exacerbate the experience of pain, and teach patients ways of safely reintroducing enjoyable activities into their lives. A substantial literature documents the efficacy of CBT for a variety of chronic pain conditions, including osteoarthritis, chronic back and neck pain (Linton & Ryberg, 2001), diabetic neuropathic pain (Otis et al., 2013), and tension headache (Holroyd et al., 2001). The evidence-base of CBT for pain management also includes a number of meta-analytic studies (Morley et al., 1999; Williams et al., 2020; Parrish et al., 2021). In a meta-analysis of 22 randomized controlled trials of psychological treatments for chronic low-back pain, cognitive-behavioral and self-regulatory treatments specifically were found to be efficacious (Hoffman et al., 2007). Further, the positive effects of CBT were noted in a recent meta-analysis examining pain in children and adolescents (Palermo et al., 2010).

When utilized within the context of managing chronic pain, ACT aims to limit the control that pain has on a person's life by teaching them to accept and live with pain, and to set goals that are consistent with their values (Roditi & Robinson, 2011). Although there is support for the use of ACT as a comparable alternative to CBT, the literature supporting ACT as an effective treatment for pain disorders is mixed. A meta-analysis examining ACT in patients with chronic pain demonstrated favorable outcomes, revealing small to medium effect sizes across pain intensity, mood and affect, physical well-being, and quality of life (Veehof et al., 2011), and a follow-up meta-analysis found small effects at posttreatment across domains of pain intensity, depression, and disability (Veehof et al., 2016). However, the Cochrane review of chronic non-cancer pain judged ACT trials to be of very low quality and determined that its benefits are uncertain (Williams et al., 2020). Thus, while the use of ACT for pain is promising, additional high-quality, disorder-specific randomized controlled trials are needed.

Credible Components of Treatments

Both CBT and ACT are composed of a number of skills that are designed to help a patient cope more effectively with their chronic pain. What follows is a description of some of the "essential elements" of treatment for both approaches.

Behavioral Goals

Patients with chronic pain often report that the experience of pain has significantly interfered with their ability to engage in daily functioning and social activities that they once found enjoyable. Patients may also avoid activities in an effort to control or reduce the potential for pain (e.g., not taking a walk for fear that it will cause an increase in pain); however, this strategy has actually been shown to increase sensitivity to and chronicity of pain symptoms (Philips, 1987). In order to address these issues, it's important for clinicians to collaborate with their patient to create a set of overall behavioral goals for therapy with the goal of decreasing the patient's avoidance of activity and reintroducing a healthy and more active lifestyle. Some patients may choose goals that involve physical functioning, such as walking, playing sports, or going to the gym; however, goals may also include activities that are far less physically demanding, such as computer work, reaching out to friends, and socializing. In situations where a patient can identify an activity that they once found enjoyable but they are no longer able to perform because of pain or other health issues (e.g., spinal instability), therapists will need to work with the patient to modify the goals so that they are realistic and consistent with their interests and abilities.

Exposure

Exposures for individuals with pain disorders may include activities such as engaging in movements believed to be painful for an individual with chronic back pain, wearing clothing items associated with pain in an individual with fibromyalgia, or eating foods that trigger pain symptoms in an individual with irritable bowel syndrome. Promisingly, research has found exposures to be an effective method for reducing pain-related fear and disability (for review, see Vlaeyen & Crombez, 2020). Relative to treatments that implement graded activity, exposure-based treatments have been shown to be equally effective at reducing pain and disability (e.g., for chronic low-back pain; Macedo et al., 2010) and possibly even more effective in the short-term (Lopez-de-Uralde-Villanueva et al., 2016). However, unlike graded activity, exposures have been shown to reduce pain-related anxiety and cognitions, such as fear-avoidance beliefs (Woods & Asmundson, 2008), pain catastrophizing (Leeuw et al., 2008), and perceived harmfulness of activities (Leeuw et al., 2008). Thus, exposures may confer additional therapeutic benefits beyond other behavioral approaches.

Activity Pacing

When engaging in activities, it is important that patients learn to balance being active with resting in order to accomplish daily activities without overdoing it and experiencing increased pain. Activity pacing is a coping strategy that aims to adjust physical activity to manageable and time-limited increments to reduce pain and fatigue associated with overexertion. Activity pacing addresses the negative impact of both underactivity (i.e., avoidance) and overactivity cycling – a maladaptive pattern of behavior in pain disorders sometimes termed *boom–bust cycling* (Antcliff et al., 2018). In activity pacing, the duration and/or intensity of activity can be gradually increased as individuals learn to manage physiological and psychological symptoms. Researchers have implemented different methods of activity pacing for pain disorders, including daily schedules alternating activity and rest, and pacing based on time- or goal-contingencies (the operant approach; Nielson et al., 2013). The latter approach teaches individuals to initiate rest periods after they reach a predetermined time-period (e.g., five minutes of activity) or quota (e.g., folding five shirts), rather than resting only after they experience an increase in pain symptoms. Although further research is needed to evaluate the relative effectiveness of different activity pacing approaches, initial studies suggest there may be slight advantages to the operant approach with certain pain disorders (Racine et al., 2019). Activity pacing is a key treatment component used by physical therapists when treating patients with chronic pain (Beissner et al., 2009), and is a common treatment component in CBT for pain disorders; however, it is also compatible with ACT when applied through the lens of acceptance, flexibility, and value-engagement. Specifically, activity pacing (and behavioral interventions more generally) is consistent with ACT principles when aimed toward engaging in meaningful activities and setting meaningful goals (Antcliff et al., 2018).

Cognitive Skills Training

Cognitive skills training is a core component of CBT for pain and aims to intervene in attentional biases and maladaptive cognitions that exacerbate the pain experience. Research shows that individuals with pain disorders may exhibit excessively fearful and catastrophic cognitions regarding anticipated or current pain (Burns et al., 2012; Sullivan et al., 2001). Catastrophizing is a cognitive distortion defined by excessively negative predictions or attributions – in other words, "thinking the worst." This cognitive style is associated with the magnification of pain sensations and is considered an important target of pain disorder treatment (Quartana et al., 2009). Cognitive change (e.g., altering catastrophic pain-related cognitions) is a therapeutic mechanism specific to CBT. Randomized controlled trials have demonstrated that CBT interventions produce significant changes in individuals' cognitive coping and appraisal skills (Morley, 1999). Accordingly, research has shown that CBT interventions that shift an individual's pain-related cognitions are linked to significantly improved outcomes (Burns, Glenn, et al., 2003; Burns, Kubilus, et al., 2003). Research has shown that reduction in pain catastrophizing following treatment is significantly associated with improved outcomes, irrespective of the treatment condition (Burns et al., 2012). This suggests that changes in pain-related cognitions may be an important mediator of treatment outcome.

Acceptance

Acceptance is a process that involves a willingness to experience pain rather than escape it. Acceptance methods promote the engagement of goal-oriented action toward unwanted experiences (e.g., pain, emotions, thoughts). The objective within ACT is to improve functioning and decrease interference of pain, using acceptance as a mediator for change (Cederberg et al., 2016). While control-oriented treatments, such as CBT, generally do not emphasize acceptance as a treatment component, efforts have been made to identify treatment mediators that could be used to improve CBT treatment outcomes. Multiple studies suggest that greater acceptance of chronic pain is associated with better psychological, physical, and social functioning (e.g., McCracken & Vowles, 2007; Vowles et al., 2007). Acceptance also appears to be a key process involved in treatment gains (Vowles et al., 2007), reduces the adverse impact of pain flares on emotional functioning (Kratz et al., 2007), and is predictive of future functioning (McCracken & Eccleston, 2005). Research on the effectiveness of ACT has demonstrated significant medium-to-large effect sizes for measures of pain acceptance (Hughes et al., 2017). Åkerblom and colleagues (2015) reported findings that highlight the role of pain-related acceptance as important to the treatment process even if it is not explicitly targeted during treatment. Based on their mediator analyses, pain-related acceptance significantly partially mediated changes in outcome measures during a CBT-based treatment program, even when other potential CBT process variables were taken into account. Previous research has examined potential process variables in CBT approaches for chronic pain (i.e., pain beliefs, perceived control over pain, coping); however, analyses indicated that changes in pain-related acceptance, which is not considered a target of traditional CBT, play an important role (Åkerblom et al., 2015). Thus, incorporating acceptance of pain as an additional treatment mechanism may enhance CBT-based treatments to improve individuals' functioning and outcomes.

Relaxation

Relaxation training is often included in interventions for pain disorders. The aim of relaxation training is to intervene on physiological factors such as increased muscle tension that may contribute to pain. Strategies include techniques such as diaphragmatic breathing, progressive muscle relaxation (PMR), visual imagery, biofeedback, or a combination thereof. A review of relaxation techniques for acute and chronic pain found some evidence for reductions in pain outcomes (Dunford & Thompson, 2010). Although research suggests that relaxation training may not confer as many lasting benefits compared to CBT (Turner, 1982), practicing relaxation and taking time to "slow the mind" and notice thoughts may facilitate the practice and development of cognitive skills (Burns et al., 2015). Further, recent research investigating the mechanisms of change in CBT for chronic pain found that change in the use of relaxation techniques was associated with changes in disability and depression, as was the use of cognitive techniques (Feldmann et al., 2021). Taken together, these findings suggest that relaxation strategies may not be adequate for producing lasting benefits on their own, but may be an impactful component of treatment packages that include other evidence-based strategies.

Mindfulness

Mindfulness practices have become widely used as self-management techniques for various long-term conditions, including chronic pain. Based on ancient eastern and Buddhist philosophy, mindfulness involves attentional control toward the present moment with acceptance, curiosity, and nonjudgment (Bishop et al., 2004; Hilton et al., 2017). For people with chronic pain, inflexible attention and lack of awareness of the present moment can lead to increased rumination and magnification of pain (Schütze et al., 2010). Mindfulness practices facilitate refocusing the mind to increase awareness of external and internal sensations, allowing individuals to self-regulate attention and reframe experiences. Research has demonstrated that mindfulness practices appear to be beneficial treatment components to management of chronic pain and are predictive of patient functioning (Kabat-Zinn et al., 1985; Sephton et al., 2007). Moreover, research suggests that the use of mindfulness approaches is associated with greater success in engaging in values-related behavior related to less distress and disability (McCracken & Yang, 2006). Mindfulness is a core component of ACT. In the context of chronic pain, awareness of physical sensations, feelings, and thoughts is needed to give rise to acceptance (Hayes et al., 2006). When attention is focused on the opportunities of the present rather than ruminating about the past or catastrophizing about the future, behavior can be directed toward realizing valued goals instead of pain control (McCracken & Vowles, 2014). While mindfulness has not been an explicit treatment component of CBT, it has been increasingly incorporated in recent years through the creation of diverse approaches such as mindfulness-based cognitive therapy (MBCT; Segal et al., 2018), MBCT for chronic pain (Day, 2017), and mindfulness-based stress reduction therapy (MBSR; Kabat-Zinn, 2003). Across these interventions, the primary focus is to remain in the present and increase awareness of emotional and physical suffering (Pardos-Gascon et al., 2021).

Psychological Flexibility

Unifying several of the processes described herein, researchers have proposed that values-based action, mindfulness, acceptance, and cognitive defusion (a strategy that involves creating space between oneself and one's thoughts and feelings) collectively comprise *psychological flexibility* (Vowles & McCracken, 2010). Psychological flexibility has been defined as the capacity to persist or to change behavior, including conscious and open contact with discomfort and other discouraging experiences, guided by goals and values (Hayes et al., 1999). Others have described this ability as "one of the foremost goals of human existence" (Kashdan & Rottenberg, 2010, p. 866). Psychological flexibility has been proposed as a model for the treatment of chronic pain ("The Psychological Flexibility Model"; McCracken & Morley, 2014) and as a mechanism of change in ACT for chronic pain (Scott & McCracken, 2015). Research suggests that psychological flexibility is both a resilience factor in chronic pain, buffering the impact of symptoms on functioning and depression (Gentili et al., 2019), and an important treatment target. Research from McCracken and Vowles (2007) found that psychological flexibility accounted for significant variance in measures of adaptive functioning among patients with chronic pain. By contrast, traditional pain management strategies, such as pacing, relaxation, and positive self-statements, did not account for significant variance on those same measures. Similarly, this research team found that treatment-related change in psychological flexibility was significantly related to improvement in several outcome measures, including pain, physical disability, psychosocial disability, and medical visits (McCracken, 2024). Taken together, these findings suggest that psychological flexibility is a key target of treatments for pain disorders and supports the effectiveness of its component parts: values-guided action, mindfulness, and acceptance.

Approaches for Youth

Psychological treatments for youth with pain disorders generally mirror those for adult populations. Thus, treatments commonly follow behavioral and cognitive-behavioral approaches, and may include exposure, acceptance, coping skills training, relaxation training, and biofeedback. Reflecting the adult literature, psychological interventions for pain disorders in youth show significant positive effects on key outcomes (e.g., pain, disability, depression), though the size of the effect and the outcomes impacted depend on the study, disorder, and treatment approach. Other research has evaluated the effects of distinct treatment approaches on youth with chronic pain. A meta-analysis of psychological treatments for children and adolescents with chronic pain (including headaches, abdominal pain, and fibromyalgia) found that CBT, relaxation therapy, and biofeedback all yielded significant positive effects on pain reduction; however, results revealed small, nonsignificant effects of treatment on disability and emotional functioning, which were included as outcomes in a subset of studies (Palermo et al., 2010). Generally, these findings reflect prior systematic reviews showing that psychological treatments – primarily brief behavioral and cognitive-behavioral interventions – resulted in significant reductions in pain symptoms in youth with chronic headaches (e.g., Eccleston et al., 2002). Promisingly, self-administered, computer-based applications (i.e., CD-ROM, internet) and face-to-face treatments were found to be similarly effective at reducing pain (Palermo et al., 2010), suggesting room for flexibility in treatment formats.

Other Variables Influencing Treatment

Assessment and Diagnosis

Prior to considering an approach for treatment, it is important to conduct a pain assessment in order to gather information about the patient's experience of pain. This will help the therapist to determine the treatment elements that will likely be of greatest benefit to the patient. For example, understanding the factors associated with the onset of the patient's pain (e.g., motor vehicle accident, assault, degenerative changes) and the anticipated chronicity of the painful condition will impact the focus of therapy.

It is also important to learn about strategies the patient has already undertaken to manage their pain. Assessment includes asking about what seems to make the pain increase and what tends to reduce it. Assessing for beliefs and expectations, coping strategies, and other cognitive processes helps to provide a full picture of an individual's strengths and vulnerabilities. The patient is the "expert" on their pain, and it is the therapist's job to find out what the patient already knows so that treatment can build upon those existing skills.

Comorbidity

Individuals with chronic pain often experience mental health problems such as anxiety, depression, posttraumatic stress, or substance use disorders. In chronic pain samples, depression prevalence rates range from 30–54% (Banks & Kerns, 1996; Elliott et al., 2003). Rates of anxiety are reported to be as high as 45% in pain populations (Kroenke et al., 2013; Staerkle et al., 2004). Comorbidity with emotional disorders can complicate the delivery of many aspects of therapy, including behavioral activities, activity engagement, cognitive training, and eliciting motivation to participate (Kerns & Haythornthwaite, 1988). Substance use may also be a way to cope with pain or its comorbidities. Substance use often interferes with the acquisition of psychotherapeutic skills, thus in cases where a substance use disorder is present, treatment of the substance use disorder should take precedence over engagement in psychological approaches for pain management.

Demographics

Research supports that there are racial and ethnic differences in the ways that people experience pain, and that race and ethnicity may also lead to differences in pain treatment preferences. In addition, there are also racial and ethnic disparities in the ways that pain treatments are provided. For example, studies indicate that people of color are more likely to have their pain underestimated by providers, are less likely to receive opioids as part of their pain management regimen, and receive less aggressive pain treatment than do White patients (Meints et al., 2019). While many studies exist documenting the benefits of psychological approaches to pain management for children and adults, fewer studies have involved older adults. A recent meta-analysis involving 22 studies with 2,208 participants with a mean age of 71.9 years concluded that psychological therapies have a small but statistically significant benefit for reducing pain and catastrophizing beliefs and improving self-efficacy for managing pain in older adults (Niknejad et al., 2018). Overall, studies support that individuals of all ages can benefit from learning strategies for managing their pain.

Medication

Pain medications can be helpful in many circumstances, including reducing pain intensity for individuals with acute pain, facilitating patient participation in rehabilitation efforts, and allowing patients with chronic pain to gain greater quality of life. The use of pain medication is not an exclusion criterion for participation in psychological treatment for pain. However, there are situations in which the use of pain medications is not desirable. For example, some patients may experience negative side effects from pain medication, such as constipation or dizziness. There may also be situations in which a patient with a history of substance use disorder will feel that the use of any pain medication may place them at risk for relapse. When working with a patient who is taking pain medications, therapists can talk openly about the ways that psychological therapies can provide them with more "tools" in their arsenal for managing pain, and that therapy can be used as an alternate to medication or in conjunction with pharmacological approaches to allow prescribed pain medications to work more effectively (Jamison & Mao, 2015).

Conclusion

Chronic pain is a highly prevalent condition that can have tremendous negative impacts on multiple domains in life, causing patients and their families significant distress and causing interference in daily functioning. Fortunately, several psychological approaches have now been developed that have garnered large evidence bases over the past few decades. CBT- and ACT-based approaches to treat chronic pain are comprised of some distinct and some overlapping skills aimed at helping patients gain greater capability in managing their pain. Importantly, therapists should tailor their treatments to individual patients with flexibility, rather than being wed to one particular protocol. Skills such as relaxation and mindfulness, cognitive skills, activity pacing, acceptance, behavioral activation, and exposure can all be used interchangeably depending on the needs of the patient. With a thorough assessment of the variables maintaining pain, and by considering comorbidities and other demographic variables that might influence treatment outcome, clinicians can thoughtfully and sensitively design a treatment plan that will yield the most positive outcomes.

Useful Resources

- Dahl, J., Lundgren, T., & Hayes, S. C. (2006). *Living beyond your pain: Using acceptance and commitment therapy to ease chronic pain*. New Harbinger Publications.
- Otis, J. D. (2007). *Managing chronic pain: A cognitive-behavioral therapy approach, therapist guide*. Treatments that Work Series. Oxford University Press.
- Thorn, B. (2017). *Cognitive therapy for chronic pain, second edition: A step-by-step guide*. The Guilford Press.

References

Åkerblom, S., Perrin, S., Rivano Fischer, M., & McCracken, L. M. (2015). The mediating role of acceptance in multidisciplinary cognitive-behavioral therapy for chronic pain. *The Journal of Pain*, 16(7), 606–615. https://doi.org/10.1016/j.jpain.2015.03.007.

American Psychological Association. (2022). *Diagnostic and statistical manual of mental disorders, 5th edition-text revision.* American Psychiatric Publications Inc.

Antcliff, D., Keeley, P., Campbell, M., et al. (2018). Activity pacing: Moving beyond taking breaks and slowing down. *Quality of Life Research*, 27(7), 1933–1935.

Bahar N., Bolier, R., Henderson C. R., et al. (2018). Association between psychological interventions and chronic pain outcomes in older adults: A systematic review and meta-analysis. *JAMA Internal Medicine*, 178(6), 830–839. https://doi.org/jamainternmed.2018.0756.

Banks, S. M., & Kerns, R. D. (1996). Explaining high rates of depression in chronic pain: A diathesis–stress framework. *Psychological Bulletin*, 119(1), 95–110.

Beissner, K., Henderson Jr, C. R., Papaleontiou, M., et al. (2009). Physical therapists' use of cognitive–behavioral therapy for older adults with chronic pain: A nationwide survey. *Physical Therapy*, 89(5), 456–469.

Bishop, S. R., Lau, M., Shapiro, S., et al. (2004). Mindfulness: A proposed operational definition. *Clinical Psychology: Science and Practice*, 11(3), 230.

Burns, J. W., Day, M. A., & Thorn, B. E. (2012). Is reduction in pain catastrophizing a therapeutic mechanism specific to cognitive-behavioral therapy for chronic pain? *Translational Behavioral Medicine*, 2(1), 22–29.

Burns, J. W., Glenn, B., Bruehl, S., Harden, R. N., & Lofland, K. (2003). Cognitive factors influence outcome following multidisciplinary chronic pain treatment: A replication and extension of a cross-lagged panel analysis. *Behaviour Research and Therapy*, 41(10), 1163–1182.

Burns, J. W., Kubilus, A., Bruehl, S., Harden, R. N., & Lofland, K. (2003). Do changes in cognitive factors influence outcome following multidisciplinary treatment for chronic pain? A cross-lagged panel analysis. *Journal of Consulting and Clinical Psychology*, 71(1), 81.

Burns, J. W., Nielson, W. R., Jensen, M. P., et al. (2015). Does change occur for the reasons we think it does? A test of specific therapeutic operations during cognitive-behavioral treatment of chronic pain. *The Clinical Journal of Pain*, 31(7), 603–611.

Cederberg, J. T., Cernvall, M., Dahl, J., von Essen, L., & Ljungman, G. (2016). Acceptance as a mediator for change in acceptance and commitment therapy for persons with chronic pain? *International Journal of Behavioral Medicine*, 23(1), 21–29. https://doi.org/10.1007/s12529-015-9494-y.

Crombez, G., Vlaeyen, J. W., Heuts, P. H., & Lysens, R. (1999). Pain–related fear is more disabling than pain itself: evidence on the role of pain–related fear in chronic back pain disability. *Pain*, 80(1–2), 329–339.

Day, M. A. (2017). *Mindfulness-based cognitive therapy for chronic pain: A clinical manual and guide.* Wiley-Blackwell.

Deary, V., Chalder, T., & Sharpe, M. (2007). The cognitive behavioural model of medically unexplained symptoms: A theoretical and empirical review. *Clinical Psychology Review*, 27(7), 781–797.

den Hollander, M., Goossens, M., de Jong, J., et al. (2016). Expose or protect? A randomized controlled trial of exposure in vivo vs pain-contingent treatment as usual in patients with complex regional pain syndrome type 1. *Pain*, 157(10), 2318–2329.

Du, S., Dong, J., Jin, S., Zhang, H., & Zhang, Y. (2021). Acceptance and Commitment Therapy for chronic pain on functioning: A systematic review of randomized controlled trials. *Neuroscience & Biobehavioral Reviews*, 131, 59–76.

Dunford, E., & Thompson, M. (2010). Relaxation and mindfulness in pain: A review. *Reviews in Pain*, 4(1), 18–22.

Eccleston, C., Morley, S., Williams, A., Yorke, L., & Mastroyannopoulou, K. (2002). Systematic review of randomised controlled trials of psychological therapy for chronic pain in children and adolescents, with a subset meta-analysis of pain relief. *Pain*, 99(1–2), 157–165.

Elliott, T. E., Renier, C. M. & Palcher, J. A. (2003). Chronic pain, depression, and quality of life: correlations and predictive value of the SF–36. *Pain Medicine* 4(4), 331–339.

Feldmann, M., Hein, H. J., Voderholzer, U., et al. (2021). Cognitive change and relaxation as key mechanisms of treatment outcome in chronic pain: Evidence from routine care. *Frontiers in Psychiatry*, 12, 617871. https://doi.org/10.3389/fpsyt.2021.617871.

Gatchel, R. J. (2004). Comorbidity of chronic pain and mental health disorders: The biopsychosocial perspective. *American Psychologist*, 59(8), 795–805.

Gatchel, R. J., & Howard, K. (2008). The biopsychosocial approach. *Practical Pain Management*, 8(4), 98–104.

Gatchel, R. J., & Maddrey, A. M. (2004). The biopsychosocial perspective of pain. In J. Raczynski and L. Leviton (Eds.). *Healthcare Psychology Handbook*. Vol II (pp. 357–378). American Psychological Association Press.

Geneen, L. J., Moore, R. A., Clarke, C., et al. (2017). Physical activity and exercise for chronic pain in adults: An overview of Cochrane Reviews. *The Cochrane Database of Systematic Reviews*, 4(4), CD011279. https://doi.org/10.1002/14651858.CD011279.pub3.

Gentili, C., Rickardsson, J., Zetterqvist, V., et al. (2019). Psychological flexibility as a resilience factor in individuals with chronic pain. *Frontiers in Psychology*, 10, 2016. https://doi.org/10.3389/fpsyg.2019.02016.

Hann, K. E., & McCracken, L. M. (2014). A systematic review of randomized controlled trials of Acceptance and Commitment Therapy for adults with chronic pain: Outcome domains, design quality, and efficacy. *Journal of Contextual Behavioral Science*, 3(4), 217–227.

Harris, R. (2009). *ACT made simple: A quick-start guide to ACT basics and beyond*. New Harbinger.

Hayes, S. C., Luoma, J. B., Bond, F. W., Masuda, A., & Lillis, J. (2006). Acceptance and commitment therapy: Model, processes and outcomes. *Behaviour Research and Therapy*, 44(1), 1–25. https://doi.org/10.1016/j.brat.2005.06.006

Hayes, S. C., Strosahl, K. D., & Wilson, K. G. (1999). *Acceptance and commitment therapy: An experiential approach to behavior change*. Guilford Press.

Hedman-Lagerlöf, M., Hedman-Lagerlöf, E., Axelsson, E., et al. (2018). Internet-delivered exposure therapy for fibromyalgia. *The Clinical Journal of Pain*, 34(6), 532–542.

Hilton, L., Hempel, S., Ewing, B. A., et al. (2017). Mindfulness meditation for chronic pain: Systematic review and meta-analysis. *Annals of Behavioral Medicine*, 51(2), 199–213.

Hoffman, B. M., Papas, R. K., Chatkoff, D. K., & Kerns, R. D. (2007). Meta-analysis of psychological interventions for chronic low back pain. *Health Psychology*, 26(1), 1–9.

Holroyd, K. A., O'Donnell, F. J., Stensland, M., et al. (2001). Management of chronic tension-type headache with tricyclic antidepressant medication, stress-management therapy, and their combination: A randomized controlled trial. *JAMA*, 285, 2208–2215.

Hughes, L. S., Clark, J., Colclough, J. A., Dale, E., & McMillan, D. (2017). Acceptance and commitment therapy (ACT) for chronic pain. *The Clinical Journal of Pain*, 33(6), 552–568.

Jamison, R. N., & Mao, J. (2015). Opioid Analgesics. *Mayo Clinic Proceedings*, 90(7), 957–968. https://doi.org/10.1016/j.mayocp.2015.04.010.

Kabat-Zinn, J. (2003). Mindfulness-based stress reduction (MBSR). *Constructivism in the Human Sciences*, 8(2), 73–107.

Kabat-Zinn, J., Lipworth, L., & Burney, R. (1985). The clinical use of mindfulness meditation for the self-regulation of chronic pain. *Journal of Behavioral Medicine*, 8(2), 163–190. https://doi.org/10.1007/BF00845519.

Kashdan, T. B., & Rottenberg, J. (2010). Psychological flexibility as a fundamental aspect of health. *Clinical Psychology Review*, 30(7), 865–878.

Kerns, R. D., & Haythornthwaite, J. A. (1988). Depression among chronic pain patients: cognitive–behavioral analysis and effect on rehabilitation outcome. *Journal of Consulting and Clinical Psychology*, 56(6), 870–876.

Kratz, A. L., Davis, M. C., & Zautra, A. J. (2007). Pain acceptance moderates the relation between pain and negative affect in female osteoarthritis and fibromyalgia patients. *Annals of Behavioral Medicine*, 33(3), 291–301.

Kroenke, K., Outcalt, S., Krebs, E., et al. (2013). Association between anxiety, health-related quality of life and functional impairment in primary care patients with chronic pain. *General Hospital Psychiatry*, 35(4), 359–365.

Leeuw, M., Goossens, M. E., van Breukelen, G. J., et al. (2008). Exposure in vivo versus operant graded activity in chronic low back pain patients: Results of a randomized controlled trial. *Pain*, 138(1), 192–207.

Linton, S. J., & Ryberg, M. (2001). A cognitive-behavioral group intervention as prevention for persistent neck and back pain in a non-patient population: A randomized controlled trial. *Pain*, 90, 83–90.

Ljótsson, B., Hesser, H., Andersson, E., et al. (2014). Provoking symptoms to relieve symptoms: A randomized controlled dismantling study of exposure therapy in irritable bowel syndrome. *Behaviour Research and Therapy*, 55, 27–39.

López-de-Uralde-Villanueva, I., Munoz-Garcia, D., Gil-Martinez, A., et al. (2016). A systematic review and meta-analysis on the effectiveness of graded activity and graded exposure for chronic nonspecific low back pain. *Pain Medicine*, 17(1), 172–188.

Macedo, L. G., Smeets, R. J., Maher, C. G., Latimer, J., & McAuley, J. H. (2010). Graded activity and graded exposure for persistent nonspecific low back pain: A systematic review. *Physical Therapy*, 90(6), 860–879.

McCracken, L. M. (2024). Psychological flexibility, chronic pain, and health. *Annual Review of Psychology*, 75, 601–624.

McCracken, L. M., & Eccleston, C. (2005). A prospective study of acceptance of pain and patient functioning with chronic pain. *Pain*, 118(1–2), 164–169.

McCracken, L. M., & Morley, S. (2014). The psychological flexibility model: A basis for integration and progress in psychological approaches to chronic pain management. *The Journal of Pain*, 15(3), 221–234.

McCracken, L. M., & Vowles, K. E. (2007). Psychological flexibility and traditional pain management strategies in relation to patient functioning with chronic pain: An examination of a revised instrument. *The Journal of Pain*, 8(9), 700–707.

McCracken, L. M., & Vowles, K. E. (2014). Acceptance and commitment therapy and mindfulness for chronic pain: model, process, and progress. *American Psychologist*, 69(2), 178–187.

McCracken, L. M., & Yang, S.-Y. (2006). The role of values in a contextual cognitive-behavioral approach to chronic pain. *Pain*, 123(1–2), 137–145. https://doi.org/10.1016/j.pain.2006.02.021.

Meints S. M., Cortes, A., Morais, C. A., Edwards, R. R. (2019). Racial and ethnic differences in the experience and treatment of noncancer pain. *Pain Manag.* 9(3), 317–334. https://doi.org/10.2217/pmt-2018-0030. Epub 2019 May 29. PMID: 31140916; PMCID: PMC6587104.

Merskey H., Bogduk N. (1994). *Classification of chronic pain.* 2nd ed. IASP Press

Morley, S., Eccleston, C., & Williams, A. (1999). Systematic review and meta-analysis of randomized controlled trials of cognitive behaviour therapy and behaviour therapy for chronic pain in adults, excluding headache. *Pain*, 80(1–2), 1–13.

Nielson, W. R., Jensen, M. P., Karsdorp, P. A., & Vlaeyen, J. W. (2013). Activity pacing in chronic pain: Concepts, evidence, and future directions. *The Clinical Journal of Pain*, 29(5), 461–468.

Otis, J. D., Sanderson, K., Hardway, C., et al. (2013). A randomized controlled pilot study of a cognitive behavioral therapy approach for painful diabetic peripheral neuropathy. *Journal of Pain*, 14(5), 475–482.

Palermo, T. M., Eccleston, C., Lewandowski, A. S., Williams, A. C. D. C., & Morley, S. (2010). Randomized controlled trials of psychological therapies for management of chronic pain in children and adolescents: An updated meta-analytic review. *Pain*, 148(3), 387–397.

Pardos-Gascón, E. M., Narambuena, L., Leal-Costa, C., & van-der Hofstadt-Román, C. J. (2021). Differential efficacy between cognitive-behavioral therapy and mindfulness-based therapies for chronic pain: Systematic review. *International Journal of Clinical and Health Psychology*, 21(1), 100197. https://doi.org/10.1016/j.ijchp.2020.08.001.

Parrish, J. M., Jenkins, N. W., Parrish, M. S., et al. (2021) The influence of cognitive behavioral therapy on lumbar spine surgery outcomes: A systematic review and meta-analysis. *European Spine Journal*, 30, 1365–1379.

Philips, H. C. (1987). Avoidance behaviour and its role in sustaining chronic pain. *Behaviour Research and Therapy*, 25(4), 273–279.

Quartana, P. J., Campbell, C. M., & Edwards, R. R. (2009). Pain catastrophizing: A critical review. *Expert Review of Neurotherapeutics*, 9(5), 745–758.

Racine, M., Jensen, M. P., Harth, M., Morley-Forster, P., & Nielson, W. R. (2019). Operant learning versus energy conservation activity pacing treatments in a sample of patients with fibromyalgia syndrome: A pilot randomized controlled trial. *The Journal of Pain*, 20(4), 420–439.

Rikard, S. M., Strahan, A. E., Schmit, K. M., & Guy, G. P. (2023). Chronic pain among adults: United States, 2019–2021. www.cdc.gov/mmwr/volumes/72/wr/mm7215a1.htm#:~: text=health%20status%20characteristics.-,During%202021%2C%20an%20estimated% 2020.9%25%20of%20U.S.%20adults%20(51.6,experienced%20high%2Dimpact% 20chronic%20pain.

Roditi, D., & Robinson, M. E. (2011). The role of psychological interventions in the management of patients with chronic pain. *Psychology Research and Behavior Management*, 4, 41–49.

Schütze, R., Rees, C., Preece, M., & Schütze, M. (2010). Low mindfulness predicts pain catastrophizing in a fear-avoidance model of chronic pain. *Pain*, 148(1), 120–127.

Scott, W., & McCracken, L. M. (2015). Psychological flexibility, acceptance and commitment therapy, and chronic pain. *Current Opinion in Psychology*, 2, 91–96.

Segal, Z., Williams, M., & Teasdale, J. (2018). *Mindfulness-based cognitive therapy for depression*. Guilford Publications.

Sephton, S. E., Salmon, P., Weissbecker, I., et al. (2007). Mindfulness meditation alleviates depressive symptoms in women with fibromyalgia: Results of a randomized clinical trial. *Arthritis and Rheumatism*, 57(1), 77–85. https://doi.org/10.1002/art.22478.

St Sauver, J. L., Warner, D. O., Yawn, B. P., et al. (2013). Why patients visit their doctors: Assessing the most prevalent conditions in a defined American population. *Mayo Clinical Proceedings*, 88, 56–67.

Staerkle, R., Mannion, A. F., Elfering, A., et al. (2004). Longitudinal validation of the fear-avoidance beliefs questionnaire (FABQ) in a Swiss-German sample of low back pain patients. *European Spine Journal*, 13(4), 332–340.

Sullivan, M. J., Thorn, B., Haythornthwaite, J. A., et al. (2001). Theoretical perspectives on the relation between catastrophizing and pain. *The Clinical Journal of Pain*, 17(1), 52–64.

Tolin, D. F., McKay, D., Forman, E. M., Klonsky, E. D., & Thombs, B. D. (2015). Empirically supported treatment: Recommendations for a new model. *Clinical Psychology: Science and Practice*, 22(4), 317–338. https://doi.org/10.1111/cpsp.12122.

Turner, J. A. (1982). Comparison of group progressive-relaxation training and cognitive-behavioral group therapy for chronic low back pain. *Journal of Consulting and Clinical Psychology*, 50(5), 757.

Urits, I., Hubble, A., Peterson, E., et al. (2019). An update on cognitive therapy for the management of chronic pain: A comprehensive review. *Current Pain and Headache Reports*, 23(8), 1–7.

Veehof, M. M., Oskam, M. J., Schreurs, K. M., & Bohlmeijer, E. T. (2011). Acceptance–based interventions for the treatment of chronic pain: A systematic review and meta-analysis. *Pain*, 152(3), 533–542.

Veehof, M. M., Trompetter, H. R., Bohlmeijer, E. T., & Schreurs, K. (2016). Acceptance–and mindfulness–based interventions for the treatment of chronic pain: A meta–analytic review. *Cognitive Behaviour Therapy*, 45(1), 5–31

Vlaeyen, J. W., & Crombez, G. (2020). Behavioral conceptualization and treatment of chronic pain. *Annual Review of Clinical Psychology*, 16, 187–212.

Vlaeyen, J. W., & Linton, S. J. (2000). Fear–avoidance and its consequences in chronic musculoskeletal pain: A state of the art. *Pain*, 85(3), 317–332.

Vowles, K. E., & McCracken, L. M. (2008). Acceptance and values-based action in chronic pain: A study of treatment effectiveness and process. *Journal of Consulting and Clinical Psychology*, 76(3), 397–407.

Vowles, K. E., & McCracken, L. M. (2010). Comparing the role of psychological flexibility and traditional pain management coping strategies in chronic pain treatment outcomes. *Behaviour Research and Therapy*, 48(2), 141–146.

Vowles, K. E., McNeil, D. W., Gross, R. T., et al. (2007). Effects of pain acceptance and pain control strategies on physical impairment in individuals with chronic low back pain. *Behavior Therapy*, 38(4), 412–425.

Vowles, K. E., Sowden, G., Hickman, J., & Ashworth, J. (2019). An analysis of within-treatment change trajectories in valued activity in relation to treatment outcomes following interdisciplinary Acceptance and Commitment Therapy for adults with chronic pain. *Behaviour Research and Therapy*, 115, 46–54.

Williams, A. C., Eccleston, C., & Morley, S. (2012). Psychological therapies for the management of chronic pain (excluding headache) in adults. *The Cochrane Database of Systematic Reviews*, 11(11), CD007407. https://doi.org/10.1002/14651858.CD007407.pub3.

Williams, A. C., Fisher, E., Hearn, L., & Eccleston, C. (2020). Psychological therapies for the management of chronic pain (excluding headache) in adults. *Cochrane Database of Systematic Reviews*, 8(8). CD007407. https://doi.org/10.1002/14651858.CD007407.pub4.

Woods, M. P., & Asmundson, G. J. (2008). Evaluating the efficacy of graded in vivo exposure for the treatment of fear in patients with chronic back pain: A randomized controlled clinical trial. *Pain*, 136(3), 271–280.

9

Eating Disorders

Jamie M. Loor, Jennifer A. Battles, Brooke L. Bennett,
Danae L. Hudson, and Brooke L. Whisenhunt

Eating disorders are characterized by a variety of symptoms, including disruption in normative eating behaviors, body-image disturbance, and/or maladaptive attempts to control weight and shape. The *Diagnostic and Statistical Manual of Mental Disorders, 5th Edition, Text Revision* (DSM–5-TR; American Psychiatric Association, 2022) includes four primary eating disorders most common in adults: anorexia nervosa (AN), bulimia nervosa (BN), binge eating disorder (BED), and other specified feeding and eating disorder (OSFED). The lifetime prevalence of eating disorders is high, with approximately 1 in 5 females and 1 in 7 males meeting criteria for an eating disorder by age 40 (Ward et al., 2019). The most common age for developing an eating disorder is 21 years old, with 95% of first-time cases occurring by age 25 (Ward et al., 2019). Although most eating disorders consist of a single episode, a significant subset of individuals will have recurrent episodes throughout adulthood (22% of male patients and 29% of female patients; Ward et al., 2019). Additionally, eating disorders are associated with a high level of impairment and reduced quality of life (van Hoeken & Hoek, 2020), underscoring the importance of science-based treatments for eating disorder pathology.

AN is characterized by restriction of caloric intake resulting in significant weight loss. Intense fear of weight gain is present and interferes with the individual's ability to sufficiently increase caloric intake in order to gain weight. Other key features of AN include an overvaluation of weight and shape, a disturbance in the perception of weight and shape, and persistent lack of recognition of the ramifications of pursuing and achieving a low-weight status. Both BN and BED are marked by repeated binge eating episodes in which an objectively large amount of food is eaten within a relatively short period of time (i.e., two hours or less), accompanied by a sense of loss of control over eating. During binge eating episodes, the individual may feel uncomfortably full, eat rapidly, or eat in the absence of hunger. Eating may occur in isolation due to embarrassment or guilt, and a feeling of disgust with oneself often follows the binge episode. The distinguishing factor between BN and BED is that in BN the individual attempts to "compensate" for the binge eating through behaviors such as self-induced vomiting, fasting, excessive exercise, or misusing medications such as laxatives, diuretics, or diet pills. In contrast, individuals with BED do not typically engage in compensatory behaviors following a binge episode. Although overvaluation of weight and shape is required for BN and not BED, research suggests that individuals with BED who also experience overvaluation of weight and shape have poorer treatment outcomes and more severe symptoms than do those who do not overvalue weight and shape (Grilo et al., 2013). The DSM-5-TR also includes an OSFED category. This category was designed to capture distressing and impairing eating disturbances that do not fit the other specific diagnostic categories. For example, OSFED can include individuals at or above a normal weight who otherwise meet criteria for AN, individuals experiencing subthreshold BN in terms of the frequency of binge eating and compensatory behaviors, individuals engaging in purging without binge eating, and individuals who experience night eating.

Etiology and Theoretical Underpinnings of Treatment

The Transdiagnostic Theory of Eating Disorders, first posed by Fairburn and col-leagues (2003) in the context of Enhanced Cognitive Behavioral Therapy (CBT-E), suggests that the processes maintaining each eating disorder are largely the same across disorders. As a result, there is considerable overlap in symptom presentation and targets for interventions. For example, a fundamental characteristic of both AN and BN is the overvaluation and disturbed perception of weight and shape (APA, 2022), a feature which must be addressed in treatment regardless of the specific diagnosis or type of treatment implemented. Additionally, binge eating among those with BN and BED is often triggered by negative mood and is maintained by temporary relief from undesired mood; therefore, binge eating can be targeted in treatment with similar approaches across these diagnoses. The transdiagnostic approach, as asserted by the most recent version of CBT-E, suggests that the symptom overlap, shared characteristics, and diagnostic fluidity across eating disorders makes emphasis on the specific diagnosis (i.e., AN versus BN) unnecessary in a treatment setting (Fairburn et al., 2003; Fairburn et al., 2008). A network analysis provided additional support for this approach in that symptoms related to overeating, food avoidance, fullness, and overvaluation of weight and shape were stable across ages for all eating disorders (Christian et al., 2020).

In addition to the specific eating and body image symptoms, more distal factors such as interpersonal difficulties are common among patients with eating disorders (Murphy et al., 2012). These experiences often interact with eating disorder and body image symptoms and contribute to the development or perpetuation of disordered eating. Research findings are unclear on directionality, but the data has consistently demonstrated that individuals with eating disorders endorse less social support than others (Grisset & Norvell, 1992; Raykos et al., 2014; Tiller et al., 1997). One proposed pathway suggests that the nature of eating disorders (i.e., eating disorders thrive in secrecy and often are associated with low self-esteem) contributes to social isolation and therefore less social support over time. Alternatively, it has been proposed that because the average age of onset is so young (Fairburn et al., 2007), individuals may not have sufficient time to develop appropriate interpersonal relationships prior to their illness. Social support has been identified as an important factor in treating eating disorders as it is associated with both illness severity (Leonidas & dos Santos, 2014) and recovery trajectory (Goodrick et al., 1999). Additionally, social support has been highlighted as a key factor in maintaining change following treatment (Linville et al., 2012), underscoring its importance as a treatment target.

Interpersonal difficulties can also contribute to the perpetuation of eating disorders in multiple ways. For example, struggling to develop and maintain intimate and social relationships can worsen self-esteem, which can in turn increase an individual's efforts to change their eating behaviors, shape, or weight in order to regain feelings of control (Fairburn et al., 2003). Additionally, several specific maladaptive eating behaviors have been associated with difficult social situations. For example, episodes of binge eating increase following the experience of interpersonal stressors (Goldschmidt et al., 2014), and dietary restraint increases along with daily and life event stress (Woods et al., 2010).

Brief Overview of Treatments

Currently, there are three primary evidence-based treatments for eating disorders in adults: cognitive-behavioral therapy (CBT), interpersonal psychotherapy (IPT), and family-based treatment (FBT). Outpatient CBT for eating disorders typically takes place over the course of 6 months and includes approximately 20 sessions with the patient (Fairburn, 2008; Waller et al., 2007). Early stages of treatment focus heavily on behavioral change to achieve weight restoration or weight stabilization. Focus is placed on establishing regular eating and reducing other maladaptive weight control behaviors such as over-exercising or purging. Regular components of treatment include meal planning, in-session weighing, self-monitoring, and psychoeducation. After weight has stabilized and disordered eating behaviors have decreased, the therapist and the patient review progress and focus on more complex patient-specific treatment goals. These objectives are often identified during the joint formulation at the beginning of treatment and are informed by the transdiagnostic theory by identifying the factors that maintain a patient's overvaluation of weight and shape, such as low self-esteem, perfectionism, difficulties with interpersonal functioning, and/or poor mood-regulation strategies (Fairburn et al., 2003). Finally, relapse prevention and treatment termination are discussed.

There is *strong* research support for CBT as an effective treatment for both BN (Division 12 of the American Psychological Association, 2016a) and BED (Division

12 of the American Psychological Association, 2016b; Hilbert et al., 2019). A recent literature review and meta-analysis found that CBT was more efficacious than other psychotherapies for individuals with BN and BED (Linardon et al., 2017). This meta-analysis involving CBT strengthens the approaches' evidence base to be more consistent with the Tolin criteria (Tolin et al., 2015). Linardon and colleagues (2017) found greater improvements with CBT compared to IPT for behavioral (e.g., bingeing and/or purging episodes) and cognitive (e.g., concern about weight, shape, or eating) symptoms at posttreatment, and for cognitive symptoms longitudinally. Additionally, CBT was found to be more effective in decreasing behavioral symptoms in BED than was behavioral weight loss (Linardon et al., 2017). However, a subsequent meta-analysis found IPT to produce the highest abstinence rates (Linardon, 2018). In addition, the results of this meta-analysis indicated that race or ethnicity was not associated with the cessation of binge eating, thus suggesting BED has good effects with underrepresented groups, another important aspect of the Tolin criteria (Cougle & Grubaugh, 2022; Tolin et al., 2015).

The research support for AN is less consistent. Currently, the research support for CBT for AN is classified as *modest* for post-hospitalization relapse prevention but *controversial* for acute weight gain (Division 12 of the American Psychological Association, 2016c). Instead, a recent literature review suggests enhanced cognitive-behavioral therapy (CBT-E) may be promising for individuals with AN. More specifically, Atwood and Friedman (2020) found that CBT-E was efficacious and effective at reducing eating disorder behaviors across all diagnostic categories and for increasing BMI in individuals with AN. However, there was not strong evidence to establish superiority of CBT-E over comparison treatments, particularly in the long-term (Atwood & Friedman, 2020). Overall, additional research is needed, ideally studies that address the Tolin criteria, to clarify the effectiveness for specific eating disorders and improve the overall efficacy of CBT for eating disorders.

Family-based treatment (FBT) is another treatment option for eating disorders. FBT for AN and BN has considerable research support confirming its efficacy for treating adolescents (Lock, 2011; Lock, 2015). However, recent studies have examined the possibility of adapting FBT for use with young adults (FBTY) and have found some support (Chen et al., 2016). For FBT with young adults, there is more flexibility in choosing a nonparent support figure to be in charge of refeeding (i.e., in order to achieve weight restoration, set amounts of foods are fed at scheduled times during the day), and developmentally appropriate levels of independence are considered. In both FBT and FBTY, the focus is on weight restoration, which is achieved through parental empowerment. A nonblaming stance and an intentional separation of the illness from the patient are both hallmarks of FBT (Lock & Le Grange, 2015). Typically, outpatient treatment lasts for 20 sessions and consists of three phases. In phase 1, parents are put in charge of weight restoration. In phase 2, the patient gradually takes over control of their eating, and phase 3 focuses on fostering autonomy. Currently, FBT for AN is considered to have *strong* research support (Division 12 of the American Psychological Association, 2016f) while FBT for BN is considered to have *modest* research support (Division 12 of the American Psychological Association, 2016g). However, the majority of the research support is for traditional FBT designed for adolescents. Initial research examining its efficacy in young adults has shown promise (Chen et al., 2016), though more research is needed.

Interpersonal Psychotherapy (IPT) is a treatment that does not focus on the symptoms of the ED, but instead on interpersonal difficulties in a patient's life as it is thought that these difficulties contribute to the onset and maintenance of the eating disorder (Wilson et al., 2010). IPT was originally created for patients with depression, with a focus on four domains: role disputes, role transitions, interpersonal deficits, and unresolved grief. Instead of a focus on disorder-specific symptoms, the focus of IPT is on the interpersonal context and is hypothesized to promote positive changes by increasing social support, reducing interpersonal stress, promoting emotional processing, and enhancing interpersonal skills (Lipsitz & Markowitz, 2013). Outpatient IPT typically lasts 20 weeks, can be administered in an individual or group format, and consists of three primary phases. In phase 1, the patient and therapist work together to identify which interpersonal problems should be the focus of treatment. In phase 2, the emphasis is on the patient taking the lead in facilitating interpersonal change. Phase 3 is focused on maintenance of improvements and relapse prevention. Currently, there is *strong* research support for the efficacy of IPT for BN (Division 12 of the American Psychological Association, 2016d) and BED (Division 12 of the American Psychological Association, 2016e). While CBT produced greater initial changes, a literature review found that IPT led to improvements occurring later and maintained over time for patients with BN (Miniati et al., 2018). Additionally, research has shown that group IPT for BED is effective in reducing binge episodes posttreatment and longitudinally (Miniati et al., 2018).

Credible Components of Treatments

Psychoeducational Strategies

Psychoeducation is utilized across CBT-E, FBT, and IPT as a tool to (1) explain the etiology of the condition and provide a rationale for the treatment approach, and (2) build motivation. In both CBT-E and FBT, patients and/or families are educated on the causes of eating disorders and the severity of ED symptoms (Dalle Grave et al., 2019; Fairburn, 2008). For CBT-E, this information is used to collaboratively create an individualized case formulation of the patient's eating disorder symptoms (Fairburn 2008). This formulation emphasizes the role of overvaluation of weight and shape in the maintenance of problematic eating behaviors (e.g., restriction, bingeing). This formulation may also incorporate the influence of individuals' mood and adverse life events in the maintenance cycle of eating disorders. It is key that patients understand their individualized case formulations (Bailey-Straebler et al., 2022). Patients are encouraged to see their eating disorder as something they can control, and case formulations are used to show patients how they can gain control over the course of treatment.

For FBT, initial psychoeducation on the eating disorder presentation serves as a reminder of the seriousness of the eating disorder and is used as a call for action with the parents of the patient (Dalle Grave et al., 2019). Emphasis is placed on seeing the eating disorder as separate from the patient. The patient is seen as not in control of their eating disorder. This approach contrasts with CBT's approach to psychoeduca-tion, and it allows parents to work on treating the eating disorder rather than the patient while helping reduce blame on the parents or the patient. Parents are encour-aged to take control of the patient's eating during the initial stages of treatment until healthy eating patterns can be established.

IPT diverges from FBT and CBT-E by emphasizing current interpersonal problems that maintain eating disorder symptoms rather than discussing the onset of the eating disorder (Murphy et al., 2012). Research on interpersonal models for eating disorders has found that interpersonal problems and low self-esteem are associated with eating pathology (Ivanova et al., 2015; Lampard et al., 2011; Raykos et al., 2017). Therefore, initial psychoeducation focuses on how interpersonal problems can exacerbate eating disorder symptoms such as bingeing or restriction. Patients are informed that adverse interpersonal events can lead to worsened self-esteem, which contributes to eating disorder symptoms over time. Consequently, resolving interpersonal problems rather than the eating disorder symptoms is the focus of IPT. Patients receive information about common interpersonal problems that lead to eating disorder symptoms such as grief, interpersonal role disputes, role transitions, interpersonal deficits, and life goals.

Nutritional/Dietary Strategies

Nutritional/dietary strategies comprise a key domain of most effective psychothera-pies for eating disorders, with some dietitians advocating for even more focus on malnutrition and dietary care within treatment manuals (Jeffrey & Heruc, 2020). Because IPT indirectly targets eating behavior, dietary strategies are not utilized in treatment. In contrast, both CBT-E and FBT utilize dietary strategies early in treat-ment with the goal of weight stabilization and reinforcement of regular eating (Dalle Grave et al., 2019). In CBT-E, patients begin monitoring their eating behavior within the first few treatment sessions (Fairburn, 2008). Self-monitoring of eating is seen as an essential component of CBT-E (Bailey-Straebler et al., 2022) and one of the primary mechanisms of change in reducing binge eating frequency because it increases awareness of eating behavior patterns and provides data that helps therapists

Box 9.1 Body Checking and Body Avoidance

For many patients, body checking and body avoidance play a major role in the maintenance of disordered eating (Nikodijevic et al., 2018). Body checking behaviors include activities such as frequent weighing, looking in the mirror, or feeling and pinching areas of the body. Regardless of the information gained from these behaviors (e.g., lost or gained weight), individuals with eating disorders interpret information in a way that strengthens their overreliance on weight and shape as primary determinants of their mood and self-esteem. For example, if weight has increased, they may feel guilty and anxious and make plans to further restrict their eating, and if weight has decreased, they may become more determined to engage in more restriction and body check more frequently. Body avoidance can include not looking in mirrors, wearing only baggy clothing, and avoiding being weighed. These behaviors also maintain disordered eating by enhancing anxiety and fear associated with body weight and shape.

work effectively with patients to establish regular eating schedules (Sivyer et al., 2020). Patients monitor their daily food intake (i.e., amount eaten and when; however, patients do not monitor caloric intake) and frequency of binges or purges. Each eating event is monitored in the context of time of day and thoughts and feelings associated with eating (Fairburn, 2008). Therapists often work with patients to establish a regular schedule of eating (e.g., three meals a day with two snacks) with the goal of disrupting previously held dietary rules.

In FBT, parents have the primary control of changing their adolescent's eating patterns. It is largely up to the parents how and when adolescents eat, and the therapist serves as a consultant as needed (Kosmerly et al., 2015). Weight restoration is the first goal established in FBT, and parents are encouraged to use whatever means they find helpful to change the adolescent's eating. While parents can choose to record their adolescent's eating behavior, it is not required. Once weight has been restored, adolescents regain control over their eating patterns.

Behavioral Strategies

Behavioral strategies form a fundamental component of effective eating disorder treatments. While numerous behavioral techniques are used, there are three core strategies: exposure therapy, social support and in-session weighing.

Exposure Therapy

Exposure interventions have been demonstrated to be an effective component of eating disorder treatments and have been linked to decreased body dissatisfaction, decreased food-related anxiety, and increased BMI in those with AN (Butler & Heimberg, 2020). Exposures may encompass a variety of formats and targets depending on a patient's presentation. For example, body-image-focused exposures can incorporate mirrors or videos where individuals view themselves and confront negative thoughts, emotions, and body sensations that arise (Griffen et al., 2018). These exposures support more realistic body size perceptions, improve body image, and reduce body checking and avoidance (Butler & Heimberg, 2020; Griffen et al., 2018). These improvements are important as seeing one's body in a more flexible way instead of avoiding disliked areas is tied to better treatment outcome (Pellizzer et al., 2018). Food exposures involve highly feared or avoided foods and/or eating situations. Studies from across the fields of anxiety and eating disorders have demonstrated that individuals must experience exposure to feared situations while reducing their use of safety behaviors to maximize the effectiveness of exposure therapy (Butler & Heimberg, 2020; Reilly et al., 2021). Therefore, therapists help patients to eat feared foods while limiting the use of safety behaviors (e.g., cutting food into small pieces, counting calories, avoiding certain types of foods). Many studies on food exposures are conducted with patients enrolled in more intensive hospitalization-based programs and are associated with positive outcomes (e.g., increased caloric intake/BMI and decreased anxiety; Butler & Heimberg, 2020). Virtual reality exposures have been increasingly used to expose individuals to a variety of environments, such as places where individuals typically binge eat or places that contain foods that provoke high anxiety. Further research is needed to determine how this approach functions compared to corresponding in vivo therapeutic approaches (Butler & Heimberg, 2020).

Social Support

Many therapeutic approaches incorporate an individual's social network by actively involving family and significant others in the treatment. This strategy is used especially when family members or significant others might be of particular help to patients or when they are making changes more difficult for patients (Fairburn, 2008). Family members or significant others involved in treatment can learn ways to best support patients in treatment, strategies for handling repeated reassurance-seeking, and approaches to help patients with decisions about when and what to eat (Fairburn, 2008; Mason et al., 2016).

FBT in particular has a more central role for family and significant others, and although FBT was originally designed for the treatment of adolescent eating disorders, it is also used with young adults with several adaptations. Adaptations include allowing individuals to choose a support adult to be involved in treatment that may or may not be a parent (Chen et al., 2016). Support adults are involved throughout treatment and assist in actively planning and eating meals with patients. Although weight restoration is still a primary objective, young adults in this treatment generally have more choice compared to adolescents in making decisions such as returning to activities like college, where to have meals, and options for individual therapy sessions, although support adults take a more active role when weight restoration goals are not being met (Chen et al., 2016).

In-Session Weighing

In-session weighing is a common component across effective treatments for eating disorders, while some treatments emphasize its use to a greater degree (e.g., central and nonnegotiable aspect in most treatments for AN, and "advisable" in IPT for BED; Waller & Mountford, 2015). Typically, patients are asked not to weigh without the presence of a treatment provider. Patients are generally weighed weekly or at every session depending on their severity. The weight or change in weight from the previous weighing is shared with the patient with an emphasis on interpreting several sessions' readings in order to focus on trends rather than overinterpretation of individual readings, which may vary for a variety of reasons (e.g., recency of eating, water intake, proximity to next menstrual cycle, etc.; Fairburn, 2008). Regular weighing allows therapists to best address patient safety and understand changes in eating patterns (Waller & Mountford, 2015). Additionally, this approach reduces anxiety associated with weight and modifies unhelpful cognitions regarding weight (e.g., "regular meals and/or eating certain types of foods will lead to immense unstoppable weight gain"; Waller & Mountford, 2015).

Cognitive Strategies

Cognitive strategies utilized in eating disorder treatments focus on noticing and changing negative thought patterns, typically about the importance of shape and weight (Palmieri et al., 2021; Tatham et al., 2015). Biases in thinking, such as black-and-white thinking, are common, and a therapist works with a patient to identify these unhelpful patterns and find more effective ways to approach difficult situations such as mealtimes. In particular, CBT-E focuses less on cognitive approaches (e.g., conventional thought records, identifying core beliefs) and more on helping patients make and sustain behavioral changes (Fairburn, 2008). This is especially true for earlier stages of treatment where gaining or stabilizing weight is the number one priority. After weight has been stabilized, more attention is then focused on how thinking patterns contribute to eating disorder symptoms.

A primary goal of effective treatments for eating disorders is to reduce the importance of shape and weight in a patient's life. In CBT-E, patients create a pie chart to illustrate the areas of their lives that impact their self-evaluation (e.g., family, work, school; Fairburn, 2008; see also Geller et al., 1997). Those with eating disorders typically have their self-evaluations primarily driven by their shape, weight, and eating. Once represented visually, the consequences of an overreliance on shape, weight, and eating are discussed. For example, patients may identify consequences such as how their lives feel controlled by shape and weight to the point where other formerly important aspects do not seem to matter anymore. Next, goals are set for reducing the importance of shape and weight, along with increasing the importance of other domains (e.g., strengthening interpersonal relationships, gaining or returning to hobbies).

Relapse Prevention Strategies

The final stage in eating disorder treatment across modalities typically includes a focus on relapse prevention. This focus is particularly important for those recovering from eating disorders given the higher rates of relapse and potential triggers following treatment (Heruc et al., 2020; Mares et al., 2022; Steinglass et al., 2022). First, the therapist and patient collaboratively take stock of progress made in treatment. Next, they create a plan to help the patient maintain positive changes once treatment ends. Relapse prevention plans are frequently multifaceted. They include the identification of relevant disordered behaviors or changes in patient functioning that would indicate risk of relapse such as frequent body checking, rigid dietary rules, or unhealthy weight control behaviors (Fairburn, 2008; Le Grange & Lock, 2007). Next, they work together to identify upcoming life events or potential scenarios that might be high-risk for weight or eating related concerns (e.g., food-driven holiday celebrations, or wearing a swimsuit at a community pool). The therapist and patient work together to create a plan for how the patient will use skills learned in therapy to manage the events and reduce overall risk of relapse.

Approaches for Youth

Adolescents treated for eating disorders tend to have better outcomes than do individuals entering treatment as adults, perhaps because of their shorter duration of illness (Lock, 2015; Mairs & Nicholls, 2016). While many components of efficacious approaches are similar for children, adolescents, and adults, there are also some important distinctions and areas of focus. FBT is the leading and most widely researched approach for adolescents (Dalle Grave et al., 2019; Lock & Le Grange, 2019; Mairs & Nicholls, 2016). FBT for children and adolescents focuses on parents taking charge of a child's eating, with initial goals of weight restoration or stabilization and the disruption of eating disorder behaviors (Lock & Le Grange, 2015). Compared to adult treatment, FBT for children and adolescents relies more on parental control over their child's eating with a gradual shift of independence back to the child that takes appropriate developmental trajectories into account. In FBT, adolescents are viewed as being separate from and controlled by the eating disorder, which results in the individual appearing to function as a much younger child in terms of emotional and social development. Instead of being blamed for causing the eating disorder, parents are seen as allies in fighting back against the eating disorder (Lock & Le Grange, 2015). The body of efficacy research on FBT has led most clinical guidelines to recommend FBT as the first line of treatment for child and adolescent eating disorders (Lock & Le Grange, 2019).

Newer evidence suggests that CBT-E adapted for adolescents is an effective alternative treatment to FBT (Dalle Grave et al., 2021; Le Grange et al., 2020). Although more research in adolescent samples is still needed, including randomized controlled trials, initial results are promising. CBT-E for adolescents is mostly similar to CBT-E for adults, in that eating disorders are viewed as belonging to the individual, and patients are actively involved in treatment from the onset and encouraged to take back control over their lives using cognitive and behavioral strategies (Dalle Grave & Calugi, 2020; Dalle Grave et al., 2019). Compared to CBT-E for adults, parents play a larger role, although their role is limited to helping the adolescent pursue goals toward behavior change (Dalle Grave et al., 2019).

Other Variables Influencing Treatment

Assessment and Diagnosis

Assessment measures are used for eating disorder screening, diagnosis, and evaluation of treatment progress. Assessments may be administered as either structured or semistructured interviews or paper-and-pencil formats. Challenges of eating disorder assessment include the stigma, ambivalence about symptom reduction, and secretive nature of eating disorders that can prompt denying, hiding, or minimizing symptoms. Furthermore, the selection of appropriate eating disorder assessment measures and careful review of results is important to consider, especially when measures are used across different groups. For example, many eating disorder measures were developed using fairly homogenous samples and may be more or less useful when applied to men or non-White groups where symptom presentation and appearance ideals may differ (Belon et al., 2015; Darcy & Lin, 2012; Kelly et al., 2012). Sufficient and accurate assessment prior to and during treatment is crucial for correctly identifying the severity of the disorder and providing appropriate recommendations about the level of care needed. Finally, regular assessment of treatment progress throughout treatment is essential. Regular assessments are used to determine if a patient's symptoms are improving, and this data influences treatment by identifying areas in need of focus in treatment. Additionally, assessment data is used to make decisions on when treatment should be terminated.

Patients may have features of an eating disorder without necessarily meeting criteria for an eating disorder diagnosis. Assessment is used to distinguish subclinical versus clinically significant eating disorders to assist with treatment planning. In many patients with subclinical eating disorders, individual and intensive psychotherapy may not be warranted, and a stepped-care model is more favorable (Le Grange et al., 2021; Wilson et al., 2000). For example, subclinical BED may be effectively treated with guided self-help CBT-E (Traviss-Turner et al., 2017). Patients read self-help materials while meeting infrequently (e.g., once every few weeks) with a therapist. Guided self-help CBT-E has also been adopted for delivery over telehealth increasing patient access to treatment (Jensen et al., 2020). Patients with subclinical eating disorders may also be an appropriate fit for outpatient group treatment (Fairburn, 2008); however, many factors will influence patients' decision to pursue group intervention (e.g., patient preference, group availability).

Comorbidity

Comorbidity is seen as the rule rather than the exception within eating disorders (Fairburn, 2008; Momen et al., 2022). The most recent literature shows a high prevalence of comorbid mood and anxiety disorders, substance use (Keski-Rahkonen, 2021), PTSD (Ferrell et al., 2022), and obsessive-compulsive disorder (Mandelli et al., 2020) among patients across the lifespan (Convertino & Blashill, 2021). Consequently, a thorough psychiatric assessment is recommended prior to beginning eating disorder treatment. When comorbid disorders are identified or suspected, it is helpful to discern which features of these comorbid disorders are treatment-interfering versus those that may be alleviated post-eating-disorder intervention. For example, Fairburn (2008) recommends that if clinically significant depression is identified during the CBT-E assessment, depression treatment should precede eating disorder intervention. There are specific features of depression (e.g., poor concentration) that directly interfere with treatment adherence and may be best addressed prior to working with the eating disorder. However, there are no data to suggest which order of treatment would be most effective with comorbid depression and eating disorders. Some comorbid disorders do not necessarily interfere with eating disorder treatment, and in these situations it is recommended that the therapist and patient work together to prioritize treatment goals. For example, patients diagnosed with comorbid PTSD may decide to complete trauma-related treatment first depending on the functional impact of trauma versus eating disorder symptoms.

Demographics

For many decades, eating disorders were believed to primarily exist within White, young, wealthy females. Emerging evidence shows that eating disorders exist among patients of every age, race/ethnicity, gender, socioeconomic status, sexual orientation, ability status, and so forth (Mitchison et al., 2014). Unfortunately, the assessment of eating disorders is only now catching up to this new evidence. Many of the commonly used diagnostic measures (e.g., the Eating Disorder Examination – Questionnaire) were exclusively validated within a homogenous population (Fairburn & Beglin, 1994). Recent research shows that the cut-off scores for several of these measures may need to be adjusted based on demographic variables (Schaefer et al., 2018). Therefore, it is important to research the most up-to-date norms on commonly used measures and use norms specific to patients' demographics. Clinicians should also acknowledge the limitations of these assessments as many may not capture culturally relevant influences on diagnostic criteria. For example, in some Black communities, a larger body size is seen as more beautiful (Awad et al., 2015; Watson et al., 2019); however, many assessments for eating disorders primarily ask about a drive for thinness. Researchers are beginning to understand that eating disorder symptomatology varies greatly across populations and further work is needed to adapt assessment procedures accordingly.

Medication

Research into pharmacotherapy has been met with mixed levels of support for different EDs. First, there are no current medications approved for the treatment of AN and no medication has been found to be effective to either promote sustained weight gain or to alleviate underlying psychopathology (de Vos et al., 2014; Mayer, 2017). In contrast, research has supported the use of medications for the treatment of BN. Specifically, antidepressant medications (selective serotonin reuptake inhibitors [SSRIs]) have been shown to decrease symptoms and reduce frequency of binge–purge cycles (Mayer, 2017; Svaldi et al., 2019). Due to potential side effects of medications, psychotherapy alone is often recommended as a first line treatment for BN, followed by combined psychotherapy with medication. Finally, medications for BED have differing levels of efficacy depending on which outcome goals are considered. While the primary goal is often to reduce binge eating, treatments may or may not also be effective at promoting weight loss. These points are important to consider as individuals with BED who seek treatment have higher BMIs and often express weight loss as a treatment goal (Goldschmidt et al., 2011). Currently, two medications have been shown to be effective for both reducing binge eating and weight loss: one is an antiepileptic (topiramate) and the other is a psychostimulant (lisdexamfetamine; Bello & Yeomans, 2018; Hudson & Pope, 2017). Additionally, some antidepressant medications have shown some efficacy in reducing binge eating but not in promoting weight loss (Hudson & Pope, 2017). Regarding the utility of combining psychological and pharmacological treatments, only a small minority of randomized controlled trials have shown a benefit for combining treatments (e.g., Reas & Grilo, 2021). However, these studies do not provide the level of analysis needed to indicate how medication(s) may moderate the effects of therapy.

Conclusion

Currently, the most studied and efficacious treatments appear to be CBT-E, IPT, and FBT. Treatments include a number of effective behavioral and cognitive components, especially focused on strategies addressing nutritional/dietary concerns and weight restoration. Treatment components also aim to decrease the overemphasis individuals place on weight, shape, and eating, and allow them to re-engage with other areas of their lives, including interpersonal relationships. Next steps for these treatments would include attempts to evaluate the research findings fully against the Tolin criteria and provide a clear recommendation of *very strong*, *strong*, or *weak*, using the transparent grading guidelines (Tolin et al., 2015).

Useful Resources

Websites

* Association for Size Diversity and Health: https://asdah.org/health-at-every-size-haes-approach/
* Australia & New Zealand Academy For Eating Disorders: www.anzaed.org.au/
* The National Eating Disorders Association: www.nationaleatingdisorders.org/

Books

* Bacon L. (2010). *Health at every size: The surprising truth about your weight* (Revised & updated ed.). BenBella Books.
* Brown H. (2010). *Brave girl eating: A family's struggle with anorexia*. William Morrow.
* Covington Armstrong, S. (2009). *Not all Black girls know how to eat: A story of bulimia*. Lawrence Hill Books.
* Fairburn, C. G. (2008). *Cognitive behavior therapy and eating disorders*. Guilford Press.
* Fairburn, C. G. (2013). *Overcoming binge eating: The proven program to learn why you binge and how you can stop (second ed.)*. Guilford Press.
* Forsberg, S., Lock, J., & Le Grange D. (2018). *Family based treatment for restrictive eating disorders: A guide for supervision and advanced clinical practice*. Taylor and Francis.
* Waller, G., Turner, H. M., Tatham, M., Mountford, V., & Wade, T. (2019). *Brief cognitive behavioural therapy for non-underweight patients: CBT-T for eating disorders*. Routledge.

References

American Psychiatric Association. (2022). *Diagnostic and statistical manual of mental disorders* (5th ed., text revision). American Psychiatric Association Publishing.

Atwood, M. E., & Friedman, A. (2020). A systematic review of enhanced cognitive behavioral therapy (CBT-E) for eating disorders. *International Journal of Eating Disorders*, 53(3), 311–330.

Awad, G. H., Norwood, C., Taylor, D. S., et al. (2015). Beauty and body image concerns among African American college women. *Journal of Black Psychology*, 41(6), 540–564. https://doi.org/10.1177/0095798414550864.

Bailey-Straebler, S., Cooper, Z., Dalle Grace, R., Calugi, S., & Murphy, R. (2022). Development of the CBT-E components checklist: A tool for measuring therapist self-rated adherence to CBT-E. *Italian Journal of Eating Disorders and Obesity*, 4, 6–10. https://doi.org/10.32044/ijedo.2022.0.

Bello, N. T., & Yeomans, B. L. (2018). Safety of pharmacotherapy options for bulimia nervosa and binge eating disorder. *Expert Opinion on Drug Safety*, 17(1), 17–23. https://doi.org/10.1080/14740338.2018.1395854.

Belon, K. E., McLaughlin, E. A., Smith, J. E., et al. (2015). Testing the measurement invariance of the eating disorder inventory in nonclinical samples of Hispanic and Caucasian women. *International Journal of Eating Disorders*, 48(3), 262–270. https://doi.org/10.1002/eat.22286.

Butler, R. M., & Heimberg, R. G. (2020). Exposure therapy for eating disorders: A systematic review. *Clinical Psychology Review*, 78, 1–12. https://doi.org/10.1016/j.cpr.2020.101851.

Chen, E. Y., Weissman, J. A., Zeffiro, T. et al. (2016). Family-based therapy for young adults with anorexia nervosa restores weight. *International Journal of Eating Disorders*, 49(7), 701–707. https://doi.org/10.1002/eat.22513.

Christian, C., Perko, V. L., Vanzhula, I. A., et al. (2020). Eating disorder core symptoms and symptom pathways across developmental stages: A network analysis. *Journal of Abnormal Psychology*, 129(2), 177.

Convertino, A. D., & Blashill, A. J. (2021). Psychiatric comorbidity of eating disorders in children between the ages of 9 and 10. *Journal of Child Psychology and Psychiatry*, 63(5), 519–526. https://doi.org/10.1111/jcpp.13484.

Cooper, Z., & Dalle Grave, R. (2017). Eating disorders: Transdiagnostic theory and treatment. In S. G. Hofmann & G. J. G. Asmundson (Eds.), *The science of cognitive behavioral therapy* (pp. 337–357). Elsevier Academic Press. https://doi.org/10.1016/B978-0-12-803457-6.00014-3.

Cougle, J. R., & Grubaugh, A. L. (2022). Do psychosocial treatment outcomes vary by race or ethnicity? A review of meta-analyses. *Clinical Psychology Review*, 102192.

Dalle Grave, R., & Calugi, S. (2020). *Cognitive behavior therapy for adolescents with eating disorders*. Guilford Press.

Dalle Grave, R., Conti, M., Sartirana, M., Sermattei, S., & Calugi, S. (2021). Enhanced cognitive behaviour therapy for adolescents with eating disorders: A systematic review of current status and future perspectives. *Italian Journal of Eating Disorders and Obesity*, 3(3), 1–11. https://doi.org/10.32044/ijedo.2021.01.

Dalle Grave, R., Eckhardt, S., Calugi, S., & Le Grange, D. (2019). A conceptual comparison of family-based treatment and enhanced cognitive behavior therapy in the treatment of adolescents with eating disorders. *Journal of Eating Disorders*, 7(1), 1–9. https://doi.org/10.1186/s40337-019-0275-x.

Darcy, A. M., & Lin, I. H. J. (2012). Are we asking the right questions? A review of assessment of males with eating disorders. *Eating Disorders*, 20(5), 416–426. https://doi.org/10.1080/10640266.2012.715521.

de Vos, J., Houtzager, L., Katsaragaki, G., et al. (2014). Meta analysis on the efficacy of pharmacotherapy versus placebo on anorexia nervosa. *Journal of Eating Disorders*, 2(1), 1–14. https://doi.org/10.1186/s40337-014-0027-x.

Division 12 of the American Psychological Association. (2016a). Cognitive Behavioral Therapy for Bulimia Nervosa. https://div12.org/treatment/cognitive-behavioral-therapy-for-bulimia-nervosa/.

Division 12 of the American Psychological Association. (2016b). Cognitive Behavioral Therapy for Binge Eating Disorder. https://div12.org/treatment/cognitive-behavioral-therapy-for-binge-eating-disorder/

Division 12 of the American Psychological Association. (2016c). Cognitive Behavioral Therapy for Anorexia Nervosa. https://div12.org/treatment/cognitive-behavioral-therapy-for-anorexia-nervosa/

Division 12 of the American Psychological Association. (2016d). Interpersonal Psychotherapy for Bulimia Nervosa. https://div12.org/treatment/interpersonal-psychotherapy-for-bulimia-nervosa/

Division 12 of the American Psychological Association. (2016e). Interpersonal Psychotherapy for Binge Eating Disorder. https://div12.org/treatment/interpersonal-psychotherapy-for-binge-eating-disorder/

Division 12 of the American Psychological Association. (2016f). Family-Based Treatment for Anorexia Nervosa. https://div12.org/treatment/family-based-treatment-for-anorexia-nervosa/

Division 12 of the American Psychological Association. (2016g). Family-Based Treatment for Bulimia Nervosa. https://div12.org/treatment/family-based-treatment-for-bulimia-nervosa/

Fairburn, C. G. (2008). *Cognitive behavior therapy and eating disorders*. Guilford Press.

Fairburn, C. G., & Beglin, S. J. (1994). Assessment of eating disorders: Interview or self-report questionnaire? *International Journal of Eating Disorders*, 16(4), 363–370.

Fairburn, C. G., Cooper, Z., & Shafran, R. (2003). Cognitive behaviour therapy for eating disorders: A "transdiagnostic" theory and treatment. *Behaviour Research and Therapy*, 41, 509–528.

Fairburn, C. G., Cooper, Z., Bohn, K., et al. (2007). The severity and status of eating disorder NOS: Implications for DSM-V. *Behaviour Research and Therapy*, 45(8), 1705–1715.

Fairburn, C. G., Cooper, Z., Shafran, R., & Wilson, T.G. (2008). Eating disorders: A transdiagnostic protocol. In D. H. Barlow (4th ed.), *Clinical handbook of psychological disorders: A step-by-step treatment manual* (578–614). The Guilford Press.

Ferrell, E. L., Russin, S. E., & Flint, D. D. (2022). Prevalence estimates of comorbid eating disorders and posttraumatic stress disorder: A quantitative synthesis. *Journal of Aggression, Maltreatment & Trauma*, 31(2), 264–282. https://doi.org/10.1080/10926771.2020.1832168.

Geller, J., Johnston, C., & Madsen, K. (1997). The role of shape and weight in self-concept: The shape and weight based self-esteem inventory. *Cognitive Therapy and Research*, 21, 5–24.

Goldschmidt, A. B., Le Grange, D., Powers, P., et al. (2011). Eating disorder symptomatology in normal-weight vs. obese individuals with binge eating disorder. *Obesity*, 19(7), 1515–1518. https://doi.org/10.1038/oby.2011.24.

Goldschmidt, A. B., Wonderlich, S. A., Crosby, R. D., et al. (2014). Ecological momentary assessment of stressful events and negative affect in bulimia nervosa. *Journal of Consulting and Clinical Psychology*, 82(1), 30–39.

Goodrick, G. K., Pendleton, V. R., Kimball, K. T., et al. (1999). Binge eating severity, self-concept, dieting self-efficacy and social support during treatment of binge eating disorder. *International Journal of Eating Disorders*, 26(3), 295–300.

Griffen, T. C., Naumann, E., & Hildebrandt, T. (2018). Mirror exposure therapy for body image disturbances and eating disorders: A review. *Clinical Psychology Review*, 65, 163–174. https://doi.org/10.1016/j.cpr.2018.08.006.

Grilo, C. M., White, M. A., Gueorguieva, R., Wilson, G. T., & Masheb, R. M. (2013). Predictive significance of the overvaluation of shape/weight in obese patients with binge eating disorder: Findings from a randomized controlled trial with 12-month follow-up. *Psychological Medicine*, 43(6), 1335–1344. https://doi.org/10.1017/S003329171 2002097.

Grisset, N. I., & Norvell, N. K. (1992). Perceived social support, social skills, and quality of relationships in bulimic women. *Journal of Consulting and Clinical Psychology*, 60(2), 293.

Heruc, G., Hurst, K., Casey, A., et al. (2020). ANZAED eating disorder treatment principles and general clinical practice and training standards. *Journal of Eating Disorders*, 8(1), 1–9. https://doi.org/10.1186/s40337-020-00341-0.

Hilbert, A., Petroff, D., Herpertz, S., et al. (2019). Meta-analysis of the efficacy of psychological and medical treatments for binge-eating disorder. *Journal of Consulting and Clinical Psychology*, 87(1), 91–105. https://doi.org/10.1016/j.eatbeh.2019.101311.

Hudson, J. I., & Pope, H. G. (2017). Psychopharmacological treatment of binge eating disorder. In K. D. Brownell & B. T. Walsh (Eds.), *Eating disorders and obesity: A comprehensive handbook* (3rd ed., pp. 308–313). Guilford.

Ivanova, I. V., Tasca, G. A., Proulx, G., & Bissada, H. (2015). Does the interpersonal model apply across eating disorder diagnostic groups? A structural equation modeling approach. *Comprehensive Psychiatry*, 63, 80–87. https://doi.org/10.1016/j.comppsych.2015.08.009.

Jeffrey, S., & Heruc, G. (2020). Balancing nutrition management and the role of dietitians in eating disorder treatment. *Journal of Eating Disorders*, 8(1), 1–3.

Jensen, E. S., Linnet, J., Holmberg, T. T., et al. (2020). Effectiveness of internet-based guided self-help for binge-eating disorder and characteristics of completers versus noncompleters. *International Journal of Eating Disorders*, 53(12), 2026–2031. https://doi.org/10.1002/eat.23384.

Kelly, N. R., Mitchell, K. S., Gow, R. W., et al. (2012). An evaluation of the reliability and construct validity of eating disorder measures in white and black women. *Psychological Assessment*, 24(3), 608–617. https://doi.org/10.1037/a0026457.

Keski-Rahkonen, A. (2021). Epidemiology of binge eating disorder: Prevalence, course, comorbidity, and risk factors. *Current Opinion in Psychiatry*, 34(6), 525–531. https://doi.org/10.1097/YCO.0000000000000750.

Kosmerly, S., Waller, G., & Robinson, A. L. (2015). Clinician adherence to guidelines in the delivery of family-based therapy for eating disorders. *International Journal of Eating Disorders*, 48(2), 223–229. https://doi.org/10.1002/eat.22276.

Lampard, A. M., Byrne, S. M., & McLean, N. (2011). Does self-esteem mediate the relationship between interpersonal problems and symptoms of disordered eating? *European Eating Disorders Review*, 19(5), 454–458. https://doi.org/10.1002/erv.1120.

Le Grange, D., & Lock, J. (2007). New and emerging treatment options for adolescent bulimia nervosa. *Clinical Practice*, 4(6), 841–849.

Le Grange, D., Eckhardt, S., Dalle Grave, R., et al. (2020). Enhanced cognitive-behavior therapy and family-based treatment for adolescents with an eating disorder: A non-randomized effectiveness trial. *Psychological Medicine*, 1–11. https://doi.org/10.1017/S0033291720004407.

Le Grange, D., Pradel, M., Pogos, D., et al. (2021). Family-based treatment for adolescent anorexia nervosa: Outcomes of a stepped-care model. *International Journal of Eating Disorders*, 54(11), 1989–1997. https://doi.org/10.1002/eat.23629.

Leonidas, C., & Dos Santos, M. A. (2014). Social support networks and eating disorders: An integrative review of the literature. *Neuropsychiatric Disease and Treatment*, 10, 915–927.

Linardon, J. (2018). Rates of abstinence following psychological or behavioral treatments for binge-eating disorder: Meta-analysis. *International Journal of Eating Disorders*, 51(8), 785–797.

Linardon, J., Wade, T. D., De la Piedad Garcia, X., & Brennan, L. (2017). The efficacy of cognitive-behavioral therapy for eating disorders: A systematic review and meta-analysis. *Journal of Consulting and Clinical Psychology*, 85(11), 1080.

Linville, D., Brown, T., Sturm, K., & McDougal, T. (2012). Eating disorders and social support: perspectives of recovered individuals. *Eating Disorders*, 20(3), 216–231.

Lipsitz, J. D., & Markowitz, J. C. (2013). Mechanisms of change in interpersonal therapy (IPT). *Clinical Psychology Review*, 33(8), 1134–1147. https://doi.org/10.1016/j.cpr.2013.09.002.

Lock, J. (2011). Evaluation of family treatment models for eating disorders. *Current Opinion in Psychiatry*, 24, 274–279.

Lock, J. (2015). An update on evidence-based psychosocial treatments for eating disorders in children and adolescents. *Journal of Clinical Child & Adolescent Psychology*, 44, 707–721.

Lock, J., & La Via, M. C. (2015). Practice parameter for the assessment and treatment of children and adolescents with eating disorders. *Journal of the American Academy of Child & Adolescent Psychiatry*, 54(5), 412–425. https://doi.org/10.1016/j.jaac.2015.01.018.

Lock, J., & Le Grange, D. (2015). *Treatment manual for anorexia nervosa: A family-based approach*. Guilford Publications.

Lock, J., & Le Grange, D. (2019). Family-based treatment: Where are we and where should we be going to improve recovery in child and adolescent eating disorders. *International Journal of Eating Disorders*, 52(4), 481–487.

Mairs, R., & Nicholls, D. (2016). Assessment and treatment of eating disorders in children and adolescents. *Archives of Disease in Childhood*, 101(12), 1168–1175. https://doi.org/10.1136/archdischild-2015-309481.

Mandelli, L., Draghetti, S., Albert, U., De Ronchi, D., & Atti, A. R. (2020). Rates of comorbid obsessive-compulsive disorder in eating disorders: A meta-analysis of the literature. *Journal of Affective Disorders*, 277, 927–939. https://doi.org/10.1016/j.jad.2020.09.003.

Mares, S. H., Burger, J., Lemmens, L. H., van Elburg, A. A., & Vroling, M. S. (2022). Evaluation of the cognitive behavioural theory of eating disorders: A network analysis investigation. *Eating Behaviors*, 44, 1–8. https://doi.org/10.1016/j.eatbeh.2021.101590.

Mason, T. B., Lavender, J. M., Wonderlich, S. A., et al. (2016). The role of interpersonal personality traits and reassurance seeking in eating disorder symptoms and depressive symptoms among women with bulimia nervosa. *Comprehensive Psychiatry*, 68, 165–171. https://doi.org/10.1016/j.comppsych.2016.04.013.

Mayer, L. (2017). Psychopharmacological treatment of anorexia nervosa and bulimia nervosa. In K. D. Brownell & B. T. Walsh (Eds.), *Eating disorders and obesity: A comprehensive handbook* (3rd ed., pp. 302–307). Guilford.

Miniati, M., Callari, A., Maglio, A., & Calugi, S. (2018). Interpersonal psychotherapy for eating disorders: Current perspectives. *Psychology Research and Behavior Management*, 11, Article 353–369.

Mitchison, D., Hay, P., Slewa-Younan, S., & Mond, J. (2014). The changing demographic profile of eating disorder behaviors in the community. *BMC Public Health*, 14(1), 1–9. www.biomedcentral.com/1471-2458/14/943.

Momen, N. C., Plana-Ripoll, O., Yilmaz, Z et al. (2022). Comorbidity between eating disorders and psychiatric disorders. *International Journal of Eating Disorders*, 55(4), 505–517. https://doi.org/10.1002/eat.23687.

Murphy, R., Straebler, S., Basden, S., Cooper, Z., & Fairburn, C. G. (2012). Interpersonal psychotherapy for eating disorders. *Clinical Psychology & Psychotherapy*, 12(2), 150–158. https://doi.org/10.1002/cpp.1780.

Nikodijevic, A., Buck, K., Fuller-Tyszkiewicz, M., de Paoli, T., & Krug, I. (2018). Body checking and body avoidance in eating disorders: Systematic review and meta-analysis. *European Eating Disorders Review*, 26(3), 159–185. https://doi.org/10.1002/erv.2585.

Palmieri, S., Mansueto, G., Ruggiero, G. M., et al. (2021). Metacognitive beliefs across eating disorders and eating behaviours: A systematic review. *Clinical Psychology & Psychotherapy*, 28(5), 1254–1265. https://doi.org/10.1002/cpp.2573.

Pellizzer, M. L., Waller, G., & Wade, T. D. (2018). Body image flexibility: A predictor and moderator of outcome in transdiagnostic outpatient eating disorder treatment. *International Journal of Eating Disorders*, 51(4), 368–372. https://doi.org/10.1002/eat.22842.

Raykos, B. C., McEvoy, P. M., & Fursland, A. (2017). Socializing problems and low self-esteem enhance interpersonal models of eating disorders: Evidence from a clinical sample. *International Journal of Eating Disorders*, 50(9), 1075–1083. https://doi.org/10.1002/eat.22740.

Raykos, B. C., McEvoy, P. M., Carter, O., Fursland, A., & Nathan, P. (2014). Interpersonal problems across restrictive and binge-purge samples: Data from a community-based eating disorders clinic. *Eating Behaviors*, 15(3), 449–452.

Reas, D. L., & Grilo, C. M. (2021). Psychotherapy and medications for eating disorders: Better together? *Clinical therapeutics*, 43(1), 17–39.

Reilly, E. E., Bohrer, B., Sullivan, D., et al. (2021). Registered report: Initial development and validation of the eating disorders safety behavior scale. *International Journal of Eating Disorders*, 54(4), 660–667. https://doi.org/10.1002/eat.23479.

Schaefer, L. M., Smith, K. E., Leonard, R., et al. (2018). Identifying a male clinical cutoff on the Eating Disorder Examination-Questionnaire (EDE-Q). *International Journal of Eating Disorders*, 51(12), 1357–1360. https://doi.org/10.1002/eat.22972.

Sivyer, K., Allen, E., Cooper, Z., Bailey-Straebler, S., et al. (2020). Mediators of change in cognitive behavior therapy and interpersonal psychotherapy for eating disorders: A secondary analysis of a transdiagnostic randomized controlled trial. *International Journal of Eating Disorders*, 53(12), 1928–1940. https://doi.org/10.1002/eat.23390.

Steinglass, J. E., Attia, E., Glasofer, D. R., et al. (2022). Optimizing relapse prevention and changing habits (REACH+) in anorexia nervosa. *International Journal of Eating Disorders*. https://doi.org/10.1002/eat.23724.

Svaldi, J., Schmitz, F., Baur, J., et al. (2019). Efficacy of psychotherapies and pharmacotherapies for bulimia nervosa. *Psychological Medicine*, 49(6), 898–910. https://doi.org/10.1017/S0033291718003525.

Tatham, M., Turner, H., Mountford, V. A., et al. (2015). Development, psychometric properties and preliminary clinical validation of a brief, session-by-session measure of eating disorder cognitions and behaviors: The ED-15. *International Journal of Eating Disorders*, 48(7), 1005–1015. https://doi.org/10.1002/eat.22430.

Tiller, J. M., Sloane, G., Schmidt, U., et al. (1997). Social support in patients with anorexia nervosa and bulimia nervosa. *International Journal of Eating Disorders*, 21(1), 31–38.

Tolin, D. F., McKay, D., Forman E. M., Klonsky, D., & Thombs, B. D. (2015). Empirically supported treatment: Recommendations for a new model. *Clinical Psychology Science and Practice*, 25(4), 317–338. https://doi.org/10.1111/cpsp.12122.

Traviss-Turner, G. D., West, R. M., & Hill, A. J. (2017). Guided self-help for eating disorders: A systematic review and metaregression. *European Eating Disorders Review*, 25(3), 148–164. https://doi.org/10.1002/erv.2507.

van Hoeken, D., & Hoek, H. W. (2020). Review of the burden of eating disorders: Mortality, disability, costs, quality of life, and family burden. *Current Opinion in Psychiatry*, 33(6), 521. https://doi.org/10.1097/YCO.0000000000000641.

Waller, G., & Mountford, V. A. (2015). Weighing patients within cognitive-behavioural therapy for eating disorders: How, when and why. *Behaviour Research and Therapy*, 70, 1–10. https://doi.org/10.1016/j.brat.2015.04.004.

Waller, G., Cordery, H., Corstorphine, E., et al. (2007). *Cognitive behavioral therapy for eating disorders: A comprehensive treatment guide*. Cambridge University Press.

Ward, Z. J., Rodriguez, P., Wright, D. R., Austin, S. B., & Long, M. W. (2019). Estimation of eating disorders prevalence by age and associations with mortality in a simulated nationally representative US cohort. *JAMA Network Open*, 2(10), e1912925–e1912925.

Watson, L. B., Lewis, J. A., & Moody, A. T. (2019). A sociocultural examination of body image among Black women. *Body Image*, 31, 280–287. https://doi.org/10.1016/j.bodyim.2019.03.008.

Wilson, G. T., Vitousek, K. M., & Loeb, K. L. (2000). Stepped care treatment for eating disorders. *Journal of Consulting and Clinical Psychology*, 68(4), 564. https://doi.org/10.1037/0022-006X.68.4.564.

Wilson, G. T., Wilfley, D. E., Agras, W. S., & Bryson, S. W. (2010). Psychological treatments for binge eating disorder. *Archives of General Psychiatry*, 67, 94–101.

Woods, A. M., Racine, S. E., & Klump, K. L. (2010). Examining the relationship between dietary restraint and binge eating: Differential effects of major and minor stressors. *Eating Behaviors*, 11(4), 276–280.

10

Insomnia Disorder

Parky Lau, Onkar Marway, and Colleen Carney

Insomnia Disorder (ID) is characterized by trouble falling asleep, staying asleep, or both, occurring three nights a week or more. The sleep disturbance must be accompanied by impairment in functioning or distress about the sleep issue. ID is conceptualized as a 24-hour disorder, or a "sleep-wake" disorder (i.e., ID causes problems in the daytime in addition to the nighttime). Importantly, ID is chronic, so the issues must be present for three months or more to meet criteria for the condition as outlined in the DSM-5-TR (American Psychological Association, 2022). The target symptom is the sleep complaint, as well its impact on daytime functioning, but the target behaviors are derived from what causes chronic insomnia. Science-based treatments operate by targeting behaviors and cognitions that are theorized to perpetuate insomnia. We will discuss these targets in greater detail in the ensuing etiology section, but briefly, to address chronic insomnia, treatment aims to re-associate the bed with sleeping, decrease sleep effort behavior, restore sleep self-efficacy, increase the drive for deep sleep, regulate the circadian system, and modify beliefs that get in the way of sleep unfolding naturally.

Etiology and Theoretical Underpinnings of Treatment

Several models have been helpful in understanding insomnia; these include the cognitive model of insomnia and the 3P model. The cognitive model of insomnia (Harvey, 2002) theorizes that people with insomnia tend to be excessively worried about their sleep and the potential daytime consequences of not getting enough sleep. This negatively toned cognitive activity increases autonomic arousal and distress, which leads to selectively attending to and monitoring of external and internal evidence of sleep deficit (e.g., feeling tired, poor concentration). As a well-intentioned attempt to compensate for perceived sleep deficits and reduce anxiety, people with insomnia engage in counterproductive safety behaviors (e.g., thought control, limiting/canceling plans and activities, going to bed early). Unfortunately, these behaviors maintain anxiety and disrupt the natural processes that govern sleep, which perpetuates the sleep problem. There is ample literature to suggest that higher negative cognitions lead to more sleep disturbances (for a review, see Hiller et al., 2015) and one reason for this may be a result of safety behaviors (Woodley & Smith, 2006). These perpetuating factors are further elaborated upon in the 3P model proposed by Spielman and colleagues (1987). The 3Ps are predisposing, precipitating, and perpetuating factors. Predisposing factors are variables that make a person more vulnerable to developing chronic sleep problems, such as high trait anxiety and perfectionism. These factors interact with precipitating factors (i.e., stressful events that trigger initial sleep disturbance) to produce acute insomnia (short-term sleep disturbances). Acute insomnia can become chronic insomnia because of perpetuating factors that maintain sleep disturbances. Specifically, there are physiological (bedtime hyperarousal), psychological (unhelpful beliefs about sleep), and behavioral (e.g., more time spent resting and reduced activity) factors that occur during the switch from acute to chronic insomnia (e.g., Bonnet & Arand, 2010; Gehrman et al., 2016; Kay et al., 2016; Riedner et al., 2016). Psychological interventions are primarily focused on changing specific behaviors and thoughts that maintain these perpetuating factors, rather than on predisposing or precipitating factors. The main perpetuating factors in ID are conditioned arousal, a dysregulated clock, and engaging in safety behaviors during the day to help conserve energy. The model is well-supported through efficacy data in therapies that employ this model to inform its treatment recommendations, such as SRT (Spielman et al., 2016).

Treatment of chronic insomnia has been conceptualized and refined based on our understanding of sleep and wake processes, and its relation with perpetuating factors of ID. Behavioral sleep medicine leverages this knowledge to target proposed causes of chronic sleep problems. For example, in the case of ID, perpetuating factors include diffused homeostatic pressure in the sleep/wake system (i.e., not enough wakefulness activity during the day to support recovery sleep), irregular circadian input, and cognitive hyperarousal – the latter of which can contribute to a learned association between the bed and wakefulness through excessive time spent in bed awake in a hyperactive state (Perlis et al., 2011). Given this understanding, behavioral interventions were developed to put pressure on the homeostatic system (e.g., sleep restriction), regularize the circadian clock (by keeping to regular bed and rise times), and reduce basal and conditioned arousal (e.g., relaxation techniques and stimulus control). It is unsurprising that science-based behavioral treatments of insomnia have demonstrated high levels of efficacy and durability because they treat insomnia by disrupting factors that maintain chronic sleep disturbance.

Brief Overview of Treatments

There are several consensus statements and clinical guidelines available for ID, and although there are some minor differences across these statements, all support that the front-line evidence-based therapy for ID is cognitive-behavioral therapy (CBT-I). For instance, Boness and colleagues (2020) applied the "Tolin Criteria" (Tolin et al., 2015) to a systematic review evaluating efficacy of CBT-I. Based on the high-quality evidence found in support of CBT-I in producing clinically significant effects on insomnia and other sleep-related outcomes, a *strong* recommendation toward the use of CBT-I was merited (see also p. 402 of this book). The most recent clinical guideline comes from one of the leading authorities on clinical sleep medicine: the American Academy of Sleep Medicine (AASM) (e.g., Edinger et al., 2021). This taskforce employed the Grading of Recommendations Assessment, Development and Evaluation (GRADE) methodology (Guyatt et al., 2008) to systematically evaluate and grade evidence for psychological treatments for ID. Only those meeting a certain rigor and those with plausible primary mechanisms made the final list of recommendations, and, of those 11 therapies, CBT-I was the one strong recommendation made by the taskforce.

There is strong evidence to support the efficacy and durability of CBT-I (e.g., Blom et al., 2016; Johnson et al., 2016). Furthermore, patients prefer psychological intervention over medication (McHugh et al., 2013), and CBT-I is generally preferred to other types of behavioral interventions for insomnia (Sidani et al., 2009). The cognitive components of CBT-I consist of restructuring unhelpful and rigidly held beliefs about sleep and can consist of the use of thought records, Socratic questioning/guided self-discovery, and behavioral experiments to challenge beliefs. The behavioral components of CBT-I consist of sleep restriction therapy (SRT), stimulus control, sleep hygiene, and occasionally relaxation therapy. The first session of CBT-I generally consists of psychoeducation of the sleep systems (i.e., the two-process model of sleep regulation; Achermann, 2004) and how we can leverage this knowledge to help the individual get their sleep back on track. Specifically, the two-process model includes Process S, which refers to the homeostatic sleep/wake system that builds up pressure for sleep the longer we are awake, and Process C, the circadian pacemaker that reflects our internal daily rhythms over a near 24-hour cycle and is independent of sleep/wake history. When harmonized, these processes interact to produce robust timing of sleep and waking. Each session is guided by continuous sleep diaries kept by the patient between sessions. SRT primarily consists of matching an individual's time in bed to their average total sleep time (Glovinsky & Spielman, 1991). This is done in an attempt to increase the individual's sleep efficiency. Stimulus control consists of breaking the conditioned association between bed and wakefulness (Bootzin, 1972) by being in bed only when asleep, or when sleep is likely to occur. Relaxation therapies (e.g., progressive muscle relaxation, guided imagery meditations) have also been used to combat hyperarousal to support a physical state that is more compatible with sleep.

Credible Components of Treatments

Stimulus Control

Stimulus control was originally a single-component behavioral therapy for chronic insomnia designed to extinguish the association between the bed/bedroom and wakefulness to restore the association of bed/bedroom with sleep (Bootzin, 1972). The associated set of instruction include: (1) go to bed only when sleepy, (2) get out of bed when unable to sleep, (3) use the bed/bedroom for sleep and sex, (4) wake up at the same time every morning irrespective of the previous night's sleep, and (5) refrain from daytime naps. Stimulus control was created using learning principles to address research-derived maintaining factors (e.g., conditioning). For example, stimulus control leverages principles of associative learning by instructing the person to go to bed only when sleepy and to get out of bed when sleep is not coming. Through these principles, the bed reacquires stimulus value for sleep (Perlis et al., 1997). In support of the theoretical utility for stimulus control, empirical data implicate the existence of a maladaptive paired association between the bed and arousal in ID. For example, Robertson et al. (2007) found that people with insomnia tend to report more cognitive arousal and less sleepiness within the bedroom environment at lights out (i.e., bedtime) compared to good sleepers. Consequently, there is a need to restore paired associations in the bedroom environment that are conducive to sleep rather than wake.

Beyond principles of learned associations, stimulus control instructions also leverage the circadian system by creating a regular rise time. This also leverages the homeostatic system by delaying bedtime until sleepy and increasing time out of bed. These two behaviors indirectly increase pressure for sleep by reducing resting behavior.

There is strong theoretical backing to support stimulus control as a treatment of chronic insomnia, and empirical data supports its efficacy. Initial practice parameters (Chesson et al., 1999) found the strongest evidence for stimulus control, and subsequent reviews of the evidence have continued to recommend stimulus control as a treatment for ID (Morgenthaler et al., 2006). Randomized controlled trials indicate that stimulus control is an effective intervention for improving sleep indices (e.g., sleep latency, wake after sleep onset) (Lacks et al., 1983; Ladouceur & Gros-Louis, 1986) and sleep quality (Harris et al., 2012), in addition to perceived insomnia severity (Sidani et al., 2019). The AASM GRADE assessment of stimulus control found low-quality evidence for its efficacy, due to imprecision (i.e., confidence intervals not meeting clinical significance) and risk of bias, such as issues of blinding, allocation concealment, and selective reporting of results (Edinger et al., 2021). More up-to-date high-quality research is needed to support stimulus control as an effective monotherapy for ID, but it is currently considered one of the main effective components of CBT-I.

Sleep Restriction Therapy

Numerous studies have shown support for SRT as a treatment for insomnia. Early studies compared SRT to other components of CBT-I in RCTs and, generally, these studies repeatedly showed that SRT was comparable to CBT-I or other components of CBT-I and superior to sleep hygiene (Epstein et al., 2012; Fernando et al., 2013; Friedman et al., 2000). SRT and stimulus control are both highly effective, but combining them into a multicomponent CBT-I produces the best remission rates and largest effects (Maurer & Kyle, 2022). At the same time, there is research to the contrary. For example, Sidani et al. (2019) conducted a randomized controlled trial comparing sleep hygiene, stimulus control, SRT, and CBT-I which combines all treatment methods studied. The researchers found that individuals in the sleep hygiene group showed the least response to treatment and that stimulus control and SRT showed higher rates of remission relative to multiple-component therapy.

SRT is hypothesized to function by increasing homeostatic pressure to sleep by limiting time in bed to an individual's mean total sleep time. This increased sleep pressure decreases sleep onset latency and wake after sleep onset. It may also, indirectly, reduce pre-sleep arousal by increasing sleep pressure (Maurer et al., 2022). Although establishing a regular time in bed can be seen as leveraging the circadian system, Maurer et al. (2020) found that compared to setting a regular bedtime and rise time, SRT produces superior reductions in insomnia symptoms.

Relaxation Therapies

Relaxation therapies are occasionally included in CBT-I when patients report trouble with high cognitive arousal or somatic tension. Patients are encouraged to use relaxation strategies throughout the day, outside of the bedroom environment, to help decrease symptoms of daytime anxiety. These methods may include progressive muscle relaxation (PMR), breathing exercises, or guided imagery. Studies support the use of relaxation therapies as a potentially beneficial component of CBT-I. There are several studies supporting relaxation therapies for insomnia (e.g., PMR, meditation, and autogenic training) (Greeff & Conradie, 1998; Means et al., 2000; Nicassio & Bootzin, 1974; Woolfolk et al.,1976).

There are few studies comparing relaxation therapies directly to CBT-I or other components of CBT-I. Espie and colleagues (1989) reported that patients receiving PMR did not improve as much as did those receiving stimulus control; similarly, Morin and Azrin (1988) reported that stimulus control was superior to imagery training in reducing wake after sleep onset. Edinger et al. (2001) reported that CBT-I significantly outperformed PMR, and those in the CBT-I condition showed a greater reduction in wake after sleep onset and increase in sleep efficiency at posttreatment. Rybarczyk et al. (2002) compared CBT-I to a relaxation-based treatment and waitlist control in 28 older adults with insomnia. The CBT group fared better, with 54% of individuals in the CBT

Box 10.1 Components Requiring Further Research

Some components that require further research include mindfulness, intensive sleep retraining, paradoxical intention, and sleep hygiene. Mindfulness approaches are used as a form of meditation, which emphasizes a nonjudgmental state of complete awareness of one's internal and external experience in the present moment. Meta-analytic results suggest that mindfulness meditation may significantly improve certain sleep indices (e.g., sleep quality, total wake time) but not others (e.g., subjective insomnia severity, unhelpful beliefs about sleep, total sleep time) (Gong et al., 2016). One study found that incorporating mindfulness meditation with behavioral strategies (e.g., SRT) led to greater rates of insomnia remission and response compared to mindfulness-based stress reduction (Ong et al., 2014). Consequently, mindfulness meditation may be particularly helpful as part of a multicomponent therapy.

Intensive Sleep Retraining (ISR) is a newly described treatment designed to markedly increase homeostatic sleep pressure using acute sleep deprivation to reduce sleep onset difficulties and sleep-state misperception (Edinger et al., 2021; Lack et al., 2019). After the use of an acute sleep deprivation, the treatment facilitates a series of rapid sleep onsets to counteract the conditioned insomnia response. The theory is that people with insomnia will begin to better recognize feelings of sleepiness and see the bed as opportunity to obtain much needed sleep rather than a place of fear. Given the relative novelty of this treatment, there is less empirical evidence regarding its efficacy, though research is promising. For example, preliminary investigations have found that ISR significantly improves nighttime and daytime symptoms of insomnia (Harris et al., 2007).

In paradoxical intention, the patient purposefully engages with the feared activity (i.e., staying awake) to reduce performance anxiety and conscious intent to sleep that counterintuitively impacts the desired outcome (i.e., falling asleep). One study found a reduction in sleep onset latency and number of nighttime awakenings in favor of the paradoxical intention group (Ascher & Turner, 1979), but other studies have not provided support (Lacks et al., 1983). Overall, a GRADE assessment of "very low" for quality of evidence supporting this treatment was provided by the AASM (Edinger et al., 2021). The current data does not support paradoxical intention as a stand-alone intervention for chronic insomnia, though paradoxical intention is listed by the American Psychological Association Division 12 Task Force as having "strong research support" under the original (1993) criteria (Division 12, 2022).

Sleep hygiene is integrated into CBT-I but does not have an empirical base as a stand-alone treatment for insomnia. Studies repeatedly show that sleep hygiene is inferior to SRT, stimulus control, and CBT-I as a whole (Chung et al., 2018). Sleep hygiene consists of education about several factors or habits that can be sleep disruptive or interfering, such as curbing intake of substances with effects on sleep microarchitecture (e.g., caffeine, alcohol, cannabis) close to bedtime and having a sleep environment that is conducive to sleep (e.g., comfortable temperature, dark, limited noise). Because of the poor evidence base, despite an unfortunate common use as a monotherapy (e.g., Moss et al., 2013), the AASM advises against its use for ID.

group experiencing a clinically significant reduction in their insomnia symptoms compared to only 35% and 6% in the relaxation and control conditions, respectively. Thus, CBT-I is considered a preferable first choice, with the option of combining relaxation with CBT-I, but relaxation remains an alternative with weaker effects.

Approaches for Youth

Whereas the evidence and treatment described so far has been established in adults, the approaches for treating childhood sleep problems are similar in their behavioral methods. There is support for several behavioral treatments, including unmodified extinction and preventive parent education, graduated extinction, bedtime fading/positive routines, and scheduled awakenings (Meltzer & Mindell, 2014). Unmodified extinction consists of ignoring negative behaviors from lights out until lights on in the morning. Graduated extinction consists of a brief caregiver check-in after lights out, which decreases in frequency until ignoring negative behavior after lights out until a set time in the morning. Parental education/prevention provides caregivers with the sleep information needed to regulate the child's sleep. Bedtime fading/positive routines involve a positive bedtime routine, moving the child's bedtime later to match when they fall asleep, and stimulus control. Scheduled awakenings involve waking a child 15–30 minutes before their habitual awakening time and consoling the child. A meta-analytic review of behavioral interventions in children supports its efficacy, although perhaps not in those with special needs as available studies were low (n=2) and statistically significant findings on sleep outcomes were not found (Meltzer & Mindell, 2014). In pediatric insomnia the treatment relies on the caregiver for implementing the treatment plan. In general, work with adolescents involves a delicate balance between parental involvement and the teen implementing the strategies. CBT-I in teens often involves modifications/additions, such as including mindfulness meditation (Bruin et al., 2020), focusing on bedtime electronic habits (Clarke et al., 2015), or greater parental assistance in treatment (Loring et al., 2016). Because some studies exclude participants with comorbidities (e.g., Clarke et al., 2015), our understanding of whether CBT-I is effective in cases where insomnia is not the only problem is limited. Lastly, because pubescent shifts in circadian rhythms require special attention when treating sleep disruptions in adolescents (Roenneberg et al., 2004), other treatments have emerged to address the full range of problems teens encounter. One such treatment is the Transdiagnostic Sleep and Circadian Intervention (TranS-C), which combines components of CBT-I along with components of circadian interventions like Interpersonal Social Rhythm Therapy – IPSRT (Harvey et al., 2016), which regularizes daily routines (e.g., sleep/wake cycles, mealtimes, rest and activity) to strengthen the circadian clock. Randomized controlled trials of TranS-C in youth have shown promising results (Harvey, 2016; Harvey et al., 2018), including in a free self-management app called Doze (Carmona et al., 2021).

Other Variables Influencing Treatment

Assessment and Diagnosis

Amalgamating data from semi-structured interviews and prospective sleep diaries are helpful in the assessment of ID. The Consensus Sleep Diary (Carney et al., 2012) is an integral part of subjective assessment of a subjective disorder. Whereas retrospective measures such as the Pittsburgh Sleep Quality Index (PSQI; Buysse et al., 1989) have affective recall biases (Hartmann et al., 2015), prospective measures capture the variability inherent in sleep. They assess both habits and subjective experience, which are key in CBT-I. Reliable data can be obtained from two weeks of sleep diaries (Wohlgemuth et al., 1999). Questionnaires like the Insomnia Severity Index (ISI; Morin, 1993) are popular patient-reported outcome measures that can be used to help track the progress of symptoms throughout and after treatment. Subjective reports of symptoms are the gold standard because insomnia is a subjective disorder of sleep complaint. Polysomnography (PSG) data are typically not required or helpful for the assessment of insomnia. Sleep studies are burdensome and oftentimes lead to over- or underestimations of sleep disturbance. On one hand, individuals may sleep better in a sleep lab than at home (McCall & McCall, 2012) and this could be because conditioned arousal is absent in a novel environment. On the other hand, research has also shown that individuals may sleep more poorly in a laboratory setting (Edinger et al., 1997) compared to at home. Furthermore, because ID is primarily a disorder of sleep complaint, PSG data does not contain the presenting complaint: a subjective dissatisfaction with sleep quality. PSG studies are helpful for differential/additional diagnosis only (e.g., sleep apnea, restless legs syndrome).

CBT-I is a treatment meant to address ID only, so diagnosis is an important first step in deciding whether to use it. Diagnostic interviews for sleep disorders, such as the Duke Structured Interview for Sleep Disorders (DSISD; Edinger et al., 2006), offer a reliable and valid approach to differentiating between sleep disorders. This is important as certain sleep disorders can present with symptoms that are similar to insomnia, but would not respond to insomnia treatment because the cause of the problem is different. For example, Delayed Sleep Phase Disorder (DSPD) can appear similar to initial insomnia, as in both sleep problems can lead to difficulty falling asleep; however, difficulty falling asleep in DSPD is because of a mismatch between when a person attempts sleep and their body's circadian preference for a later bedtime rather than an insomnia problem. CBT-I is not an effective treatment option for DSPD (Figueiro, 2016; van Geijlswijk et al., 2010). Other sleep disorders, such as restless legs syndrome and sleep apnea, can also present with similar symptoms as insomnia but require a different treatment approach.

Comorbidity

Insomnia has been described as a prodromal symptom for mental disorders, a feature of them, and also as a residual symptom that lingers after successful treatment and can contribute to risk of relapse (Benson, 2015; Fang et al., 2019; Cox & Olatunji, 2020). Meta-analytic studies indicate that the efficacy of CBT-I on insomnia remains robust across populations with insomnia with comorbid psychiatric and medical conditions (Wu et al., 2015). However, there are certain comorbidities in which components of CBT-I, such as sleep restriction, can exacerbate health issues. For example, sleep restriction is contraindicated in epilepsy because the initial sleep deprivation from sleep restriction can increase risk for epileptic seizures (Dell'Aquila & Soti, 2022). Sleep restriction has also been contraindicated in bipolar disorders because acute sleep deprivation may result in (hypo)manic symptoms (Colombo et al., 1999). However, research studying the use of SRT in bipolar disorder does not support behavioral treatments of insomnia as being harmful to patients with a bipolar disorder diagnosis (Kaplan & Harvey, 2013). Insomnia is also frequently comorbid with other sleep disorders. One of the most frequently studied comorbidities is sleep apnea (Sweetman et al., 2019a). Recent investigations show that insomnia and sleep apnea can be successfully treated concurrently and that CBT-I may help increase adherence to sleep apnea treatment (i.e., continuous positive airway pressure machine use) (Sweetman et al., 2019b; Sweetman et al., 2020).

Demographics

CBT-I is effective across populations and has demonstrated efficacy across the lifespan. For example, studies have found improved sleep and health outcomes in youth (Ma et al., 2018), adults (Natsky et al., 2020), and older adults (Rybarczyk et al., 2005). Moreover, sex does not appear to impact CBT-I's efficacy (Cheng et al., 2019), though more research is needed to understand the interaction between gender/sex and insomnia. A burgeoning line of research has become focused on treatment outcomes in minoritized populations, especially considering the impact of race on health disparities at all levels (Barr, 2014; Simmons et al., 2021). In insomnia, studies have found that racial discrimination is a significant mediator for sleep health disparities (Cheng et al., 2020). Although existing research is promising and suggests that CBT-I demonstrates comparable efficacy across ethnic/racial groups (Cheng et al., 2019), a fulsome investigation into the role of discrimination in sleep health and treatment outcomes is needed. Further research should evaluate whether inclusion of direct therapy work in CBT-I regarding the role of discrimination on sleep health adds unique value in marginalized populations.

Medication

Although behavioral treatments are considered first-line, it is important to mention pharmacotherapy as a treatment for insomnia and other sleep disorders. Research indicates that sleep medications are comparable in efficacy to CBT-I in the short-term (Mitchell et al., 2012); however, CBT-I's effect is more durable and is preferred by patients when given a choice (Cheung et al., 2018; Mitchell et al., 2012). Generally, medication does not influence the process and outcome of psychotherapy (Morin et al., 2009); however, medication use is recommended to be kept consistent, rather than contingent, in its use. Using medication at a similar time and dose supports positive sleep self-efficacy by avoiding situations where the patient takes medication reactively to thoughts of not being able to sleep.

In some sleep disorders, however, sleep medication is the first-line recommended treatment, such as restless legs syndrome (Earley & Silber, 2010) and narcolepsy (Thorpy, 2007).

Conclusion

Insomnia is a burdensome and costly condition, and CBT-I is a relatively short-term treatment with high potential impact. Indeed, CBT-I is the gold-standard treatment for insomnia and there is a strong empirical base supporting its efficacy. Moreover, there is support for its mechanisms. The etiological underpinnings of ID are that conditioned arousal, reduced sleep drive, and a dysregulated clock perpetuate chronic insomnia, and stimulus control and SRT have effects across these factors. SRT and sleep hygiene are the two behavioral components of CBT-I with some support as monotherapies, albeit not as strong as combining them in a multicomponent treatment. Sleep hygiene is not a recommended treatment and there is no empirical base for its recommendation as a stand-alone treatment for insomnia. CBT-I has been shown to be effective in children and adolescents and across several common comorbidities. With respect to the assessment of insomnia, subjective patient reports are the gold standard, as how patients perceive their symptoms is what matters. Burdensome objective measures of sleep disturbance don't necessarily relate to the patients' experience and the disorder is subjective.

Useful Resources

- American Academy of Sleep Medicine: www.aasm.org
- Association for Behavioral and Cognitive Therapies: www.abct.org
- Canadian Sleep Society: www.css-scs.ca
- Society for Behavioral Sleep Medicine: www.behavioralsleep.org

References

Achermann, P. (2004). The two-process model of sleep regulation revisited. *Aviation, Space, and Environmental Medicine*, 75(3), A37–A43.

American Psychological Association Division 12. (2022). Brief Summary Paradoxical Intention for Insomnia. https://div12.org/treatment/paradoxical-intention-for-insomnia/ (accessed February 22, 2023).

American Psychological Association. (2022). *Diagnostic and statistical manual of mental disorders: DSM-5-TR*. American Psychiatric Publications Inc.

Ascher, L. M., & Turner, R. M. (1979). Paradoxical intention and insomnia: an experimental investigation. *Behavior Research and Therapy*, 17(4), 408–411.

Barr, D. A. (2014). *Health disparities in the United States: Social class, race, ethnicity, and health*. Johns Hopkins University Press.

Benson K. L. (2015). Sleep in Schizophrenia: Pathology and Treatment. *Sleep Medicine Clinics*, 10(1), 49–55. https://doi.org/10.1016/j.jsmc.2014.11.001.

Blom, K., Jernelöv, S., Rück, C., Lindefors, N., & Kaldo, V. (2016). Three-year follow-up of insomnia and hypnotics after controlled internet treatment for insomnia. *Sleep*, 39(6), 1267–1274.

Boness, C. L., Hershenberg, R., Kaye, J., et al. (2020). An evaluation of cognitive behavioral therapy for insomnia: A systematic review and application of Tolin's Criteria for empirically supported treatments. *Clinical Psychology: Science and Practice*, 27(4), e12348.

Bonnet, M. H., & Arand, D. L. (2010). Hyperarousal and insomnia: state of the science. *Sleep Medicine Reviews*, 14(1), 9–15.

Bootzin, R. R. (1972). Stimulus control treatment for insomnia. *Proceedings of the American Psychological Association*, 7, 395–396.

Buysse, D. J., Reynolds III, C. F., Monk, T. H., Berman, S. R., & Kupfer, D. J. (1989). The Pittsburgh Sleep Quality Index: A new instrument for psychiatric practice and research. *Psychiatry Research*, 28(2), 193–213. https://doi.org/10.1016/0165-1781(89) 90047-4.

Carmona, N. E., Usyatynsky, A., Kutana, S., et al. (2021). A transdiagnostic self-management web-based app for sleep disturbance in adolescents and young adults: Feasibility and acceptability study. *JMIR Formative Research*, 5(11), e25392.

Carney, C. E., Buysse, D. J., Ancoli-Israel, S., et al. (2012). The consensus sleep diary: Standardizing prospective sleep self-monitoring. *Sleep*, 35(2), 287–302.

Cheng, P., Cuellar, R., Johnson, D. A., et al. (2020). Racial discrimination as a mediator of racial disparities in insomnia disorder. *Sleep Health*, 6(5), 543–549.

Cheng, P., Luik, A. I., Fellman-Couture, C., et al. (2019). Efficacy of digital CBT for insomnia to reduce depression across demographic groups: A randomized trial. *Psychological Medicine*, 49(3), 491–500.

Chesson Jr, A. L., Anderson, W. M., Littner, M., et al. (1999). Practice parameters for the nonpharmacologic treatment of chronic insomnia. *Sleep*, 22(8), 1128–1133.

Cheung, J. M., Bartlett, D. J., Armour, C. L., Saini, B., & Laba, T. L. (2018). Patient preferences for managing insomnia: A discrete choice experiment. *The Patient-Patient-Centered Outcomes Research*, 11(5), 503–514.

Chung, F., Abdullah, H. R., & Liao, P. (2016). STOP-Bang Questionnaire: A Practical Approach to Screen for Obstructive Sleep Apnea. *Chest*, 149(3), 631–638. https://doi.org/ 10.1378/chest.15-0903.

Chung, K. F., Lee, C. T., Yeung, W. F., et al. (2018). Sleep hygiene education as a treatment of insomnia: A systematic review and meta-analysis. *Family Practice*, 35(4), 365–375.

Clarke, G., McGlinchey, E. L., Hein, K., et al. (2015). Cognitive-behavioral treatment of insomnia and depression in adolescents: A pilot randomized trial. *Behaviour Research and Therapy*, 69, 111–118.

Colombo, C., Benedetti, F., Barbini, B., Campori, E., & Smeraldi, E. (1999). Rate of switch from depression into mania after therapeutic sleep deprivation in bipolar depression. *Psychiatry Research*, 86(3), 267–270.

Cox, R. C., & Olatunji, B. O. (2020). Sleep in the anxiety-related disorders: A meta-analysis of subjective and objective research. *Sleep Medicine Reviews*, 51, 101282. https://doi.org/10.1016/j.smrv.2020.101282.

de Bruin, E. J., Meijer, A., & Bögels, S. M. (2020). The contribution of a body scan mindfulness meditation to effectiveness of internet-delivered CBT for insomnia in adolescents. *Mindfulness*, 11, 872–882.

Dell'Aquila, J. T., & Soti, V. (2022). Sleep deprivation: A risk for epileptic seizures. *Sleep Science*, 15(2), 245–249.

Earley, C. J., & Silber, M. H. (2010). Restless legs syndrome: understanding its consequences and the need for better treatment. *Sleep Medicine*, 11(9), 807–815.

Edinger, J. D., Arnedt, J. T., Bertisch, S. M., et al. (2021). Behavioral and psychological treatments for chronic insomnia disorder in adults: An American Academy of Sleep Medicine clinical practice guideline. *Journal of Clinical Sleep Medicine*, 17(2), 255–262.

Edinger, J. D., Fins, A. I., Sullivan, R. J., Jr, et al. (1997). Sleep in the laboratory and sleep at home: Comparisons of older insomniacs and normal sleepers. *Sleep*, 20(12), 1119–1126. https://doi.org/10.1093/sleep/20.12.1119.

Edinger, J. D., Kirby, A. C., Lineberger, M. D. et al. (2006). Duke Structured Interview Schedule for DSM-IV-TR and International Classification of Sleep Disorders, Second Edition, Sleep Disorders Diagnoses. Veterans Affairs and Duke University Medical Centers.

Edinger, J. D., Wohlgemuth, W. K., Radtke, R. A., Marsh, G. R., & Quillian, R. E. (2001). Cognitive behavioral therapy for treatment of chronic primary insomnia: A randomized controlled trial. *JAMA*, 285(14), 1856–1864. https://doi.org/10.1001/jama.285.14.1856.

Epstein, D. R., Sidani, S., Bootzin, R. R., & Belyea, M. J. (2012). Dismantling multicomponent behavioral treatment for insomnia in older adults: A randomized controlled trial. *Sleep*, 35(6), 797–805. https://doi.org/10.5665/sleep.1878.

Espie, C. A., & Lindsay, W. R. (1987). Cognitive strategies for the management of severe sleep-maintenance insomnia: A preliminary investigation. *Behavioral and Cognitive Psychotherapy*, 15(4), 388–395.

Espie, C. A., Lindsay, W. R., Brooks, D. N., Hood, E. M., & Turvey, T. (1989). A controlled comparative investigation of psychological treatments for chronic sleep-onset insomnia. *Behavior Research and Therapy*, 27(1), 79–88.

Fang, H., Tu, S., Sheng, J., & Shao, A. (2019). Depression in sleep disturbance: A review on a bidirectional relationship, mechanisms and treatment. *Journal of Cellular and Molecular Medicine*, 23(4), 2324–2332. https://doi.org/10.1111/jcmm.14170.

Fernando III, A., Arroll, B., & Falloon, K. (2013). A double-blind randomised controlled study of a brief intervention of bedtime restriction for adult patients with primary insomnia. *Journal of Primary Health Care*, 5(1), 5–10.

Figueiro, M. G. (2016). Delayed sleep phase disorder: clinical perspective with a focus on light therapy. *Nature and Science of Sleep*, 8, 91–106.

Friedman, L., Benson, K., Noda, A., et al. (2000). An actigraphic comparison of sleep restriction and sleep hygiene treatments for insomnia in older adults. *Journal of Geriatric Psychiatry and Neurology*, 13(1), 17–27. https://doi.org/10.1177/089198870001300103.

Gehrman, P. R., Hall, M., Barilla, H., et al. (2016). Stress reactivity in insomnia. *Behavioral Sleep Medicine*, 14(1), 23–33.

Glovinsky, P. B., & Spielman, A. J. (1991). Sleep restriction therapy. In P. J. Hauri (Ed.), *Case studies in insomnia* (pp. 49–63). Springer.

Gong, H., Ni, C. X., Liu, Y. Z., et al. (2016). Mindfulness meditation for insomnia: A meta-analysis of randomized controlled trials. *Journal of Psychosomatic Research*, 89, 1–6.

Greeff, A. P., & Conradie, W. S. (1998). Use of progressive relaxation training for chronic alcoholics with insomnia. *Psychological Reports*, 82(2), 407–412. https://doi.org/10.2466/pr0.1998.82.2.407.

Guyatt, G. H., Oxman, A. D., Vist, G. E., et al. (2008). GRADE: An emerging consensus on rating quality of evidence and strength of recommendations. *BMJ*, 336(7650), 924–926.

Harris, J., Lack, L., Kemp, K., Wright, H., & Bootzin, R. (2012). A randomized controlled trial of intensive sleep retraining (ISR): A brief conditioning treatment for chronic insomnia. *Sleep*, 35(1), 49–60.

Harris, J., Lack, L., Wright, H., Gradisar, M., & Brooks, A. (2007). Intensive sleep retraining treatment for chronic primary insomnia: A preliminary investigation. *Journal of Sleep Research*, 16(3), 276–284.

Hartmann, J. A., Carney, C. E., Lachowski, A., & Edinger, J. D. (2015). Exploring the construct of subjective sleep quality in patients with insomnia. *The Journal of Clinical Psychiatry*, 76(6), e768–e773. https://doi.org/10.4088/JCP.14m09066.

Harvey, A. G. (2000). Sleep hygiene and sleep-onset insomnia. *Journal of Nervous and Mental Disease*, 188(1), 53–55.

Harvey, A. G. (2002). A cognitive model of insomnia. *Behavior Research and Therapy*, 40(8), 869–893.

Harvey, A. G. (2016). A transdiagnostic intervention for youth sleep and circadian problems. *Cognitive Behavioral Practice*, 23(3), 341–355.

Harvey, A. G., Hein, K., Dolsen, M. R., et al. (2018). Modifying the impact of eveningness chronotype ("night-owls") in youth: A randomized controlled trial. *Journal of the American Academy of Child and Adolescent Psychiatry*, 57(10), 742–754. https://doi.org/10.1016/j.jaac.2018.04.020.

Harvey, A. G., Hein, K., Dong, L., et al. (2016). A transdiagnostic sleep and circadian treatment to improve severe mental illness outcomes in a community setting: study protocol for a randomized controlled trial. *Trials*, 17(1), 606. https://doi.org/10.1186/s13063-016-1690-9.

Hiller, R. M., Johnston, A., Dohnt, H., Lovato, N., & Gradisar, M. (2015). Assessing cognitive processes related to insomnia: A review and measurement guide for Harvey's cognitive model for the maintenance of insomnia. *Sleep Medicine Reviews*, 23, 46–53.

Johnson, J. A., Rash, J. A., Campbell, T. S., et al. (2016). A systematic review and meta-analysis of randomized controlled trials of cognitive behavior therapy for insomnia (CBT-I) in cancer survivors. *Sleep Medicine Reviews*, 27, 20–28.

Kaplan, K. A., & Harvey, A. G. (2013). Behavioral treatment of insomnia in bipolar disorder. *American Journal of Psychiatry*, 170(7), 716–720.

Kay, D. B., Karim, H. T., Soehner, A. M., et al. (2016). Sleep-wake differences in relative regional cerebral metabolic rate for glucose among patients with insomnia compared with good sleepers. *Sleep*, 39(10), 1779–1794.

Lack, L., Scott, H., & Lovato, N. (2019). Intensive sleep retraining treatment of insomnia. *Sleep Medicine Clinics*, 14(2), 245–252.

Lacks, P., Bertelson, A. D., Sugerman, J., & Kunkel, J. (1983). The treatment of sleep-maintenance insomnia with stimulus-control techniques. *Behavior Research and Therapy*, 21(3), 291–295.

Ladouceur, R., & Gros-Louis, Y. (1986). Paradoxical intention vs stimulus control in the treatment of severe insomnia. *Journal of Behavior Therapy and Experimental Psychiatry*, 17(4), 267–269.

Loring, W. A., Johnston, R., Gray, L., Goldman, S., & Malow, B. (2016). A brief behavioral intervention for insomnia in adolescents with autism spectrum disorders. *Clinical Practice in Pediatric Psychology*, 4(2), 112–124.

Ma, Z. R., Shi, L. J., & Deng, M. H. (2018). Efficacy of cognitive behavioral therapy in children and adolescents with insomnia: A systematic review and meta-analysis. *Brazilian Journal of Medical and Biological Research*, 51(6), e7070.

Maurer, L. F., & Kyle, S. D. (2022). Efficacy of multicomponent CBT-I and its single components. *Cognitive-Behavioural Therapy For Insomnia (CBT-I) Across The Life Span: Guidelines and Clinical Protocols for Health Professionals*, 42–50.

Maurer, L. F., Espie, C. A., Omlin, X., Emsley, R., & Kyle, S. D. (2022). The effect of sleep restriction therapy for insomnia on sleep pressure and arousal: a randomized controlled mechanistic trial. *Sleep*, 45(1), zsab223. https://doi.org/10.1093/sleep/zsab223.

Maurer, L. F., Espie, C. A., Omlin, X., et al. (2020). Isolating the role of time in bed restriction in the treatment of insomnia: A randomized, controlled, dismantling trial comparing sleep restriction therapy with time in bed regularization. *Sleep*, 43(11), zsaa096. https://doi.org/10.1093/sleep/zsaa096.

McCall, C., & McCall, W. V. (2012). Objective vs. subjective measurements of sleep in depressed insomniacs: First night effect or reverse first night effect? *Journal of Clinical Sleep Medicine*, 8(1), 59–65. https://doi.org/10.5664/jcsm.1664.

McHugh, R. K., Whitton, S. W., Peckham, A. D., Welge, J. A., & Otto, M. W. (2013). Patient preference for psychological vs pharmacologic treatment of psychiatric disorders: A meta-analytic review. *The Journal of Clinical Psychiatry*, 74(6), 13979.

Means, M. K., Lichstein, K. L., Epperson, M. T., & Johnson, C. T. (2000). Relaxation therapy for insomnia: Nighttime and day time effects. *Behavior Research and Therapy*, 38(7), 665–678. https://doi.org/10.1016/s0005-7967(99)00091-1.

Meltzer, L. J., & Mindell, J. A. (2014). Systematic review and meta-analysis of behavioral interventions for pediatric insomnia. *Journal of Pediatric Psychology*, 39(8), 932–948.

Mitchell, M. D., Gehrman, P., Perlis, M., & Umscheid, C. A. (2012). Comparative effectiveness of cognitive behavioral therapy for insomnia: A systematic review. *BMC Family Practice*, 13(1), 1–11.

Morgenthaler, T., Kramer, M., Alessi, C., et al. (2006). Practice parameters for the psychological and behavioral treatment of insomnia: An update. An American academy of sleep medicine report. *Sleep*, 29(11), 1415–1419.

Morin, C. M. (1993). *Insomnia: Psychological assessment and management.* Guilford Press.

Morin, C. M. (2006). Cognitive-behavioral therapy of insomnia. *Sleep Medicine Clinics*, 1(3), 375–386.

Morin, C. M., & Azrin, N. H. (1988). Behavioral and cognitive treatments of geriatric insomnia. *Journal of Consulting and Clinical Psychology*, 56(5), 748–753. https://doi.org/10.1037//0022-006x.56.5.748.

Morin, C. M., Vallières, A., Guay, B., et al. (2009). Cognitive behavioral therapy, singly and combined with medication, for persistent insomnia: a randomized controlled trial. *JAMA*, 301(19), 2005–2015.

Moss, T. G., Lachowski, A. M., & Carney, C. E. (2013). What all treatment providers should know about sleep hygiene recommendations. *The Behavior Therapist*. 36(4), 76–83.

Natsky, A. N., Vakulin, A., Chai-Coetzer, C. L., et al. (2020). Economic evaluation of cognitive behavioral therapy for insomnia (CBT-I) for improving health outcomes in adult populations: A systematic review. *Sleep Medicine Reviews*, 54, 101351.

Nicassio, P., & Bootzin, R. (1974). A comparison of progressive relaxation and autogenic training as treatments for insomnia. *Journal of Abnormal Psychology*, 83(3), 253–260. https://doi.org/10.1037/h0036729.

Ong, J. C., Manber, R., Segal, Z., et al. (2014). A randomized controlled trial of mindfulness meditation for chronic insomnia. *Sleep*, 37(9), 1553–1563.

Perlis, M. L., Giles, D. E., Mendelson, W. B., Bootzin, R. R., & Wyatt, J. K. (1997). Psychophysiological insomnia: The behavioral model and a neurocognitive perspective. *Journal of Sleep Research*, 6(3), 179–188.

Perlis, M., Shaw, P. J., Cano, G., & Espie, C. A. (2011). Models of insomnia. *Principles and Practice of Sleep Medicine*, 5(1), 850–865.

Riedner, B. A., Goldstein, M. R., Plante, D. T., et al. (2016). Regional patterns of elevated alpha and high-frequency electroencephalographic activity during nonrapid eye movement sleep in chronic insomnia: A pilot study. *Sleep*, 39(4), 801–812.

Robertson, J. A., Broomfield, N. M., & Espie, C. A. (2007). Prospective comparison of subjective arousal during the pre-sleep period in primary sleep-onset insomnia and normal sleepers. *Journal of Sleep Research*, 16(2), 230–238.

Roenneberg, T., Kuehnle, T., Pramstaller, P. P., et al. (2004). A marker for the end of adolescence. *Current Biology: CB*, 14(24), R1038–R1039. https://doi.org/10.1016/j.cub.2004.11.039.

Rybarczyk, B., Lopez, M., Benson, R., Alsten, C., & Stepanski, E. (2002). Efficacy of two behavioral treatment programs for comorbid geriatric insomnia. *Psychology and Aging*, 17(2), 288–298.

Rybarczyk, B., Stepanski, E., Fogg, L., et al. (2005). A placebo-controlled test of cognitive-behavioral therapy for comorbid insomnia in older adults. *Journal of Consulting and Clinical Psychology*, 73(6), 1164.

Sateia, M. J., Buysse, D. J., Krystal, A. D., Neubauer, D. N., & Heald, J. L. (2017). Clinical practice guideline for the pharmacologic treatment of chronic insomnia in adults: An American Academy of Sleep Medicine clinical practice guideline. *Journal of Clinical Sleep Medicine*, 13(2), 307–349.

Sidani, S., Epstein, D. R., Bootzin, R. R., Moritz, P., & Miranda, J. (2009). Assessment of preferences for treatment: Validation of a measure. *Research in Nursing & Health*, 32(4), 419–431.

Sidani, S., Epstein, D. R., Fox, M., & Collins, L. (2019). Comparing the effects of single-and multiple-component therapies for insomnia on sleep outcomes. *Worldviews on Evidence-Based Nursing*, 16(3), 195–203.

Simmons, A., Chappel, A., Kolbe, A. R., Bush, L., & Sommers, B. D. (2021). Health disparities by race and ethnicity during the Covid-19 pandemic: Current evidence and policy approaches. *Washington, DC: Office of the Assistant Secretary for Planning and Evaluation, US Department of Health and Human Services.*

Spielman, A. J., Caruso, L. S., & Glovinsky, P. B. (1987). A behavioral perspective on insomnia treatment. *Psychiatric Clinics of North America*, 10(4), 541–553.

Spielman, A. J., Yang, C. M., & Glovinsky, P. B. (2016). Insomnia: Sleep restriction therapy. In S. Buysse, (Ed.) *Insomnia* (pp. 293–305). CRC Press.

Sweetman, A., Lack, L., & Bastien, C. (2019a). Co-morbid insomnia and sleep apnea (COMISA): Prevalence, consequences, methodological considerations, and recent randomized controlled trials. *Brain Sciences*, 9(12), 371. https://doi.org/10.3390/brainsci9120371.

Sweetman, A., Lack, L., Catcheside, P. G., et al. (2019b). Cognitive and behavioral therapy for insomnia increases the use of continuous positive airway pressure therapy in obstructive sleep apnea participants with comorbid insomnia: A randomized clinical trial. *Sleep*, 42(12), zsz178. https://doi.org/10.1093/sleep/zsz178.

Sweetman, A., Lack, L., McEvoy, R. D., et al. (2020). Cognitive behavioral therapy for insomnia reduces sleep apnoea severity: a randomised controlled trial. *ERJ Open Research*, 6(2), 00161–2020. https://doi.org/10.1183/23120541.00161-2020.

Thorpy, M. (2007). Therapeutic advances in narcolepsy. *Sleep Medicine*, 8(4), 427–440.

Tolin, D. F., McKay, D., Forman, E. M., Klonsky, E. D., & Thombs, B. D. (2015). Empirically supported treatment: Recommendations for a new model. *Clinical Psychology: Science and Practice*, 22(4), 317.

van Geijlswijk, I. M., Korzilius, H. P., & Smits, M. G. (2010). The use of exogenous melatonin in delayed sleep phase disorder: a meta-analysis. *Sleep*, 33(12), 1605–1614.

Wilson, S. J., Nutt, D. J., Alford, C., et al. (2010). British Association for Psychopharmacology consensus statement on evidence-based treatment of insomnia, parasomnias and circadian rhythm disorders. *Journal of Psychopharmacology*, 24(11), 1577–1601.

Wohlgemuth, W. K., Edinger, J. D., Fins, A. I., & Sullivan Jnr., R. J. (1999). How many nights are enough? The short-term stability of sleep parameters in elderly insomniacs and normal sleepers. *Psychophysiology*, 36(2), 233–244.

Woodley, J., & Smith, S. (2006). Safety behaviors and dysfunctional beliefs about sleep: Testing a cognitive model of the maintenance of insomnia. *Journal of Psychosomatic Research*, 60(6), 551–557.

Woolfolk, R. L., Carr-Kaffashan, L., McNulty, T. F., & Lehrer, P. M. (1976). Meditation training as a treatment for insomnia. *Behavior Therapy*, 7(3), 359–365.

Wu, J. Q., Appleman, E. R., Salazar, R. D., & Ong, J. C. (2015). Cognitive behavioral therapy for insomnia comorbid with psychiatric and medical conditions: A meta-analysis. *JAMA Internal Medicine*, 175(9), 1461–1472.

11

Sexual Dysfunctions

Amy D. Lykins and Marta Meana

Sexuality was at the center of early psychodynamic theorizing about the etiology of psychological conflict, but it was not until Masters and Johnson (1970) introduced sex therapy that sexual dysfunction became the specific target of treatment. Equipped with their model of the sexual response cycle as consisting of the distinct and sequential stages of excitement, plateau, orgasm, and resolution, they proceeded to develop interventions specific to the challenges therein. Kaplan (1979) later introduced desire as a first motivational stage and pared the model down to three phases: desire, arousal, and orgasm. It is this triphasic model that has been the organizing principle behind the seven sexual dysfunctions not directly attributable to a substance or medication in the latest version of the *Diagnostic and Statistical Manual of Mental Disorders* (DSM-5-TR; American Psychiatric Association, 2022) and those that preceded it (see Pukall, 2023 for a critique of these early conceptualizations). A heterogeneous group of disorders with varying etiologies and gender-specific manifestations, they are clustered together as a function of their interference with sexual activity, responsivity, and/or pleasure, as well as associated distress with said interference. Using the three morbidity criteria in the DSM-5 (6-month persistence, experienced on 75–100% of sexual encounters, and causing significant distress), most dysfunctions are relatively prevalent when assessed for their presence in the past year (population prevalence rates range from 5.2% to 25.0%[1]) and can result in significant relationship challenges.

Disorders of desire are characterized by deficient or absent sexual thoughts, fantasies, and/or desire for sexual activity. In men, this problem is diagnosed as male hypoactive sexual desire disorder (MHSDD; 5.2% prevalence rate), with low estimated prevalence rates in young men that increase with age (Corona et al., 2013); in women, low desire and arousal problems (lack of response to sexual cues and/or absent or reduced physical sensations) are combined under the diagnostic criteria for

---

[1] Please note that all prevalence rates have been reported as per Mitchell et al.'s (2016) population-based assessment of sexual function problems.

female sexual interest/arousal disorder (FSIAD), a much more commonly presenting disorder (9.1% prevalence rate; Mitchell et al., 2013, 2016). The disorder of arousal specific to men is erectile disorder (ED; 14.1% prevalence rate), characterized by significant difficulty in obtaining or maintaining an erection, and/or a marked decrease in erectile rigidity, a dysfunction with an increasing prevalence rate as men age (Lewis et al., 2010). Disorders relating to orgasm are also gender specific. Delayed ejaculation (DE) (5.5% prevalence rate) and female orgasmic disorder (FOD) (11.6% prevalence rate) entail problems achieving orgasm, including reduced intensity of orgasmic sensations. Men can also be diagnosed with premature (early) ejaculation (PE) (11.6% prevalence rate) when orgasm occurs within one minute of vaginal penetration (and before the person wishes it). Finally, genito-pelvic pain/ penetration disorder (GPPPD) (25.0% prevalence rate) combines the old DSM-IV diagnoses of dyspareunia and vaginismus and encompasses a number of conditions (e.g., vulvodynia, age-related vaginal atrophy) that can cause pain with penetration, as well as a phobic anxiety and fear of penetration most commonly associated with vaginismus in the past. It is a relatively common disorder currently diagnosed only in women (Christensen et al., 2011; Pukall et al., 2016).

Etiology and Theoretical Underpinnings of Treatment

Historically, etiological factors for impaired sexual performance have swung from psychological to physical explanations and back again, finally settling on the more holistic biopsychosocial approach (Meana & Hall, 2023). The etiological drivers of sexual dysfunctions are as multifaceted as their clinical presentations (e.g., Bancroft, 2009) and are generally multifactorial; all potential biological, psychological, and relational factors should be considered as part of a comprehensive clinical assessment. The DSM-5-TR (APA, 2022) specifies five areas of consideration for assessment, as they are known to be associated with sexual functioning: (1) partner factors, including comorbid partner dysfunction or physical health issues; (2) relationship factors, such as poor communication and discrepant desire; (3) intrapersonal factors, such as poor body image, histories of abuse, comorbid psychological problems, and high levels of stress; (4) the client's cultural and religious context, as it affects sexual scripts and the value placed on sexual pleasure; and (5) common medical problems (e.g., injuries, infections, cardiovascular diseases) that can impact sexual function.

Masters and Johnson's groundbreaking new sex therapy approached treatment from a cognitive-behavioral perspective and included components of psychoeducation (based on the premise that many sexual problems were the result of a lack of sexual knowledge), along with cognitive interventions and behavioral exercises. In positing that performance anxiety lay at the heart of sexual dysfunction, therapy aimed to remove goal-based performance and replace it with a focus on pleasure, using both behavioral and, to a lesser degree, cognitive techniques. Components of systematic desensitization, guided practice, and cognitive restructuring remain important elements of treatment for sexual dysfunctions 50 years later. Growing recognition of the relevance of physiological factors also led to the rise of sexual medicine and the integration of pharmaceutical and physiological treatments into therapies for sexual dysfunction. Best practice recommendations advise that these multidisciplinary treatment approaches be implemented concurrently for optimal outcomes (Binik & Meana, 2009).

Brief Overview of Treatments

Due to the heterogeneous nature of the disorders classified as sexual dysfunctions, there is no "one-size-fits-all" treatment package for intervention. A woman experiencing pain with intercourse will be treated very differently than a man experiencing erectile difficulties. On the other hand, it is likely that, despite radically different etiologies to their problem, both are engaging in thoughts and behaviors that maintain or compound the problem. It is also likely that patterns of communication between them and their partners have become dysregulated around this specific issue, further complicating the situation. Consequently, there are significant commonalities across treatment packages as they target the cognitive, emotional, behavioral, and relational dynamics that can either hinder or facilitate treatment progress.

The overall level of research support for the psychological treatment of sexual dysfunctions is poor. Despite Masters and Johnson's early claims of high efficacy with brief, time-limited interventions, these results have either failed to be replicated or have simply not been revisited with today's more rigorous research standards (see Fruhauf et al., 2013 for systematic review and meta-analysis). Psychological interventions for most disorders would not have met the criteria for "well established" efficacy as defined by Chambless et al. (1998), not to mention the far more stringent standards of the Tolin et al. (2015) criteria. Relatively few randomized control trials (RCTs) have been conducted on psychological interventions for sexual dysfunctions, and they are of varying quality (Fruhauf et al., 2013). As per the aforementioned review, there is good evidence for the effectiveness of psychological interventions for sexual desire and orgasm problems in women; however, no consistent reductions in symptom severity for ED, PE, or vaginismus were observed in their analyses. Most of the more recent RCTs have assessed the efficacy of treatment for GPPPD, in which surgical (Landry et al., 2008) and physical therapy (Morin et al., 2017) interventions continue to evidence the best outcomes.

The relative lack of high-quality RCTs for sexual dysfunctions makes it difficult to draw conclusions on psychological treatment efficacy with any confidence. As discussed by Meana and colleagues (2020), the reasons for this gap are likely both practical and philosophical. Research on sex therapy interventions is notably underfunded, particularly in the United States. The preference for a simple pill, and the financial incentive for pharmaceutical companies to develop and deliver said pill, far outweighs any monetary motivation for outcome assessments of psychological interventions. As a result, most of the RCTs for sexual dysfunctions have investigated the treatment efficacy of available pharmaceutical options, leaving the efficacy of psychotherapeutic interventions relatively uncharted.

Perhaps most importantly, a consistent and agreed-upon definition for outcome success in sexual dysfunction intervention is evasive. Restoring "function" in someone with a "dysfunction" can sometimes be clear: a man with PE can now have sex for longer than one minute, a woman previously experiencing pain during intercourse no longer does so, or a man with ED can obtain an erection sufficiently rigid for penetration. In other cases, despite improvements, the man may still not last as long as he or his partner desires, or intercourse pain may not completely remit, or desire may have increased but continues to pale in comparison to a partner's. Where does the treatment success line lie? A growing number of therapists and researchers are banking on sexual satisfaction and the reduction of distress as the only truly viable treatment outcome measures, as originally proposed by Rosen and Bachman (2008). This may seem a capitulation to treatment indeterminacy but, arguably, increasing sexual satisfaction can, in turn, have a powerful impact on function when it can be restored. In cases in which it cannot, such as age-related changes that are not easily amenable to change, finding alternate ways to achieve sexual satisfaction can be fruitful outcome goals. Additionally, given the multifactorial nature of sexual dysfunction etiology, there are a variety of issues that could present as sexual problems that may require techniques that do not address sexual functioning specifically, including increasing self-esteem and body image, reducing life stressors, and addressing problematic relationship dynamics. If these lead to greater sexual and relationship satisfaction even in the face of unremitting or reduced function problems, this would be considered a "success" by many psychotherapists and clients. Ultimately, sexuality is not about plumbing as much as it is about pleasure and human connection, both of which happily can arise in many ways.

Credible Components of Treatments

In 2009, Binik and Meana provided a detailed table that matched the major components of psychotherapy interventions that are implemented in the treatment of sexual dysfunctions. Their goal was twofold: first, to emphasize the many commonalities across the treatment of different dysfunctions, and second, to demonstrate that most interventions are well within the toolkit of general therapists who might want to join the effort to treat these highly prevalent problems. These interventions, covered in the following section, remain the most commonly utilized, as well as ones that have demonstrated treatment efficacy, if not always as rigorously as would be optimal.

Psychoeducation

Delivery of psychoeducation on the basic features of sexual response and skills is typically the first step in therapy for sexual dysfunctions, though the focus of this information is guided by the person's presenting problems. Psychoeducation was more prominent when sex therapy was in its early years and the public did not have access to the vast resources that are today available from a personal computer, tablet, or phone. However, the general public still struggles to obtain reliable sex information, and myths about sexual performance continue to abound in media depictions and pornography.

Normalizing desire discrepancies in couples (Herbenick et al., 2014), explaining how women's sexual desire may more often be responsive rather than appetitive (Basson, 2000), and deconstructing the myth that men's sexual desire should be unwavering are important psychoeducation points. Communicating information on the physiology of erectile function, as well as normative age- and health-related declines, can help normalize erectile problems and reduce stigma (Kalogeropoulos & Larouche, 2020). Specifically, communicating how physical (e.g., cardiovascular diseases) and mental (e.g., depression, anxiety, stress) health conditions and relationship conflict can affect erectile function may also support lifestyle changes and the inclusion of additional mental health support.

For women with difficulties attaining orgasm, basic education on sexual anatomy and response, as well as information about types of stimulation that are likely to lead to orgasm, may be helpful (Carvalheira & Leal, 2013; Meana, 2012). Informing clients that most women cannot reach orgasm with vaginal penetration alone (Mintz, 2017) can normalize their experience and lead partners to alternate forms of stimulation. Encouraging genital self-exploration can help women learn what they find pleasurable, which they can then direct their partners to do (Meana, 2012). For men with PE, simply knowing what normative intravaginal ejaculatory latency times are can go a long way toward dispelling misconceptions about how long men should "last." Genital self-exploration can also be useful for women experiencing GPPPD to identify locations of pain (Bergeron et al., 2020), and psychoeducation about the multifactorial nature of pain – how anxiety, hypervigilance, catastrophizing, and solicitous partner responses can serve to maintain it (Rosen & Bergeron, 2019) – is effective, as evidenced in outcome studies (Meana & Binik, 2022).

Cognitive Restructuring/Emotional Regulation

Consistent with cognitive-behavioral approaches for many nonsexual psychological disorders, cognitive restructuring and emotional regulation practices are commonly employed in sexual dysfunction intervention. Theories of, and a great deal of supporting empirical data on, the development of sexual dysfunction point to performance anxiety and/or cognitive distraction as major drivers of sexual difficulties (Barlow, 1986; McCabe, 2005; Nobre & Pinto-Gouveia, 2008). Understanding and targeting cognitive distortions and schemas that contribute to performance anxiety and negative automatic and maladaptive thoughts is an important component of psychotherapy for sexual dysfunctions. Poor body image and negative attitudes about sex (e.g., guilt and shame) have been shown to contribute to FSIAD (Brotto et al., 2016); cognitive psychotherapeutic techniques are used to challenge these negative thoughts and promote the development of more positive thoughts and attitudes. ED in men can be addressed with the use of positive visualization techniques to overcome existing anxiety (such as imagining successfully obtaining an erection) and addressing myths and misconceptions about men's virility (e.g., "real men are always ready and able to obtain an erection") (Kalogeropoulos & Larouche, 2020). Similarly, targeting other types of maladaptive thoughts and beliefs (e.g., "all men can put off orgasming as long as they want") and reducing high emotional reactivity has shown efficacy in treating PE (Rowland & Cooper, 2017). Addressing cognitive distraction by working to bring attention back to the physical pleasure experienced during sexual encounters is a common component of sexual dysfunction interventions, including for FSIAD (Brotto, 2018; Meana, 2012), FOD (Meana, 2012), and GPPPD (Meana et al., 2023) in women, and ED (Rowland, 2012) and DE (Meana et al., 2023) in men.

Cognitive restructuring and emotion regulation are of particular importance in the treatment of women who experience pain during sex. Rosen and Bergeron (2019) proposed the Interpersonal Emotion Regulation Model of women's sexual dysfunction, and provided a particularly in-depth exploration of how this model applies to the multifaceted experiences of women's genito-pelvic pain. In this model, both proximal and distal factors are posited to influence how the couple experiences difficulties with emotional awareness, expression, and experience, and how their use of more adaptive (e.g., reappraisal, approach, acceptance, mindfulness, problem-solving, disclosure) or less adaptive (e.g., avoidance, suppression, catastrophizing, emotional outbursts) emotion regulation strategies can result in different outcomes with respect to genito-pelvic pain and overall sexual and relationship satisfaction. Accordingly, cognitive and emotion regulation therapy techniques may be used to encourage positive, adaptive coping strategies, as well as to manage relevant proximal and distal factors contributing to the development and maintenance of these poor emotion regulation strategies (Bergeron et al., 2020; Rosen & Bergeron, 2019). Given that this is a relatively new theoretical model, empirical data are scant at this time but starting to accumulate. For example, in one recent study, Bergeron and colleagues (2021) found that perceived partner emotional responsiveness was associated with greater sexual function and sexual satisfaction in women with GPPPD.

Stimulus Control/Desensitization

Many of the behavioral techniques used to complement the cognitive and emotional components of therapy for sexual dysfunctions comprise different versions of stimulus control or desensitization. Some methods have general applicability, whereas others have been designed for specific disorders.

Sensate focus exercises are generally considered relevant to the treatment of all sexual dysfunctions. Sensate focus typically involves a temporary ban on intercourse followed by a graduated series of exercises moving from nongenital sensual massage to sensual genital touching, with intercourse only being reintroduced after these earlier sessions have been completed. This process aims to remove any existing goal-oriented performance anxiety and cognitive distraction, and to allow space for focusing on pleasurable sensations. Recent reviews have supported the efficacy of sensate focus exercises in treating sexual problems, though it should be noted that most of these studies have combined sensate focus with other intervention methods (e.g., cognitive-behavioral therapy, mindfulness) (Avery-Clark et al., 2019; Linschoten et al., 2016).

Directed masturbation is often recommended for both male and female orgasm disorders, as well as ED. Following psychoeducation and genital exploration, treatment success for directed masturbation for women with lifelong FOD ranges from 60–90% (Laan et al., 2013). When highly prescribed and/or unusual methods of masturbation are considered to be contributing to DE in men, it is recommended that men work to shape their masturbation patterns to more closely approximate the speed and friction provided by intercourse (Perelman, 2004). Kalogeropoulos and Larouche (2020) also recommend directed masturbation to be used in the treatment of ED by bringing more awareness to one's sexual response and helping to build confidence and perceptions of control.

When GPPPD is related to penetration anxiety, the Fear-Avoidance Model has been useful in providing a "map" for understanding potential etiological and maintenance factors that can be targeted in treatment (ter Kuile et al., 2010). Briefly, this model proposes that negative beliefs about or experiences with vaginal penetration predispose a woman toward pain catastrophizing, resulting in fear, hypervigilance, and, ultimately, avoidance. Research has shown that when penetration is attempted, penetration-related fear and associated pelvic floor tension can be such that penetration either cannot occur or is experienced as painful (thus reinforcing the fear and avoidance) (Lahaie et al., 2015; Reissing et al., 2004). Accordingly, exposure-based interventions have been trialed and found to be effective (ter Kuile et al., 2013). These exposure exercises typically involve gradual exposure to increasingly larger sized dilators (or fingers) used for vaginal penetration (ter Kuile & Reissing, 2020).

Finally, several techniques have been developed specifically for the treatment of PE; these include the "squeeze" and the "stop-start" techniques. The squeeze technique involves the man indicating to his partner when he feels ejaculation is imminent, at which point sexual stimulation stops and the partner applies pressure to the glans until arousal lessens. The stop-start technique is performed as described above; however, the couple simply pauses sexual stimulation. The goal of these techniques is to help the client become more aware of different levels of excitement so that he can attain better control over ejaculation (Althof, 2020). Though later efficacy assessments have not reached the levels of success reported by Masters and Johnson, these techniques continue to be used in the treatment of PE (Meana & Hall, 2023).

Behavioral, Situational, and Contextual Modifications

Important components of behavioral, situational, and contextual modifications are regularly utilized in the treatment of sexual dysfunctions. In women with FSIAD and men with MHSDD, this may involve a greater consideration and modification of contextual conditions (e.g., timing, environment) to ensure that they facilitate desire and arousal. Women with FOD may be asked to role-play losing control to lessen pre-existing anxiety associated with orgasm (Laan et al., 2013). Men with DE may be asked to discontinue masturbating altogether (Meana et al., 2023), and men with ED may be asked to address lifestyle factors that contribute to erectile problems (e.g., lose weight, stop smoking) (Harte & Meston, 2013; Silva et al., 2017). Assessing and modifying restricted sexual scripts and behavioral repertoires is worth considering for all sexual problems.

Mindfulness

More recently, third-wave therapeutic techniques have been trialed in the treat-ment of some female sexual dysfunctions, with promising results. According to Brotto and Heiman (2007), mindfulness-based interventions aim to promote and nurture active, nonjudgmental, and compassionate awareness of the body and its sensations, resembling some aspects of older sensate focus techniques in com-bination with more recently developed mindfulness intervention techniques. This body of literature is in the early stages, but three randomized controlled studies have shown success in increasing sexual desire, arousal, and relationship satis-faction, and decreasing sexual distress in women with FSIAD (Brotto et al., 2021); improving sexual function and satisfaction, and reducing sexual distress in women with FOD (Adam et al., 2020); and reducing pain in women with GPPPD (Brotto et al., 2019), indicating that mindfulness may be a useful addition to the sex therapy toolkit.

Relationship Skills-Building

Most people seeking sex therapy are in some type of relationship, and difficulties therein can serve as etiological factors for sexual dysfunctions (and vice versa) (McCabe & Cobain, 1998; Velten & Margraf, 2017). As such, relationship skills-building exercises are common components of psychotherapeutic interventions for sexual dysfunction. Therapy should address any obvious discord present in the relationship, which may include hostility, resentment, and relationship insecurity (Perelman & Rowland, 2006; Rowland & Cooper, 2017). Couples may need to learn how to navigate desire discrepancies without increasing hostility and conflict (Meana, 2012), highlighting the importance of communication training. Issues related to communication become particularly relevant when managing pain during intercourse, as interaction patterns may develop that are, ironically, pain-reinforcing (Meana et al., 2023). Partner responses to pain can vary from solicitous (e.g., attention, sympathy), to negative (e.g., hostility, frustration), to facilitative (e.g., affection and adaptive coping); research has indicated that facilitative responses are associated with lower reports of genito-pelvic pain, and greater sexual and relationship satisfaction (Rosen & Bergeron, 2019).

Other Variables Influencing Treatment

Assessment and Diagnosis

As with any psychological disorder, it is important to conduct a comprehensive clinical assessment prior to the commencement of treatment. This is especially salient in the case of sexual dysfunctions, given their generally multifactorial etiologies. A detailed case conceptualization – comprising predisposing, precipitating, perpetuating, and protective factors from a biopsychosocial perspective – will help to provide a holistic understanding of how the sexual problem started, what factors are involved in the maintenance cycle, and strengths to draw upon in treatment. Ideally, this assessment is conducted with both members of a couple if the presenting client is partnered. Notable rule-outs include medical conditions that have caused the dysfunction (APA, 2022); a physician's assessment may assist with eliminating these potential explanations. Although even medically induced sexual dysfunctions often have psychological components, psychotherapy alone in these cases is likely inappropriate. Several standardized and freely available sexual dysfunction screening questionnaires exist that may be useful in clinical assessment, though they should never be fully relied upon for diagnosis. The Female Sexual Function Inventory (FSFI; Rosen et al., 2000) is a useful measure for women, and the International Index of Erectile Function (IIEF; Rosen et al., 1997) is a valid screener for male sexual dysfunctions (not just erectile dysfunction, despite its title). If indicated, daily diaries may be used to record the frequency of sexual activity and associated experiences. Additionally, in the case

Box 11.1 Comprehensive Sex Education for Youth

A number of different methods for youth sex education have been developed over the years, which typically vary by different definitions, goals, and philosophies (Goldfarb & Lieberman, 2021). Large review studies have concluded that *prevention programs*, such as abstinence-only education, largely do not appear to reduce unprotected sexual activity, youth pregnancy rates, or rates of sexually transmitted infections (Chin et al., 2012), and may even contribute to higher rates of teen pregnancy (Stanger-Hall & Hall, 2011).

Because abstinence-only programs have proved to be only marginally more effective than no education at all, and not especially effective even in their intended aims (e.g., Hall et al., 2016), sex educators are more likely to promote the use of *comprehensive sex education programs*. This approach involves education on "the sexual knowledge, beliefs, attitudes, values, and behaviors of individuals. Its various dimensions involve the anatomy, physiology, and biochemistry of the sexual response system; identity, orientation, roles, and personality; and thoughts, feelings, and relationships" (SIECUS, 2018, para 1). A review by Goldfarb and Lieberman (2021) concludes that there is "substantial evidence" supporting comprehensive sex education that begins in primary school and is scaffolded in a developmentally appropriate manner across K–12 educational programs. In addition to reducing rates of teen pregnancy over no sex education, which abstinence-only education does not do (Kohler et al., 2008), the more positive and rights-based comprehensive sex education programs have been found to lower homophobia and reduce homophobic bullying; expand a student's understanding of gender and gender norms; promote the recognition of gender equity, rights, and social justice; improve knowledge and attitudes about, and reporting of, both dating and intimate partner violence; decrease intimate violent behavior and victimization; promote healthy relationships by increasing knowledge, attitudes, and communication skills in relationships; and contribute to child sex abuse prevention (Goldfarb & Lieberman, 2021). In summary, it appears that the best prevention of negative outcomes in teen sexuality and relationships is knowledge rather than prohibition.

of ED, sexual psychophysiological assessment (i.e., Penile Doppler ultrasound) may be indicated, along with a referral to a urologist.

To ensure that sexual symptoms are not transient and are simply reflective of normal fluctuations in sexual functioning, the diagnosis of sexual dysfunction (other than substance/medication-induced sexual dysfunction) requires that the symptoms have persisted for at least six months. Three types of diagnostic specifiers must also be identified in diagnosis. A *lifelong* problem has been present from the beginning of a person's sexual experiences, whereas *acquired* problems begin after a period of normal sexual functioning. *Generalized* sexual problems are not limited to certain types of stimulation, situations, or partners, whereas *situational* problems are. Lastly, the severity of the client's distress about the presenting problem(s) must be rated as *mild*, *moderate*, or *severe*. *Distress* is probably the most relevant of the diagnostic criteria; if distress is not present, neither a diagnosis nor treatment is indicated.

Other diagnostic issues of note include the shift in disorder definitions and diagnostic criteria across different versions of the *DSM*. In moving from the fourth to the fifth edition, the diagnostic criteria for women, in particular, underwent significant revision. As mentioned, previous diagnoses of hypoactive sexual desire disorder and female sexual arousal disorder were collapsed into one diagnosis of FSIAD. Similarly, previous diagnoses of dyspareunia and vaginismus were collapsed into a diagnosis of GPPPD. Thus, much of the research prior to 2013 may have assessed components of the current diagnoses, but how well they address treatment outcome for the currently defined disorders requires further investigation.

Comorbidity

Given how important satisfying sexual relationships are to overall relationship satisfaction, it should come as no surprise that sexual dysfunctions often present comorbid with other psychological, sexual, and medical difficulties. Perhaps most commonly, sexual dysfunctions present as comorbid with other sexual dysfunctions or with partner sexual dysfunction (Mitchell et al., 2016; Nobre et al., 2006). Persistent desire and orgasm difficulties are commonly comorbid in both men (both premature and delayed ejaculation) and women (Mitchell et al., 2016). Low desire and deficient arousal can also exacerbate intercourse pain in women with GPPPD, as these conditions can result in reduced vaginal lubrication, thereby increasing the potential for pain. A variety of medical problems (e.g., cardiovascular diseases, diabetes) and mood disorders (e.g., depression, anxiety) also frequently present along with various sexual problems (Laurent & Simons, 2009; Polland et al., 2018; van Lankveld & Grotjohann, 2000). Comorbidity studies are generally correlational and cannot directly address causality but, in the case of mental health problems, it is reasonable to posit that their relationship with sexual dysfunction is bidirectional.

Demographics

Critically, the DSM-5-TR (APA, 2022) notes that gender-diverse people may not fit neatly into the binary gender constructs that currently separate some sexual dysfunction diagnoses. Unless specifically defined by anatomy (e.g., ED, PE, DE, GPPPD), diagnoses can be applied to gender-diverse individuals as judged to be clinically relevant. Also worth noting are the normative age-related declines in sexual functioning which can contribute to desire, arousal, and orgasm difficulties;

a comprehensive diagnostic assessment will help delineate between the consequences of normative aging processes and clinical disorders. Lastly, the great
majority of the research conducted on sexual function has been conducted on
members of so-called "WEIRD" (i.e., Western, educated, industrialized, rich, and
democratic) societies, which represent only 12% of the world's population (Henrich
et al., 2010). As Hall and Graham (2020) have noted, culture exacts a significant
influence on sexual behaviors, norms, and expectations. Studies investigating the
prevalence and experiences of sexual dysfunctions cross-culturally have found
a great deal of variation in what people report as problematic. Furthermore, given
that much of sex therapy was developed in these WEIRD societies, their utility in
more diverse communities is currently unknown (Hall & Graham, 2020). This gap
in knowledge requires targeted investigation to ensure that we are conducting sex
research with diverse populations and delivering sex therapy interventions in
a humble and culturally responsive manner.

Medication

Given the biopsychosocial nature of sexual dysfunctions, multiple treatment options
may be required to target different aspects of these experiences. Concurrent multidisciplinary treatment modalities have shown efficacy in intervention for several sexual
dysfunctions, although more research on this team approach is needed (Binik &
Meana, 2009). While multimethod treatments delivered by a coordinated team of
specialists is not a novel idea, the power in these interventions derives from their
concurrent (rather than serial) implementation, so that treatment gains in one area can
reinforce those in others.

Outcome research has revealed good efficacy of concurrent psychotherapeutic
and medical interventions. A combined psychotherapy and medical approach for
treating PE – typically involving medications known to delay orgasm (e.g.,
selective serotonin reuptake inhibitors) or topical agents that reduce penile
sensitivity – have shown superior efficacy to either method alone (Althof,
2020). Likewise, the recommended approach for the treatment of ED involves
psychotherapy delivered with a PDE-5 inhibitor (e.g., sildenafil), as in one study,
while both PDE-5 inhibitor alone and PDE-5 inhibitor plus cognitive-behavioral
sex therapy showed efficacy in improving erectile function, only the combined
treatment also resulted in improved couple sexual satisfaction and female sexual
function (Boddi et al., 2015). Recommended treatment protocols for women with
GPPPD involve psychotherapy, pelvic floor physical therapy, and, if indicated,
vestibulectomy (i.e., excision of the posterior hymen and painful mucosa in the
posterior and anterior vestibule) (Landry et al., 2008; Meana & Binik, 2022;
Morin et al., 2017). To date, research has not examined the extent to which
somatic treatments help or hinder psychological therapy for GPPPD.

Conclusion

Sex therapy continues to thrive despite the paucity of sound empirical studies attesting to its effectiveness. The treatment components covered here represent the core of clinical practice, some with direct empirical support from studies on participants with sexual dysfunction and others with empirical support from the larger body of cognitive-behavioral therapy applied to any number of disorders. In the absence of funding for treatment outcome studies, sex therapists continue to respond to their clients' appeals for help with theoretically sound practices that represent reasonable choices. The Masters and Johnson promise of highly effective short treatments did not pan out quite as simply as they claimed, but they drew much-needed attention to sexual concerns and laid a foundation that has persisted to a large extent. In order to confidently assert sex therapy's efficacy for different dysfunctions, we would have to witness a dramatic increase in RCTs. However, that is not to say that current practice is not effective; we simply do not know the extent to which it is effective in the case of most sexual dysfunctions. On the other hand, the core elements of psychoeducation, cognitive restructuring/emotional regulation, stimulus control, behavioral/contextual/ situational modification, mindfulness, and relationship skill building are hardly esoteric. They are at the heart of current cognitive-behavioral therapy practice and they boast empirical support in the treatment of a large number of psychological challenges. Their importation into the sex therapy enterprise seems wise as we await further empirical validation.

The undeniably physical component of the sexual response also challenges sex therapists to collaborate with physical therapists, gynecologists, and urologists to build treatment teams that can simultaneously target all reasonably identified etiological factors. This will no doubt complicate the treatment outcome research effort, but there is little sense in testing only one component of what in many cases will be a multidisciplinary treatment. An additional challenge is the definition of treatment success across dysfunctions and the roles of sexual satisfaction and distress reduction versus improvements in actual function. Looking ahead, treatment for sexual dysfunctions will also have to grapple with socioeconomic and cultural considerations, not to mention the more complex sexual and gender identity landscape that we now know to be more characteristic of our clients than we previously appreciated. Thus, clinical practice continues in the face of these challenges, and in light of these opportunities to broaden the horizon of treatment for sexual dysfunctions. The scientific enterprise in support of sex therapy is likely to continue lagging behind the highly needed practice of sex therapy. We cannot wait for science to catch up, as clients' distress is in the here and now. We can, however, continue to adhere to evidence-based treatments that should reasonably transfer to the aid of sexual challenges.

Useful Resources

- Brotto, L. A., & Nagoski, E. (2018). *Better sex through mindfulness: How women can cultivate desire*. Greystone Books.
- Goldstein, A., Pukall, C. F., & Goldstein I. (2020). *Female sexual pain disorders evaluation and management* (2nd ed.). Wiley-Blackwell.
- Hall, K. S. K., & Binik, Y. M. (2020). *Principles and practice of sex therapy* (6th ed.). Guilford Press.
- McCarthy, B. W., & McCarthy, E. J. (2021). *Contemporary male sexuality: Confronting myths and promoting change*. Routledge.
- Meana, M. (2012). *Sexual dysfunction in women*. Hogrefe Publishing.
- Perel, E. (2007). *Mating in captivity: Unlocking erotic intelligence)*. Harper.
- Rowland, D. (2012). *Sexual dysfunction in men*. Hogrefe Publishing.

References

Adam, F., De Sutter, P., Day, J., & Grimm, E. (2020). A randomized study comparing video-based mindfulness-based cognitive therapy with video-based traditional cognitive behavioral therapy in a sample of women struggling to achieve orgasm. *Journal of Sexual Medicine*, 17(2), 312–324.

Althof, S. (2020). Treatment of premature ejaculation: Psychotherapy, pharmacotherapy, and combined therapy. In: K. S. K. Hall & Y. M. Binik (Eds.), *Principles and practice of sex therapy* (6th ed.) (pp. 134–155). Guilford Press.

American Psychiatric Association (2022). *Diagnostic and statistical manual of mental disorders* (5th ed., text revision). American Psychiatric Association.

Avery-Clark, C., Weiner, L. & Adams-Clark, A. A. (2019). Sensate focus for sexual concerns: An updated, critical literature review. *Current Sexual Health Reports*, 11, 84–94.

Bancroft, J. (2009). *Human sexuality and its problems* (3rd ed.). Elsevier.

Barlow, D. H. (1986). Causes of sexual dysfunction: The role of anxiety and cognitive interference. *Journal of Consulting and Clinical Psychology*, 54, 140–148.

Basson, R. (2000). The female sexual response: A different model. *Journal of Sex & Marital Therapy*, 26(1), 51–65.

Bergeron, S., Paquet, M., Steben, M., & Rosen, N. O. (2021). Perceived partner responsiveness is associated with sexual well-being in couples with genito-pelvic pain. *Journal of Family Psychology*, 35, 628–638.

Bergeron, S., Rosen, N. O., Pukall, C. F., & Corsini-Munt, S. (2020). Genital pain in women and men. In K. S. K. Hall & Y. M. Binik (Eds.), *Principles and practice of sex therapy* (6th ed.) (pp. 180–201). The Guilford Press.

Binik, Y. M., & Meana, M. (2009). The future of sex therapy: Specialization or marginalization? *Archives of Sexual Behavior*, 38(6), 1016–1027.

Boddi, V., Castellini, G., Casale, H., et al. (2015). An integrated approach with vardenafil orodispersible tablet and cognitive-behavioral sex therapy for treatment of erectile dysfunction: A randomized controlled pilot study. *Andrology*, 3(5), 909–918.

Brotto, L. A. (2018). *Better sex through mindfulness*. Greystone.

Brotto, L. A., Attallah, S., Johnson-Agbakwu, C., et al. (2016). Psychological and interpersonal dimensions of sexual function and dysfunction. *Journal of Sexual Medicine*, 13, 538–571.

Brotto, L. A., Bergeron, S., Zdaniuk, B., et al. (2019). A comparison of mindfulness-based cognitive therapy vs cognitive behavioral therapy for the treatment of provoked vestibulodynia in a hospital setting. *Journal of Sexual Medicine*, 16(6), 909–923.

Brotto, L. A., & Heiman, J. R. (2007). Mindfulness in sex therapy: Applications for women with sexual difficulties following gynecologic cancer. *Sexual and Relationship Therapy*, 22, 3–11.

Brotto, L. A., Zdaniuk, B., Chivers, M. L., et al. (2021). A randomized control trial comparing group mindfulness-based cognitive therapy with group supportive sex education and therapy for the treatment of female sexual interest/arousal disorder. *Journal of Consulting and Clinical Psychology*, 89(7), 626–639.

Carvalheira, A., & Leal, I. (2013). Masturbation among women: Associated factors and sexual response in a Portuguese community. *Journal of Sex and Marital Therapy*, 39(4), 347–367.

Chambless, D. L., Baker, M. J., Baucom, D. H., et al. (1998). Update on empirically validated therapies. II. *The Clinical Psychologist*, 51(1), 3–16.

Chin, H. B., Sipe, T. A., Elder, R., et al. (2012). The effectiveness of group-based comprehensive risk-reduction and abstinence education interventions to prevent or reduce the risk of adolescent pregnancy, human immunodeficiency virus, and sexually transmitted infections: Two systematic reviews for the Guide to Community Preventative Services. *American Journal of Preventative Medicine*, 42, 272–294.

Christensen, B. S., Gronbaek, M., Osler, M., et al. (2011). Sexual dysfunctions and difficulties in Demark: Prevalence and associated sociodemographic factors. *Archives of Sexual Behavior*, 40, 121–132.

Corona, G., Rastrelli, G., Ricca, V., et al. (2013). Risk factors associated with primary and secondary reduced libido in male patients with sexual dysfunction. *Journal of Sexual Medicine*, 10, 1074–1089.

Fruhauf, S., Gerger, H., Maren Schmidt, H., Munder, T., & Barth, J. (2013). Efficacy of psychological interventions for sexual dysfunction: A systematic review and meta-analysis. *Archives of Sexual Behavior*, 42, 915–933.

Goldfarb, E. S., & Lieberman, L. D. (2021). Three decades of research: The case for comprehensive sex education. *Journal of Adolescent Health*, 2021, 13–27.

Hall, K. S. K., & Graham, C. A. (2020). The privileging of pleasure: Sex therapy in global cultural context. In K. S. K. Hall & Y. M. Binik (Eds.), *Principles and practice of sex therapy* (6th ed.) (pp. 180–201). The Guilford Press.

Hall, S. K., Males, J. M., Komro, K. A., & Santelli, J. (2016). The state of sex education in the United States. *Journal of Adolescent Health*, 58, 595–597.

Harte, C. B., & Meston, C. M. (2013). Association between cigarette smoking and erectile tumescence: The mediating role of heart rate variability. *International Journal of Impotence Research*, 25(4), 155–159.

Henrich, J., Heine, S. J., & Norenzayan, A. (2010). The weirdest people in the world? *Behavioral and Brain Sciences*, 32(2/3), 1–75.

Herbenick, D., Mullinax, M., & Mark, K. (2014). Sexual desire discrepancy as a feature, not a bug, of long-term relationships: Women's self-reported strategies for modulating sexual desire. *Journal of Sexual Medicine*, 11(9), 2196–2206.

Kalogeropoulos, D., & Larouche, J., (2020). An integrative biopsychosocial approach to the conceptualization and treatment of erectile disorder. In: K. S. K. Hall & Y. M. Binik (Eds.), *Principles and practice of sex therapy* (6th ed.) (pp. 87–108). The Guilford Press.

Kaplan, H. S. (1979). *Disorders of sexual desire and other new concepts and techniques in sex therapy.* Brunner/Mazel.

Kohler, P. K., Manhart, L. E., & Lafferty, W. E. (2008). Abstinence-only and comprehensive sex education and the initiation of sexual activity and teen pregnancy. *Journal of Adolescent Health*, 42, 344–351.

Laan, E., Rellini, A. H., & Barnes, T. (2013). Standard operating procedures for female orgasmic disorder: Consensus of the International Society for Sexual Medicine. *Journal of Sexual Medicine*, 10, 74–82.

Lahaie, M. A., Amsel, R., Khalife, S., et al. (2015). Can fear, pain, and muscle tension discriminate vaginismus from dyspareunia/ provoked vestibulodynia? Implications for the new DSM-5 diagnosis of genito-pelvic pain/penetration disorder. *Archives of Sexual Behavior*, 44, 1537–1550.

Landry, T., Bergeron, S., Dupuis, M.-J., & Desrochers, G. (2008). The treatment of provoked vestibulodynia: A critical review. *Clinical Journal of Pain*, 24, 155–171.

Laurent, S. E., & Simons, A. D. (2009). Sexual dysfunction in depression and anxiety: Conceptualizing sexual dysfunction as part of an internalizing dimension. *Clinical Psychology Review*, 29, 573–585.

Lewis, R. W., Fugl-Meyer, K. S., Corona, G., et al. (2010). Definitions/epidemiology/risk factors for sexual dysfunction. *Journal of Sexual Medicine*, 7(4), 1598–1607.

Linschoten, M., Weiner, L., & Avery-Clark, C. (2016). Sensate focus: A critical literature review. *Sexual and Relationship Therapy*, 31, 230–247.

Masters, W. H., & Johnson, V. E. (1966). *Human sexual response.* Little, Brown

Masters, W. H., & Johnson, V. E. (1970). *Human sexual inadequacy.* Little, Brown.

McCabe, M. (2005). The role of performance anxiety in the development and maintenance of sexual dysfunction in men and women. *International Journal of Stress Management*, 12, 379–388.

McCabe, M. P., & Cobain, M. J. (1998). The impact of individual and relationship factors on sexual dysfunction among males and females. *Sexual and Marital Therapy*, 13, 131–143.

Meana, M. (2012). *Sexual dysfunction in women.* Hogrefe Press.

Meana, M., & Binik, Y. M. (2022). The biopsychosocial puzzle of painful sex. *Annual Review of Clinical Psychology*, 18, 471–495.

Meana, M., & Hall, K. (2023). Sexual dysfunctions. In T. L. Leong, J. Callahan, C. Eubanks, & M. Constantino (Eds.), *APA handbook of psychotherapy.* American Psychological Association.

Meana, M., Hall, K., & Binik, Y. M. (2020). Conclusion: Where is sex therapy going? In K. S. K. Hall & Y. M. Binik (Eds.), *Principles and practice of sex therapy* (6th ed.) (pp. 505–522). The Guilford Press.

Meana, M., Nobre, P., & Tavares, I. (2023). Sexual dysfunctions. In A. Tasman et al. (Eds.) *Tasmin's Psychiatry* (5th ed.). Springer.

Metz, M. E., & Epstein, N. (2002). Assessing the role of relationship conflict in sexual dysfunction. *Journal of Sex & Marital Therapy*, 28, 139–164.

Mintz, L. (2017). *Becoming cliterate: Why orgasm equality matters – A guide for survivors of sexual abuse.* Avon.

Mitchell, K. R., Mercer, C. H., Ploubidis, G. B., et al. (2013). Sexual function in Britain: Findings from the Third National Survey of Sexual Attitudes and Lifestyles (NATSAL-3). *Lancet*, 382, 1817–1829.

Mitchell, K. R., Jones, K.G., Wellings, K., et al. (2016). Estimating the prevalence of sexual function problems: The impact of morbidity criteria. *Journal of Sex Research*, 53(8), 955–967.

Morin, M., Carroll, M.-S., & Bergeron, S. (2017). Systematic review of the effectiveness of physical therapy modalities in women with provoked vestibulodynia. *Sexual Medicine Reviews*, 5(3), 295–322.

Nobre, P. G., & Pinto-Gouveia, J. (2008). Differences in automatic thoughts presented during sexual activity between sexually functional and dysfunctional men and women. *Cognitive Therapy and Research*, 32, 37–49.

Nobre, P. J., Pinto-Gouveia, J., & Gomes, F. A. (2006). Prevalence and comorbidity of sexual dysfunctions in a Portuguese clinical sample. *Journal of Sex & Marital Therapy*, 32(2), 173–182.

Perelman, M. A. (2004). Regarded ejaculation. In J. Mulhull (Ed.), *Current sexual health reports* (pp. 95–101). Current Science.

Perelman, M. A., & Rowland, D. L. (2006). Retarded ejaculation. *World Journal of Urology*, 24(6), 645–652.

Polland, A., Davis, M., Zeymo, A., & Venkatesen, K. (2018). Comparison of correlated comorbidities in male and female sexual dysfunction: Findings from the Third National Survey of Sexual Attitudes and Lifestyles (NATSAL-3). *Journal of Sexual Medicine*, 15(5), 678–686.

Pukall, C. F. (2023). Sexual issues. In S. Hupp & C. L. Santa Maria (Eds.), *Pseudoscience in therapy: A skeptical field guide* (pp. 162–178). Cambridge University Press.

Pukall, C. F., Goldstein, A. T., Bergeron, S., et al. (2016). Vulvodynia: Definition, prevalence, impact, and pathophysiological factors. *Journal of Sexual Medicine*, 13(3), 291–304.

Reissing, E. D., Binik, Y. M., Khalife, S., Cohen, D., & Amsel, R. (2004). Vaginal spasm, pain, and behavior: An empirical investigation of the diagnosis of vaginismus. *Archives of Sexual Behavior*, 33, 5–17.

Rosen, N. O., & Bergeron, S. (2019). Genito-pelvic pain through a dyadic lens: Moving toward an interpersonal emotional regulation model of women's sexual dysfunction. *The Journal of Sex Research*, 56(4), 440–461.

Rosen, R. C., & Bachman, G. A. (2008). Sexual well-being, happiness, and satisfaction in women. The case for a new conceptual paradigm. *Journal of Sex and Marital Therapy*, 34, 291–297.

Rosen, R. C., Brown, C., Heiman, J., et al. (2000). The Female Sexual Function Index (FSFI): A multidimensional self-report instrument for the assessment of female sexual function. *Journal of Sex and Marital Therapy*, 26(2), 191–208.

Rosen, R. C., Riley, A., Wagner, G., et al. (1997). The International Index of Erectile Function (IIEF): A multidimensional scale for assessment of erectile dysfunction. *Urology*, 49, 822–830.

Rowland, D. L. (2012). *Sexual dysfunction in men*. Hogrefe Press.

Rowland, D. L., & Cooper, S. E. (2017). Treating men's orgasmic difficulties. In Z. D. Peterson (Ed.), *The Wiley handbook of sex therapy* (pp. 72–97). Wiley-Blackwell.

SIECUS (2018). Position statements. Sexuality Information and Education Council of the United States. https://siecus.org/wp-content/uploads/2018/07/Position-Statements-2018.pdf (accessed March 29, 2023).

Silva, A. B., Sousa, N., Azevedo, L. F., & Martins, C. (2017). Physical activity and exercise for erectile dysfunction: Systematic review and meta-analysis. *British Journal of Sports Medicine*, 51, 1419–1424.

Stanger-Hall, K. F., & Hall, D. W. (2011). Abstinence-only education and teen pregnancy rates: Why we need comprehensive sex education in the US. *PLoS One*, e24658.

ter Kuile, M. M., Both, S., & van Lankveld, J. J. (2010). Cognitive-behavioral therapy for sexual dysfunctions in women. *Psychiatric Clinics of North America*, 33, 595–610.

ter Kuile, M. M., Melles, R., de Groot, H. E., Tuijnman-Raasveld, C. C., & van Lankveld, J. J. (2013). Therapist-aided exposure for women with lifelong vaginismus: A randomized waiting-list controlled trial of efficacy. *Journal of Consulting and Clinical Psychology*, 81, 1127–1136.

ter Kuile, M. M., & Reissing, E. D. (2020). Lifelong inability to experience intercourse (vaginismus). In K. S. K. Hall & Y. M. Binik (Eds.), *Principles and practice of sex therapy* (6th ed.) (pp. 202–223). Guilford Press.

Tolin, D. F., McKay, D., Forman, E. M., Klonsky, E. D., & Thombs, B. D. (2015). Empirically supported treatment: Recommendations for a new model. *Clinical Psychology: Science and Practice*, 22, 317–338.

van Lankveld, J. D. M., & Grotjohann, Y. (2000). Psychiatric comorbidity in heterosexual couples with sexual dysfunction assessed with the Composite International Diagnostic Interview. *Archives of Sexual Behavior*, 29, 479–498.

Velten, J., & Margraf, J. (2017). Satisfaction guaranteed? How individual, partner, and Relationship factors impact sexual satisfaction within partnerships. *PLoS One*, e0172855.

12

Substance Use Disorders

Victoria E. Stead, Andrew B. Lumb, Jennifer Brasch, and James MacKillop

Substance use disorders (SUDs) are among the most common psychiatric conditions and are major global causes of morbidity and mortality. Diagnostically, SUDs are defined differently in the *Diagnostic and Statistical Manual, 5th Edition, Text Revision* (DSM-5-TR) and the *International Statistical Classification of Diseases and Related Health Problems, 11th revision* (ICD-11) (APA, 2013; WHO, 2019). Both nosological systems include symptoms related to loss of control over substance use and substance use taking over other activities, resulting in life-long health problems, tolerance, and physiological withdrawal effects (APA, 2013; WHO, 2019). The DSM-5-TR uses a single continuous polythetic diagnosis – substance use disorder – with three levels of severity (mild, moderate, and severe), whereas ICD-11 has two diagnoses – harmful pattern of use and substance dependence – with the former being less severe. These diagnoses clinically operationalize the colloquial term "addiction," although the construct of addiction generally connotes more severe manifestations (i.e., severe substance use disorder, substance dependence) (McLellan et al., 2022).

Etiology and Theoretical Underpinnings of Treatment

Contemporary theories of SUDs emphasize a highly multifactorial etiology and an integrative biopsychosocial approach (MacKillop & Ray, 2018). The primary focus here is on psychological determinants; however, there is a recognition of important biological factors such as genetic liability (Goldman et al., 2006) and neuroadaptive changes based on persistent exposure to the drug's pharmacological actions (Koob, 2006). Similarly, social and sociocultural factors, such as drug policy (e.g., taxation, minimum age of legal access, legal status) and presence of prevention programming, are also established as affecting SUD risk (MacKillop et al., 2022).

From a psychological standpoint, these biological and sociocultural processes are integrated into a perspective that emphasizes behavioral and cognitive factors

193

that underlie SUDs. A major theme in contemporary psychological theories of SUDs is the application of learning theory, which posits that excessive and problematic substance use reflects a form of maladaptive learning. The earliest perspective, and one that is still influential, is an operant (instrumental) learning perspective (Bigelow, 2001). Specifically, this approach theorizes SUDs to be maladaptive instrumental learning that is governed by the positively and negatively reinforcing psychoactive effects of the drug that have become excessively dominant and often displace more salutary nondrug alternative reinforcers. This approach is supported by an extensive evidence base, from human laboratory studies demonstrating drug self-administration conforming to operant predictions to observational and clinical studies implicating overvaluation of immediate reinforcement, persistently high drug reinforcing value, and a dearth of alternative reinforcers (Acuff et al., 2019; González-Roz et al., 2019; MacKillop et al., 2011; Martínez-Loredo et al., 2021). The most recent incarnation of a reinforcement-based formulation is referred to as the reinforcer pathology approach, which integrates these psychological principles with concepts and methods from microeconomics (Bickel et al., 2014; Mackillop, 2016).

A second learning-based account of addiction emphasizes social learning theory (Monti & O'Leary, 1999; Bandura, 1977; Monti, 2002) and emerged as an application of the broader cognitive-behavioral approach in clinical psychology. Rather than emphasizing reinforcing value per se, this perspective theorizes that substance use is maintained by skills deficits (e.g., difficulty resisting social pressures to use) and maladaptive cognitions (e.g., equating a single lapse with full relapse). A social learning account emphasizes that individuals with SUDs lack the skills to cope with affectively negative experiences (e.g., stress, sadness, cravings, withdrawal symptoms), as well as other situations associated with substance use (e.g., being around others using substances). Substance use becomes a prepotent maladaptive coping strategy for managing diverse antecedents.

A final important element in a contemporary psychological approach to SUDs pertains to motivation for recovery. In contrast to lay notions that individuals with SUDs are uniformly in "denial," there is extensive evidence that many individuals are indeed motivated or actively trying to change. Moreover, motivation for change, for individuals with SUDs and other psychiatric conditions, is increasingly understood to be fluid (state-like versus trait-like), and existing on a spectrum, from resistance to high desire for and action toward change. This is the transtheoretical stages of change model that emphasizes a sequential progression from precontemplation, reflecting minimal motivation, to action and maintenance, reflecting meaningful efforts toward behavior change (DiClemente et al., 2004; Prochaska & DiClemente, 1983, 1992). As important has been the insight that, rather than needing to "break through" denial, empathy and a client-centered approach is critical for change (Miller & Rose, 2009). This is a brief overview of contemporary psychological theories of SUDs, and these learning and motivational perspectives provide a theoretical foundation for science-based components of treatment that are reviewed below.

Brief Overview of Treatments

A number of psychological treatments for SUDs have robust scientific support. First, cognitive-behavioral therapy (CBT) for SUDs is considered a first-line psychotherapy and is an extension of the broader "second wave" cognitive-behavioral movement in psychotherapy (Beck et al., 1993; Ray et al., 2020). Second, motivational interviewing and motivational enhancement therapy (MET) are client-centered treatment approaches that aim to strengthen a client's intrinsic motivation for and commitment to healthier behavior change through exploring and resolving ambivalence (Miller & Rollnick, 2012). Using the Chambless criteria for empirically supported treatments (Chambless & Hollon, 1998), the Society of Clinical Psychology (n.d.) designated motivational interviewing, MET, and MET + CBT as all being well-established treatments for SUDs in general. Third and fourth are two forms of reinforcement-based treatment – contingency management and the community reinforcement approach – both of which have been extensively supported. Contingency management is a behavioral treatment using direct incentives to reinforce treatment engagement and behavior change, whereas the Community Reinforcement Approach (CRA) is a comprehensive psychosocial intervention to develop alternative competing reinforcers that decrease the reinforcing values of substance use (for a review, see Pfund et al., 2022).

To date, a few treatments have been evaluated using the Tolin criteria for empirically supported treatments (Tolin et al., 2015). First, a recent systematic review evaluated five meta-analyses of CBT for SUDs and endorsed a *strong recommendation* (but not yet a *very strong recommendation*) for CBT for SUDs based on the outcomes, quality of evidence, and other important contextual considerations (e.g., efficacy in diverse populations, cost, flexibility of delivery, etc.) (Boness et al., 2023). Of note, CBT was determined to be most effective at short-term (1–6 months) versus long-term (8+ months) follow-up (Boness et al., 2023). Second, a recent systematic review and meta-analysis evaluated five meta-analyses of contingency management (Pfund et al., 2022). Two were rated as "moderate quality," with the other three rated as "low–critically low quality." In these studies, contingency management was evaluated against active treatment, placebo, treatment as usual, and inactive/no treatment, with the primary outcome being abstinence. Contingency management was given a *strong recommendation* and deemed most effective (i.e., "moderate quality") when compared with all control groups on measures of abstinence and follow-up abstinence (Pfund et al., 2022). See also page 402 of this book's Postscript.

Box 12.1 Mutual Support Organizations

Traditional mutual support organizations (MSOs), like Alcoholic Anonymous (AA) or Narcotics Anonymous (NA), use a twelve-step program that comprises regular group meetings, fellowship from others, and a spiritual model toward recovery. Though ubiquitous in the treatment community, MSOs are grassroots self-help organizations rather than empirically supported interventions per se and, until relatively recently, research on the utility of these programs was methodologically poor (Kelly et al., 2017; Sparks, 2014). More recent research has shown AA participation, and treatments designed to simulate participation in AA (i.e., Twelve-Step Facilitation [TSF]), to be beneficial (Kelly et al., 2020). Indeed, even when compared to theoretically driven, empirically supported interventions, TSF tends to produce as-good or better outcomes, particularly for sustained abstinence and remission, in randomized controlled trials (Kelly et al., 2020). Although how MSOs help patients is not fully understood, similar mechanisms to empirically supported treatments and long-term social support are hypothesized to drive positive outcomes for those who deeply engage with these programs (Connery et al., 2020; Kelly et al., 2021). Importantly, MSOs, and TSFs in particular, are not necessarily a good fit for all patients, as some do not resonate with the emphasis on spirituality, the twelve-step tenets, or abstinence as the principal definition of successful recovery. Finally, a relatively novel MSO is Self-Management and Recovery Training (SMART), which includes elements of motivational interviewing and CBT in a mutual support group format has been found to provide positive effects (Beck et al., 2017; Connery et al., 2020).

Credible Components of Treatments

Skills Training

Promoting the development of new skills to reduce substance use is a cornerstone of CBT for SUDs. CBT approaches emphasize instrumental and social learning theory, meaning this approach targets an individual's learning history and environment in determining behavior (Liese & Beck, 2022). Within the CBT model for SUDs, substance use is typically understood as being a maladaptive coping strategy that individuals use in response to internal and external triggers (e.g., interpersonal conflict, boredom, withdrawal symptoms, environmental cues). Broadly speaking, CBT for SUDs targets cognitive, affective, and environmental risk factors for substance use and incorporates training in coping skills to ultimately help individuals reduce the harms associated with their use and/or maintain abstinence. The overall goal of treatment is to help individuals learn skills to address the factors that lead to their substance use (i.e., antecedents of their use). Ongoing case conceptualization of proximal and distal factors associated with clients' use is considered an essential aspect of CBT for SUDs. This is to help individuals ultimately be better able to anticipate and thus better able to cope with identified factors that might make them more vulnerable to using. Concurrently, individuals also learn how and when to employ different, more adaptive, coping strategies (e.g., refusal skills, distract and delay) (Daley & Douaihy, 2019; Marlatt & Donovan, 2005). As individuals expand their repertoire of coping strategies, the aim is for them to become less reliant on using substances as a primary means to cope.

In terms of empirical support, an early meta-analysis by Magill and Ray (2009) examined the efficacy of CBT across studies targeting substance use, finding that 58% of patients who received CBT showed significantly better outcomes (i.e., performed better than median score for the comparison group, ranging from minimal treatment to non-CBT treatment-as-usual). Of note, the benefit of CBT was largest in studies on cannabis use, and female patients showed better outcomes than males. An updated meta-analysis by Magill et al. (2019) examined CBT across SUDs in a larger group of more heterogeneous studies, albeit finding a more modest effect size of benefit relative to minimal treatment. When examining the efficacy of CBT compared to other therapies (e.g., motivational interviewing and contingency management), the outcomes were equivalent. Taken together, CBT appears to be efficacious in general, and similar in benefits to other evidence-based strategies (Magill et al., 2019, 2020; McHugh et al., 2010).

Though there is general evidence supporting the use of CBT for SUDs, not all CBT-based approaches have been rigorously tested across all substances to date (Liese & Beck, 2022; Magill et al., 2019). Indeed, a challenge within the current literature is the substantial heterogeneity across studies relating to the substances targeted, co-occurring clinical presentations, length of intervention, format of interventions (individual versus group), comparison groups/treatments, combination of treatment modalities (e.g., addition of pharmacotherapy and/or other evidence-based modalities), methods employed, and mechanisms of treatment change assessed (Magill et al., 2019, 2020; Ray et al., 2020). As a result, rather than being a singular set of elements, CBT for SUDs can be thought of as a genus comprising a number of species.

The earliest and most widely implemented CBT-based approaches include relapse prevention (Marlatt & Gordon, 1985), which emphasizes the identification and prevention of high-risk situations, and coping/communication skills training (e.g., substance refusal skills, developing social nonsubstance supports, etc.) (Monti & O'Leary, 1999; Monti et al., 2001), which focuses on addressing deficits that are commonly present among individuals with SUDs. The CBT approach has also been adapted into behavioral couples therapy (McCrady et al., 2009), which has been supported for both short- and long-term outcomes (Klostermann et al., 2011; McCrady et al., 2009; Powers et al., 2008). Other important outcomes for behavioral couple therapy (BCT) include increased adjustment for children of parents with alcohol use disorder (AUD) receiving BCT (Kelley & Fals-Stewart, 2002; Lam, Fals-Stewart, & Kelley, 2008). Additionally, two preliminary studies supported BCT for treating dual-AUD couples (McCrady et al., 2009; Rotunda et al., 2008), a challenging subpopulation.

In addition to the coping skills noted here, a more recently developed component of CBT for SUDs is mindfulness training in the form of mindfulness-based relapse prevention (MBRP). This approach combines mindfulness practices (i.e., purposefully paying attention to the present moment without judgment; Kabat-Zinn, 1994) and conventional relapse-prevention skills training (Bowen et al., 2014). The main goals of MBRP are to promote attentional awareness of internal and external cues related to substance use, thus reducing automatic engagement of substance use, but also, critically, to enhance tolerance for uncomfortable and painful emotional states rather than relief via substance use (Korecki et al., 2020). Initial evidence for MBRP supports its efficacy in significantly lowering levels of substance use and cravings, while increasing acceptance and awareness of the present moment, and self regulation and emotion regulation (Li et al., 2017), though results have been mixed (Zgierska et al., 2019).

A gap in knowledge for CBT for SUDs pertains to evidence supporting individual specific skills training as opposed to the omnibus packages that are typically delivered. In other words, there is limited evidence for each of the specific components of treatment. Dismantling studies and studies specifically investigating individual skills as mechanisms of behavior change are a priority for determining the value of individual domains and potentially optimizing outcomes.

Motivational Enhancement

Enhancing and sustaining motivation for changing substance use is the superordinate goal of motivational interviewing. This is based on the contemporary understanding that motivation for change is malleable and fluctuating in SUDs. In other words, patients shouldn't be categorized as "motivated" or "unmotivated" because motivation is a dynamic, continuous psychological process, not a dichotomous one. Originally, motivational interviewing comprised four core principles – expressing empathy, developing discrepancy, supporting self-efficacy, and rolling with resistance (Miller & Rollnick, 2002) – but it has evolved to focus on motivational interviewing spirit and specific fundamental processes (Miller & Rollnick, 2012). The spirit is defined as a therapeutic alliance that is a collaborative partnership fostering an autonomy-supportive, nonjudgmental, and compassionate atmosphere that affirms clients' values and strengths (Miller & Rollnick, 2012). The fundamental processes include: (1) *engaging*, where a working relationship with clients is established by building trust through accurately understanding their perspective; (2) *focusing*, where therapist and client come to a shared idea about the main focus in session, akin to agenda setting; (3) *evoking*, where therapists help clients explore their own reasons for change ("change talk") and amplify the strength and frequency of change talk; and (4) *planning*, where therapists help clients consider a menu of options and collaboratively plan how they will go about change. These fundamentals are intended to be initially sequential, but more broadly recursive, with the focus shifting as priorities warrant during treatment.

In terms of empirical support, a review by Lundahl and Burke (2009) revealed that motivational interviewing produced 10–20% greater improvement on outcomes compared to no treatment and that motivational interviewing was generally equal to other active treatments for alcohol, cannabis, tobacco, and use of other illicit drugs (cocaine, heroin). More recently, a review (DiClemente et al., 2017) of 34 review articles revealed the strongest evidence for motivational interviewing and brief motivational interviewing interventions (e.g., one 15-minute session, one hour-long session, to four or more one-hour long sessions) on substance use outcomes and treatment engagement in the areas of alcohol, tobacco, and cannabis use. For these substances, motivational interviewing was more effective than no treatment and equal to other active treatments.

In terms of individual processes, an extensive literature has investigated therapist and client behaviors, as these are essential to understand the underlying mechanisms and efficacy of motivational interviewing. Generally, it is proposed that behavior consistent with motivational interviewing will elicit and reinforce client language in favor of change, which will result in improved outcomes (Miller, 1983; Miller & Rollnick, 2012). Findings reveal that therapist behaviors that are consistent with motivational interviewing increase client change talk (Apodaca & Longabaugh, 2009; Romano & Peters, 2016), increase realization of the discrepancy between values and behaviors, and decrease resistance (Apodaca & Longabaugh, 2009). Increased change talk is, in turn, related to reductions in substance use at follow-up (Magill et al., 2018, 2019; Romano & Peters, 2016). Interestingly, behaviors consistent with motivational interviewing increase both change and sustain talk (Magill et al., 2018). Clinically, this may not be surprising, as the process of resolving ambivalence may at first simultaneously heighten change and sustain talk, followed by resolution, wherein clients strengthen their language in favor of change. A systematic review by Romano and Peters (2016) revealed that a higher ratio of therapist reflections to questions and more use of affirmations predicted positive outcomes most consistently. Therapist empathy and spirit of motivational interviewing have also been shown to increase client change and sustain talk, increase therapist behaviors that are consistent with motivational interviewing, and decrease behaviors that are inconsistent with motivational interviewing (Pace et al., 2017). Conversely, therapist behaviors that are inconsistent with motivational interviewing lead to more sustain talk and worse outcomes (Apodaca & Longabaugh, 2009; Magill et al., 2018; Pace et al., 2017).

Access to Nondrug Alternative Reinforcement

Often, social learning and operant learning perspectives are broadly classed together as CBT treatment of SUDs because of the common emphasis on a person's learning history. However, there is a distinction because traditional CBT (as discussed earlier) emphasizes intraindividual factors (e.g., coping skills), whereas operant (reinforcement-based) treatments emphasize modifying extraindividual (environmental) factors, specifically in the form of increasing nondrug alternative reinforcement. The two operant treatment approaches that use this perspective are the community reinforcement approach (CRA; Hunt & Azrin, 1973), which is a comprehensive psychosocial intervention that works with the client to develop alternative competing sources of reinforcement that are mutually exclusive with substance use, and contingency management (Stitzer & Petry, 2006), a strategy that directly reinforces treatment-related behaviors, such as abstinence or treatment attendance, using direct incentives. These approaches are premised on the foundational behavioral evidence that addictive substances are powerful positive and negative reinforcers, and, for individuals with SUDs, a substance's reinforcing value becomes persistently elevated, disrupting other meaningful activities and creating a vicious cycle in which substance use becomes one of the few reinforcing behaviors available in a person's life.

There is considerable empirical support for the efficacy of both CRA and contingency management. Importantly, CRA has been adapted into an intervention for families of individuals with SUDs – community reinforcement approach family training (CRAFT) – which has also been found to be efficacious (Dutcher et al., 2009; Kirby et al., 1999; Meyers et al., 2002; Miller et al., 1999; Sisson & Azrin, 1986). There is a similarly strong empirical literature supporting the efficacy of contingency management (Dougherty et al., 2014; Higgins et al., 2000; Ledgerwood et al., 2014; McCaul et al., 1984; Petry et al., 2000, 2013). An early meta-analysis of more than 40 randomized controlled trials supported the efficacy of this treatment (Prendergast et al., 2006), and subsequent ones have been similarly supportive (Bentzley et al., 2021; Bolívar et al., 2021; Brown & DeFulio, 2020; Notley et al., 2019; Winters et al., 2021). Furthermore, contingency management has been shown to be beneficial in complex populations, such as individuals with SUDs and common comorbidities (Destoop et al., 2021; Secades-Villa et al., 2020) and younger patients (Stanger & Budney, 2019). Finally, given the inherent financial cost of vouchers, it also bears mentioning that cost-effectiveness analyses have been supportive of contingency management (González-Roz et al., 2021; Lott & Jencius, 2009; Olmstead & Petry, 2009; Sindelar et al., 2007).

Two important distinctions are worth noting about contingency management. First, unlike CRA, which has a relatively codified treatment package, the exact format of contingency management varies substantially from study to study. This is a deliberate feature of contingency management insofar as it is intended to be mapped onto the different priorities across programs and populations, but it means that there is a high degree of heterogeneity in formats. Formats using both the voucher reinforcement method and the prize-based reinforcement method have both been shown to be efficacious (Benishek et al., 2014; Lussier et al., 2006). As such, although the balance of evidence supports contingency management as being

Box 12.2 Harm Reduction

Harm reduction refers to strategies aimed at reducing adverse health and social outcomes associated with substance use without necessarily identifying abstinence as the goal (Thomas., 2005). Harm reduction can take many forms, including both public health strategies (e.g., drug testing, naloxone kits, needle exchanges) and clinical strategies (e.g., focusing on a reduction or moderation outcome rather than complete abstinence). Harm reduction has been shown to reduce the risk of overdose and other harmful consequences (morbidity and mortality) associated with use, as well as to improve treatment initiation, adherence, and retention (Denis-Lalonde et al., 2019; Hawk et al., 2017; Hunt et al., 2003; Kimmel et al., 2021). Although abstinence typically remains a priority outcome in clinical research evaluating efficacious treatments, contemporary perspectives emphasize a patient-centered approach in clinical practice. This would include a spectrum of outcomes, from no change in use with minimization of harms to a reduction in consumption without abstinence to complete abstinence. Moreover, these outcomes need not be mutually exclusive over time. For example, lack of success with a moderation goal may evolve into an abstinence goal, or successful long-term abstinence may be followed by the goal of resuming moderation.

beneficial, implementation of contingency management should be based on the evidence that comes from the most germane settings, conditions, and populations. Second, it is important to note that contingency management is typically not intended to be a stand-alone treatment, but to be one element in a broader treatment package (González-Roz et al., 2021; Lott & Jencius, 2009; Olmstead & Petry, 2009; Sindelar et al., 2007).

A gap in the literature pertains to which specific features of both CM and CRA are essential for clinical benefits. For CM, there is some evidence that larger magnitude rewards are more effective (Businelle et al., 2009; Petry et al., 2004; Regnier et al., 2022), but also evidence that magnitude has a ceiling (Carroll et al., 2002; Petry et al., 2015). Incentive amount received and spending have also been found to be predictive of benefits (Lake et al., 2023; Petry & Roll, 2011), but how to optimize CM is by no means definitive. For CRA, the status is similar to CBT insofar as the evidence for the package is robust, but less is known about which specific alternative reinforcers are most potent or important for promoting positive outcomes.

Approaches for Youth

Substance use most often initiates during adolescence (UNODC, 2020), and the peak prevalence of SUDs is during emerging adulthood, spanning ages 18–25 years (Grant et al., 2015; Hasin, 2018; Sarvet & Hasin, 2016). This transition from childhood to adulthood is marked by numerous physiological, academic, vocational, interpersonal, and neurobiological changes that increase the likelihood for substance use and, in turn, risk for negative substance-related outcomes (Arnett, 2000; Dawson et al., 2007). Adolescents and emerging adults are also more likely to engage in polysubstance use (Kelly et al., 2015; Zuckermann et al., 2019, 2020), which is associated with worse physical and mental health problems and more risky behaviors (e.g., risky sexual behaviors, driving under the influence) (Bohnert et al., 2014; Connell et al., 2009). Adolescents who engage in substance use earlier on and/or use multiple substances show worse academic performance, have lower rates of high school completion, and can experience negative long-term effects on their overall cognitive functioning (Bohnert et al., 2014; Morin et al., 2019). Importantly, those who initially engage in substance use during early adolescence are also more likely to go on to develop SUDs in young adulthood and adulthood (Choi et al., 2018; Merrin et al., 2018; Zuckermann et al., 2020). Importantly, substance use during these developmental periods is not a benign experimentation but, rather, is a leading cause of disability among individuals during this time (Erskine et al., 2015). For example, alcohol is implicated in a quarter of deaths among Americans aged 20–34 (Esser et al., 2022). Collectively, there is a strong need for intervention because of the high rates of morbidity and mortality, but also to interrupt adverse trajectories that may affect an individual across the lifespan.

Few of the treatments for SUDs have been specifically tested for adolescents and young adults (Catchpole & Brownlie, 2016). Because substance use is typically illegal for adolescents, prevention and abstinence-based interventions have been the primary approach, but this approach can be stigmatizing, demotivating, and leave young people at an increased risk for relapse and overdose (Corace et al., 2018; Faggiano et al., 2014; Stigler et al., 2011). It has been recommended that, instead, the full range of treatment options should be available to young people, including harm reduction (Bruneau et al., 2018; Corace et al., 2019). Even without extensive developmentally specific research, adaptations of the psychological approaches detailed herein – such as the Adolescent CRA, ecological family-based treatment, individual CBT, and group CBT – are generally beneficial in adolescent and young adult populations (Godley et al., 2014; Silvers et al., 2019; Waldron et al., 2007). There has been less research on behavioral family-based treatment and motivational interviewing, but both approaches appear to be moderately efficacious (Hogue et al., 2019). In addition, emotional regulation skill-based interventions, informed by dialectical behavior therapy, have been shown to be promising for youth with concurrent disorders (Hawkins, 2009; Henderson et al., 2019). Importantly, it has been demonstrated that incorporating young adult perspectives in the development of SUD services enhances overall treatment uptake, engagement, and satisfaction (Hawke et al., 2019).

Other Variables Influencing Treatment

Assessment and Diagnosis

Assessment plays a critical role in treatment in a number of ways, including screening for and diagnosing SUDs, identifying co-occurring conditions, identifying functional relationships that maintain substance use, defining and prioritizing specific treatment outcomes, providing patients with objective feedback about substance use, and evaluating progress over the course of treatment. Idiographic assessment using a battery of psychometrically validated tests is a foundational component of empirically supported psychological treatment.

Commonly used screening tools include the Alcohol Use Disorders Identification Test (AUDIT; WHO, 2001), the Cannabis Use Disorders Identification Test (CUDIT; Adamson et al., 2010), the Drug Use Disorders Identification Test (DUDIT; Berman et al., 2005), the Drug Abuse Screen Test (DAST; Skinner, 1982), and the Alcohol, Smoking and Substance Involvement Screening Test (ASSIST; NIDA, 2009). Following initial screening, comprehensive assessments that incorporate diagnostic and multidimensional approaches are necessary, and are particularly important for differential diagnosis of SUDs and other psychiatric conditions (APA, 2013; Daley & Douaihy, 2019; Liese & Beck, 2022; Reus et al., 2018). For example, patients commonly endorse depressive symptoms, but these may be the result of negative consequence from substance use, withdrawal symptoms, or fully independent symptoms reflecting major depressive disorder, requiring careful assessment for disambiguation. Thus, a fulsome assessment of history and onset of use, patterns of use (frequency, amount, route of administration), negative consequences from use, physiological dependence (features of tolerance and withdrawal), psychiatric symptoms and history, and medical history is warranted. This may be obtained using an integrated assessment, such as the Addiction Severity Index, or a bespoke battery of validated measures. Accurate diagnostic evaluations are also necessary to identify the most appropriate level of care depending on presenting substance use (or polysubstance use), and symptom severity (e.g., withdrawal management for acute withdrawal versus outpatient treatment versus residential inpatient treatment).

In terms of treatment process, functional analysis is strongly recommended to understand the patterns of active substance use, drugs of choice (i.e., primary/secondary substances), and functional profiles of use to prioritize treatment targets with patients. Understanding the antecedents (i.e., prepotent internal and external cues and triggers), behavioral patterns, and consequences through the lens of positively and negatively reinforcing motivational functions provides a blueprint for the most appropriate credible treatment components (e.g., relevant coping skills, need for motivational enhancement, availability of alternative reinforcers). Increasingly, a measurement-based care (MBC) approach is being applied to SUDs (Clarke et al.,

2021; Marsden et al., 2019), which refers to structured repeated assessment of key process mechanisms (e.g., motivation, self-efficacy, cravings) that can be thought of as "recovery vital signs" and substance use itself and comorbid symptoms. This ongoing process and outcome measurement provides quantitative metrics that can reveal positive patient progress (and be incorporated therapeutically), but can also be used to change direction or implement a new component if the trajectory is unfavorable. Importantly, MBC is a framework, not a single protocol, and can take many forms, akin to the many ways contingency management can be configured for specific clinical questions (Lewis et al., 2019). The use of standardized validated measures is the common recommendation across MBC protocols. Furthermore, MBC-based approaches offer an opportunity to develop practice-based evidence about clinical innovations in real-world clinical settings.

Comorbidity

A major factor affecting SUD treatment response is the presence of co-occurring psychiatric disorders, referred to by several terms including concurrent disorders, dual diagnosis, and dual disorders. The presence of an SUD with one or more other comorbidities is clinically common (Keen et al., 2022; Rush et al., 2008; Skinner et al., 2004) and is associated not only with poorer treatment outcomes but also with increased risk of suicidal behavior, interpersonal violence, hospitalization, traumatic brain injury, criminal justice system involvement, and overdose death (Connery et al., 2020; Keen et al., 2022). The most commonly prevalent co-occurring disorders are mood, anxiety, and stress-related disorders, but there are numerous possible combinations of co-occurring SUD and other psychiatric disorders (Keen et al., 2022). Heterogeneous clinical presentations, combined with the varying severity of co-occurring disorders, and the degree of available psychosocial supports further complicates the clinical picture (Drake et al., 2007; McKee, 2017; Mueser et al., 2003). Currently, there are few well-validated integrated treatment protocols for specific combinations, although promising examples exist, including concurrent treatment of SUD with major depressive disorder (Daughters et al., 2018; Samokhvalov et al., 2018) and with posttraumatic stress disorder (Back et al., 2019). More generally, integrated treatment offering evidence-based approaches that target both the SUDs and mental health symptoms simultaneously is the recommended strategy (Magill et al., 2020; McKee, 2017; Mueser et al., 2003).

Demographics

There is robust epidemiological evidence that specific demographic subpopulations are at a greater risk for SUDs, including individuals experiencing socioeconomic adversity and discrimination, sexual minorities, those with lower educational attainment, males, and adolescents and young adults (Medley et al., 2016; SAMHSA, 2020; Witkiewitz et al., 2022). At present, however, there is limited evidence that would specifically recommend (or contraindicate) the preceding evidence-based components for specific demographic subpopulations. Rather, a common theme to all of the components is the importance of a thorough idiographic assessment and incorporation of these important features of identity and personal history into a treatment plan. For example, a functional analysis in CBT should fully incorporate demographic considerations, including a person's sex and gender, race and ethnicity, and socioeconomic factors, as potential determinants of substance use. As noted, the most fulsome example of this is that many treatments were not developed for or validated in youth specifically but are nonetheless implemented with incorporation of youth considerations. Furthermore, recent research has started to investigate subpopulation-specific interventions, such as a "two-eyed seeing" approach for Indigenous people that incorporates the historical context and experiences of Indigenous people (Hawke et al., 2019; Marsh et al., 2015). A challenge, of course, is that there is substantial heterogeneity within subpopulations, so tailoring of interventions has to be careful not to assume that all individuals of a certain identity will experience common determinants. Nonetheless, there is no question that demographic factors such as race, sex, and sexual orientation are implicated in SUD risk and need to be incorporated into SUD treatment.

Medication

When approved medications are available, integrated psychological and pharmacological treatment is warranted (MacKillop et al., 2018), unless a patient has a medical contraindication or strong preference to the contrary. Unless a pharmacotherapy is available in an over-the-counter format, this is typically via collaborative care with a physician. For opioid use disorder, buprenorphine (a partial opioid agonist combined with naltrexone to deter intravenous use) and methadone (a full opioid agonist) are first-line treatments to alleviate withdrawal (Bruneau et al., 2018; Perry et al., 2022; Soyka & Franke, 2021). For tobacco use disorder, nicotine replacement therapy (NRT) is an over-the-counter first-line treatment that is available in multiple formulations, including patch, gum, lozenge, oral spray, and intranasal inhaler. It is typically used in a dual-formulation strategy (i.e., slow-acting transdermal patch plus a faster-acting formulation for breakthrough cravings) (Rigotti et al., 2022). Varenicline and buprenorphine XL are medications that have also been shown to be efficacious (Rigotti et al., 2022), typically in combination with a behavioral treatment program. For moderate-to-severe AUD, both naltrexone (a partial μ opioid receptor antagonist) and acamprosate (an *N*-methyl-D-aspartic acid receptor modulator) are recommended first-line medications (Reus et al., 2018). Disulfiram, which disrupts alcohol metabolism and produces an aversive reaction if alcohol is consumed, has inconsistent efficacy and is only recommended for individuals who are seeking abstinence, have not responded to naltrexone and acamprosate, and are capable of understanding the potential risks of drinking while taking disulfiram (Reus et al., 2018). Topiramate and gabapentin are also second-line options (Reus et al., 2018).

Most germane to psychological treatment, in a recent meta-analysis, CBT and other specific therapies in combination with pharmacotherapies were found to produce significantly improved overall treatment outcomes when compared to psychological treatment or medication alone (Ray et al., 2020). Beyond concurrently offering psychological and pharmacological treatment, however, it is not clear how medication integration effects psychotherapy process or outcome. Direct synergistic integration of pharmacological and psychological treatment has been demonstrated in early-stage proof-of-concept studies (e.g., MacKillop et al., 2015), but research in this area is nascent and the standard-of-care is parallel pharmacological and psychological treatment.

Conclusion

A core portfolio of psychological treatments is available for treating SUDs. These interventions – CBT, motivational interviewing, and reinforcement-based approaches – are premised on robust theoretical and etiological frameworks and supported by methodologically rigorous intervention research. Although there are important nuances in the treatment outcome literature, the balance of the evidence supports these approaches. From these approaches come core competencies for clinical psychologists, and standard training in these techniques is warranted, akin to other common psychiatric conditions. Given that only a small minority of individuals with SUDs receive treatment and in many treatment programs empirically supported practices are often not employed (Knudsen & Roman, 2016; Olmstead et al., 2012), expanding training in these competencies and increasing the workforce of mental health providers implementing these strategies is critical.

Useful Resources

Book/Manual

- Daley, D. C., & Douaihy, A. B. (2019). *Managing your substance use disorder: Client workbook* (3rd ed.). Oxford University Press.
- Miller, W. R. (2004). *Combined behavioral intervention manual: A clinical research guide for therapists treating people with alcohol abuse and dependence.* National Institutes of Health.

Websites

- National Harm Reduction Coalition: Overdose prevention: https://harmreduction.org/issues/overdose-prevention/
- NIAAA Core Resource on Alcohol: www.niaaa.nih.gov/health-professionals-communities/core-resource-on-alcohol
- NIAAA Treatment Navigator: https://alcoholtreatment.niaaa.nih.gov/
- SMART Recovery: www.smartrecovery.org/
- Surgeon General's Report on Addiction: https://addiction.surgeongeneral.gov/sites/default/files/surgeon-generals-report.pdf
- Veterans Affairs: www.healthquality.va.gov/

References

Acuff, S. F., Dennhardt, A. A., Correia, C. J., & Murphy, J. G. (2019). Measurement of substance-free reinforcement in addiction: A systematic review. *Clinical Psychology Review*, 70, 79–90

Adamson, S. J., Kay-Lambkin, F. J., Baker, A. L., et al. (2010). An improved brief measure of cannabis misuse: The Cannabis Use Disorders Identification Test-Revised (CUDIT-R). *Drug and Alcohol Dependence*, 110(1–2), 137–143.

American Psychiatric Association (APA). (2013). *Diagnostic and statistical manual of mental disorders* (5th ed.). American Psychiatric Association.

Apodaca, T. R., & Longabaugh, R. (2009). Mechanisms of change in motivational interviewing: A review and preliminary evaluation of the evidence. *Addiction*, 104(5), 705–715. https://doi.org/10.1111/j.1360-0443.2009.02527.x

Arnett, J. J. (2000). Emerging adulthood: A theory of development from the late teens through the twenties. *American Psychologist*, 55(5), 469–480.

Back, S. E., Killeen, T., Badour, C. L., et al. (2019). Concurrent treatment of substance use disorders and PTSD using prolonged exposure: A randomized clinical trial in military veterans. *Addictive Behaviors*, 90, 369–377. https://doi.org/10.1016/J.ADDBEH.2018.11.032.

Bandura, A. (1977). Self-efficacy: Toward a unifying theory of behavioral change. *Psychological Review*, 84, 191–215.

Baskin-Sommers, A., & Sommers, I. (2006). The co-occurrence of substance use and high-risk behaviors. *Journal of Adolescent Health*, 38(5), 609–611.

Beck, A. K., Forbes, E., Baker, A. L., et al. (2017). Systematic review of SMART Recovery: Outcomes, process variables, and implications for research. *Psychology of Addictive Behaviors*, 31(1), 1–20.

Beck, A. T., Wright, F. D., Newman, C. F., & Liese, B. S. (1993). *Cognitive therapy of substance abuse*. Guilford Press.

Benishek, L. A., Dugosh, K. L., Kirby, K. C., et al. (2014). Prize-based contingency management for the treatment of substance abusers: A meta-analysis. *Addiction*, 109(9), 1426–1436.

Bentzley, B. S., Han, S. S., Neuner, S., et al. (2021). Comparison of treatments for cocaine use disorder among adults: A systematic review and meta-analysis. *JAMA Network Open*, 4(5), e218049.

Berman, A., Bergman, H., Palmstierna, T., & Schlyter, F. (2005). *Drug use disorders identification test manual*. Karolinska Institute.

Bickel, W. K., Johnson, M. W., Koffarnus, M. N., MacKillop, J., & Murphy, J. G. (2014). The behavioral economics of substance use disorders: Reinforcement pathologies and their repair. *Annual Review of Clinical Psychology*, 10(1), 641–677. https://doi.org/10.1146/annurev-clinpsy-032813-153724

Bigelow, G. E. (2001). An operant behavioral perspective on alcohol abuse and dependence. In N. Heather, T. J. Peters, & T. Stockwell (Eds.), *International handbook of alcohol dependence and problems* (pp. 299–315). John Wiley & Sons.

Bohnert, K. M., Walton, M. A., Resko, S., et al. (2014). Latent class analysis of substance use among adolescents presenting to urban primary care clinics. *American Journal of Drug and Alcohol Abuse*, 40(1), 44–50. https://doi.org/10.3109/00952990.2013.844821.

Bolívar, H. A., Klemperer, E. M., Coleman, S. R. M., et al. (2021). Contingency management for patients receiving medication for opioid use disorder: A systematic review and meta-analysis. *JAMA Psychiatry*, 78(10), 1092–1102. https://doi.org/10.1001/jamapsychiatry.2021.1969.

Boness, C. L., Votaw, V. R., Schwebel, F. J., et al. (2023). An evaluation of cognitive behavioral therapy for substance use disorders: A systematic review and application of the Society of Clinical Psychology criteria for empirically supported treatments. *Clinical Psychology: Science and Practice*, 30(2), 129–142. https://doi.org/10.1037/cps0000131.

Bowen, S., Witkiewitz, K., Clifasefi, S. L., et al. (2014). Relative efficacy of mindfulness-based relapse prevention, standard relapse prevention, and treatment as usual for substance use disorders: A randomized clinical trial. *JAMA Psychiatry*, 71(5), 547–556.

Brown, H. D., & DeFulio, A. (2020). Contingency management for the treatment of methamphetamine use disorder: A systematic review. *Drug and Alcohol Dependence*, 216, 108307. https://doi.org/10.1016/j.drugalcdep.2020.108307.

Bruneau, J., Ahamad, K., Goyer, M. È., et al. (2018). Management of opioid use disorders: A national clinical practice guideline. *Canadian Medical Association Journal*, 190(9), E247–E257.

Businelle, M. S., Rash, C. J., Burke, R. S., & Parker, J. D. (2009). Using vouchers to increase continuing care participation in veterans: Does magnitude matter? *The American Journal on Addictions*, 18(2), 122–129. https://doi.org/10.1080/10550490802545125.

Carroll, K. M., Sinha, R., Nich, C., Babuscio, T., & Rounsaville, B. J. (2002). Contingency management to enhance naltrexone treatment of opioid dependence: A randomized clinical trial of reinforcement magnitude. *Experimental and Clinical Psychopharmacology*, 10(1), 54–63. https://doi.org/10.1037//1064-1297.10.1.54.

Catchpole, R. E., & Brownlie, E. B. (2016). Characteristics of youth presenting to a Canadian youth concurrent disorders program: Clinical complexity, trauma, adaptive functioning and treatment priorities. *Journal of the Canadian Academy of Child and Adolescent Psychiatry*, 25(2), 106.

Chambless, D. L., & Hollon, S. D. (1998). Defining empirically supported therapies. *Journal of Consulting and Clinical Psychology*, 66(1), 7–18. https://doi.org/10.1037/0022-006X.66.1.7.

Choi, H. J., Lu, Y., Schulte, M., & Temple, J. R. (2018). Adolescent substance use: Latent class and transition analysis. *Addictive Behaviors*, 77, 160–165.

Clarke, D. E., Ibrahim, A., Doty, B., et al. (2021). Addiction Medicine Practice-Based Research Network (AMNet): Assessment tools and quality measures. *Substance Abuse and Rehabilitation*, 12, 27–39. https://doi.org/10.2147/SAR.S305972.

Connell, C. M., Gilreath, T. D., & Hansen, N. B. (2009). A multiprocess latent class analysis of the co-occurrence of substance use and sexual risk behavior among adolescents. *Journal of Studies on Alcohol and Drugs*, 70(6), 943–951.

Connery, H. S., McHugh, R. K., Reilly, M., Shin, S., & Greenfield, S. F. (2020). Substance use disorders in global mental health delivery: epidemiology, treatment gap, and implementation of evidence-based treatments. *Harvard Review of Psychiatry*, 28(5), 316–327. https://doi.org/10.1097/HRP.0000000000000271.

Corace, K., Willows, M., Schubert, N., Overington, L., & Howell, G. (2018). Youth require tailored treatment for opioid use and mental health problems: A comparison with adults. *Canadian Journal of Addiction*, 9(4), 15–24.

Daley, D. C., & Douaihy, A. B. (2019). *Managing substance use disorder: Practitioner guide*. Oxford University Press.

Daughters, S. B., Magidson, J. F., Anand, D., et al. (2018). The effect of a behavioral activation treatment for substance use on post-treatment abstinence: A randomized controlled trial. *Addiction (Abingdon, England)*, 113(3), 535–544. https://doi.org/10.1111/ADD.14049.

Dawson, D. A., Grant, B. F., & Li, T. K. (2007). Impact of age at first drink on stress-reactive drinking. *Alcoholism: Clinical and Experimental Research*, 31(1), 69–77.

Denis-Lalonde, D., Lind, C., & Estefan, A. (2019). Beyond the buzzword: A concept analysis of harm reduction. *Research and Theory for Nursing Practice*, 33(4), 310–323.

Destoop, M., Docx, L., Morrens, M., & Dom, G. (2021). Meta-analysis on the effect of contingency management for patients with both psychotic disorders and substance use disorders. *Journal of Clinical Medicine*, 10(4), 1–14. https://doi.org/10.3390/jcm10040616.

DiClemente, C. C., Corno, C. M., Graydon, M. M., Wiprovnick, A. E., & Knoblach, D. J. (2017). Motivational interviewing, enhancement, and brief interventions over the last decade: A review of reviews of efficacy and effectiveness. *Psychology of Addictive Behaviors*, 31(8), 862.

DiClemente, C. C., Schlundt, D., & Gemmell, L. (2004). Readiness and stages of change in addiction treatment. *American Journal on Addictions*, 13(2), 103–119.

Dougherty, D. M., Hill-Kapturczak, N., Liang, Y., et al. (2014). Use of continuous transdermal alcohol monitoring during a contingency management procedure to reduce excessive alcohol use. *Drug and Alcohol Dependence*, 142, 301–306. https://doi.org/10.1016/j.drugalcdep.2014.06.039.

Drake, R., Mueser, K., & Brunette, M. F. (2007). Management of persons with co-occurring severe mental illness and substance use disorder: Program implications. *World Psychiatry*, 6(3), 131.

Dutcher, L. W., Anderson, R., Moore, M., et al. (2009). Community reinforcement and family training (CRAFT): An effectiveness study. *Journal of Behavior Analysis in Health, Sports, Fitness and Medicine*, 2(1), 80–93.

Erskine, H. E., Moffitt, T. E., Copeland, W. E., et al. (2015). A heavy burden on young minds: the global burden of mental and substance use disorders in children and youth. *Psychological Medicine*, 45(7), 1551–1563.

Esser, M. B., Leung, G., Sherk, A., et al. (2022). Estimated deaths attributable to excessive alcohol use among US adults aged 20 to 64 Years, 2015 to 2019. *JAMA Network Open*, 5(11), e2239485–e2239485.

Faggiano, F., Minozzi, S., Versino, E., & Buscemi, D. (2014). Universal school-based prevention for illicit drug use. *Cochrane Database of Systematic Reviews*, *12*, CD003020.

Godley, S. H., Smith, J. E., Passetti, L. L., & Subramaniam, G. (2014). The Adolescent Community Reinforcement Approach (A-CRA) as a model paradigm for the management of adolescents with substance use disorders and co-occurring psychiatric disorders. *Substance Abuse*, 35(4), 352–363. https://doi.org/10.1080/08897077.2014.936993.

Goldman, D., Oroszi, G., & Ducci, F. (2006). The genetics of addictions: Uncovering the genes. *Focus*, 6(3), 521–415.

González-Roz, A., Jackson, J., Murphy, C., Rohsenow, D. J., & MacKillop, J. (2019). Behavioral economic tobacco demand in relation to cigarette consumption and nicotine dependence: A meta-analysis of cross-sectional relationships. *Addiction*, 114(11), 1926–1940.

González-Roz, A., Weidberg, S., García-Pérez, Á., Martínez-Loredo, V., & Secades-Villa, R. (2021). One-year efficacy and incremental cost-effectiveness of contingency management for cigarette smokers with depression. *Nicotine and Tobacco Research*, 23(2), 320–326. https://doi.org/10.1093/ntr/ntaa146.

Grant, B. F., Goldstein, R. B., Saha, T. D., et al. (2015). Epidemiology of DSM-5 alcohol use disorder: Results from the National Epidemiologic Survey on Alcohol and Related Conditions III. *JAMA Psychiatry*, 72(8), 757. https://doi.org/10.1001/JAMA PSYCHIATRY.2015.0584.

Hasin, D. S. (2018). US eEpidemiology of cannabis use and associated problems. *Neuropsychopharmacology*, 43(1), 195–212. https://doi.org/10.1038/npp.2017.198.

Hawk, M., Coulter, R. W., Egan, J. E., et al. (2017). Harm reduction principles for healthcare settings. *Harm Reduction Journal*, 14, 1–9.

Hawke, L. D., Mehra, K., Settipani, C., et al. (2019). What makes mental health and substance use services youth friendly? A scoping review of literature. *BMC Health Services Research*, 19(1), 257. https://doi.org/10.1186/s12913-019-4066-5.

Hawkins, E. H. (2009). A tale of two systems: Co-occurring mental health and substance abuse disorders treatment for adolescents. *Annual Review of Psychology*, 60, 197–227.

Henderson, J. L., Brownlie, E. B., McMain, S., et al. (2019). Enhancing prevention and intervention for youth concurrent mental health and substance use disorders: The Research and Action for Teens study. *Early Intervention in Psychiatry*, 13(1), 110–119. https://doi.org/10.1111/eip.12458.

Higgins, S. T., Wong, C. J., Badger, G. J., Ogden, D. E., & Dantona, R. L. (2000). Contingent reinforcement increases cocaine abstinence during outpatient treatment and 1 year of follow-up. *Journal of Consulting and Clinical Psychology*, 68(1), 64–72.

Hogue, A., Bobek, M., Dauber, S., et al. (2019). Core elements of family therapy for adolescent behavior problems: Empirical distillation of three manualized treatments. *Journal of Clinical Child and Adolescent Psychology*, 48(1), 29–41. https://doi.org/10.1080/15374416.2018.1555762.

Hunt, G. M., & Azrin, N. H. (1973). A community-reinforcement approach to alcoholism. *Behaviour Research and Therapy*, 11(1), 91–104.

Hunt, N., Ashton, M., Lenton, S., et al. (2003). Review of the evidence-base for harm reduction approaches to drug use. www.hri.global/files/2010/05/31/HIVTop50Documents11.pdf.

Kabat-Zinn, J. (1994). *Mindfulness meditation for everyday life*. Hyperion.

Keen, C., Kinner, S. A., Young, J. T., et al. (2022). Prevalence of co-occurring mental illness and substance use disorder and association with overdose: A linked data cohort study among residents of British Columbia, Canada. *Addiction*, 117(1), 129–140.

Kelley, M. L., & Fals-Stewart, W. (2002). Couples- versus individual-based therapy for alcohol and drug abuse: Effects on children's psychosocial functioning. *Journal of Consulting and Clinical Psychology*, 70(2), 417–427. https://doi.org/10.1037/0022-006X.70.2.417.

Kelly, A. B., Chan, G. C. K., Mason, W. A., & Williams, J. W. (2015). The relationship between psychological distress and adolescent polydrug use. *Psychology of Addictive Behaviors*, 29(3), 787–793. https://doi.org/10.1037/adb0000068.

Kelly, J. F., Abry, A., Ferri, M., & Humphreys, K. (2020). Alcoholics anonymous and 12-step facilitation treatments for alcohol use disorder: A distillation of a 2020 Cochrane review for clinicians and policy makers. *Alcohol and Alcoholism*, 55(6), 641–651.

Kelly, J. F., Bergman, B. G., Hoeppner, B. B., Vilsaint, C., & White, W. L. (2017). Prevalence and pathways of recovery from drug and alcohol problems in the United States population: Implications for practice, research, and policy. *Drug and Alcohol Dependence*, 181, 162–169.

Kelly, P. J., McCreanor, K., Beck, A. K., et al. (2021). SMART Recovery International and COVID-19: Expanding the reach of mutual support through online groups. *Journal of Substance Abuse Treatment*, 131, 108568. https://doi.org/10.1016/j.jsat.2021.108568.

Kimmel, S. D., Gaeta, J. M., Hadland, S. E., Hallett, E., & Marshall, B. D. (2021). Principles of harm reduction for young people who use drugs. *Pediatrics*, 147(Supplement 2), S240–S248.

Kirby, K. C., Marlowe, D. B., Festinger, D. S., Garvey, K. A., & LaMonaca, V. (1999). Community reinforcement training for family and significant others of drug abusers: A unilateral intervention to increase treatment entry of drug users. *Drug and Alcohol Dependence*, 56, 85–96. https://doi.org/10.1016/S0376-8716(99)00022-8.

Klostermann, K., Chen, R., Kelley, M. L., et al. (2011). Coping behavior and depressive symptoms in adult children of alcoholics. *Substance Use and Misuse*, 46(9), 1162–1168. https://doi.org/10.3109/10826080903452546.

Knudsen, H. K., & Roman, P. M. (2016). Service delivery and pharmacotherapy for alcohol use disorder in the era of health reform: Data from a national sample of treatment organizations. *Substance Abuse*, 37(1), 230–237. https://doi.org/10.1080/08897077.2015.1028699.

Koob, G. F. (2006). The neurobiology of addiction: A neuroadaptational view relevant for diagnosis. *Addiction*, 101, 23–30.

Korecki, J. R., Schwebel, F. J., Votaw, V. R., & Witkiewitz, K. (2020). Mindfulness-based programs for substance use disorders: A systematic review of manualized treatments. *Substance Abuse Treatment, Prevention, and Policy*, 15(1), 1–37.

Lake, M. T., Krishnamurti, T., Murtaugh, K. L., van Nunen, L. J., Stein, D. J., & Shoptaw, S. (2023). Decision-making tendencies and voucher spending independently support abstinence within contingency management for methamphetamine use disorder. *Experimental and Clinical Psychopharmacology*, 31(2), 324–329. https://doi.org/10.1037/PHA0000574.

Lam, W. K., Fals-Stewart, W., & Kelley, M. L. (2008). Effects of parent skills training with behavioral couples therapy for alcoholism on children: A randomized clinical pilot trial. *Addictive Behaviors*, 33(8), 1076–1080.

Ledgerwood, D. M., Arfken, C. L., Petry, N. M., & Alessi, S. M. (2014). Prize contingency management for smoking cessation: A randomized trial. *Drug and Alcohol Dependence*, 140, 208–212. https://doi.org/10.1016/j.drugalcdep.2014.03.032

Lewis, C. C., Boyd, M., Puspitasari, A., et al. (2019). Implementing measurement-based care in behavioral health: A review. *JAMA Psychiatry*, 76(3), 324–335. https://doi.org/10.1001/JAMAPSYCHIATRY.2018.3329.

Li, W., Howard, M. O., Garland, E. L., McGovern, P., & Lazar, M. (2017). Mindfulness treatment for substance misuse: A systematic review and meta-analysis. *Journal of Substance Abuse Treatment*, 75, 62–96.

Liese, B. S., & Beck, A. T. (2022). *Cognitive-behavioral therapy of addictive disorders*. Guilford Publications.

Lott, D. C., & Jencius, S. (2009). Effectiveness of very low-cost contingency management in a community adolescent treatment program. *Drug and Alcohol Dependence*, 102(1–3), 162–165. https://doi.org/10.1016/J.DRUGALCDEP.2009.01.010

Lundahl, B., & Burke, B. L. (2009). The effectiveness and applicability of motivational interviewing: A practice-friendly review of four meta-analyses. *Journal of Clinical Psychology*, 65(11), 1232–1245.

Lussier, J. P., Heil, S. H., Mongeon, J. A., Badger, G. J., & Higgins, S. T. (2006). A meta-analysis of voucher-based reinforcement therapy for substance use disorders. *Addiction*, 101(2), 192–203.

MacKillop, J, Few, L., Stojek, M. K., et al. (2015) D-cycloserine to enhance extinction of cue-elicited craving for alcohol: A translational approach. *Translational Psychiatry*, 5(4), e544. https://doi.org/10.1038/tp.2015.41.

MacKillop, J. (2016). The behavioral economics and neuroeconomics of alcohol use disorders. *Alcoholism: Clinical and Experimental Research*, 40(4), 672–685.

MacKillop, J., & Ray, L. A. (2018). The etiology of addiction: A contemporary biopsychosocial approach. In J. MacKillop, G. Kenna, L. Leggio, & L. A. Ray (Eds.), *Integrating psychological and pharmacological treatments for addictive disorders: An evidence-based guide* (pp. 32–53). Routledge/Taylor & Francis Group.

MacKillop, J., Agabio, R., Feldstein Ewing, S. W., et al. (2022). Hazardous drinking and alcohol use disorders. *Nature Reviews Disease Primers*, 8(1), 80.

MacKillop, J., Amlung, M. T., Few, L. R., et al. (2011). Delayed reward discounting and addictive behavior: A meta-analysis. *Psychopharmacology*, 216(3), 305–321. https://doi.org/10.1007/s00213-011-2229-0.

MacKillop, J., VanderBroek-Stice, L., & Munn, C. (2018). Enhancing motivation. In S. C. Hayes & S. G. Hoffman (Eds.), *Process-Based CBT: The Science and Core Clinical Competencies of Cognitive Behavioral Therapy* (pp. 389–402). Context Press.

Magill, M., & Ray, L. A. (2009). Cognitive-behavioral treatment with adult alcohol and illicit drug users: A meta-analysis of randomized controlled trials. *Journal of Studies on Alcohol and Drugs*, 70(4), 516–527.

Magill, M., Apodaca, T. R., Borsari, B., et al. (2018). A meta-analysis of motivational interviewing process: Technical, relational, and conditional process models of change. *Journal of Consulting and Clinical Psychology*, 86(2), 140–157. https://doi.org/10.1037/ccp0000250.

Magill, M., Ray, L., Kiluk, B., et al. (2019). A meta-analysis of cognitive-behavioral therapy for alcohol or other drug use disorders: Treatment efficacy by contrast condition. *Journal of Consulting and Clinical Psychology*, 87(12), 1093–1105. https://doi.org/10.1037/ccp0000447.

Magill, M., Tonigan, J. S., Kiluk, B., et al. (2020). The search for mechanisms of cognitive behavioral therapy for alcohol or other drug use disorders: A systematic review. *Behaviour Research and Therapy*, 131, 103648. https://doi.org/10.1016/j.brat.2020.103648.

Marlatt, G. A. Gordon, J.R. (1985). *Relapse prevention*. Guilford Press.

Marlatt, G. A., & Donovan, D. M. (Eds.). (2005). *Relapse prevention: Maintenance strategies in the treatment of addictive behaviors*. Guilford Press.

Marsden, J., Tai, B., Ali, R., et al. (2019). Measurement-based care using DSM-5 for opioid use disorder: Can we make opioid medication treatment more effective? *Addiction*, 114(8), 1346–1353. https://doi.org/10.1111/ADD.14546.

Marsh, T. N., Cote-Meek, S., Toulouse, P., et al. (2015). The application of two-eyed seeing decolonizing methodology in qualitative and quantitative research for the treatment of intergenerational trauma and substance use disorders. *International Journal of Qualitative Methods*, 14(5), 1609406915618046.

Martínez-Loredo, V., González-Roz, A., Secades-Villa, R., Fernández-Hermida, J. R., & MacKillop, J. (2021). Concurrent validity of the Alcohol Purchase Task for measuring the reinforcing efficacy of alcohol: An updated systematic review and meta-analysis. *Addiction*, 116(10), 2635–2650.

McCaul, M. E., Stitzer, M. L., Bigelow, G. E., & Liebson, I. A. (1984). Contingency management interventions: effects on treatment outcome during methadone detoxification *Journal of Applied Behavior Analysis*, 17(1), 35–43. https://doi.org/10.1901/jaba.1984.17-35.

McCrady, B. S., Epstein, E. E., Cook, S., Jensen, N., & Hildebrandt, T. (2009). A randomized trial of individual and couple behavioral alcohol treatment for women. *Journal of Consulting and Clinical Psychology*, 77(2), 243–256. https://doi.org/10.1037/a0014686.

McHugh, R. K., Hearon, B. A., & Otto, M. W. (2010). Cognitive behavioral therapy for substance use disorders. *Psychiatric Clinics*, 33(3), 511–525.

McKee, S. A. (2017). Concurrent substance use disorders and mental illness: Bridging the gap between research and treatment. *Canadian Psychology/Psychologie Canadienne*, 58(1), 50.

McLellan, A. T., Koob, G. F., & Volkow, N. D. (2022). Preaddiction – a missing concept for treating substance use disorders. *JAMA Psychiatry*, 79(8), 749–751.

Medley G., Lipari R., Bose J., et al. (2016). Sexual orientation and estimates of adult substance use and mental health: Results from the 2015 National Survey on Drug Use and Health. Substance Abuse and Mental Health Services Administration, US Department of Health and Human Services.

Merrin, G. J., Thompson, K., & Leadbeater, B. J. (2018). Transitions in the use of multiple substances from adolescence to young adulthood. *Drug and Alcohol Dependence*, 189, 147–153. https://doi.org/10.1016/j.drugalcdep.2018.05.015.

Meyers, R. J., Miller, W. R., Smith, J. E., & Tonigan, J. S. (2002). A randomized trial of two methods for engaging treatment-refusing drug users through concerned significant others. *Journal of Consulting and Clinical Psychology*, 70(5), 1182.

Miller, W. R. (1983). Motivational interviewing with problem drinkers. *Behavioural and Cognitive Psychotherapy*, 11(2), 147–172.

Miller, W. R., & Rollnick, S. (2002). *Motivational interviewing: Preparing people for change* (2nd ed.). Guilford Press.

Miller, W. R., & Rollnick, S. (2012). Meeting in the middle: Motivational interviewing and self-determination theory. *International Journal of Behavioral Nutrition and Physical Activity*, 9, 25. https://doi.org/10.1186/1479-5868-9-25.

Miller, W. R., & Rose, G. S. (2009). Toward a theory of motivational interviewing. *American Psychologist*, 64(6), 527. https://doi.org/10.1037/a0016830.

Miller, W. R., Meyers, R. J., & Hiller-Sturmhofel, S. (1999). The community-reinforcement approach. *Alcohol Research and Health*, 23(2), 116–121.

Monti, P. M. (Ed.). (2002). *Treating alcohol dependence: A coping skills training guide*. Guilford Press.

Monti, P. M., & O'Leary, T. A. (1999). Coping and social skills training for alcohol and cocaine dependence. *Psychiatric Clinics*, 22(2), 447–470.

Monti, P. M., Rohsenow, D. J., Swift, R. M., et al. (2001). Naltrexone and cue exposure with coping and communication skills training for alcoholics: treatment process and 1-year outcomes. *Alcoholism: Clinical and Experimental Research*, 25(11), 1634–1647.

Morin, J. F. G., Afzali, M. H., Bourque, J., et al. (2019). A population-based analysis of the relationship between substance use and adolescent cognitive development. *American Journal of Psychiatry*, 176(2), 98–106. https://doi.org/10.1176/appi.ajp.2018.18020202.

Mueser, K. T., Noordsy, D. L., Drake, R. E., & Fox, L. (2003). *Integrated treatment for dual disorders: A guide to effective practice*. Guilford Press.

National Institute on Drug Abuse (2009). NIDA Modified Alcohol, Smoking and Substance Involvement Screening Test (ASSIST). www.samhsa.gov/resource/ebp/nida-modified-assist-nm-assist-clinicians-screening-tool-drug-use-general-medical.

National Institute on Drug Abuse. (2017). *Trends & statistics*. National Institute of Health.

National Institute on Drug Abuse. (2018). *Drugs, brains, and behavior: The Science of Addiction*.

Notley, C., Gentry, S., Livingstone-Banks, J., et al. (2019). Incentives for smoking cessation. *Cochrane Database of Systematic Reviews*, 2019(7). https://doi.org/10.1002/14651858.CD004307.pub6.

Olmstead, T. A., & Petry, N. M. (2009). The cost-effectiveness of prize-based and voucher-based contingency management in a population of cocaine- or opioid-dependent outpatients. *Drug and Alcohol Dependence*, 102(1–3), 108–115. https://doi.org/10.1016/j.drugalcdep.2009.02.005.

Olmstead, T. A., Cohen, J. P., & Petry, N. M. (2012). Health-care service utilization in substance abusers receiving contingency management and standard care treatments. *Addiction*, 107(8), 1462–1470.

Pace, B. T., Dembe, A., Soma, C. S., et al. (2017). A multivariate meta-analysis of motivational interviewing process and outcome. *Psychology of Addictive Behaviors*, 31(5), 524–533. https://doi.org/10.1037/adb0000280.

Perry, C., Liberto, J., Milliken, C., et al. (2022). The management of substance use disorders: synopsis of the 2021 US Department of Veterans Affairs and US Department of Defense clinical practice guideline. *Annals of Internal Medicine*, 175(5), 720–731. https://doi.org/10.7326/M21-4011.

Petry, N. M., & Roll, J. M. (2011). Amount of earnings during prize contingency management treatment is associated with posttreatment abstinence outcomes. *Experimental and Clinical Psychopharmacology*, 19(6), 445–450. https://doi.org/10.1037/A0024261.

Petry, N. M., Alessi, S. M., & Rash, C. J. (2013). A randomized study of contingency management in cocaine-dependent patients with severe and persistent mental health disorders. *Drug and Alcohol Dependence*, 130(1–3), 234–237. https://doi.org/10.1016/j.drugalcdep.2012.10.017.

Petry, N. M., Alessi, S. M., Barry, D., & Carroll, K. M. (2015). Standard magnitude prize reinforcers can be as efficacious as larger magnitude reinforcers in cocaine-dependent methadone patients. *Journal of Consulting and Clinical Psychology*, 83(3), 464–472. https://doi.org/10.1037/A0037888.

Petry, N. M., Martin, B., Cooney, J. L., & Kranzler, H. R. (2000). Give them prizes and they will come: Contingency management for treatment of alcohol dependence. *Journal of Consulting and Clinical Psychology*, 68(2), 250–257.

Petry, N. M., Tedford, J., Austin, M., et al. (2004). Prize reinforcement contingency management for treating cocaine users: How low can we go, and with whom? *Addiction*, 99(3), 349–360. https://doi.org/10.1111/J.1360-0443.2003.00642.X.

Pfund, R. A., Ginley, M. K., Boness, C. L., et al. (2022). Contingency management for drug use disorders: Meta-analysis and application of Tolin's criteria. *Clinical Psychology: Science and Practice*. https://doi.org/10.1037/cps0000121.

Powers, M. B., Vedel, E., & Emmelkamp, P. M. (2008). Behavioral couples therapy (BCT) for alcohol and drug use disorders: A meta-analysis. *Clinical Psychology Review*, 28(6), 952–962. https://doi.org/10.1016/j.cpr.2008.02.002.

Prendergast, M., Podus, D., Finney, J., Greenwell, J., & Roll, J. (2006). Contingency management for treatment of substance use disorders: A meta-analysis. *Addiction*, 101, 1546–1560.

Prochaska, J. O., & DiClemente, C. C. (1992). Stages of change in the modification of problem behaviors. *Progress in Behavior Modification*, 28, 183–218. https://pubmed.ncbi.nlm.nih.gov/1620663/.

Prochaska, J. O., DiClemente, C. C., Velicer, W. F., & Rossi, J. S. (1992). Criticisms and concerns of the transtheoretical model in light of recent research. *British Journal of Addiction*, 118(1), 825–828. https://doi.org/10.1111/j.1360-0443.1992.tb01973.x.

Prochaska, J. Q., & Diclemente, C. C. (1983). Stages and processes of self-change of smoking: Toward an Integrative model of change. *Journal of Consulting and Clinical Psychology*, 51(3), 390–395.

Ray, L. A., Meredith, L. R., Kiluk, B. D., et al. (2020). Combined pharmacotherapy and cognitive behavioral therapy for adults with alcohol or substance use disorders: A systematic review and meta-analysis. *JAMA Network Open*, 3(6), e208279–e208279. https://doi.org/10.1001/jamanetworkopen.2020.8279.

Regnier, S. D., Strickland, J. C., & Stoops, W. W. (2022). A preliminary investigation of schedule parameters on cocaine abstinence in contingency management. *Journal of the Experimental Analysis of Behavior*, 118(1), 83–95. https://doi.org/10.1002/JEAB.770.

Reus, V. I., Fochtmann, L. J., Bukstein, O., et al. (2018). The American Psychiatric Association Practice Guideline for the pharmacological treatment of patients with alcohol use disorder, *American Journal of Psychiatry* 175(1), 86–90. https://Doi.Org/10.1176/Appi.Ajp.2017.1750101.

Rigotti, N. A., Kruse, G. R., Livingstone-Banks, J., & Hartmann-Boyce, J. (2022). Treatment of tobacco smoking: A review. *JAMA*, 327(6), 566–577. https://doi.org/10.1001/JAMA.2022.0395.

Romano, M., & Peters, L. (2016). Understanding the process of motivational interviewing: A review of the relational and technical hypotheses. *Psychotherapy Research*, 26(2), 220–240.

Rotunda, R. J., O'Farrell, T. J., Murphy, M., & Babey, S. H. (2008). Behavioral couples therapy for comorbid substance use disorders and combat-related posttraumatic stress disorder among male veterans: An initial evaluation. *Addictive Behaviors*, 33, 180–187.

Rush, B., Urbanoski, K., Bassani, D., et al. (2008). Prevalence of co-occurring substance use and other mental disorders in the Canadian population. *Canadian Journal of Psychiatry*, 53(12), 800–809. https://doi.org/10.1177/070674370805301206.

Samokhvalov, A. V., Probst, C., Awan, S., et al. (2018). Outcomes of an integrated care pathway for concurrent major depressive and alcohol use disorders: A multisite prospective cohort study. *BMC Psychiatry*, 18(1). https://doi.org/10.1186/S12888-018-1770-3.

Sarvet, A. L., & Hasin, D. (2016). The natural history of substance use disorders. *Current Opinion in Psychiatry*, 29(4), 250–257. https://doi.org/10.1097/YCO.0000000000000257.

Secades-Villa, R., Aonso-Diego, G., García-Pérez, Á., & González-Roz, A. (2020). Effectiveness of contingency management for smoking cessation in substance users: A systematic review and meta-analysis. *Journal of Consulting and Clinical Psychology*, 88(10), 951–964. https://doi.org/10.1037/ccp0000611.

Silvers, J. A., Squeglia, L. M., Rømer Thomsen, K., Hudson, K. A., & Feldstein Ewing, S. W. (2019). Hunting for what works: Adolescents in addiction treatment. *Alcoholism, Clinical and Experimental Research*, 43(4), 578–592. https://doi.org/10.1111/ACER.13984.

Sindelar, J. L., Olmstead, T. A., & Peirce, J. M. (2007). Cost-effectiveness of prize-based contingency management in methadone maintenance treatment programs. *Addiction*, 102(9), 1463–1471. https://doi.org/10.1111/j.1360-0443.2007.01913.x.

Sisson, R. W., & Azrin, N. H. (1986). Family-member involvement to initiate and promote treatment of problem drinkers. *Journal of Behavior Therapy and Experimental Psychiatry*, 17(1), 15–21.

Skinner, H. A. (1982). The drug abuse screening test. *Addictive Behaviors*, 7(4), 363–371.

Skinner, W., O'Grady, C., Bartha, C., & Parker, C. (2004). *Concurrent substance use and mental health disorders*. Centre for Addiction and Mental Health.

Society of Clinical Psychology (n.d.). Mixed substance abuse/dependence. https://div12.org/diagnosis/mixed-substance-abuse-dependence/.

Soyka, M., & Franke, A. G. (2021). Recent advances in the treatment of opioid use disorders – Focus on long-acting buprenorphine formulations. *World Journal of Psychiatry*, 11(9), 543–552. https://doi.org/10.5498/WJP.V11.I9.543.

Sparks, R. D. (2014). Broadening the base of treatment for alcohol problems, a 1990 report for the institute of medicine: Personal reflections. In W. L. White & T. F. McGovern (Eds.), *Alcohol problems in the United States: Twenty years of treatment perspective* (pp. 227–231). Routledge.

Stahler, G. J., Mennis, J., & DuCette, J. P. (2016). Residential and outpatient treatment completion for substance use disorders in the US: Moderation analysis by demographics and drug of choice. *Addictive Behaviors*, 58, 129–135.

Stanger, C., & Budney, A. J. (2019). Contingency management: Using incentives to improve outcomes for adolescent substance use disorders. *Pediatric Clinics of North America*, 66(6), 1183–1192. https://doi.org/10.1016/j.pcl.2019.08.007.

Stigler, M. H., Neusel, E., & Perry, C. L. (2011). School-based programs to prevent and reduce alcohol use among youth. *Alcohol Research & Health*, 34(2), 157.

Stitzer, M., & Petry, N. (2006). Contingency management for treatment of substance abuse. *Annual Review of Clinical Psychology*, 2, 411–434.

Substance Abuse and Mental Health Services Administration (SAMHSA). (2020). *Key substance use and mental health indicators in the United States: Results from the 2019 National Survey on Drug Use and Health (HHS Publication No. PEP20-07-01-001, NSDUH Series H-55)*. Center for Behavioral Health Statistics and Quality, Substance Abuse and Mental Health Services Administration. www.samhsa.gov/data/.

Thomas, G. (2005). *Harm reduction policies and programs involved for persons involved in the criminal justice system*. Canadian Centre on Substance Use.

Tolin, D. F., McKay, D., Forman, E. M., Klonsky, E. D., & Thombs, B. D. (2015). Empirically supported treatment: Recommendations for a new model. *Clinical Psychology: Science and Practice*, 22(4), 317–338. https://doi.org/10.1111/cpsp.12122.

United Nations Office on Drugs and Crime (UNODC), World Drug Report 2020 (United Nations publication, Sales No. E.21.XI.8).

Waldron, H. B., Kern-Jones, S., Turner, C. W., Peterson, T. R., & Ozechowski, T. J. (2007). Engaging resistant adolescents in drug abuse treatment. *Journal of Substance Abuse Treatment*, 32(2), 133–142. https://doi.org/10.1016/j.jsat.2006.07.007.

WHO (2001). AUDIT: The Alcohol Use Disorders Identification Test. www.who.int/publications/i/item/WHO-MSD-MSB-01.6a.

Winters, K. C., Mader, J., Budney, A. J., et al. (2021). Interventions for cannabis use disorder. *Current Opinion in Psychology*, 38, 67–74. https://doi.org/10.1016/j.copsyc.2020.11.002.

Witkiewitz, K., Pfund, R. A., & Tucker, J. A. (2022). Mechanisms of behavior change in substance use disorder with and without formal treatment. *Annual Review of Clinical Psychology*, 18, 497–525. https://doi.org/10.1146/annurev-clinpsy-072720.

World Drug Report (2020). (United Nations publication, Sales No. E.20.XI.6). https://wdr.unodc.org/wdr2020/en/index2020.html.

World Health Organization (2019). International Statistical Classification of Diseases and Related Health Problems (11th ed.). World Health Organization.

Zgierska, A. E., Burzinski, C. A., Mundt, M. P., et al. (2019). Mindfulness-based relapse prevention for alcohol dependence: Findings from a randomized controlled trial. *Journal of Substance Abuse Treatment*, 100, 8–17. https://doi.org/10.1016/j.jsat.2019.01.013.

Zuckermann, A. M., Williams, G. C., Battista, K., et al. (2020). Prevalence and correlates of youth poly-substance use in the COMPASS study. *Addictive Behaviors*, 107, 106400. https://doi.org/10.1016/j.addbeh.2020.106400.

Zuckermann, A. M., Williams, G., Battista, K., et al. (2019). Trends of poly-substance use among Canadian youth. *Addictive Behaviors Reports*, 10, 100189. https://doi.org/10.1016/j.abrep.2019.100189.

13

Cognitive Loss

Claudia Drossel

Behavioral health providers and trainees will likely encounter individuals who present with subjective cognitive complaints that may emerge from the sequelae of multiple etiologies. As time spent living generates risk factors such as injuries, exposure to neurotoxins, and chronic diseases, subjective cognitive complaints are common in midlife and represent a significant public health concern (Taylor et al., 2018). The cognitive repertoires at risk of decline are foundational to building and maintaining relationships across home, work, school, or leisure settings. These repertoires include attending, perceiving (e.g., spatial relations), planning, reasoning, organizing, problem-solving, comprehending, learning, remembering, communicating, self-reflection, and taking perspectives different from one's own.

Corresponding to the World Health Organization's (2019) distinction between cognitive decline and dementia, the American Psychiatric Association (2022) distinguishes mild from major neurocognitive disorders (NCDs) as syndromes across a spectrum of severity (see Bermejo-Pareja et al. [2021] for the distinction between "mild NCD" and an alternative construct, "mild cognitive impairment"). While both mild and major NCD diagnoses require a decline from a previous baseline functional status confirmed by objective evidence (such as neuropsychological data), the diagnosis of mild NCD characterizes subtle inefficiencies, greater effort or more errors during task completion, or the use of new compensatory strategies with continued independence in activities of daily living and decision-making. When cognitive decline is sufficient to disrupt instrumental activities of daily living, such as meal preparation, financial management, medication adherence, and household chores, it meets criteria for major NCD (formerly "dementia") if delirium or other acute conditions are not present. About 11% of adults older than 45 years of age voice subjective complaints (Taylor et al., 2018). Of individuals older than 65 years of age, about 22% meet the criteria for mild cognitive impairment, and 10% meet the criteria

Author Note: Thank you to Thomas Waltz, Jacqueline Pachis, and Kayla Rinna for comments on an earlier draft of this chapter.

for major NCD (Manly et al., 2022). However, inconsistent diagnostic definitions and methodological limitations call into question the accuracy of current global estimates (Pais et al., 2020).

Etiology and Theoretical Underpinnings of Treatment

A proper diagnostic workup is essential to determine the nature of cognitive decline. In addition to neurodegenerative diseases, such as Alzheimer's disease (AD) or Lewy body disease (LBD), causes of cognitive loss include physical trauma (e.g., related to motor vehicle accidents, falls, or assaults), long-term metabolic disturbances (e.g., poorly managed diabetes, thyroid disease), cardiovascular or cerebrovascular events (e.g., cardiac arrest or stroke), exposure to neurotoxins (e.g., mood-altering substances, pesticides), neoplasms (e.g., brain tumors), and certain medical treatments (e.g., radiation or chemotherapy, long-term antiretroviral therapies) (for an introduction, see Miller & Boeve, 2017).

The progression from subjective complaints to mild NCD, and from mild to major NCD, is poorly understood. Population-based studies suggest that some individuals with mild NCD maintain their cognitive status, others recover baseline functioning (Overton et al., 2020), and yet others progress to irreversible neurodegenerative diseases. Some NCD subtypes are further classified by dominant behavioral changes, such as marked impulsivity and neglect of social mores, or progressive language deficits (i.e., variants of frontotemporal lobar degeneration) (Boeve et al., 2022). Recently, emotional and behavioral changes, specifically irritability and apathy (Roberto et al., 2021), have received attention as predictors of progression. The absence of uniform diagnostic criteria for clinical trials and variability in ruling out reversible sources of cognitive loss remain persistent threats to the validity of research in this area (but see McKeith et al., 2020), and the intervention literature that takes into account specific etiologies is slowly expanding.

Empirically based principles of behavior change to guide effective, individually tailored practice with individuals with NCD have been examined for more than half a century (Lindsley, 1964), often with small-N research designs. The operant model, emphasizing that the meaning of behavior (B) emerges when its probabilistic antecedents (A) and consequences (C) are analyzed across time, has been disseminated as the functional approach (Bourgeois & Hickey, 2009), the contextual model (Fisher et al., 2007; McCurry & Drossel, 2011), or as the ABCs (i.e., antecedents-behavior-consequences), within caregiver intervention packages and cognitive behavior therapies for people with NCD (Ehrhardt et al., 1998). According to the philosophy of behavior analysis (Baum, 2017; Chiesa, 1994), a functional model interprets the emotional and behavioral changes that accompany and often precede detectable cognitive decline as predictable and changeable results of subtle and seemingly inexplicable disruptions of one's social life and routines (see also

Kitwood & Brooker, 2019). Rather than describing individuals with cognitive loss as intentionally withdrawing or becoming hostile, a functional model views persons as continuing to value active task or community engagement, human connection, and intimacy, regardless of the degree to which cognitive decline has become a barrier to being effective. Interventions occur across interrelated social–cognitive–behavioral–affective domains, depending on the person's history and current needs.

Brief Overview of Treatments

Effective treatments for emotional and behavioral changes associated with cognitive loss understand these changes in terms of their current consequences or impact (What does the behavior accomplish? For example, does a given behavior aid the person in withdrawing from a difficult situation?) and antecedents – the person's interpersonal coping history and current social circumstances, such as role shifts and interpersonal demands. They eschew default physiological explanations (i.e., blanket attributions of emotional and behavioral changes to the NCD per se). Instead, they apply Hussian's (1981) seminal observation that when emotional and behavioral problems are uncharacteristic of the person and severe enough to consult a behavioral health specialist, they should lead to a systematic and thorough investigation of a potential acute change in physical status and of the possibility of adverse or coercive social interactions. Even when cognitive loss is moderate to severe, emotional and behavioral changes can be understood in terms of these events, and quality of life can be achieved by building appropriate social and instrumental supports. Focusing on idiographic assessment and related behavioral processes (e.g., stimulus control, reinforcement) rather than topographies (e.g., patient personality, caregiver style) allows for more nuanced and individualized assessment and linked interventions when complexity is high.

Description of Treatment Packages

Depending on the severity of cognitive loss, treatment packages whose primary targets are emotional and behavioral changes may involve the person with NCD, or they may consist of caregiver interventions that exclude the person with NCD from assessment and intervention and rely solely on the care partners' reports. Existing cognitive-behavioral therapies have been adapted for individuals with mild to moderate cognitive loss (for adaptation strategies, see Gallagher et al., 2019) and sometimes involve informal or formal care partners to ensure carryover and implementation of between-session assignments (Orgeta et al., 2022). However, to the extent that these adaptations maintain their original psychopathological models (e.g., foci on maladaptive beliefs or lack of psychological flexibility), they are at risk of being unresponsive to the actual social and instrumental challenges posed by cognitive decline that require active advocacy and targeted problem-solving (for an alternative approach, see Hayes et al., 2020).

Additionally, a distinct class of treatments targeting improvements in cognition or activities of daily living as primary outcomes is also available (Tulliani et al., 2022), with a parallel neglect of emotional and behavioral status as potential barrier to or facilitator of engagement (but see Kurz et al., 2012; Tonga et al., 2021). These treatments are characterized as "remediation," an umbrella term for interventions targeting cognitive or functional status: (1) *training* via learning and memory techniques that aim to improve specific cognitive domains; (2) *rehabilitation* via compensatory or adaptive strategies that do not target improvements in cognition but scaffold daily task completion; and (3) *stimulation* via social engagement and games or preferred activities, such as gardening or cooking – effectively, activity scheduling with a cognitive rationale, to reduce loneliness and improve quality of life (Tulliani et al., 2022). Notably, rather than applying comprehensive idiographic functional assessment and treatment strategies across closely related cognitive (activities of daily living) and emotional-behavioral targets, most intervention packages for the person with NCD tend to be siloed within specific status domains (i.e., emotional/behavioral– cognitive–functional).

When cognitive loss is moderate to severe, multicomponent caregiver interventions predominate to improve the quality of life of both care partners and the person about whom they care, and to mitigate care partners' physical and emotional strain (Xu et al., 2020). Care partners often are unprepared to understand the range with which neurological diseases affect a person's functioning, to act as assessors and interventionists to appropriately scaffold repertoires, and to complete nursing tasks. Many family care partners provide extensive assistance under untenable conditions of financial losses and lack of specialized respite services (Gaugler & Kane, 2015; Glenn, 2010). For this reason, treatment modules broadly cover education, stress management strategies, problem-solving, and essential behavioral skills to manage care recipients' emotional or behavioral changes.

Behavioral skills training components of well-studied and translated intervention packages (such as Resources for Enhancing Alzheimer's Caregivers Health, REACH II; e.g., Belle et al., 2006) or Staff Training in Assisted Living Residences (STAR; e.g., Teri et al., 2005) represent consistent efforts to disseminate and implement a science-based approach to emotional and behavioral changes in the context of cognitive loss, by teaching functional "ABCs" to formal or informal caregivers (Moniz Cook et al., 2012). Ideally, caregivers learn to systematically monitor behavior and emotion in their antecedent and consequent situational contexts, and to design and evaluate interventions based on the resulting patterns. Components such as interventions based on stimulus control or differential reinforcement inherent in these treatment packages, are detailed in the "Credible Components of Treatments" section of this chapter.

Overall Level of Research Support

Despite the unequivocal call for nonpharmacological interventions across inter-national practice guidelines, the state of the evidence could still be improved after almost 30 years of research on individual psychological interventions (Orgeta et al., 2022) and 50 years of research on caregiver interventions (Cheng et al., 2022; Meng et al., 2021). Cognitive-behavioral interventions involving persons with mild or major NCD produce small effects on depression, with moderate-certainty evidence (Orgeta et al., 2022), and details related to active components have not been sufficiently investigated. Among cognitive remediation strategies, only cognitive rehabilitation (Jeon et al., 2021; Kudlicka et al., 2023) and stimulation (Woods et al., 2023) have empirical support for improving functional status and quality of life, respectively. Cognitive training, which consists of practicing specific cognitive tasks, enhances task performance and global cognition for individuals with mild to moderate cognitive loss (Bahar-Fuchs et al., 2019). It is unclear whether cognitive training generalizes to everyday situations, and it is currently not recommended for individuals with major NCD (National Institute for Health and Care Excellence, 2018; Sala & Gobet, 2019; von Bastian et al., 2022).

The effects of multicomponent caregiver interventions go beyond those of phar-macotherapies for emotional and behavioral changes associated with NCD (Gerlach & Kales, 2020). Caregiver interventions consistently produce small (Cheng et al., 2022; Meng et al., 2021) or small to moderate benefits on care partner competency/knowledge, well-being, burden, and mood, and on care recipient behavioral/emo-tional status (Walter & Pinquart, 2020).

Overall, continued population heterogeneity due to new and evolving diagnostic categories, failure to distinguish etiological subtypes of NCD, or including both mild – and thereby potentially reversible – and major NCD; heterogeneity in targeted domains and outcome measures; uncertainty about the degree to which care partner outcomes generalize to care recipient well-being; and complexity in terms of comor-bidities and sedative medication status still hamper an answer to the question for whom, when, and under what conditions particular treatments work (Paul, 1967).

Functional-contextual approaches are individually tailored and tend to be evaluated within small-N designs or integrated in multicomponent interventions. To date, large-N trials of functional-contextual interventions are lacking (Holle et al., 2017; Moniz Cook et al., 2012), and systematic dismantling studies have not been conducted. However a study that omitted "ABC" training from an empirically supported inter-vention for caregivers (Prick et al., 2016) failed to replicate the original study's effects on care recipient behavior, health, or mood (Teri et al., 2003). While Prick et al. attributed the failure to replicate to translational and cultural issues, it is as likely that the eliminated experimental ABC training would have equipped caregivers with the problem-solving needed to implement interventions flexibly, tailored to the individual situation (contrast with Kurz et al., 2012, who did attribute their lack of intervention effects to a failure to individualize treatment goals).

Credible Components of Treatments

Credible components of treatments are those that effectively educate the person with NCD and their care partners about the specifics of cognitive loss and its intersection with the person's life. In line with disability advocacy, they counteract narrowing repertoires and re-engage the person with NCD in a range of meaningful activities, whether intentionally rehabilitative in nature or important for maintaining that specific person's quality of life. Because NCDs represent a heterogeneous collection of individual strengths and weaknesses that interact with a person's social and medical histories and current circumstances, individualized functional assessments often are necessary for flexible problem-solving within a person's given context. Interventions that suggest a multipronged one-size-fits-all approach may be effective some of the time but are at risk of missing important contextual determinants of individual well-being, such as social consequences that are distributed in time and only become visible with repeated systematic observations (for an analysis of coercive processes in the family, see Patterson, 1982). Particularly when problems appear intractable and not amenable to nonpharmacological solutions, repeated systematic observations detect contingencies that elude snapshot assessments and suggest points of intervention.

The intervention components that follow are contained within existing treatment packages to varying degrees. They may target the person with NCD directly, or indirectly via the care partner.

The Basics

Reducing Vascular Risk Factors and Preventing Excess Disability

Health conditions whose poor management may exacerbate or contribute to cognitive decline are often overlooked. In 1996, The American Academy of Neurology Ethics and Humanities Subcommittee recommended medical and behavioral health follow-up for all individuals with NCD, to decrease concurrent vascular risk factors and to prevent excess disability (i.e., functional decline exceeding that predicted by a given neurodegenerative disease alone) (Kahn, 1965; Ngandu et al., 2015). Throughout the course of NCD, lifestyle factors and concurrent conditions that may contribute to cognitive, emotional, or behavioral decline must be taken into account, including optimizing nutrition and hydration; addressing bowel and urinary concerns to prevent restlessness and agitation; maximizing sleep; carefully limiting the number and dosage of medications; treating comorbid medical conditions (e.g., hypo- or hyperglycemic episodes; pulmonary disease; see Frederiksen & Waldemar, 2021); managing acute or chronic pain or discomfort; addressing hearing and vision to facilitate communication and prevent misperceptions (Littlejohn et al., 2021); decreasing substance use; and increasing physical activity and enhancing outdoor mobility.

Any abrupt decline in functioning should lead to the systematic investigation of adverse events that may disrupt cognition further, such as stroke or seizures, or failure to tolerate novel or previously tolerated medications (see also the related literature of delirium occurring in cases of those with cognitive impairment; Oh et al., 2017). Individuals with cognitive loss who have access to academic or larger healthcare settings will find many of the needed services within one health system; however, many community-dwelling adults in suburban or rural areas may need to put together a healthcare team and coordinate communication across team members.

Education and Healthcare Navigation

If cognitive losses do not interfere with self-management and goal-directed behavior, individuals may participate in all aspects of assessment and related medical and behavioral health services without care partner support. However, such autonomy can become problematic when decline is progressive and irreversible. For example, if a person with mild NCD and insulin-dependent diabetes later develops difficulties measuring blood glucose levels and calculating the sliding-scale insulin dose, when and how will the care partner take over the task? Many care partners learn about diabetes management from the person with NCD at a point when reporting has become unreliable (Feil et al., 2009; Munshi, 2017). The risks of misremembering and unreliable reporting suggest that care partners best learn about the person's medical and behavioral health needs and routines before self-direction is disrupted. Moreover, an NCD diagnosis may lead a care partner to attribute behavioral and emotional changes to cognitive decline rather than frequent undetected or poorly managed medical conditions. For this reason, education and medical care navigation are important components of interventions for NCD, and should be tailored to the individual (e.g., managing common comorbidities of specific neurological diseases, such as constipation or REM sleep behavior disorder with LBD) and involve a care partner early. The completion of advance directives (e.g., for healthcare or for research) aids care partners' and providers' consideration of individuals' values and preferences throughout the care trajectory (Reamy et al., 2013). Care partners must learn about care fragmentation to effectively coordinate services across multiple providers and receive advocacy for accessing third-party care. For some care partners, assertiveness training may be necessary to shape an accurate description of the dyad's functional status and needs for assistance, and to solicit support across agencies that may cover different functional domains. Many care partners must acquire the skills to hire and manage third-party carers (Bieber et al., 2019) or to direct the person with NCD's care in institutionalized settings or at the end of life.

Advanced Problem-Solving: Applications of Behavioral Science

The following subsections represent the application of structured and systematic, yet flexible functional analysis-based problem-solving (Haynes & O'Brien, 1990; Haynes et al., 2011).

Problem-Solving Stance and Application

Problem-solving strategies are essential to service provision involving persons with cognitive loss (e.g., Areán et al., 2010). Initial repertoires for effective problem-solving are the problem orientation (i.e., detecting the need for change) and a problem definition (clearly delineating the target of change) (D'Zurilla & Goldfried, 1971). The stigma of cognitive loss combined with sociocultural pressures for conformity, and ableist or often ageist assumptions, require detailed attention to the questions "What is the problem, and whose problem is it?" If, for example, a person who walks five miles per day develops difficulties finding their way home, and the family responds by restricting the person's mobility (e.g., discouraging or preventing leaving the house), whose problem are the resulting restlessness and difficulty sleeping? These questions are compounded in residential settings that severely restrict choices and thereby not only disrupt individuals' lifelong routines but also compromise or violate individuals' values and preferences. Social demands directing the person to "gain insight" into their difficulties (e.g., losing one's way) are often demands to relinquish activities (e.g., stop going for walks) when they become inconvenient and cumbersome because they cannot be self-directed or executed without assistance. For an introduction to ethics in geropsychology, see Bush et al. (2017).

Providers who teach problem-solving strategies to the person with cognitive loss and/or their care partner must be aware of their own biases and assumptions (e.g., the contraindicated stance that one must "slow down" with age or after a diagnosis) and of the tension inherent in dyads when the person with cognitive loss seeks continuity of usual activities and habits under new circumstances and thereby disrupts routine arrangements, such as walking alone. Problem-solving then focuses on finding acceptable scaffolding or assistance, soliciting friends or communal support (e.g., walking group), and advocating to maintain quality of life by engaging in valued activities. Whether an individual solution works is an experimental question: If not, then further problem-solving considering removal of encountered barriers is required. Barriers are best viewed as opportunities for learning and not as signs of unchangeability. Sociocultural beliefs related to disability and intersecting aspects of diversity (e.g., gendered or age-dependent role expectations) should be specifically explored when building a problem orientation and defining the problem. Subsequent collaborative and constructive problem-solving will maintain quality of life and prevent the experience of NCD as one of innumerable losses.

Systematic Observations

Persons with NCD as well as their care partners may be unreliable historians, and survey tools assessing caregiver needs perform poorly in areas of construct validity, test–retest reliability, and sensitivity to change (Kipfer & Pihet, 2020). For this reason, systematic observations play a significant role in services for people with NCD, providing the data needed to link assessment to intervention. Systematic observations, by self (self-monitoring) or others, are analytical tools for detecting the probabilistic functional relations between context (antecedents and consequences) and emotional or behavioral changes (Bridges-Parlet et al., 1994; Cohen-Mansfield et al., 2017). Data collection forms the prerequisite for function-based behavioral management (see "Function-Based Behavioral Management") and examining the outcome of interventions.

When cognitive decline prevents regular self-monitoring, the care partner may assist the person with NCD, or wearable devices may fill the gap if the provider can present the data to the client in a user-friendly format (e.g., a printout of a graph showing activity level as a function of weekdays versus weekends when family members tend to visit). Self-monitoring of, for example, the relation between mood and care demands, or sleep and mood, is also important for care partners, who tend to encounter unrealistic and untenable social expectations about their ability to serve as the sole source of support for the person with NCD for years or decades (for digital monitoring with feedback, see van Knippenberg et al., 2018).

Function-Based Behavioral Management

Stimulus Control Interventions. The term "stimulus control" describes a probabilistic relationship between behavior and its context, particularly that behavior is more likely in one situation than another. Here, a "stimulus" or situation is conceptualized broadly; for example, a person might routinely drink coffee in the morning (temporal stimulus control), differentially disclose personal information (audience stimulus control), or be more likely to eat sweets when working late at night (stimulus control by physiological factors, such as time since last meal or fatigue). Nervous-system insults tend to result in marked sensory alterations, making it difficult to discern and thus respond to situational cues. Many problems arise from that breakdown of stimulus control – the failure of the context to occasion appropriate behavior. Among these breakdowns are olfactory alterations with resulting food selectivity, refusal to eat, or lack of engagement in personal care (for a review of anosmia, see Boesveldt et al. (2017)); visuo-spatial alterations with resulting misperceptions, visual disturbances, and refusal to enter certain spaces such as uniformly tiled bathrooms (Weil & Lees, 2021); and alterations in binaural hearing with resulting preference for one-on-one interactions or refusal to engage with multiple speakers (Li et al., 2021; Littlejohn et al., 2021).

Many behavioral changes associated with cognitive loss can be understood as normal reactions to a breakdown in stimulus control. Idiographic assessment can suggest systematic changes to the antecedent context, with the goal to decrease confusion and facilitate the person's detection of situational cues and engagement in behavior appropriate to that situation. An example is a daughter who notices that her dad, who lives independently, has stopped reheating his cherished morning coffee, which she prepares for him in advance. He vaguely complains about the microwave. Observations show that he approaches the microwave but fails to locate the recessed button that opens the door. Verbal prompting ("press this button to open" – verbal stimulus control) is effective but does not carry over to the next morning. However, placing a red sticker onto the recessed button works: Dad picks up his routine again. This simple example of visual stimulus control illustrates that teaching the person with NCD or the care partner how to re-establish cues by making them more salient, or how to shift to novel and effective cues, can prevent premature dependence and interpersonal strain.

Many interventions rely on stimulus control as a behavioral process but do not explicitly identify as such. For ease of dissemination, stimulus control interventions are integrated within caregiver training packages (e.g., within the antecedent part of the antecedent–behavior–consequence ABC training) or in cognitive rehabilitation approaches as environmental modifications (e.g., introducing digital calendar apps to aid temporal orientation; painting the floor of the bathtub and its walls in different colors to facilitate spatial navigation), making it difficult to assess their independent effects. Moreover, across these packages, measured outcomes vary: Target repertoires are individualized in caregiver training, where care partners are encouraged to examine situations that pose new difficulties and require extra efforts from the person with NCD, or in which emotional responding, withdrawal, and refusal are common. Sleep interventions for people with NCD also contain some stimulus control strategies, such as establishing regular sleep/wake times with activity during the day and wind-down routines in the evening, or reducing sleep disruptors such as noise, light, or screens. In cognitive rehabilitation, targets generally reflect the degree to which activities of daily living are self-directed, albeit with assistance or scaffolding. Thus, the applicability of stimulus control as a behavioral process is broad and a keystone in most multicomponent interventions. It is understudied as a stand-alone intervention.

To what extent a person is affected by sensory changes must be examined on a case-by-case basis. Because of heterogeneous presentations and the integration of stimulus control in multicomponent interventions, evidence for stimulus control interventions specifically comes from small-N designs (for a detailed review, see Spira & Edelstein, 2006). The disambiguation of situational cues, based on individual functional assessment and response to intervention (assessed via outcome monitoring), can alleviate common behavioral and emotional changes associated with cognitive loss.

Re-establishing Chains and Sequences. As noted, interventions that re-engage individuals in everyday activities fall under the umbrella of "cognitive rehabilitation" (Jeon et al., 2021). Most activities – from dressing, laundry, meal preparation and medication management to operating technical equipment or computers – are comprised of sequences or behavioral chains. The outcome or consequence of one step of the chain automatically becomes the antecedent for the next step (e.g., closing the door of the microwave sets the occasion for setting the cooking time, which then occasions pressing start). A disruption of this functional switch from consequent to antecedent may generate inexplicable performance failure and confusion. People often say they seem to be "drawing a blank." Increased reaction times and latencies to the next step are common and can also appear in verbal behavior when an utterance trails off or a person "loses their thread." Self-directed, effortful, explicit problem-solving may be necessary to get back on track and complete the task in question. Implementing daily structure and routines may help to maintain the automaticity of habits.

When in-the-moment problem-solving fails, task analyses and self-prompting routines – from least to most intrusive or physical prompts – may re-establish some or parts of the chain. Alternatively, procedures that re-establish sequencing, such as errorless learning procedures (also called the procedure of vanishing cues), may be indicated (de Werd et al., 2013). A recent randomized controlled trial (Voigt-Radloff et al., 2017) did not find a benefit of errorless over trial-and-error learning (i.e., both approaches resulted in the reacquisition of instrumental repertoires selected by the participants with NCD). However, the development of individualized errorless learning procedures is an advanced skill and adequate treatment fidelity evaluations do not exist. Systematic reviews of cognitive remediation for mild to moderate cognitive losses suggest that – in addition to re-establishing the repertoire selected for training (high-certainty evidence at the end of treatment; Kudlicka et al., 2023) – continued engagement might have an antidepressant effect, lifting the mood of the person with NCD (Chan et al., 2020).

When the person with cognitive loss ceases to initiate the independent use of prompts (e.g., Post-It notes are present but do not guide the relevant behavioral steps), then external or third-party prompting becomes necessary. Caregiver skills training in the use of task analyses and prompting hierarchies prevents premature dependence on others for task completion (Beck et al., 1997; Engelman et al., 1999). Here, too, a highly individualized approach – determining what works for each person at a given time to maximize engagement – is recommended. Goal selection must consider the person's status, starting with steps that are achievable and thereby preventing frustration and agitation associated with a failure to progress.

Access to Meaningful Events (Reinforcers). The film *Alive Inside: A Story of Music and Memory* (Rossato-Bennett, 2014) fascinated audiences by documenting that individuals with severe major NCD continued to enjoy music. The erroneous conclusion by many was that music would have the same effect on all people with NCD, regardless of personal preferences, history, and current status. Indeed, activity scheduling is somewhat of a misnomer in that activity per se is insufficient. Selected activities must connect to the person's history: that is, ideally, they are meaningful in some way, continuous with a person's identities, match the person's skill level, fit into the person's larger sociocultural context, and consider the available social and material resources and program assistive problem-solving when needed (Teri et al., 1997; Tierney & Beattie, 2020).

For many adults with NCD, opportunities that are linked to cognition are especially meaningful. Social and physical activities introduced under the premise of "cognitive stimulation" (e.g., trivia, card games, walking, social support groups) may affect general mood and well-being rather than cognition per se (Woods et al., 2023). Similarly, reminiscence therapy – with an emphasis on personal interaction and life story – may improve particularly the quality of life of adults with NCD in long-term service settings (low-certainty evidence; Woods et al., 2018). Because of conceptual confusion regarding what is meant by person-centered or individually tailored meaningful activities and other methodological problems (e.g., heterogeneity of population and procedures), systematic reviews so far have produced low-certainty evidence that individually tailored and meaningful activities may prevent behavioral and emotional difficulties and increase quality of life when cognitive losses are mild to moderate and people with NCD reside at home (Möhler et al., 2020). Given an impoverished environment plagued by staffing difficulties and lack of appropriate choices, empirical support is lacking for individuals residing in long-term service settings (Kim & Park, 2017; Möhler et al., 2023). Here, small-N studies suggest effectiveness (e.g., LeBlanc et al., 2006). In general, implementation efforts at the individual level should be evaluated.

Differential Reinforcement or Noncontingent Access. Differential reinforcement or noncontingent access are techniques that break the contingent relationship between a target (i.e., NCD-related) behavior and an outcome. These techniques maintain the valued outcome or consequence but alter the means by which the outcome is achieved. From this perspective, the outcome or consequence is valid, and the person's right to meaningful engagement is preserved (for an application, see Gitlin et al., 2008). Small-N studies lend support and suggest that, regardless of the severity of NCD, a person's behavior remains sensitive to its consequences (e.g., Buchanan & Fisher, 2002; Heard & Watson, 1999; Noguchi et al., 2013).

Intervening on Social Contingencies. Rate-decreasing behavioral processes, such as inadvertent extinction and punishment delivered by family and friends, are plausible culprits in producing premature functional decline. Evidence from correlational studies support the notion that the quality of social interactions plays a role in the rate of decline, and that inadvertent punishment and extinction may be ubiquitous. First, individuals with higher educational levels commonly experience a steeper verbal decline (Cadar et al., 2015), implying more opportunities for extinction but also potentially a stronger reaction to the loss of abilities by families, friends, and colleagues. Secondly, "elder speak," defined as a conversational partner's changes in pitch, covaries with disengagement, such that decreased verbal output and increased refusal of care are common in settings in which older adults are likened to children and engaged in activities that are not age-appropriate – patronizing at best, infantilizing at worst (Garrison-Diehn et al., 2022). Third, care partners commonly resort to coercive techniques, such as yelling, threatening, or using more force than necessary, when encountering refusal of assistance or refusal to engage or to follow a care partner's rules (Patterson, 1982; Thoma et al., 2004), and abuse is common in long-term service settings (Mileski et al., 2019).

Advocacy and problem-solving predominate when a person's decline is mild. Later interventions consist of providing caregivers with communicative strategies (e.g., "Do not argue"; McCurry, 2006) and behavioral skills to engage in monitoring of contextual determinants and functional problem-solving. Communication skills training improves care partners' skills and knowledge, but to date methodological limitations prohibit strong conclusions as to effects on dyadic quality of life (Morris et al., 2018). Further, as study designs have not focused on the quality of relationships as primary outcomes, empirical support for targeting improvements in the relationship between the care partner and the person with NCD is still limited (Rausch et al., 2017).

Cognitive Reframing. Interventions targeting verbal behavior (i.e., thoughts, beliefs, or attitudes) assume that "nothing's either good or bad, just thinking makes it so" (Clark & Wright, 1989, p. 1022). The person has been observed to have the skills and the resources to be effective in a given situation, but verbalizations ("I will wake up one morning not knowing who I am"; "I shouldn't have to do this"; "These are supposed to be the golden years"; "She's just stubborn as a mule"; "This is never going to work") may keep the person from deploying skills or resources that would improve the situation in the long run. Noticing and identifying unhelpful interpretations, without acting directly upon them (defusing) or challenging them (cognitive restructuring), are the goals of such interventions (Farmer & Chapman, 2016; Losada et al., 2015). While not examined in isolation and based on low-quality evidence, cognitive reframing as part of multicomponent interventions for care partners has empirical support, showing effects on measures of care partner anxiety, depression, and distress (Vernooij-Dassen et al., 2011).

Distress Tolerance Skills. When active, problem-focused coping is not available as an option, distress tolerance skills may be temporarily employed until a solution is found (Linehan, 1993). Acceptance, distraction, relaxation, arousal reduction, and other escape or avoidance strategies may increase well-being in the short run but must be balanced with active problem-solving in the long run, often requiring collaboration with other members of the family and coordination with employers or additional service agencies. While relaxation or distress tolerance skills are contained in many multicomponent interventions for caregivers (see, for example, Steffen (2000) for anger management), the evidence for stand-alone treatments such as mindfulness-based stress reduction, characterized as promising in terms of temporary reduction of depression and anxiety, is of low to very low quality (Liu et al., 2018). To the extent that studies of multicomponent psychosocial interventions have failed to identify specific caregiver stressors (e.g., competing workplace or family demands, financial strain, medical comorbidities) and to detail necessary treatment components to increase resilience and effective coping, the current state of the evidence cannot lend empirical support to specific effects (Gilhooly et al., 2016).

Other Variables Influencing Treatment

Assessment and Diagnosis

The heterogeneity of cognitive loss, its etiology, and its effects on a person's life – including partners, family, friends, colleagues, and neighbors – requires special attention to assessment. As noted earlier, assessment of emotional and behavioral status should occur in the context of multiple specialty providers (e.g., primary care, neurology, neuropsychology). It is essential to remember that significant cognitive decline is not a part of aging and is always a sign of nervous system compromise. The assessment of behavioral and emotional status in this context and the selection of interventions requires additional training. Variables to consider are: (a) the severity of cognitive decline (Cary et al., 2019), or the degree to which cognitive decline is expected to remain stable, worsen, or potentially revert, varies substantially within and across NCD etiologies and may alter the appropriateness of treatment targets and modalities as well as client priorities and preferences for treatment, and (b) the extent to which a person with cognitive loss can participate in treatment and self-direct between-session assignments might suggest adaptations, including determination of whether or when care partner involvement or a caregiver intervention is warranted. The following subsections represent additional considerations during assessment.

Comorbidity

Medical Conditions

Cognitive loss is a sign of a potentially serious neurological compromise that warrants medical attention. While cognitive loss correlates with age, it is not part of aging and thus should receive a comprehensive assessment with the goal of developing a treatment plan to optimize the person's well-being (American Psychiatric Association, 2022). From a behavioral health perspective, cognitive loss is better conceptualized as an insult to the whole body than to the brain: Chronic medical conditions frequently accompany NCDs (for example, diabetes and hypertension with vascular disease [Romay et al., 2019]; bowel and urinary difficulties with LBD [Nardone et al., 2020]). Their management deteriorates as a person's self-management skills decline, and they might be overlooked or undetected when persons lose their self-descriptive skills, increasing the risk of serious adverse health events and further decline. Self-observation and reliable reporting on one's own physical, emotional, or behavioral status are sophisticated skills and often among the first to be compromised (Defrin et al., 2015), and disruptive or uncharacteristic behavior patterns are better interpreted as behavioral indices of unmet needs (Algase et al., 1996).

Whether concerns are for mild or major NCD, behavioral health providers should refer to and collaborate with neurology, neuropsychology, primary care, and other specialty care when applicable, to fully understand the person's context at the intersection of medical/neurological conditions and behavioral/emotional status and history. In academic hospital or specialty clinic settings (e.g., physical medicine and rehabilitation, geriatrics), team approaches are the standard of care. When events leading to decline have been abrupt (e.g., stroke, traumatic brain injury), acute and subacute rehabilitative services aim at the reacquisition of repertoires (Duncan et al., 2021). However, outside of these settings medical follow-up for individuals with NCD tends to be insufficient as NCDs are stigmatized (Scerri et al., 2023), and healthcare systems are unprepared to conduct the observational detective work necessitated by unreliable self-reports that can accompany cognitive decline (Frederiksen & Waldemar, 2021). Behavioral health providers who detect or hear concerns about cognitive decline from their community-dwelling clients must be prepared to become their advocates, coordination hubs, and in-session problem-solvers for collaborative treatment planning across multiple providers to improve quality of life in a fragmented healthcare system.

Psychiatric Conditions

Depression, anxiety, and apathy are most observed with NCD; indeed, withdrawal from activities, general apprehension, and failure to initiate interactions can be understood in the context of narrowing skills and repertoires; at the same time, they also are a risk factor of progression from mild to major NCD (Ma, 2020). The interventions discussed earlier are applicable to NCD comorbid with these conditions.

Anecdotally, individuals with psychiatric treatment histories, particularly involuntary hospitalizations, and other interpersonal trauma histories may be more likely to refuse services, interpret visuospatial disturbances as threatening, or engage in self-protective behaviors. When past trauma-related responses have been well managed during an individual's lifetime, cognitive decline may lead to a concomitant decrease in relevant coping and self-management skills, with a re-emergence of posttraumatic fear responding. Currently, there are no assessment tools that assist with distinguishing post-traumatic stress from other emotional and behavioral changes (Havermans et al., 2022), and population prevalence data are not available (Sobczak et al., 2021). Trauma-informed service protocols are emerging in geriatric settings (e.g., Cations et al., 2021; Couzner et al., 2022), but current evidence for their effectiveness is lacking. In general, as discussed throughout this chapter, the destigmatizing of emotional and behavioral changes and the promotion of reassurance and safety from interpersonal coercion are recommended.

Assessment should include the degree to which care partners may have longstanding behavioral or physical health difficulties that might interfere with providing instrumental assistance and warrant their referral to individual treatment; such comorbidities cannot be ignored, as they correlate with abuse and neglect of the person with cognitive loss (Pillemer et al., 2016).

Demographics

While overall risk for NCD is declining, in the United States non-Hispanic Black individuals are at a relatively greater risk of developing neurodegenerative diseases than non-Hispanic White individuals (Power et al., 2021), with Hispanic White individuals also at greater risk than non-Hispanic White individuals (Manly et al., 2022), and women at a greater risk than men. Such differences likely reflect differential risk factors (systemic oppression, education, health literacy, socioeconomic status) in the presence of health disparities (e.g., untreated hypertension, uncorrected sensory loss). These disparities continue throughout the care trajectory. During the Covid-19 pandemic, Black men with NCD, for example, were more likely to be diagnosed with new-onset schizophrenia and treated with sedatives than other resident populations in long-term service settings (Cai et al., 2022). Thus, discriminatory behavior and misconduct by providers are ongoing social justice concerns (Findley et al., 2023).

Sociocultural and familial systems differ in terms of expectations of autonomy and reliance on family members for assistance, related expectations of family care, demands on individual family members, attitudes toward third-party or residential care, and resources. These aspects must be assessed on a case-by-case basis. Recent large-N, cross-cultural studies with adequate methodology and sampling suggest – contrary to some earlier studies – that, in the United States, Black caregivers report greater psychological well-being than White ones, potentially due to familial expectations and availability of social support networks (Liu et al., 2021). When working with members of LGBTQIA+ populations, whose communities rely on mutual aid, distinct needs for advocacy and health trajectories may be identified and addressed (Singleton & Enguidanos, 2022). Notably, many members of the cohort with cognitive decline today lost friends and partners during the height of the AIDS crisis and have significant histories of criminalization and stigmatization. Suggestions as to how to deliver culturally humble and linguistically sensitive interventions are emerging.

The availability of social and financial resources affects problem-solving, including the readiness of spouses or family members to support the person with cognitive loss (e.g., current employment status, past or current relationship strain) and the availability of occasional respite or structured third-party assistance (e.g., long-term care insurance, eligibility for social services). In the United States, age at diagnosis may have a significant impact on the availability of services.

Medication

Nonpharmacological interventions are first line for behavioral and emotional changes associated with cognitive loss (e.g., Meng et al., 2021; National Institute for Health and Care Excellence, 2018). Yet, inappropriate medication use is high with NCD (Maust et al., 2017), both in community-dwelling populations (Bae-Shaaw et al., 2023) and in long-term service settings, where concerted efforts to decrease psychotropic medications are ongoing (McDermid et al., 2023). At present, central nervous system (CNS) depressants – none of which have an indicated use for restlessness or confused and self-protective behavior (e.g., warding off staff attempts to undress the person) – have been suggested only for short-term, emergency administrations (Peisah et al., 2011), after acute medical conditions, pain, adverse medication effects (Al Rihani et al., 2021), and social or other environmental factors have been ruled out and documented (Kales et al., 2019). Many healthcare providers, residential care staff, and family members, upon reaching the limit of their problem-solving abilities and when proximal "triggers" are not obvious, tend to attribute behavioral and emotional problems to the inevitable effects of the neurological disease and resort to the off-label prescription of sedating medications (Ma et al., 2020). Emerging evidence (e.g., Anderson et al., 2014) suggests that the presence of a specialist team can shift prescribing practices, even when behavioral disturbances led to hospitalization. In a vulnerable population whose central nervous system is already compromised by neurodegenerative processes, long-term use of psychotropic medication with anticholinergic or CNS-depressant properties

Box 13.1 Format and Duration

Interventions for individuals with cognitive loss and their care partners are available across a range of formats (bibliotherapy, computer-based interventions, in-person and telehealth sessions, individual and group formats) with different durations. Selection should be individualized, weighing whether a given format circumvents common barriers to accessing services (e.g., lack of transportation or respite) and offers the person opportunities for full engagement with treatment (e.g., quality of technology and connectivity; provider's ability to effectively observe and shape repertoires via behavioral skills training). When neurocognitive disorders are degenerative, the person with NCD and their family might need regular consultation for emotional and behavioral changes as functional status shifts.

increases fatigue, confusion, and fall risk (Lippert et al., 2020), and hastens decline. Thus, administration should be accompanied by systematic monitoring of whether use interferes with orientation, goal-oriented behavior, and engagement in meaningful activities.

Conclusion

Nonpharmacological interventions are first-line interventions for the emotional and behavioral changes associated with cognitive loss. They represent a high-complexity area of practice because of multiple etiologies, highly variable presentations, and the level of comorbidities. Advanced competencies in behavioral science are needed to successfully problem-solve, with individually tailored functional-analysis-based interventions to promote client well-being. Interdisciplinary care coordination is necessary to ensure that behavioral interventions are not applied to behavioral changes that communicate pain or other acute medical events. At present, multicomponent interventions incorporate functional-analysis-based behavioral management to varying degrees, and those that have removed functional analysis from their protocols have failed to produce reliable outcomes.

Useful Resources

Books

- Bush, S. S., Allen, R. S., & Molinari, V. A. (2017). *Ethical practice in geropsychology*. APA Books.
- Farmer, R. F., & Chapman, A. L. (2016). *Behavioral interventions in cognitive therapy: Practical guidance for putting theory into action* (2nd ed.). APA Books.

- Gaugler, J. E., & Kane, R. L. (Eds.). (2015). *Family caregiving in the new normal*. Academic Press.
- Haynes, S. N., O'Brien, W. H., & Kaholokula, J. (2011). *Behavioral assessment and case formulation*. John Wiley & Sons, Inc.
- Kitwood, T., & Brooker, D. (2019). *Dementia reconsidered revisited: The person still comes first* (2nd ed.). McGraw-Hill Education (UK).
- McCurry, S., & Drossel, C. (2011). *Treating dementia in context: A step-by-step guide to working with individuals and families*. APA Books.
- Miller, B. L., & Boeve, B. F. (Eds.). (2017). *The behavioral neurology of dementia* (2nd ed.). Cambridge University Press.

Websites

- American Psychological Association caregiver briefcase: www.apa.org/pi/about/publications/caregivers
- American Psychological Association Guidelines for the evaluation of dementia and age-related cognitive change: www.apa.org/practice/guidelines
- Geropsychology resources: https://gerocentral.org

Systematic Review

- Gallagher, M., McLeod, H. J., & McMillan, T. M. (2019). A systematic review of recommended modifications of CBT for people with cognitive impairments following brain injury. *Neuropsychological Rehabilitation*, 29(1), 1–21. https://doi.org/10.1080/09602011.2016.1258367

References

Al Rihani, S. B., Deodhar, M., Darakjian, L. I., et al. (2021). Quantifying anticholinergic burden and sedative load in older adults with polypharmacy: A systematic review of risk scales and models. *Drugs & Aging*, 38(11), 977–994. https://doi.org/10.1007/s40266-021-00895-x.

Algase, D. L., Beck, C., Kolanowski, A., et al. (1996). Need-driven dementia-compromised behavior: An alternative view of disruptive behavior. *American Journal of Alzheimer's Disease*, 11(6), 10–19. https://doi.org/10.1177/153331759601100603.

American Psychiatric Association. (2022). *Diagnostic and statistical manual of mental disorders* (5th ed., text rev.). https://doi.org/10.1176/appi.books.9780890425787.

Anderson, K., Bird, M., Blair, A., & MacPherson, S. (2014). Development and effectiveness of an integrated inpatient and community service for challenging behaviour in late life: From confused and disturbed elderly to Transitional Behavioural Assessment and Intervention Service. *Dementia*, 15(6), 1340–1357. https://doi.org/10.1177/1471301214559106.

Areán, P. A., Raue, P., Mackin, R. S., et al. (2010). Problem-solving therapy and supportive therapy in older adults with major depression and executive dysfunction. *American Journal of Psychiatry*, 167(11), 1391–1398. https://doi.org/10.1176/appi.ajp.2010.09091327.

Bae-Shaaw, Y. H., Shier, V., Sood, N., Seabury, S. A., & Joyce, G. (2023). Potentially inappropriate medication use in community-dwelling older adults living with dementia. *Journal of Alzheimer's Disease*, 93, 471–481. https://doi.org/10.3233/JAD-221168.

Bahar-Fuchs, A., Martyr, A., Goh, A. M. Y., Sabates, J., & Clare, L. (2019). Cognitive training for people with mild to moderate dementia. *Cochrane Database of Systematic Reviews* (3). https://doi.org/10.1002/14651858.CD013069.pub2.

Baum, W. M. (2017). *Understanding behaviorism: Behavior, culture, and evolution* (3rd ed.). John Wiley & Sons, Inc. https://doi.org/10.1002/9781119143673.

Beck, C., Heacock, P., Mercer, S. O., et al. (1997). Improving dressing behavior in cognitively impaired nursing home residents. *Nursing Research*, 46(3), 126–132. https://journals.lww.com/nursingresearchonline/Fulltext/1997/05000/Improving_Dressing_Behavior_in_Cognitively.2.aspx.

Belle, S. H., Burgio, L., Burns, R., et al. (2006). Enhancing the quality of life of dementia caregivers from different ethnic or racial groups. *Annals of Internal Medicine*, 145(10), 727–738. https://doi.org/10.7326/0003-4819-145-10-200611210-00005.

Bermejo-Pareja, F., Contador, I., del Ser, T., et al. (2021). Predementia constructs: Mild cognitive impairment or mild neurocognitive disorder? A narrative review. *International Journal of Geriatric Psychiatry*, 36(5), 743–755. https://doi.org/10.1002/gps.5474.

Bieber, A., Nguyen, N., Meyer, G., & Stephan, A. (2019). Influences on the access to and use of formal community care by people with dementia and their informal caregivers: A scoping review. *BMC Health Services Research*, 19(1), 88. https://doi.org/10.1186/s12913-018-3825-z.

Boesveldt, S., Postma, E. M., Boak, D., et al. (2017). Anosmia – A clinical review. *Chemical Senses*, 42(7), 513–523. https://doi.org/10.1093/chemse/bjx025.

Boeve, B. F., Boxer, A. L., Kumfor, F., Pijnenburg, Y., & Rohrer, J. D. (2022). Advances and controversies in frontotemporal dementia: Diagnosis, biomarkers, and therapeutic considerations. *The Lancet Neurology*, 21(3), 258–272. https://doi.org/10.1016/S1474-4422(21)00341-0.

Bourgeois, M. S., & Hickey, E. M. (2009). *Dementia: From diagnosis to management – a functional approach*. Psychology Press.

Bridges-Parlet, S., Knopman, D., & Thompson, T. (1994). A descriptive study of physically aggressive behavior in dementia by direct observation [https://doi.org/10.1111/j.1532-5415.1994.tb04951.x]. *Journal of the American Geriatrics Society*, 42(2), 192–197. https://doi.org/10.1111/j.1532-5415.1994.tb04951.x.

Buchanan, J. A., & Fisher, J. E. (2002). Functional assessment and non-contingent reinforcement in the treatment of disruptive vocalization in elderly dementia patients. *Journal of Applied Behavior Analysis*, 35(1), 99–103. https://doi.org/10.1901/jaba.2002.35-99.

Bush, S. S., Allen, R. S., & Molinari, V. A. (2017). *Ethical practice in geropsychology*. APA Books.

Cadar, D., Stephan, B. C. M., Jagger, C., et al. (2015). Is education a demographic dividend? The role of cognitive reserve in dementia-related cognitive decline: A comparison of six longitudinal studies of ageing. *The Lancet*, 386, S25. https://doi.org/10.1016/S0140-6736(15)00863-6

Cai, S., Wang, S., Yan, D., Conwell, Y., & Temkin-Greener, H. (2022). The diagnosis of schizophrenia among nursing home residents with ADRD: Does race matter? *The*

American Journal of Geriatric Psychiatry, 30(5), 636–646. https://doi.org/10.1016/j.jagp.2021.10.008.

Cary, M. P., Smith, V. A., Shepherd-Banigan, M., et al. (2019). Moderators of treatment outcomes from family caregiver skills training: Secondary analysis of a randomized controlled trial. *OBM Geriatrics*, 3(2), 049. https://doi.org/10.21926/obm.geriatr.1902049.

Cations, M., Laver, K., Couzner, L., et al. (2021). Trauma-informed care in geriatric inpatient units to improve staff skills and reduce patient distress: a co-designed study protocol. *BMC Geriatrics*, 21(1), 492. https://doi.org/10.1186/s12877-021-02441-1.

Chan, J. Y. C., Chan, T. K., Kwok, T. C. Y., et al. (2020). Cognitive training interventions and depression in mild cognitive impairment and dementia: A systematic review and meta-analysis of randomized controlled trials. *Age and Ageing*, 49(5), 738–747. https://doi.org/10.1093/ageing/afaa063.

Cheng, S.-T., Li, K.-K., Or, P. P. L., & Losada, A. (2022). Do caregiver interventions improve outcomes in relatives with dementia and mild cognitive impairment? A comprehensive systematic review and meta-analysis. *Psychology and Aging*, 37, 929–953. https://doi.org/10.1037/pag0000696.

Chiesa, M. (1994). *Radical behaviorism: The philosophy and the science*. Cambridge Center for Behavioral Studies.

Clark, W. G., & Wright, W. A. (Eds.). (1989). *The unabridged William Shakespeare: A complete library of his works*. Running Press.

Cohen-Mansfield, J., Golander, H., & Cohen, R. (2017). Rethinking psychosis in dementia: An analysis of antecedents and explanations. *American Journal of Alzheimer's Disease & Other Dementias*, 32(5), 265–271. https://doi.org/10.1177/1533317517703478.

Couzner, L., Spence, N., Fausto, K., et al. (2022). Delivering trauma-informed care in a hospital ward for older adults with dementia: An illustrative case series [Original Research]. *Frontiers in Rehabilitation Sciences*, 3. https://doi.org/10.3389/fresc.2022.934099.

D'Zurilla, T. J., & Goldfried, M. R. (1971). Problem solving and behavior modification. *Journal of Abnormal Psychology*, 78, 107–126. https://doi.org/10.1037/h0031360.

de Werd, M. M., Boelen, D., Rikkert, M. G. M. O., & Kessels, R. P. C. (2013). Errorless learning of everyday tasks in people with dementia. *Clinical Interventions in Aging*, 8, 1177–1190. https://doi.org/10.2147/CIA.S46809.

Defrin, R., Amanzio, M., De Tommaso, M., et al. (2015). Experimental pain processing in individuals with cognitive impairment: current state of the science. *Pain*, 156(8), 1396–1408.

Duncan, P. W., Bushnell, C., Sissine, M., et al. (2021). Comprehensive stroke care and outcomes: time for a paradigm shift. *Stroke*, 52(1), 385–393.

Ehrhardt, T., Hampel, H., Hegerl, U., & Möller, H. J. (1998). Das verhaltenstherapeutische Kompetenztraining VKT – eine spezifische Intervention für Patienten mit einer beginnenden Alzheimer-Demenz. *Zeitschrift fur Gerontologie und Geriatrie [Journal for Gerontology and Geriatrics]*, 31(2), 112–119. https://doi.org/10.1007/s003910050026.

Engelman, K. K., Altus, D. E., & Mathews, R. M. (1999). Increasing engagement in daily activities by older adults with dementia. *Journal of Applied Behavior Analysis*, 32(1), 107–110. https://doi.org/10.1901/jaba.1999.32-107.

Farmer, R. F., & Chapman, A. L. (2016). *Behavioral interventions in cognitive therapy: Practical guidance for putting theory into action* (2nd ed.). APA Books.

Feil, D. G., Pearman, A., Victor, T., et al. (2009). The role of cognitive impairment and caregiver support in diabetes management of older outpatients. *The International Journal of Psychiatry in Medicine*, 39(2), 199–214. https://doi.org/10.2190/PM.39.2.h.

Findley, C. A., Cox, M. F., Lipson, A. B., et al. (2023). Health disparities in aging: Improving dementia care for Black women [Perspective]. *Frontiers in Aging Neuroscience*, 15, 1107372. https://doi.org/10.3389/fnagi.2023.1107372.

Fisher, J. E., Drossel, C., Yury, C., & Cherup, S. (2007). A contextual model of restraint-free care for persons with dementia. In P. Sturmey (Ed.), *Functional analysis in clinical treatment* (pp. 211–237). Academic Press/Elsevier.

Frederiksen, K. S., & Waldemar, G. (2021). *Management of patients with dementia: The role of the physician*. Springer.

Gallagher, M., McLeod, H. J., & McMillan, T. M. (2019). A systematic review of recommended modifications of CBT for people with cognitive impairments following brain injury. *Neuropsychological Rehabilitation*, 29(1), 1–21. https://doi.org/10.1080/09602011.2016.1258367.

Garrison-Diehn, C., Rummel, C., Au, Y. H., & Scherer, K. (2022). Attitudes toward older adults and aging: A foundational geropsychology knowledge competency. *Clinical Psychology: Science and Practice*, 29, 4–15. https://doi.org/10.1037/cps0000043.

Gaugler, J. E., & Kane, R. L. (Eds.). (2015). *Family caregiving in the new normal*. Academic Press.

Gerlach, L. B., & Kales, H. C. (2020). Pharmacological management of neuropsychiatric symptoms of dementia. *Current Treatment Options in Psychiatry*, 7(4), 489–507. https://doi.org/10.1007/s40501-020-00233-9.

Gilhooly, K. J., Gilhooly, M. L. M., Sullivan, M. P., et al. (2016). A meta-review of stress, coping and interventions in dementia and dementia caregiving. *BMC Geriatrics*, 16(1), 106. https://doi.org/10.1186/s12877-016-0280-8.

Gitlin, L. N., Winter, L., Burke, J., et al. (2008). Tailored activities to manage neuropsychiatric behaviors in persons with dementia and reduce caregiver burden: A randomized pilot study. *The American Journal of Geriatric Psychiatry*, 16(3), 229–239. https://doi.org/10.1097/01.JGP.0000300629.35408.94.

Glenn, E. N. (2010). *Forced to care: Coercion and caregiving in America*. Harvard University Press.

Havermans, D. C. D., van Alphen, S. P. J., Olff, M., et al. (2022). The need for a diagnostic instrument to assess post-traumatic stress disorder in people with Dementia: Findings from a Delphi study. *Journal of Geriatric Psychiatry and Neurology*, 36(2), 129–142. https://doi.org/10.1177/08919887221103583.

Hayes, S. C., Hofmann, S. G., & Ciarrochi, J. (2020). A process-based approach to psychological diagnosis and treatment: The conceptual and treatment utility of an extended evolutionary meta model. *Clinical Psychology Review*, 82, 101908. https://doi.org/10.1016/j.cpr.2020.101908.

Haynes, S. N., & O'Brien, W. H. (1990). Functional analysis in behavior therapy. *Clinical Psychology Review*, 10(6), 649–668. https://doi.org/10.1016/0272-7358(90)90074-K.

Haynes, S. N., O'Brien, W. H., & Kaholokula, J. (2011). *Behavioral assessment and case formulation*. John Wiley & Sons.

Heard, K., & Watson, T. S. (1999). Reducing wandering by persons with dementia using differential reinforcement. *Journal of Applied Behavior Analysis*, 32(3), 381–384. https://doi.org/10.1901/jaba.1999.32-381.

Holle, D., Halek, M., Holle, B., & Pinkert, C. (2017). Individualized formulation-led interventions for analyzing and managing challenging behavior of people with dementia: An integrative review. *Aging & Mental Health*, 21(12), 1229–1247. https://doi.org/10.1080/ 13607863.2016.1247429.

Hussian, R. A. (1981). *Geriatric psychology: A behavioral perspective.* Van Nostrand Reinhold.

Jeon, Y.-H., Milne, N., Kaizik, C., & Resnick, B. (2021). Improving functional independence: Dementia rehabilitation programs. In L.-F. Low & K. Laver (Eds.), *Dementia rehabilitation* (pp. 227–261). Academic Press. https://doi.org/10.1016/ B978-0-12-818685-5.00013-1.

Kahn, R. S. (1965). Comments. In Proceedings of the York House Institute on the mentally impaired aged. Philadelphia Geriatric Center.

Kales, H. C., Gitlin, L. N., & Lyketsos, C. G. (2019). When less is more, but still not enough: Why focusing on limiting antipsychotics in people with dementia is the wrong policy imperative. *Journal of the American Medical Directors Association*, 20(9), 1074–1079. https://doi.org/10.1016/j.jamda.2019.05.022.

Kim, S. K., & Park, M. (2017). Effectiveness of person-centered care on people with dementia: a systematic review and meta-analysis. *Clinical Interventions in Aging*, 12, 381–397. https://doi.org/10.2147/CIA.S117637.

Kipfer, S., & Pihet, S. (2020). Reliability, validity and relevance of needs assessment instruments for informal dementia caregivers: A psychometric systematic review. *JBI Evidence Synthesis*, 18(4), 704–742. https://doi.org/10.11124/jbisrir-2017-003976.

Kitwood, T., & Brooker, D. (2019). *Dementia reconsidered revisited: The person still comes first* (2nd ed.). McGraw-Hill Education (UK).

Kudlicka, A., Martyr, A., Bahar-Fuchs, A., et al. (2023). Cognitive rehabilitation for people with mild to moderate dementia. *Cochrane Database of Systematic Reviews*, (6). https://doi.org/ 10.1002/14651858.CD013388.pub2.

Kurz, A., Thöne-Otto, A., Cramer, B., et al. (2012). CORDIAL: Cognitive rehabilitation and cognitive-behavioral treatment for early dementia in Alzheimer disease: A multicenter, randomized, controlled trial. *Alzheimer Dis Assoc Disord*, 26(3), 246–253. https://doi.org/ 10.1097/WAD.0b013e318231e46e.

LeBlanc, L. A., Cherup, S. M., Feliciano, L., & Sidener, T. M. (2006). Using choice-making opportunities to increase activity engagement in individuals with dementia. *American Journal of Alzheimer's Disease & Other Dementias®*, 21(5), 318–325. https://doi.org/ 10.1177/1533317506292183.

Li, S., Cheng, C., Lu, L., et al. (2021). Hearing Loss in Neurological Disorders [Review]. *Frontiers in Cell and Developmental Biology*, 9. https://doi.org/10.3389/fcell.2021 .716300.

Lindsley, O. R. (1964). Geriatric behavioral prosthetics. In R. Kastenberg (Ed.), *New thoughts on old age* (pp. 41–60). Springer Publishing Company, Inc. https://doi.org/10.1007/978-3- 662-38534-0_3.

Linehan, M. M. (1993). *Cognitive-behavioral treatment of borderline personality disorder.* Guilford Press.

Lippert, T., Maas, R., Fromm, M. F., et al. (2020). Einfluss zentralnervös dämpfender Arzneimittel auf Stürze mit Verletzungsfolgen bei Menschen mit Demenz in Pflegeheimen [Impact of sedating drugs on falls resulting in injuries among people with dementia in a nursing home setting]. *Gesundheitswesen (Bundesverband der Ärzte des Öffentlichen Gesundheitsdienstes (Germany))*, 82(1), 14–22. https://doi.org/ 10.1055/a-1071-7911.

Littlejohn, J., Bowen, M., Constantinidou, F., et al. (2021). International practice recommendations for the recognition and management of hearing and vision impairment in people with dementia. *Gerontology*, 68(2), 121–135. https://doi.org/10.1159/000515892.

Liu, C., Badana, A. N. S., Burgdorf, J., et al. (2021). Systematic review and meta-analysis of racial and ethnic differences in dementia caregivers' well-being. *The Gerontologist*, 61(5), e228–e243. https://doi.org/10.1093/geront/gnaa028.

Liu, Z., Sun, Y. Y., & Zhong, B. L. (2018). Mindfulness-based stress reduction for family carers of people with dementia. *Cochrane Database of Systematic Reviews*, (8). https://doi.org/10.1002/14651858.CD012791.pub2.

Losada, A., Márquez-González, M., Romero-Moreno, R., et al. (2015). Cognitive-behavioral therapy (CBT) versus acceptance and commitment therapy (ACT) for dementia family caregivers with significant depressive symptoms: Results of a randomized clinical trial. *Journal of Consulting and Clinical Psychology*, 83(4), 760–772. https://doi.org/10.1037/ccp0000028

Ma, D., Zhao, Y., Wan, Z., et al. (2020). Nurses' attitudes and views on the application of antipsychotics in patients with dementia: A systematic review of qualitative studies. *Geriatric Nursing*, 41(6), 669–676. https://doi.org/10.1016/j.gerinurse.2019.10.007.

Ma, L. (2020). Depression, anxiety, and apathy in mild cognitive impairment: Current perspectives. *Frontiers in Aging Neuroscience*, 12(9). https://psycnet.apa.org/doi/10.3389/fnagi.2020.00009.

Manly, J. J., Jones, R. N., Langa, K. M., et al. (2022). Estimating the prevalence of dementia and mild cognitive impairment in the US: The 2016 Health and Retirement Study Harmonized Cognitive Assessment Protocol Project. *JAMA Neurology*, 79(12), 1242–1249. https://doi.org/10.1001/jamaneurol.2022.3543.

Maust, D. T., Langa, K. M., Blow, F. C., & Kales, H. C. (2017). Psychotropic use and associated neuropsychiatric symptoms among patients with dementia in the USA. *International Journal of Geriatric Psychiatry*, 32(2), 164–174. https://doi.org/10.1002/gps.4452.

McCurry, S. M. (2006). *When a family member has dementia: Steps to becoming a resilient caregiver*. Praeger.

McCurry, S., & Drossel, C. (2011). *Treating dementia in context: A step-by-step guide to working with individuals and families*. American Psychological Association.

McDermid, J., Ballard, C., Khan, Z., et al. (2023). Impact of the Covid-19 pandemic on neuropsychiatric symptoms and antipsychotic prescribing for people with dementia in nursing home settings. *International Journal of Geriatric Psychiatry*, 38(1), e5878. https://doi.org/10.1002/gps.5878.

McKeith, I. G., Ferman, T. J., Thomas, A. J., et al. (2020). Research criteria for the diagnosis of prodromal dementia with Lewy bodies. *Neurology*, 94(17), 743–755. https://doi.org/10.1212/wnl.0000000000009323.

Meng, X., Su, J., Li, H., et al. (2021). Effectiveness of caregiver non-pharmacological interventions for behavioural and psychological symptoms of dementia: An updated meta-analysis. *Ageing Research Reviews*, 71, 101448. https://doi.org/10.1016/j.arr.2021.101448.

Mileski, M., Lee, K., Bourquard, C., et al. (2019). Preventing the abuse of residents with dementia or Alzheimer's disease in the long-term care setting: A systematic review. *Clinical Interventions in Aging*, 14, 1797–1815. https://doi.org/10.2147/CIA.S216678.

Miller, B. L., & Boeve, B. F. (Eds.). (2017). *The behavioral neurology of dementia* (2nd ed.). Cambridge University Press.

Möhler, R., Calo, S., Renom, A., Renom, H., & Meyer, G. (2023). Personally tailored activities for improving psychosocial outcomes for people with dementia in long-term care. *Cochrane Database of Systematic Reviews*, (3). https://doi.org/10.1002/14651858.CD009812.pub3.

Möhler, R., Renom, A., Renom, H., & Meyer, G. (2020). Personally tailored activities for improving psychosocial outcomes for people with dementia in community settings. *Cochrane Database of Systematic Reviews*, (8). https://doi.org/10.1002/14651858.CD010515.pub2

Moniz Cook, E. D., Swift, K., James, I., et al. (2012). Functional analysis-based interventions for challenging behaviour in dementia. *Cochrane Database of Systematic Reviews*, (2), CD006929. https://doi.org/10.1002/14651858.CD006929.pub2.

Morris, L., Horne, M., McEvoy, P., & Williamson, T. (2018). Communication training interventions for family and professional carers of people living with dementia: a systematic review of effectiveness, acceptability and conceptual basis. *Aging & Mental Health*, 22(7), 863–880. https://doi.org/10.1080/13607863.2017.1399343.

Munshi, M. N. (2017). Cognitive dysfunction in older adults with diabetes: What a clinician needs to know. *Diabetes Care*, 40(4), 461–467. https://doi.org/10.2337/dc16-1229

Nardone, R., Höller, Y., Brigo, F., Versace, V., et al. (2020). Spinal cord involvement in Lewy body-related α-synucleinopathies. *The Journal of Spinal Cord Medicine*, 43(6), 832–845.

National Institute for Health and Care Excellence. (2018). Dementia: Assessment, management, and support for people living with dementia and their carers. www.nice.org.uk/guidance/ng97.

Ngandu, T., Lehtisalo, J., Solomon, A., et al. (2015). A 2 year multidomain intervention of diet, exercise, cognitive training, and vascular risk monitoring versus control to prevent cognitive decline in at-risk elderly people (FINGER): A randomised controlled trial. *The Lancet*, 385(9984), 2255–2263. https://doi.org/10.1016/S0140-6736(15)60461-5.

Noguchi, D., Kawano, Y., & Yamanaka, K. (2013). Care staff training in residential homes for managing behavioural and psychological symptoms of dementia based on differential reinforcement procedures of applied behaviour analysis: A process research. *Psychogeriatrics*, 13(2), 108–117. https://doi.org/10.1111/psyg.12006.

Oh, E. S., Fong, T. G., Hshieh, T. T., & Inouye, S. K. (2017). Delirium in older persons: Advances in diagnosis and treatment. *JAMA*, 318(12), 1161–1174. https://doi.org/10.1001/jama.2017.12067.

Orgeta, V., Leung, P., del-Pino-Casado, R., et al. (2022). Psychological treatments for depression and anxiety in dementia and mild cognitive impairment. *Cochrane Database of Systematic Reviews*, (4), CD009125. https://doi.org/10.1002/14651858.CD009125.pub3.

Overton, M., Pihlsgård, M., & Elmståhl, S. (2020). Diagnostic stability of mild cognitive impairment, and predictors of reversion to normal cognitive functioning. *Dementia and Geriatric Cognitive Disorders*, 48(5–6), 317–329. https://doi.org/10.1159/000506255.

Pais, R., Ruano, L. P., Carvalho, O., & Barros, H. (2020). Global cognitive impairment prevalence and incidence in community dwelling older adults: A systematic review. *Geriatrics*, 5(4), 84. www.mdpi.com/2308-3417/5/4/84.

Patterson, G. R. (1982). *Coercive family process*. Castalia Publication Company.

Paul, G. L. (1967). Strategy of outcome research in psychotherapy. *Journal of Consulting Psychology*, 31, 109–118. https://doi.org/10.1037/h0024436.

Peisah, C., Chan, D. K. Y., McKay, R., Kurrle, S. E., & Reutens, S. G. (2011). Practical guidelines for the acute emergency sedation of the severely agitated older patient. *Internal Medicine Journal*, 41(9), 651–657. https://doi.org/10.1111/j.1445-5994.2011.02560.x.

Pillemer, K., Burnes, D., Riffin, C., & Lachs, M. S. (2016). Elder abuse: global situation, risk factors, and prevention strategies. *The Gerontologist*, 56(Suppl_2), S194–S205.

Power, M. C., Bennett, E. E., Turner, R. W., et al. (2021). Trends in relative incidence and prevalence of dementia across non-Hispanic Black and White individuals in the United States, 2000-2016. *JAMA Neurology*, 78(3), 275–284. https://doi.org/10.1001/jamaneurol.2020.4471.

Prick, A.E., de Lange, J., Scherder, E., Twisk, J., & Pot, A. M. (2016). The effects of a multicomponent dyadic intervention on the mood, behavior, and physical health of people with dementia: A randomized controlled trial. *Clinical Interventions in Aging*, 11, 383–395. https://doi.org/10.2147/CIA.S95789.

Rausch, A., Caljouw, M. A. A., & van der Ploeg, E. S. (2017). Keeping the person with dementia and the informal caregiver together: a systematic review of psychosocial interventions. *International Psychogeriatrics*, 29(4), 583–593. https://doi.org/10.1017/S1041610216002106.

Reamy, A. M., Kim, K., Zarit, S. H., & Whitlatch, C. J. (2013). Values and preferences of individuals with dementia: Perceptions of family caregivers over time. *The Gerontologist*, 53(2), 293–302. https://doi.org/10.1093/geront/gns078.

Roberto, N., Portella, M. J., Marquié, M., et al. (2021). Neuropsychiatric profiles and conversion to dementia in mild cognitive impairment, a latent class analysis. *Scientific Reports*, 11(1), 6448. https://doi.org/10.1038/s41598-021-83126-y.

Romay, M. C., Toro, C., & Iruela-Arispe, M. L. (2019). Emerging molecular mechanisms of vascular dementia. *Current Opinion in Hematology*, 26(3), 199–206.

Rossato-Bennett, M. (2014). *Alive inside: A story of music and memory*. www.aliveinside.us/#land.

Sala, G., & Gobet, F. (2019). Cognitive training does not enhance general cognition. *Trends in Cognitive Sciences*, 23(1), 9–20. https://doi.org/10.1016/j.tics.2018.10.004.

Scerri, A., Innes, A., & Scerri, C. (2023). Healthcare professionals' perceived challenges and solutions when providing rehabilitation to persons living with dementia: A scoping review. *Journal of Clinical Nursing*, 32, 5493–5513.

Singleton, M. C., & Enguidanos, S. M. (2022). Exploration of demographic differences in past and anticipated future care experiences of older sexual minority adults. *Journal of Applied Gerontology*, 41(9), 2045–2055. https://doi.org/10.1177/07334648221098996.

Sobczak, S., Olff, M., Rutten, B., Verhey, F., & Deckers, K. (2021). Comorbidity rates of posttraumatic stress disorder in dementia: A systematic literature review. *European Journal of Psychotraumatology*, 12(1), 1883923. https://doi.org/10.1080/20008198.2021.1883923.

Spira, A. P., & Edelstein, B. A. (2006). Behavioral interventions for agitation in older adults with dementia: An evaluative review. *International Psychogeriatrics*, 18(2), 195–225. https://doi.org/10.1017/S1041610205002747.

Steffen, A. M. (2000). Anger management for dementia caregivers: A preliminary study using video and telephone interventions. *Behavior Therapy*, 31(2), 281–299. https://doi.org/10.1016/S0005-7894(00)80016-7.

Taylor, C. A., Bouldin, E. D., & McGuire, L. C. (2018). Subjective cognitive decline among adults aged ≥45 years – United States, 2015-2016. *MMWR Morbidity and Mortality Weekly Report*, 67(27), 753–757. https://doi.org/10.15585/mmwr.mm6727a1.

Teri, L., Gibbons, L. E., McCurry, S. M., et al. (2003). Exercise plus behavioral management in patients with Alzheimer disease: A randomized controlled trial. *JAMA*, 290(15), 2015–2022. https://doi.org/10.1001/jama.290.15.2015.

Teri, L., Logsdon, R. G., Uomoto, J., & McCurry, S. M. (1997). Behavioral treatment of depression in dementia patients: A controlled clinical trial. *The Journals of Gerontology: Series B*, 52B(4), P159–P166. https://doi.org/10.1093/geronb/52B.4.P159.

Teri, L., McCurry, S. M., Logsdon, R., & Gibbons, L. E. (2005). Training community consultants to help family members improve dementia care: A randomized controlled trial. *The Gerontologist*, 45(6), 802–811. https://doi.org/10.1093/geront/45.6.802.

The American Academy of Neurology Ethics and Humanities Subcommittee. (1996). Ethical issues in the management of the demented patient. *Neurology*, 46(4), 1180–1183. https://doi.org/10.1212/wnl.46.4.1180.

Thoma, J., Zank, S., & Schacke, C. (2004). Gewalt gegen demenziell Erkrankte in der Familie: Datenerhebung in einem schwer zugänglichen Forschungsgebiet. *Zeitschrift für Gerontologie undGeriatrie [Journal for Gerontology and Geriatrics]*, 37(5), 349–350. https://doi.org/10.1007/s00391-004-0256-8.

Tierney, L., & Beattie, E. (2020). Enjoyable, engaging and individualised: A concept analysis of meaningful activity for older adults with dementia. *International Journal of Older People Nursing*, 15(2), e12306. https://doi.org/10.1111/opn.12306.

Tonga, J. B., Šaltytė Benth, J., Arnevik, E. A., et al. (2021). Managing depressive symptoms in people with mild cognitive impairment and mild dementia with a multicomponent psychotherapy intervention: A randomized controlled trial. *International Psychogeriatrics*, 33(3), 217–231. https://doi.org/10.1017/S1041610220000216.

Tulliani, N., Bissett, M., Fahey, P., Bye, R., & Liu, K. A.-O. (2022). Efficacy of cognitive remediation on activities of daily living in individuals with mild cognitive impairment or early-stage dementia: a systematic review and meta-analysis. *Systematic Reviews*, 11(1), 156. https://doi.org/10.1186/s13643-022-02032-0.

van Knippenberg, R. J. M., de Vugt, M. E., Ponds, R. W., Myin-Germeys, I., & Verhey, F. R. J. (2018). An experience sampling method intervention for dementia caregivers: Results of a randomized controlled trial. *The American Journal of Geriatric Psychiatry*, 26(12), 1231–1243. https://doi.org/10.1016/j.jagp.2018.06.004.

Vernooij-Dassen, M., Draskovic, I., McCleery, J., & Downs, M. (2011). Cognitive reframing for carers of people with dementia. *Cochrane Database of Systematic Reviews*, (11). https://doi.org/10.1002/14651858.CD005318.pub2.

Voigt-Radloff, S., de Werd, M. M. E., Leonhart, R., et al. (2017). Structured relearning of activities of daily living in dementia: The randomized controlled REDALI-DEM trial on errorless learning. *Alzheimer's Research & Therapy*, 9(1), 22. https://doi.org/10.1186/s13195-017-0247-9.

von Bastian, C. C., Belleville, S., Udale, R. C., et al. (2022). Mechanisms underlying training-induced cognitive change. *Nature Reviews Psychology*, 1(1), 30–41. https://doi.org/10.1038/s44159-021-00001-3.

Walter, E., & Pinquart, M. (2020). How effective are dementia caregiver interventions? An updated comprehensive meta-analysis. *The Gerontologist*, 60(8), e609–e619. https://doi.org/10.1093/geront/gnz118.

Weil, R. S., & Lees, A. J. (2021). Visual hallucinations. *Practical Neurology*, 21(4), 327–332. https://doi.org/10.1136/practneurol-2021-003016.

14

Antisocial Behavior

Devon L. L. Polaschek

Antisocial behavior is defined as behavior that violates common social mores or legislation by infringing on the rights of others, or otherwise offending or harming others (Skeem & Cooke, 2010). Antisocial personality disorder (AsPD) and conduct disorder (CD) are diagnoses for people whose behavior is frequently, persistently, and diversely antisocial (APA, 2022). Although many criminal behaviors contribute to meeting the criteria for these diagnoses, so too do behaviors that may not be criminally sanctionable, but are commonly considered immoral, unethical, or negligent.

People whose pattern of antisocial behavior *starts* in adulthood may be diagnosed with CD, but alternatively their presentation may be labeled adult antisocial behavioral syndrome (AABS; Ehlers et al., 2022). CD is most often diagnosed in people under the age of 18, and symptoms may emerge as early as the preschool years. Regardless of age, CD requires "A repetitive and persistent pattern of behavior in which the basic rights of others or major age-appropriate societal norms or rules are violated, as manifested by the presence of at least three of … 15 criteria in the past 12 months … with at least one criterion present in the past 6 months" (APA, 2022, p. 530). The criteria are organized into four categories: aggression to people and animals, destruction of property, deceitfulness and theft, and serious violations of rules; criteria from any category meet diagnostic requirements.

AsPD requires "a pervasive pattern of disregard for and violation of the rights of others, occurring since age 15 years" (APA, 2022, p. 748). AsPD symptoms include behavior that is grounds for arrest, deception or lying, impulsivity, irritability, aggressiveness, recklessness or irresponsible behavior, or a failure to show remorse for those harmed. Behaviors typifying evidence of AsPD vary widely in their severity and criminality; a substantial proportion of those with AsPD may have seldom or never broken the law, while others may have long conviction histories (NCCMH, 2009).

Diagnostic criteria for AsPD have varied considerably over the evolving versions of the *Diagnostic and Statistical Manual of Mental Disorders* (DSM), sometimes with little overlap from one to the next (Cunningham & Reidy, 1998), in an effort to

246

produce a reliable and valid way of capturing "criminal personality" (Gurley, 2009) even though, in reality, the personalities of people involved in crime are diverse (Blackburn, 1988). Since the DSM-III, reliance primarily on behavior as symptoms has concealed heterogeneity in the underlying personality traits, because the same behavior can result from diverse traits (Brazil et al., 2018). The picture is further complicated by conflation in the text surrounding the criteria with a more serious and rarer disorder, psychopathy, that is not included in the DSM. A minority of people with AsPD meet criteria for psychopathy (Brazil et al., 2018). Psychopathy will not be further covered in this chapter, but clinicians most often use one of the Hare Psychopathy Checklist measures (e.g., the Psychopathy Checklist-Revised; Hare, 2003) to identify levels and components of psychopathy.

Lifetime prevalence estimates of AsPD in community samples range from 1% to 4%; the disorder is 3–5 times more common in men than in women (Werner et al., 2015). People with antisocial behavior presenting mainly in adulthood (AABS, or adult-onset CD) are much more numerous (Ehlers et al., 2022). On average, a quarter to a half of male prisoners and about 20% of female prisoners have been diagnosed with AsPD, depending on the institution and jurisdiction (Fazel & Danesh, 2002).

The relevance of these diagnoses to treatment varies substantially, depending on the setting. Diagnosis is typically important in health settings. However, most treatment for people with extended histories of antisocial behavior occurs in the criminal justice system, where these diagnoses are often not used at all. Bringing together health and justice knowledge of antisocial behavior to create the most informative picture of how to approach psychotherapy is a major focus of this chapter.

Etiology and Theoretical Underpinnings of Treatment

In principle, diagnosis gathers together people whose difficulties share a common etiology that guides treatment. But with its emphasis strongly on behavior, a diagnosis of AsPD gathers together a heterogeneous group of people with regard to personality traits and comorbidity; some have even suggested that, as a group, people with AsPD have little in common other than their antisocial behavior (Cox et al., 2013). Unpacking this heterogeneity into more homogeneous subtypes could lead to a better understanding both of etiology and of treatment effectiveness (McKinley et al., 2018). But, to date, subtyping research does not directly inform treatment.

Instead, the etiology of AsPD is typically discussed in very general terms that do not reflect whether there are meaningful differences within the diagnosed population. AsPD etiology is usually described as "biopsychosocial," reflecting the contributions of various domains of phenomena or experiences to clinical presentations (Glenn et al., 2013). Furthermore, most studies of etiology have examined people with a history of antisocial behavior, rather than specifically those who meet AsPD criteria, making the etiological relevance of meeting the diagnostic criteria difficult to evaluate.

Biopsychosocial models bring together biological, psychological, and both social and physical environmental factors (Thomson, 2019). About half of the variance in antisocial behavior is attributed to heritable or genetic factors (Tuvblad, 2014), including temperamental tendencies that facilitate rule breaking, and various subtle neuropsychological deficits that may be evident in infancy (e.g., Moffitt, 2007). Longitudinal studies have also identified a plethora of other psychological and environmental factors that increase the risk of AsPD from conception and into childhood, including prenatal maternal malnutrition or substance use, birth complications, maternal withdrawal, neglect, child abuse and maternal-partner-violence victimization, erratic and punitive parental discipline, subtle neuropsychological deficits, modeling and reinforcement for antisocial behavior, family poverty, and crime-riddled neighborhoods (DeLisi et al., 2019; Farrington et al., 2017; Moffitt, 2007).

Two distinct paradigms guide the treatment of AsPD: medical or mental health models, and correctional psychology. Each paradigm views etiology similarly, but medical model approaches emphasize genetic and biological factors more (Brazil et al., 2018; NCCMH, 2019) while correctional psychological approaches draw on both criminological theories and longitudinal research on the development of antisocial propensity, and so give somewhat less emphasis to genetics and biology (Bonta & Andrews, 2016; Farrington, 2003).

The medical approach to treatment is not logically connected to the emphasis on biological and genetic mechanisms in etiology; instead, it is "mainly rooted in tradition" (i.e., generic psychiatric treatment traditions: psychotropic and psychosocial; Bateman et al., 2015, p. 736). Drug treatment is not recommended due to a lack of evidence of effectiveness but may be effective for comorbid disorders (Bateman et al., 2015). Various schools of psychotherapy used with personality disorders in general (e.g., dialectical behavior therapy, schema therapy, social problem-solving therapy, psychodynamic and client-centered psychotherapy; van den Bosch et al., 2018) have been used with AsPD.

The correctional psychology approach has eschewed medical diagnosis; treatment reflects the severity of the person's propensity for antisocial behavior, based on estimates of their risk of future crime. The foci of treatment are psychological and social characteristics that conceptually and empirically underpin that propensity: the number, type, and extent of these "symptoms" (i.e., the dynamic risk factors). Relevant theories and models of antisocial propensity explain the development and maintenance of these presenting symptoms and how they contribute to antisocial and criminal behavior. Treatment uses the most effective approaches to improving both symptoms and behavior (i.e., reducing dynamic risk factors): social learning, behavioral, and cognitive approaches (Bonta & Andrews, 2016). Although both medical and correctional approaches primarily focus on psychological and environmental aspects of intervention, we cannot assume that biology or gene expression are thus unaltered. Although treatment effects on these aspects are poorly understood and seldom researched, psychosocial approaches may lead to alterations in these substrates (Thomson, 2019).

Brief Overview of Treatments

Mental-health-based commentary on treatment currently concludes that, at best, there is "little or no evidence of effective treatments" (van den Bosch et al., 2018, p. 72) for adult patients with AsPD (Gibbon et al., 2020). Meta-analyses of treatments for persistently antisocial adults outside of health settings tell a different story (Lipsey et al., 2007), meaning that this section and the next are informed largely by research and treatment with people in the criminal justice system. Cognitive-behavioral approaches have the strongest empirical support for effectiveness (e.g., Lipsey et al., 2007; Smith et al., 2009). The following paragraphs present three representative examples of "branded" programs under this umbrella.

First, developed in the mid-eighties, Reasoning and Rehabilitation (R&R; Ross et al., 1988) aims to remediate widespread cognitive skill deficits associated with antisocial behavior (Robinson & Porporino, 2004). It focuses primarily on cognitive skills, including meta-cognition (e.g., reflecting on *how* people think informs *what* they think and do) and self-control (e.g., stopping to consider consequences before acting), critical reasoning, and developing better values to live by (e.g., appreciating other people's values, attitudes, and needs). It is provided in structured small group discussion format and has been widely used internationally with people in the criminal justice system. A narrative review and meta-analysis of 16 evaluations – 26 separate comparisons – from 4 countries found that R&R completion was associated with an average 14% decrease in the likelihood of reconviction (Tong & Farrington, 2006). The evaluation designs were typical of those used to determine intervention effectiveness with offender rehabilitation programs; a mix of randomized controlled trials and quasi-experimental evaluations compared samples of R&R attendees with untreated control samples (Tong & Farrington, 2006).

Second, alongside evidence of skill deficits in *how* people think, there is also substantial research evidence of an association between *what* people think – referred to by various terms (e.g., attitudes, beliefs, values, thinking errors, moral judgments, cognitive distortions, dysfunctional automatic thoughts) – and antisocial or criminal behavior (Helmond et al., 2015). Cognitive self-change (CSC; Bush et al., 2016) is an example of a small group intervention that focuses on "thinking reports," in which each participant learns to observe and report on the content of their own specific thoughts during recent incidents. As this skill develops, they identify habitual patterns of thinking that help to generate or support criminal and violent acts, and learn how to intervene to challenge these patterns. Ultimately, summaries of the thinking habits they have identified become the basis for a plan for maintaining changes in their new thinking skills in the face of routine life challenges. Other intervention elements support CSC provision, including supportive authority by group leaders, and an emphasis on participant autonomy and choice (see Bush et al., 2016). A study of incarcerated people in Vermont compared CSC participants with a control group of similar incarcerated people who were not offered the program. Although the sample sizes were small, the results suggested that undertaking CSC led to reduced recidivism risk; 50% of CSC attendees and 71% of controls were charged with a new crime in the community in the two years following release from prison (Henning & Frueh, 1996).

Third, aggression replacement training (ART; Goldstein & Glick, 1987) was primarily developed for youth, but also used with adults. ART is directed toward theorized deficits in prosocial skills, resulting from a developmental environment in which such skills were not modeled or reinforced, in young people who instead develop an extensive antisocial and aggressive behavior repertoire. There is evidence that young people with CD may lack some of these skills: for example, poor social problem-solving and peer relationship skills (Dodge, 1993), and difficulties with cognitive and affective perspective taking (Anastassiou-Hadjicharalambous & Warden, 2008).

ART has three main components: (a) skillstreaming, comprising a curriculum of skills training for 50 prosocial behaviors; (b) anger control; and (c) moral reasoning training. ART has been widely used across all ages, and its efficacy in increasing prosocial behavior and reducing recidivism in young people has been demonstrated (Goldstein & Glick, 1994), its effectiveness has not yet been adequately researched with adults (Brännström et al., 2016).

In practice, branded treatment packages like these represent only a small proportion of the treatment programs offered to people with problematic levels of antisocial behavior. Most are not "branded"; they are constructed following a more general approach that is outlined in the next section, and are mainly delivered in adult correctional or juvenile justice settings.

The relevance of this work to the treatment of antisocial behavior in health settings has been somewhat overlooked, in part due to the "nontraditional" treatment settings (e.g., prisons), but perhaps also because the diagnosis of AsPD is seldom assigned in these contexts, and success is most often measured in terms of reduced likelihood of reconviction, rather than symptom change.

Since the 1980s, a large number of meta-analyses have examined the effectiveness of diverse interventions for antisocial behavior; McGuire (2013) listed 100 more than a decade ago. Among these, psychological treatment programs that are described as cognitive-behavioral, behavioral, or otherwise based on cognitive social learning theory (Bandura, 1986) are associated with the strongest effect sizes on average (Bonta & Andrews, 2016; Lipsey et al., 2007; Pearson et al., 2002; Wilson et al., 2005). These meta-analyses report results for both RCTs and quasi-experimental evaluations (QEEs; i.e., designs pairing statistically matched treatment and untreated samples), with the latter typically constituting the majority of individual studies. Although RCTs are in principle methodologically stronger, myriad factors can compromise the "gold standard" RCT design (Polaschek, 2019b), and effect sizes for RCTs and higher-quality QEEs are often similar (Gannon et al., 2019; see also Lipsey et al., 2007; Mackenzie & Farrington, 2015), justifying the expanded number of studies. Overall, although there is considerable heterogeneity of effect sizes for these cognitive and behavioral psychological treatment programs, recidivism rates are typically lower for the treatment conditions compared to controls (see Lipsey et al., 2007, fig. 1), whether RCTs or QEEs. Wilson et al., (2005) reported a mean effect size of 0.51 (based on standardized mean differences in the proportion of recidivists in treatment vs. control conditions). By contrast, the mean effect size for the Lipsey et al. (2007) meta-analysis was an odds ratio of 1.53; approximately equivalent to 40% of controls and 30% of treated individuals recidivating in the 12 months after intervention. These meta-analyses also confirm that treatments that are effective with antisocial behavior come from a relatively small segment of the array of psychotherapies used with psychological disorders. Although the correctional treatment field is now dominated by a variety of cognitive and behavioral interventions, older research confirms that approaches popular for other presenting problems are not effective (e.g., client-centered psychotherapy, psychodynamic psychotherapy; Andrews et al., 1990; Garrett, 1985).

Health research based only on evaluations of the (in)effectiveness of these more common generic approaches to mental health treatment (e.g., client-centered psychotherapy, psychodynamic psychotherapy; van den Bosch et al., 2018), or that use only RCTs to determine treatment effectiveness (Gibbon et al., 2020), and include studies of treatment participants only if they have been assessed as having AsPD, can, in combination, lead to erroneous conclusions about the treatment of antisocial behavior, including that little is known about "what works" – or, worse, that "nothing works." Correctional treatment is no miracle solution to the lack of well-constructed or well-informed health treatments for antisocial behavior, but accumulating empirical research has supported the promulgation over 20 years of a consistent series of principles to guide the development and delivery of interventions (e.g., Bonta & Andrews, 2016; Bourgon et al., 2009; Gendreau & Smith, 2012; McGuire, 2013). More recently, some of these practice guidelines are filtering through into health settings (e.g., NCCMH, 2009), albeit that there is still considerable work to do in these settings to ensure that they are adapted to provide the best possible service for people with antisocial behavior disorders.

Credible Components of Treatments

Scientifically credible interventions link intervention design and delivery to plausible theories of etiology, and target empirically supported change mechanisms using empirically supported change methods. They are successful in achieving symptom reduction during treatment, and beyond the end of the intervention (Hecht et al., 2018). Effective interventions for criminal behavior typically are intensive and multimodal; they target multiple features using a range of methods. And they target this extensive input at those most at risk, recognizing that here is where the most real-world impact can be achieved, but only with considerable effort. Treatment processes attend closely to common characteristics of the treatment population, and the context of treatment is also important. Treatment content, process, and context are described in Box 14.1, drawing from the empirical and theoretical literature on what works with criminal behavior (e.g., Craig et al., 2013; Latessa et al., 2020), and from the Risk-Need-Responsivity (RNR) model (Bonta & Andrews, 2016).

Developing Treatment Readiness

Readiness is enhanced by gently nudging clients toward seeing their antisocial behavior as their responsibility, as harmful, or even as problematic to their own goals. Cognitive techniques for exposing antisocial thinking (e.g., CSC) are used here. A detailed map of a recent offense process – the person's cognitive, affective and behavioral steps in the build-up, enactment, and post-offense consequences – is also useful for exposing and for reflection on ingrained habits of thinking, reacting, and acting that become the focus of later treatment. In group treatment, therapists often observe that other members may be more effective than themselves in helping to draw out the details, possibly because their perspectives are more highly valued by other group members (Wetzelaer et al., 2014). The approach is collaborative rather than aggressively confrontational (Bonta & Andrews, 2016); often, these ways of thinking and behaving have been functional at some point in the person's life, but when triggered in adulthood, they facilitate antisocial behavior (e.g., Early Maladaptive Schemas; Bernstein et al., 2007). Understanding how they developed from adverse childhood experiences can help to reduce defensiveness and promote motivation to change.

Learning Key Skills

Once the referred person begins to recognize that their offenses don't occur "out of the blue," they can identify which of their treatment needs (i.e., "symptoms") they are prepared to work on, leading into the second major content phase. Here, a variety of skills directly target common dynamic risk factors (DRFs): the "symptoms." DRFs are putatively changeable characteristics that are empirical correlates of crime (Olver et al., 2014). Besides antisocial beliefs, attitudes, and values, common targets for improvement or change include an irritable, aggressive, impulsively reactive temperament, a preference for spending time with antisocial rather than prosocial peers,

Box 14.1 Treatment Process

Clients with antisocial behavior seldom come to treatment recognizing the need for change, or having the capabilities to effect it; they may be treatment resistant (Derefinko & Widiger, 2016). The residue of childhood trauma, traumatic brain injuries, drug and alcohol use, unstable living and working circumstances, extreme views of personal autonomy, a self-focused view of the world, attentional difficulties, physical restlessness, illiteracy, learning difficulties and other comorbidities (see "Other Variables Influencing Treatment") needs to be accommodated for effective treatment. Accordingly, therapists socialize clients into the treatment process, motivate them to engage, and minimize barriers to client change. Neither psychoeducation nor insight-development therapy leads clients through what "behaving better" (i.e., more skillfully) looks and feels like; it is action-oriented, well scaffolded, and repetitive.

Often, two collaborative and supportive therapists lead a group of 8–12 clients. Group formats are preferred because antisocial behavior is often social behavior (Hollin, 2010). In groups, people's dysfunctional and self-focused patterns of thinking and behaving emerge during interaction with other group members' own treatment participation. Group members, as peers, also provide a more ecologically valid and credible audience with whom to try out ideas and practice skills.

Therapists need a well-developed manual, expert therapy skills, familiarity with antisocial clients and regular clinical supervision. Monitoring treatment fidelity – the extent to which the treatment adheres to the manual – is vital. Therapy can fail, or even enhance antisociality if therapists cannot establish a prosocial group environment, or drift away from treatment-as-designed.

Treatment also needs to be intensive, whether group-based, individual, or both. Group treatments of between 150 and 300 hours are recommended, reflecting clients' challenges in weakening entrenched habits by learning new skills whose effectiveness they may doubt. Little research informs whether recidivism outcomes or symptom changes are greater in one format over another (Gannon et al., 2019; Looman et al., 2014).

Health professionals' training seldom prepares them for working with antisocial clients. Effective therapists have a passion for the challenges of this type of clinical practice, and find it rewarding. They work hard to facilitate effective client alliances, and interact with warmth and humor, but also use a firm but fair (authoritative not authoritarian) manner. Once developed, they use the relationship to influence the client toward positive change, ignoring or occasionally disapproving of antisocial or negative behavior (Bonta & Andrews, 2016). Effective therapists use social learning principles such as modeling, supporting imitation, and shaping approximations of desired behavior through practice and contingent use of praise (Palmer, 2019; Wilson et al., 2005).

substance abuse, poor quality interpersonal relationships, and an underdeveloped work ethic (Bonta & Andrews, 2016). Treatment focuses on actively modeling, rehearsing, and reinforcing concrete skills that provide alternatives to antisocial solutions (e.g., prosocial thinking; problem-solving; managing volatile emotional reactivity and substance use; and prosocial relationships, communication, and conflict resolution; Polaschek, 2019a).

Preparing for Posttreatment Life

The last phase of treatment concentrates on consolidating and generalizing changes, and planning for posttreatment living, which typically includes developing prosocial capital and putting in place lifestyle elements that support more prosocial behavior (e.g., where one lives and works, who one socializes with), and identifying likely scenarios for failure and strategies to mitigate these high-risk situations (e.g., recognizing precursors early, seeking help from social supports, turning down risky opportunities; known as relapse prevention). The quality of release plans and relapse prevention have each been shown to lead to improved outcomes with respect to recidivism (Dickson et al., 2013; Dowden et al., 2003).

Treatment Context

The remaining important component of effective treatment is the context in which it occurs, and the processes in place for maintenance after treatment finishes. If antisocial behavior is often social behavior, then the social environment around treatment is also essential to success; the people around the treatment participant – whether institutional staff or family and friends – need to be supportive of change. Therapeutic communities are one option for institutional treatment that can achieve this support. In community-based treatment, this means involving prosocial family in aspects of the intervention in order to enhance the likelihood that they will support the client's positive changes, and to balance potential sources of reinforcement for antisocial behavior. Antisocial peers, which can include family members, are a major risk factor for ongoing antisocial behavior (Olver et al., 2014). Also desirable is for treatment to be followed by ongoing professional support to help with linking the person to other services (e.g., housing, employment, financial management, parenting) that will address associated issues, and to help with troubleshooting around future incidents of antisocial behavior, or problems that increase the likelihood of reverting to old habits. In correctional psychology this aspect is often referred to as reintegration, or supporting desistance (Polaschek, 2019a).

Approaches for Youth

Disruptive behavior or disordered conduct in childhood is also heterogeneous in presentation and etiology (Kazdin, 2015) but there is much more research informing treatment. Effective treatments strive to intervene with multiple factors from child, family, school, and neighborhood domains (Boxmeyer et al., 2018). Effective approaches for children under 12 years old have been identified in an evidence review using rigorous criteria to allocate 64 studies into "well established," "probably efficacious," "possibly efficacious," or "experimental" categories (Kaminski & Claussen, 2017). The authors concluded that parent-focused behavior therapy, whether individually or in groups, and including behavioral elements, was empirically well established (Kaminski & Claussen, 2017).

Using a similar approach to Kaminski and Claussen (2017), McCart et al. (2023) identified some treatments that have strong research support for adolescents already in contact with the criminal justice system, but less so for young people who are not. That is, all of the well-established treatments were targeted for youth involved in the juvenile justice system. They included multisystemic therapy, functional family therapy, and treatment foster care (McCart et al., 2023). The next level down – "probably efficacious" – also included interventions for youth with disruptive behavior disorders outside the criminal justice system. The most compelling evidence of effectiveness in this category was for combined therapies from two or more theoretical orientations: typically, cognitive-behavioral with another, such as family therapy or attachment therapy (McCart et al., 2023). Research on children with high callous-unemotional traits – a more severe subtype of disruptive behavior disorder – has been particularly prominent in recent years. Although callous-unemotional traits may predict poorer treatment outcome overall, promising interventions may be emerging (Polaschek & Skeem, 2018). Parent–child interaction therapy, modified to increase warm and responsive parenting, reward-based parenting, and parental coaching and reinforcement of children's emotional skills, was provided to the parents of 3–6-year-old children with callous-unemotional traits and conduct problems. The intervention was associated with large effects on parent-rated conduct problems, callous-unemotional traits and empathy, and observer-rated compliance at the end of treatment, and these changes persisted through three months of posttreatment follow-up (Kimonis et al., 2019). A recent RCT of 159 adolescents given either functional family therapy or a control intervention resulted in improvements in aggressive behavior, social skills, family cohesion, and youth-rated material support, even though callous-unemotional traits themselves did not appreciably reduce (Thøgersen et al., 2022).

Other Variables Influencing Treatment

Assessment and Diagnosis

The assessment of AsPD in health settings should use a purpose-designed instrument such as the Structured Clinical Interview for DSM-5 Personality Disorders (SCID-5-PD; First et al., 2016) though there are no established ways of judging severity on this basis, and it remains unclear whether applying dichotomously a diagnosis of AsPD is relevant to treatment outcomes for people with antisocial behavior. In correctional settings, assessment processes center around validated tools for assessing both the level of risk of the person committing further criminal offenses and their most relevant treatment targets for reducing risk (e.g., the Level of Supervision Inventory; Andrews et al., [2004]; the Violence Risk Scale; Wong & Gordon, [2006]), termed DRFs. Severity can then be judged by the number and extent to which DRFs are present, which then informs both treatment intensity and focus. Assessment of antisocial behavior problems ideally includes both client interview and interviews with key informants (e.g., residential staff, family members).

Comorbidity

Comorbidity is common in people with antisocial behavior histories. Those with AsPD, for instance, may show elevated prevalence of many other types of mental disorder, with comorbidity being the norm rather than the exception. Substance abuse disorders, anxiety, depression, and borderline personality disorder are the most common (Glenn et al., 2013; NCCMH, 2009). Although in health settings antisocial behavior leads to concern about the treatment of comorbidity and the rejection of AsPD clients from comorbid treatment (NCCMH, 2009), equally comorbidity may affect treatment progress directed at antisocial behavior change (Glenn et al., 2013).

Antisocial behavior is also associated with a host of negative life circumstances and outcomes across mental and physical health, economic success, and lifestyle stability. The Dunedin longitudinal study showed that at age 32, along with increased rates of anxiety, depression, post-traumatic stress, alcohol and drug dependence, and suicide attempts, men and women with early-onset and longstanding antisocial behavior also were in significantly poorer physical health (lung functioning, gum disease, serious injury, cardiovascular functioning) than multiple comparison groups, including one whose antisocial behavior began in adolescence and another of low-antisocial people (Odgers et al., 2008). Economically, this same antisocial group had lower incomes, more were unemployed and had no qualifications, and more lacked money for necessities (Odgers et al., 2008). Finally, people with AsPD are more likely to experience almost all forms of premature death (Krasnova et al., 2019). Associated features confirm that people with AsPD would benefit from help or intervention across multiple lifestyle areas.

Demographics

In western countries, AsPD is diagnosed in about 3% of the population; about 75% of those diagnosed are men. Few studies have examined ethnicity or race; in the US, Ehlers et al., (2022) found no differences between African, European, or Indigenous Americans, but this is clearly an area that needs more investigation, especially given wide disparities between European, non-European, and Indigenous imprisonment rates in several western nations (e.g., Canada, US, UK, Australia, NZ).

Medication

To date, trials of various medications suggest that that medication is neither helpful nor harmful in ameliorating antisocial behavior. A recent Cochrane Review (Khalifa et al., 2020) reported results for people with AsPD from four RCTs; all relevant participants were in study samples for reasons other than AsPD (e.g., substance use problems). The studies compared a placebo condition with an antiepileptic drug (phenytoin), desipramine, nortripyline (both antidepressants), and bromocriptine (a dopamine agonist that caused severe side effects). The reviewers found that no conclusions could be drawn, based on the poor methodological standards, general lack of studies, and failure to measure relevant outcomes, including reconviction. Overall, there also appears to be little rationale for *how* a particular class of drugs might be effective in reducing presenting features of AsPD. The most popular idea is that abnormalities in the serotonergic system that may cause impulsive aggressive behavior – a features of some people with AsPD – may respond to antidepressants, while others have suggested that drugs that are effective with underregulated behavior, such as anticonvulsants, may also be useful. By contrast, another recent review (Sesso & Masi, 2023) advocated for overcoming the limitations of the Khalifa review findings by "including all meaningful sources of evidence that may provide relevant details for a better definition of effective therapeutic strategies" (p. 184), but still came up with very few studies, even when focusing on RCTs for pharmacological treatment of potentially related conditions such as impulsive aggression. Sesso and Masi (2023) noted that better definitions of the aspects of AsPD (e.g., aggression or mood instability) being targeted were needed to advance pharmacological research, noting the poor quality and outdated nature of the extant research. They concluded that the treatment of first choice remans psychotherapy.

Conclusion

The development of effective interventions for adult antisocial behavior in health settings remains mired in the limitations of current relevant diagnoses. AsPD and CD diagnoses have no clear etiology, and tautologically specify symptoms that largely comprise the behavior associated with having these purported mental disorders. In health settings, AsPD has then been used to exclude people from treatment for other mental disorders, and failed attempts to use generic mental health treatments for reducing antisocial behavior has led some health professionals to conclude that "nothing works."

Parallel developments in correctional psychology interventions offer promise that is still to be fully capitalized on in health settings. But they also have significant limitations in filling the needs of health practitioners. Correctional settings differ in important ways from health settings. Those referred for correctional treatment may also differ from the referral population in a health setting, where extensive criminal convictions may not be inevitable. The focus on identifying effectiveness by reducing reconviction risk is only indirectly related to the more immediate need to focus on change in symptoms. Conceiving of symptoms as DRFs is useful, but correctional treatment outcome studies mainly need to meet accountability requirements for policy makers and politicians, to reduce recidivism. Consequently, the meaningful measurement of change within treatment is underdeveloped and not always successful (Polaschek, 2017). Also unclear are the most effective ways to work across cultures. Although people from diverse ethnicities may also benefit from conventional western psychology-based treatment approaches (Usher & Stewart, 2014) in some correctional settings, Indigenous treatment approaches or hybrids incorporating equally diverse cultural frameworks are under development and show early promise (Gutierrez et al., 2018). Finally, correctional treatment is predominantly effective when provided by cognitive-behaviorally trained psychologists or those trained by them (Bonta & Andrews, 2016; Gannon et al., 2019). That leaves unaddressed how those with other professional orientations can effectively contribute to treatment.

The UK NICE guidelines (NCCMH, 2009) begin the process of bringing together these two separate areas of practice; doing so may offer benefits for both fields. Perhaps the development of effective person-based approaches to treatment (e.g., treating a person's anxiety, substance abuse, and antisocial propensity together) may result from this union. The most pressing research area with regard to effective treatment is how best to approach those whose antisocial behavior largely excludes criminal convictions.

With empirically supported treatments, people with histories of persistent criminal behavior may be able to exit the criminal justice system more rapidly than they otherwise would. But with rare exceptions (see Coupland & Olver, 2020), treatment studies have not examined long-term functioning other than recidivism, due to the formidable challenges of follow-up studies. Future research should attend to this important question.

Even without treatment, the long-term prognosis for people with AsPD is cautiously positive. Longitudinal research suggests that much fewer people who met AsPD diagnostic criteria as young adults continue to do so later in adulthood (Black et al., 1995; Mulder et al., 1994). Research tracking people over decades shows that those involved in antisocial behavior when young do show steady, if slow, improvements in life functioning, reduced involvement in crime, and less engagement with the criminal justice system (Farrington et al., 2009; Laub & Sampson, 2003). Future research needs to examine whether the underlying personality characteristics have also improved.

Useful Resources

- The best example of integration between the health and criminal justice research literatures reviewed here is the NICE guidelines: Antisocial Personality Disorder: The NICE Guideline on Treatment Management and Prevention.
- For a succinct summary of the RNR model, see www.publicsafety.gc.ca/cnt/rsrcs/pblctns/rsk-nd-rspnsvty/index-en.aspx
- For a series of slides on "what works" for criminal behavior, see, see www.bscc.ca.gov/wp-content/uploads/Principles-of-Effective-Interventions.pdf
- For those doing individual therapy Tafrate, R. C., & Mitchell, D. (2014). *Forensic CBT: A handbook of clinical practice*. Wiley.

References

American Psychiatric Association (APA). (2022). *Diagnostic and statistical manual of mental disorders, fifth edition, text revision*. American Psychiatric Association.

Anastassiou-Hadjicharalambous, X., & Warden, D. (2008). Cognitive and affective perspective-taking in conduct-disordered children high and low on callous-unemotional traits. Child and Adolescent Psychiatry and Mental Health, 2(1), 16. https://doi.org/10.1186/1753-2000-2-16.

Andrews, D. A., Bonta, J., & Wormith, J. S. (2004). *The level of service/case management inventory (LS/CMI)*. Multi-Health Systems.

Andrews, D. A., Zinger, I., Hoge, R. D., et al. (1990). Does correctional treatment work? A clinically relevant and psychologically informed meta-analysis. *Criminology*, 28, 369–404.

Bandura, A. (1986). *Social foundations of thought and action: A social-cognitive theory*. Prentice-Hall.

Bateman, A. W., Gunderson, J., & Mulder, R. (2015). Treatment of personality disorder. *Lancet*, 385(9969), 735–743. https://doi.org/10.1016/s0140-6736(14)61394-5.

Bernstein, D. P., Arntz, A., & Vos, M. D. (2007). Schema focused therapy in forensic settings: Theoretical model and recommendations for best clinical practice. *International Journal of Forensic Mental Health*, 6(2), 169–183.

Black, D. W., Baumgard, C. H., & Bell, S. E. (1995). A 16- to 45-year follow-up of 71 men with antisocial personality disorder. *Comprehensive Psychiatry*, 36(2), 130–140. https://doi.org/10.1016/S0010-440X(95)90108-6.

Blackburn, R. (1988). On moral judgements and personality disorders: The myth of psychopathic personality revisited. *The British Journal of Psychiatry*, 153(4), 505–512.

Bonta, J., & Andrews, D. A. (2016). *The psychology of criminal conduct* (6th ed.). Routledge.

Bourgon, G., Bonta, J., Rugge, T., Scott, T., & Yessine, A. K. (2009). Translating "what works" into sustainable everyday practice: Program design, implementation and evaluation. www.publicsafety.gc.ca/cnt/rsrcs/pblctns/2009-05-pd/index-en.aspx.

Boxmeyer, C. L., Powell, N. P., Mitchell, Q., et al. (2018). Psychosocial treatment and prevention in middle childhood and early adolescence. In J. E. Lochman & W. Matthys (Eds.), *The Wiley handbook of disruptive and impulse-control disorders* (pp. 451–466). Wiley.

Brännström, L., Kaunitz, C., Andershed, A.-K., South, S., & Smedslund, G. (2016). Aggression replacement training (ART) for reducing antisocial behavior in adolescents and adults: A systematic review. *Aggression and Violent Behavior*, 27, 30–41.

Brazil, I. A., van Dongen, J. D. M., Maes, J. H. R., Mars, R. B., & Baskin-Sommers, A. R. (2018). Classification and treatment of antisocial individuals: From behavior to biocognition. *Neuroscience and Biobehavioral Reviews*, 91, 259–277.

Bush, J., Harris, D. M., & Parker, R. J. (2016). *Cognitive self-change: How offenders experience the world and what we can do about it*. Wiley.

Coupland, R. B. A., & Olver, M. E. (2020). Assessing protective factors in treated violent offenders: Associations with recidivism reduction and positive community outcomes. *Psychological Assessment*, 32(5), 493–508.

Cox, J., Edens, J. F., Magyar, M. S., et al. (2013). Using the Psychopathic Personality Inventory to identify subtypes of antisocial personality disorder. *Journal of Criminal Justice*, 41(2), 125–134.

Craig, L. A., Dixon, L., & Gannon, T. A. (Eds.). (2013). *What works in offender rehabilitation: An evidence-based approach to assessment and treatment*. Wiley.

Cunningham, M. D., & Reidy, T. J. (1998). Antisocial personality disorder and psychopathy: diagnostic dilemmas in classifying patterns of antisocial behavior in sentencing evaluations. *Behavioral Science and the Law*, 16(3), 333–351.

DeLisi, M., Drury, A. J., & Elbert, M. J. (2019). The etiology of antisocial personality disorder: The differential roles of adverse childhood experiences and childhood psychopathology. *Comprehensive Psychiatry*, 92, 902–917.

Derefinko, K. J., & Widiger, T. A. (2016). Antisocial personality disorder. In S. H. Fatemi & P. J. Clayton (Eds.), *The medical basis of psychiatry* (pp. 229–245). Springer.

Dickson, S. R., Polaschek, D. L. L., & Casey, A. R. (2013). Can the quality of high-risk violent prisoners' release plans predict recidivism following intensive rehabilitation? A comparison with risk assessment instruments. *Psychology, Crime and Law*, 19, 371–389.

Dodge, K. A. (1993). Social-cognitive mechanisms in the development of conduct disorder and depression. *Annual Review of Psychology*, 44, 559–584.

Dowden, C., Antoniwicz, D., & Andrews, D. A. (2003). The effectiveness of relapse prevention with offenders: A meta-analysis. *International Journal of Offender Therapy and Comparative Criminology*, 47, 516–528.

Ehlers, C. L., Schuckit, M. A., Hesselbrock, V., et al. (2022). The clinical course of antisocial behaviors in men and women of three racial groups. *Journal of Psychiatric Research*, 151, 319–327.

Farrington, D. P. (2003). Developmental and life-course criminology: Key theoretical and empirical issues – The 2002 Sutherland Award address. *Criminology*, 41, 221–255.

Farrington, D. P., Gaffney, H., & Ttofi, M. M. (2017). Systematic reviews of explanatory risk factors for violence, offending, and delinquency. *Aggression and Violent Behavior*, 33, 24–36.

Farrington, D. P., Ttofi, M. M., & Coid, J. W. (2009). Development of adolescence-limited, late-onset, and persistent offenders from age 8 to age 48. *Aggressive Behavior*, 35, 150–163.

Fazel, S., & Danesh, J. (2002). Serious mental disorder in 23000 prisoners: A systematic review of 62 surveys. *The Lancet*, 359, 545–550.

First, M. B., Williams, J. B. W., Benjamin, L. S., & Spitzer, R. L. (2016). *Structured clinical interview for DSM-5 personality disorders*. American Psychiatric Association.

Gannon, T. A., Olver, M. E., Mallion, J. S., & James, M. (2019). Does specialized psychological treatment for offending reduce recidivism? A meta-analysis examining staff and program variables as predictors of treatment effectiveness. *Clinical Psychology Review*, 73, 101752.

Garrett, P. (1985). Effects of residential treatment of adjudicated delinquents: a meta-analysis. *Journal of Research in Crime and Delinquency*, 22, 287–308.

Gendreau, P., & Smith, P. (2012). Assessment and treatment strategies for correctional institutions. In J. Dvoskin, J. Skeem, R. Novaco, & K. Douglas (Eds.), *Using social science to reduce violent offending* (pp. 157–177). Guilford.

Gibbon, S., Khalifa, N. R., Cheung, N. H., Völlm, B. A., & McCarthy, L. (2020). Psychological interventions for antisocial personality disorder. *Cochrane Database System Reviews*, 9(9), Cd007668.

Glenn, A. L., Johnson, A. K., & Raine, A. (2013). Antisocial personality disorder: A current review. *Current Psychiatry Reports*, 15(12), 427.

Goldstein, A. P., & Glick, B. (1987). *Aggression replacement training: A comprehensive intervention for aggressive youth*. Research Press.

Goldstein, A. P., & Glick, B. (1994). Aggression replacement training: Curriculum and evaluation. *Simulation and Gaming*, 25, 9–26.

Gurley, J. R. (2009). A history of changes to the criminal personality in the DSM. *History of Psychology*, 12(4), 285–304.

Gutierrez, L., Chadwick, N., & Wanamaker, K. A. (2018). Culturally relevant programming versus the status quo: A meta-analytic review of the effectiveness of treatment of indigenous offenders. *Canadian Journal of Criminology and Criminal Justice*, 60, 321–353.

Hare, R. D. (2003). *The Hare Psychopathy Checklist: Revised technical manual* (2nd ed.). Multi-Health Systems.

Hecht, L. K., Latzman, R. D., & Lilienfeld, S. O. (2018). The psychological treatment of psychopathy: Theory and research. In D. David, S. J. Lynn, & G. H. Montgomery (Eds.), *Evidence based psychotherapy: The state of the science and practice* (pp. 271–298). Wiley.

Helmond, P., Overbeek, G., Brugman, D., & Gibbs, J. C. (2015). A meta-analysis on cognitive distortions and externalizing problem behavior: Associations, moderators, and treatment effectiveness. *Criminal Justice and Behavior*, 42(3), 245–262.

Henning, K. R., & Frueh, B. C. (1996). Cognitive-behavioral treatment of incarcerated offenders: An evaluation of the Vermont Department of Corrections' cognitive self-change program. *Criminal Justice & Behavior*, 23, 523–541.

Hollin, C. R. (2010). Commentary directions for group process work. *Aggression and Violent Behavior*, 15, 150–151.

Kaminski, J. W., & Claussen, A. H. (2017). Evidence base update for psychosocial treatments for disruptive behaviors in children. *Journal of Clinical Child and Adolescent Psychology*, 46(4), 477–499.

Kazdin, A. E. (2015). Psychosocial treatments for conduct disorder in children and adolescents. In P. E. Nathan & J. M. Gorman (Eds.), *A guide to treatments that work* (4th ed., pp. 141–173). Oxford University Press.

Khalifa, N. R., Gibbon, S., Völlm, B. A., Cheung, N.-Y., & McCarthy, L. (2020). Pharmacological interventions for antisocial personality disorder. *Cochrane Database of Systematic Reviews* 2020 (9), 1–106.

Krasnova, A., Eaton, W. W., & Samuels, J. F. (2019). Antisocial personality and risks of cause-specific mortality: Results from the Epidemiologic Catchment Area study with 27 years of follow-up. *Social Psychiatry and Psychiatric Epidemiology*, 54(5), 617–625.

Latessa, E. J., Johnson, S. L., & Koetzle, D. (2020). *What works (and doesn't) in reducing recidivism* (2nd ed.). Routledge.

Laub, J. H., & Sampson, R. J. (2003). *Shared beginnings, divergent lives: Delinquent boys to age 70.* Harvard University Press.

Lipsey, M. W., Landenberger, N. A., & Wilson, S. J. (2007). *Effects of cognitive behavioral programs for criminal offenders.* The Campbell Collaboration.

Looman, J., Abracen, J., & Fazio, D. (2014). Efficacy of group vs. individual treatment of sex offenders. *Sexual Abuse in Australia and New Zealand*, 6(1), 48–56.

MacKenzie, D. L., & Farrington, D. P. (2015). Preventing future offending of delinquents and offenders: what have we learned from experiments and meta-analyses? *Journal of Experimental Criminology*, 11, 565–595. https://doi.org/10.1007/s11292-015-9244-9.

McCart, M. R., Sheidow, A. J., & Jaramillo, J. (2023). Evidence base update of psychosocial treatments for adolescents with disruptive behavior. *Journal of Clinical Child and Adolescent Psychology*, 52(4), 447–474.

McGuire, J. (2008). A review of effective interventions for reducing aggression and violence. *Philosophical Transactions of the Royal Society B*, 363, 2577–2497. https://doi.org/ 10.1098/rstb.2008.0035.

McGuire, J. (2013). What works to reduce reoffending: 18 years on. In L. A. Craig, L. Dixon, & T. A. Gannon (Eds.), *What works in offender rehabilitation: An evidence-based approach to assessment and treatment* (pp. 20–49). Wiley.

McKinley, S., Patrick, C. J., & Verona, E. (2018). Antisocial personality disorder: Neurophysiological mechanisms and distinct subtypes. *Current Behavioral Neuroscience Reports 5*, 72–80.

Moffitt, T. E. (2007). A review of research on the taxonomy of life-course persistent versus adolescence-limited antisocial behavior. In D. J. Flannery, A. T. Vazsonyi, & I. D. Waldman (Eds.), *The Cambridge handbook of violent behaviour and aggression.* Cambridge University Press.

Mulder, R. T., Wells, J. E., Joyce, P. R., & Bushnell, J. A. (1994). Antisocial women. *Journal of Personality Disorders*, 8(4), 279–287.

National Collaborating Centre for Mental Health (NCCMH, 2009). *Antisocial personality disorder: Treatment, management and prevention (NICE Clinical Guideline 77).* British Psychological Society and Royal College of Psychiatrists.

Odgers, C. A., Moffitt, T. E., Broadbent, J. M., et al. (2008). Female and male antisocial trajectories: From childhood origins to adult outcomes. *Development and Psychopathology*, 20, 673–716.

Olver, M. E., Stockdale, K. C., & Wormith, J. S. (2014). Thirty years of research on the Level of Service scales: A meta-analytic examination of predictive accuracy and sources of variability. *Psychological Assessment*, 26, 156–176.

Palmer, E. J. (2019). Group programmes with offenders. In P. Ugwudike, H. Graham, F. McNeill, P. Raynor, F. S. Taxman, & C. Trotter (Eds.), *The Routledge companion to rehabilitative work in criminal justice* (pp. 1117–1130). Routledge.

Pearson, F. S., Lipton, D. S., Cleland, C. M., & Yee, D. S. (2002). The effects of behavioral/cognitive-behavioral programs on recidivism. *Crime and Delinquency*, 48(3), 476–496.

Polaschek, D. L. L. (2017). Reporting change. In S. Brown, E. Bowen, & D. Prescott (Eds.), *The forensic psychologists' report writing guide* (pp. 91–102). Routledge.

Polaschek, D. L. L. (2019a). Interventions to reduce recidivism in adult violent offenders. In D. L. L. Polaschek, A. Day, & C. R. Hollin (Eds.), *The Wiley international handbook of correctional psychology*. (pp. 501–514). Wiley.

Polaschek, D. L. L. (2019b). Treatment outcome evaluations: How do we know what works. In D. L. L. Polaschek, A. Day, & C. R. Hollin (Eds.), *The Wiley international handbook of correctional psychology*. (pp. 410–426). Wiley.

Polaschek, D. L. L., & Skeem, J. L. (2018). Treatment of adults and juveniles with psychopathy. In C. J. Patrick (Ed.), *Handbook of psychopathy* (2nd ed., pp. 710–731). Guilford.

Robinson, D., & Porporino, F. J. (2004). Programming in cognitive skills: The reasoning and rehabilitation programme. In C. R. Hollin (Ed.), *The Essential Handbook of Offender Assessment and Treatment* (pp. 63–78). Wiley.

Ross, R. R., Fabiano, E. A., & Ewles, C. D. (1988). Reasoning and rehabilitation. *International Journal of Offender Therapy and Comparative Criminology*, 32, 29–36.

Sesso, G., & Masi, G. (2023). Pharmacological strategies for the management of the antisocial personality disorder. *Expert Review of Clinical Pharmacology*, 16(3), 181–194.

Skeem, J. L., & Cooke, D. J. (2010). Is criminal behavior a central component of psychopathy? Conceptual directions for resolving the debate. *Psychological Assessment*, 22(2), 433–445.

Smith, P., Gendreau, P., & Swartz, K. (2009). Validating the principles of effective intervention: A systematic review of the contributions of meta-analysis in the field of corrections. *Victims and Offenders*, 4, 148–169.

Thøgersen, D. M., Elmose, M., Viding, E., McCrory, E., & Bjørnebekk, G. (2022). Behavioral improvements but limited change in callous-unemotional traits in adolescents treated for conduct problems. *Journal of Child and Family Studies*, 31(12), 3342–3358.

Thomson, N. (2019). *Understanding psychopathy: The biopsychosocial perspective* (1st ed.). Routledge.

Tong, L. S. J., & Farrington, D. P. (2006). How effective is the "Reasoning and Rehabilitation" programme in reducing reoffending? A meta-analysis of evaluations in four countries. *Psychology, Crime & Law*, 12, 3–24.

Tuvblad, C. (2014). Genetic influences on antisocial behavior across the life-course. In M. DeLisi & M. Vaughn (Eds.), *The Routledge international handbook of biosocial criminology* (pp. 77–100). Routledge.

Usher, A. M., & Stewart, L. A. (2014). Effectiveness of correctional programs with ethnically diverse offenders: A meta-analytic study. *International Journal of Offender Therapy & Comparative Criminology*, 58(2), 209–230.

van den Bosch, L. M. C., Rijckmans, M. J. N., Decoene, S., & Chapman, A. L. (2018). Treatment of antisocial personality disorder: Development of a practice focused framework. *International Journal of Law & Psychiatry*, 58, 72–78.

Werner, K. B., Few, L. R., & Bucholz, K. K. (2015). Epidemiology, comorbidity, and behavioral genetics of Antisocial Personality Disorder and psychopathy. *Psychiatric Annals*, 45(4), 195–199.

Wetzelaer, P., Farrell, J., Evers, S.M., et al. (2014). Design of an international multicentre RCT on group schema therapy for borderline personality disorder. *BMC Psychiatry*, 14 (1), 1–15.

Wilson, D. B., Bouffard, L. A., & MacKenzie, D. L. (2005). A quantitative review of structured, group-oriented, cognitive-behavioral programs for offenders. *Criminal Justice and Behavior*, 32, 172–204.

Wong, S. C. P., & Gordon, A. (2006). The validity and reliability of the Violence Risk Scale: A treatment-friendly violence risk assessment tool. *Psychology, Public Policy, and Law*, 12, 279–309.

15

Borderline Personality and Other Personality Disorders

Joel Paris

Personality disorder (PD) is defined in the *Diagnostic and Statistical Manual* (DSM-5-TR; American Psychiatric Association, 2022) as an enduring pattern of inner experience and behavior, manifested in at least two of the following areas: cognition, affectivity, interpersonal functioning, and impulse control. PDs begin in youth and lead to difficulties in multiple contexts (work and relationships) over many years. In this way, PDs differ from diagnoses such as major depressive disorder in being a life-course pattern rather than an episode. The idea that PDs should not be diagnosed before adulthood is mistaken: an early onset of borderline personality disorder, usually in adolescence, has been confirmed by a large body of research (Chanen & McCutcheon, 2013; Sharp & Tackett, 2014). (Note: this chapter will use the convention of abbreviating PD when discussing general personality disorder and will write out any specific personality disorder that is mentioned.)

It is also important to note that most of the research on PDs, particularly as related to psychotherapy, has been on the borderline category. The idea that patients with a PD always require long courses of therapy has little research support. This idea is based on the assumption that symptoms present for a long time must require a lengthy therapy. However, there is little evidential support for that conclusion. In fact, long-term therapy for any diagnostic entity has not been well researched. Most of the research literature in psychotherapy concerns treatments that last no more than six months, and virtually all outcome studies concern therapies that last for a few months, or a year at most (Markham et al., 2021).

In spite of a lack of evidence, the history of PD treatment has been marked by advocacy for lengthy courses of therapy. Open-ended treatments, as opposed to time-limited therapies, are likely to be chosen by therapists trained in psychodynamic methods (Paris, 2019). Open-ended therapy has long been known to be associated with large drop-out rates (Skodol et al., 1983), and its efficacy has not been evaluated in randomized controlled trials (RCTs).

The absence of research on extended courses of therapy reflects the clinical reality that, in practice, most psychotherapies are brief, since longer treatments tend to be expensive and inaccessible. Yet well-targeted interventions can have rapid effects on symptoms, and many patients with borderline personality disorder who have had symptoms for years can be treated effectively within a few months (Blum & Black, 2020; Laporte et al., 2018).

The impact of therapy needs to be framed by the life course of patients. Borderline personality disorder typically begins in adolescence or early youth, and then gradually improves with time, usually remitting by age 30 or 40 (Paris, 2020; Zanarini, 2019). Instead of continuing therapy for years, treatment programs should set the goal of hastening recovery.

The situation is now changing. A number of innovative methods of treatment have been developed for borderline personality disorder, and clinicians have several choices of methods (Choi-Kain, 2020). However, the situation for other categories of PD is less encouraging – hardly any research has been carried out on these disorders, so there is little to choose from.

Etiology and Theoretical Underpinnings of Treatment

Personality disorders are complex forms of psychopathology that have a complex etiology. The best model is to frame PDs as the product of gene–environment interactions, as exemplified by a biopsychosocial model (Engel, 1980). Linehan (1993) applied a similar approach to the borderline category: a biosocial model that hypothesizes interactions between heritable traits of emotion dysregulation and an invalidating environment. The idea that borderline personality disorder is mainly due to childhood trauma is mistaken, although it is true that early adversities of that nature tend to make the disorder more severe (Yuan et al., 2023).

PDs as a whole can most usefully be understood as exaggerations of personality trait variations that have become extreme and dysfunctional. The most researched system for describing these traits is the Five Factor Model (Widiger & Costa, 2013). That is, patients with PDs tend to have higher amounts of: (1) negative affectivity, (2) detachment, (3) antagonism, (4) disinhibition, and/or (5) psychoticism. These five maladaptive traits fall on the opposite end of a continuum with more adaptive traits (i.e., emotional stability, extraversion, agreeableness, conscientiousness, and lucidity).

These relationships between disorders and traits offer some guidance for setting treatment goals. Thus, for example, patients with PDs are generally high in neuroticism but low in agreeableness and conscientiousness. This suggests that they can benefit from skills in handling emotions, in developing more persistence in the pursuit of life goals, and in managing relationships in ways that make them work.

Brief Overview of Treatments

Borderline personality disorder is marked by long-term problems in emotion regulation, interpersonal relationships, and impulsivity. Psychotherapy is the backbone of treatment for this disorder. Over the last 30 years, well-designed clinical trials have been conducted on several methods designed to treat borderline personality disorder. The results generally show that tailored and structured forms of therapy yield superior results when compared to treatment as usual. However, accessibility of these expensive therapies is problematic, and more research is needed on ways to shorten treatment (Paris, 2015, 2020).

Dialectical Behavior Therapy

Dialectical behavior therapy (DBT) is an adaptation of cognitive-behavioral therapy (CBT) combined with interventions drawn from other approaches (Linehan, 1993). The method is specifically designed to target the emotion dysregulation (mood instability) that characterizes borderline personality disorder, and to reduce impulsive behaviors that accompany that dysregulation (Crowell et al., 2009). It applies chain analysis to incidents leading to self-injury and overdoses, encouraging patients to describe the emotions that lead up to impulsive behaviors. Therapy then teaches patients alternative ways of handling dysphoric emotions. DBT also emphasizes empathic responses to distress that provide validation for the inner experience of patients with borderline personality. The program consists of individual and group psychoeducation, as well as telephone availability for coaching.

DBT was the first psychological treatment for borderline personality disorder to be tested in an RCT (Linehan et al., 1993). Its efficacy has since been replicated in studies conducted by the original research group (Linehan et al., 2006), as well as by others (Levy et al., 2018). The level of evidence for the efficacy of borderline personality disorder has been rated as *strong* by the Society for Clinical Psychology (SCP, n.d.a.).

The first trial (Linehan et al., 1993) compared one year of DBT to treatment as usual (TAU), and found DBT to be clearly superior, especially in regard to reductions in self-harm, overdosing, and hospitalization. A second clinical trial (Linehan et al., 2006) used a comparison group of "treatment by community experts" – therapists in practice who identified themselves as interested in borderline personality disorder, and whose fees were paid by the research team. The results again favored DBT, with reductions in overdoses and subsequent hospitalizations within a year, although this time there were no differences in reduction of self-harm. Replication studies in other centers have produced similarly encouraging results, as confirmed by a Cochrane Report (Storebo et al., 2020). These findings indicate that DBT is an effective and specific method that is usually superior to traditional ways of treating patients with borderline personality disorder.

There are unanswered questions about DBT. While the original cohort received therapy 20 years ago, they were never followed up for more than a year, so we do not know whether treated patients maintained their gains and/or continued to improve. Also, given the resources required to offer DBT in its original form for at least a year, this form of therapy is not widely available.

DBT needs to be dismantled and/or streamlined for greater clinical impact (Paris, 2015). One report found that a 6-month version of DBT can be effective (Stanley et al., 2007), and a larger study found 6 months of DBT to be as efficacious as a 12-month course (McMain et al., 2022). DBT can probably be further shortened, as shown by an effectiveness study that reported a good symptomatic response following a 12-week course of therapy (Laporte et al., 2018).

While the most extensive body of research concerns DBT, it is unclear whether it is a uniquely efficacious treatment, or whether other well-structured approaches yield much the same results in borderline personality disorder. To address this issue, McMain et al. (2009) administered DBT for one year, with the comparison condition being another program developed specifically for borderline personality disorder: general psychiatric management.

General Psychiatric Management

General Psychiatric Management (GPM) is an alternative method based on American Psychiatric Association guidelines for the treatment of borderline personality disorder (Oldham et al., 2001), and has been manualized (Choi-Kain, 2020). The results of a comparative trial between DBT and GPM found no differences between groups in terms of suicidality, hospitalization, or self-harm (McMain et al., 2009), and both groups were doing well two years later (McMain et al., 2012). These findings have important clinical implications, suggesting that while DBT is often better than TAU, it can be matched by other therapies that are designed for this population.

Systems Training for Emotional Predictability and Problem Solving

Systems Training for Emotional Predictability and Problem Solving (STEPPS) (Blum et al., 2008) is a program whose theory and practice closely resemble DBT. Focusing on emotional dysregulation, it offers a brief intervention conducted in groups. STEPPS is designed to supplement standard therapies, and it is therefore particularly suitable for regions where specialized treatment is not available. The method has been subject to a successful clinical trial (Blum et al., 2008) and independent replication (Bos et al., 2010). STEPPS offers an alternative to the lengthy and expensive methods of DBT.

Other Treatment Options

In addition to DBT, the Society of Clinical Psychology also lists two treatments for borderline personality disorder that can be viewed as a hybrid between CBT and psychodynamic therapy. First, mentalization-based therapy (MBT; Bateman & Fonagy, 2006) is derived from the concept that patients need to be taught to "mentalize" (i.e., to accurately observe their own feelings and those of others). As in DBT, patients are taught to recognize their emotions, to learn how to tolerate them, and to manage them in more adaptive ways. Second, schema-focused therapy (SFT; Young, 1999) aims to modify maladaptive schemas deriving from adverse experiences in childhood. However, access to SFT is not easy, especially given that it is designed to last for three years. The level of evidence for both of these hybrid approaches has been rated as *moderate* by the Society for Clinical Psychology (SCP, n.d.a.), and so they will not be discussed further.

Transference-focused psychotherapy (TFP) is a modification of psychodynamic treatment that aims to correct distortions in the patient's perception of the therapist during sessions (Clarkin et al., 2007). It differs from DBT and MBT by placing emphasis on correcting transference phenomena, with the aim of generalizing these observations to outside relationships. The level of evidence for its efficacy has been rated as *strong/controversial* by the Society for Clinical Psychology (SCP; n.d.a.). The controversial categorization was provided because of the mixed results from RCTs, and so this treatment will not be discussed further.

Credible Components of Treatments

If therapies based on so many different theories, and using very different techniques, can produce the same results, might they have something in common? The findings reviewed here show that structured therapies of any kind are most likely to be successful for patients with borderline personality disorder. Traditional therapies may have been less effective because they rely on unstructured methods that leave patients who struggle with chaotic emotions adrift.

Common Factors

The treatments described earlier all have some evidence for their efficacy. They may target different aspects of borderline personality disorder, yet the failure of comparative trials to find differences in outcome suggests that common factors must be of crucial importance (Wampold & Imel, 2015). The most important common factors in any therapy are a strong working alliance, empathy, and a practical, problem-solving approach (Markham et al., 2021).

In a complex disorder like borderline personality disorder, psychotherapy needs to maximize these common factors and to make them more specific. The best-validated methods offer a defined structure, focus on the regulation of emotions, and encourage the solution of interpersonal problems through self-observation. Moreover, structure is an essential element of treatment for patients with borderline personality disorder, who often lead unstable lives and have unstable emotions. That is probably why treatments that provide this essential element achieve better results than does unstructured TAU in the community (Linehan et al., 1993).

Empathy and validation are essential elements of any therapy, and are particularly important for patients with PDs, some of whom are sensitive to the slightest hint of invalidation (Linehan, 1993). In other words, these are patients who can easily feel that their emotions are dismissed by others. Feeling invalidated may lead to difficulty absorbing other aspects of the therapy. When one learns to observe emotions (and not be derailed by them), one can stand aside from crises and begin to think about alternative solutions to problems.

Teaching Emotion Regulation Skills

Psychotherapies designed for borderline personality disorder have earned a strong evidence base (Paris, 2020). However, it is not clear that "any old" psychotherapy will do. DBT offers an additional component: the teaching of skills that promote emotion regulation.

Patients usually come to sessions and tell stories about stressful events that have occurred over the week, and therapists usually validate their feelings. It is easy to see why this can be helpful, but many patients with borderline personality disorder misunderstand and distort their interpersonal environment. The danger is that patients will conclude that we agree with them – that is, that other people are bad, and that they are victims.

Empathy therefore has to be linked to tactful confrontations to help patients learn new ways of dealing with their problems, what Bateman and Fonagy (2006) call the capacity to "mentalize," and what Linehan (1993) calls a "dialectical" approach (i.e., understanding why it is hard to change, but encouraging patients to change anyway). Therefore, therapy needs to promote change, based on a strong enough alliance that allows patients to see their problems in a different light.

These principles help us to understand why psychodynamic therapy has often been ineffective for patients with borderline personality disorder. There are clinical trials supporting transference-focused therapy (Doering et al., 2010), but that is a major adaptation of the psychodynamic approach. Most patients who mentalize, or who are constantly in the throes of emotion dysregulation, cannot make use of procedures such as free association with a relatively silent therapist who only intervenes to make "interpretations."

Box 15.1 Self-Injurious Thoughts and Behaviors in Youth

There has been an increase in the prevalence of suicidal ideation and/or nonsuicidal self-injury (NSSI) in young people. Although many adolescents who engage in NSSIs are experimenting, those that continue to do so are more likely to develop borderline personality disorder (Biskin et al., 2021). In a systematic review, DBT has been characterized as a well-established treatment (i.e., having strong research support) for youth with both suicidal ideation and deliberate self-harm (Glenn et al., 2019). Within the DBT framework, suicidal ideation and NSSIs are viewed as ways to control emotional dysregulation when distress feels overwhelming. They can also be a way to communicate distress to others (Nock, 2009).

Present-Oriented Focus

If therapy focuses on the past rather than the present, patients are more likely to be mired down than to "work through" past events. There may also be problems in focusing excessively on re-experiencing traumatic events from childhood. Koenigsberg (2010) has shown that patients with borderline personality disorder do not habituate to stressful thoughts, but that they become increasingly activated and disturbed as they repeatably try to process them. This may help to explain the regression and increasing symptom levels so often seen in therapies that focus on traumatic events.

Therapies that are present-oriented, have a strong cognitive component, balance acceptance and change, offer a predictable structure, and in which therapists are active and engaged are more likely to succeed. They place more importance on the present than the past.

Approaches for Other Personality Disorders

The most researched PD is borderline personality disorder, as this diagnosis describes patients who often come for treatment and who place great demands on mental health practitioners. The picture is quite different in community studies that include those who meet criteria for a PD but do not usually seek therapy (Trull et al., 2010). The picture is also different in clinical settings where systematic evaluations of PD are routinely conducted. In a large outpatient clinic (n=859), Zimmerman et al. (2005) examined the clinical prevalence of the various categories of PD described in the DSM-IV. Of the total PD cases, somewhat less than half of patients, somewhat less than half of all patients, the most frequent were avoidant personality disorder, at 14.7%, followed by unspecified personality disorder at 14.1%. Other more frequent PDs included borderline personality disorder (9.3%), obsessive-compulsive personality disorder (8.7%), paranoid personality disorder (4.2%), antisocial personality disorder (3.6%), and narcissistic personality disorder (2.3%). All other categories were quite rare (less than 2% of the total).

Unspecified Personality Disorder

Unspecified personality disorder is the most common PD that clinicians see, even if this diagnosis is not always made (Zimmerman et al., 2005). What this means is that most patients do not fit into any of the DSM categories. Thus, any patient who meets the overall criteria for a PD but does not meet criteria for any specific category can qualify for this diagnosis, if one carefully follows the rules in the DSM-5-TR. The question is whether this is a meaningful entity or a "wastebasket." There are no data concerning specific treatments. The fact that so many PDs cannot be specified points to the many serious weaknesses in the DSM-5-TR system.

Avoidant Personality Disorder

Avoidant personality disorder is one of the most common disorders seen in clinics (Zimmerman et al., 2005); however, since there are no established methods for treating these patients, they may not receive psychotherapy. Avoidant personality disorder has a large overlap with social anxiety disorder, so some of the literature on treatment describes CBT methods originally developed for social anxiety (Sanislow et al., 2012). But there is no specific protocol for treating the PD, and there have been no clinical trials (a Cochrane Report was proposed at one point, but it was withdrawn for lack of research evidence).

Obsessive-Compulsive Personality Disorder

Obsessive-compulsive personality disorder (OCPD) is a trait disturbance that fades imperceptibly into high conscientiousness or to normality, but can affect interpersonal functioning (Cain et al., 2015). Inspired by DBT, Lynch (2018) has described a method for treating OCPD called radically open dialectical behavior therapy, which offers a protocol for treating disorders of over-control (as opposed to under-control). There is some evidence that this approach is useful for refractory depression (Lynch, 2018), and the method has gained approval from the Society of Clinical Psychology as having *modest* support for depression (SCP, n.d.b.), but further clinical trials are needed to fully assess its efficacy.

Antisocial Personality Disorder

Antisocial personality disorder (AsPD) has been heavily studied for etiology, course over time, and implications for criminal law (Black, 2022), but there is little evidence of effective treatments for AsPD. We do not have any strong empirical evidence that AsPD can be managed in therapy. And, given the low level of treatment-seeking, it is not clear that research on treatment would even be practical. Most of these patients are seen in forensic settings and do not ask for treatment to cope with their inner suffering; rather, they are more focused on avoiding the consequences of their behavior. Therapists who are not working in a correctional setting rarely see such patients and tend to avoid treating them if they do. For those working within a correctional setting, Chapter 14 on antisocial behavior is a good resource.

Narcissistic Personality Disorder

Although relatively uncommon in practice, a good deal of clinical literature, mostly from psychoanalysts, has focused on narcissistic personality disorder. A large handbook of narcissistic personality disorder and trait narcissism (Campbell & Miller, 2011), as well an edited book on treatment (Ogrodiczuk, 2013), have described many potential methods of therapy, but no RCTs have been conducted. Moreover, people with narcissistic traits tend to blame others for their problems, making a therapeutic alliance more difficult. In the absence of data telling clinicians what works (and what doesn't work) for narcissistic personality disorder, we may need a therapy package that is specific to this disorder, and that targets its most problematic aspect, paralleling what Linehan did for borderline personality disorder.

Dependent Personality Disorder

Dependent personality disorder is defined in the DSM-5-TR by criteria that describe the same problem in different contexts, which might lead one to ask "how many ways can people be overly dependent?" The category was close to being dropped from the DSM-5, but it was retained when the decision was made to retain all diagnoses from the previous edition, and to put Alternative Model of Personality Disorders (AMPD) into Section III of the manual. Bornstein (1992) is one of the few researchers interested in dependent personality traits which lead to major difficulties in life. There is no specific protocol for treating patients with dependent personality disorder, and as yet there has been little active research or clinical trials on this topic.

Other Personality Disorders

The other PDs listed in DSM-5-TR have attracted even less research interest. Four PDs (histrionic, schizoid, paranoid, and dependent) were removed from the original proposals for DSM-5, and although they can still be found in Section II of the manual, they are absent from the "hybrid" AMPD in Section III (APA, 2022). The retention of two other categories (avoidant personality disorder and obsessive-compulsive personality disorder) in Section II may have been based on the fact that they were examined for long-term outcome in the Collaborative Longitudinal Study of

Personality Disorders (CLPS; Gunderson et al., 2011). However, research on these diagnoses remains thin.

Schizotypal, schizoid, and paranoid PDs are generally seen as falling within a *schizophrenic spectrum*, since they are associated with a family history of psychosis, with which they share some biomarkers (Esterberg et al., 2010). The hybrid proposal in Section III of DSM-5-TR folds all of these disorders into a single category of schizotypal personality disorder.

Histrionic personality disorder belongs to the history of psychiatry and is rarely diagnosed today (Novais et al., 2015). Decades ago, "hysteria" was used to describe a wide range of patients, some of whom had personality traits associated with

---

Box 15.2 Therapy for Personality Disorders Based on Trait Dimensions

The ten categories of PD retained in Section II of DSM-5-TR do a poor job (with the important exception of borderline personality disorder) of describing the range of psychopathology described by the PD construct as a whole. They are derived from traditional labels that do not correspond to the factors identified by trait psychology. In contrast, dimensional systems tend to track the Five Factor Model of Personality (Widiger & Costa, 2013).

One of the innovations in the AMPD model in Section III of DSM-5 was the use of trait dimensional profiles to build PD diagnoses of categories (Hopwood et al., 2019). The five overall dimensions are negative affectivity, detachment, antagonism, disinhibition, and psychoticism. In principle, one might treat traits such as emotion dysregulation, impulsivity, or social avoidance with methods specific to these characteristics. At this point, no one has proposed such a protocol. Research up to now has focused on the validity and reliability of the AMPD. That could change if the model in Section III of the manual were allowed to replace the categories in Section II. However, to date, no clinical trials of psychotherapy have been based on the AMPD. Moreover, the system is fairly complex, and clinicians may be reluctant to use it unless it can be shown to aid the treatment of patients with PDs.

The *International Classification of Diseases, 11th edition* (ICD-11; World Health Organization, 2018) has introduced dimensional diagnoses for most cases of PD. It only retained one category of borderline personality disorder, which can now be rated as a "borderline pattern," to be scored on top of the general features of all PDs. The five dimensions to be scored are Negative Affectivity, Detachment, Disinhibition, Dissociality, and Anankastia (compulsivity), and clinicians can also code severity. No protocols have been developed to apply these traits to psychotherapy, and there have been no clinical trials using this system.

In the end, the DSM system remains predominant in clinical practice. One reason is that it is familiar to most clinicians; another reason is that each of the alternatives have problems of their own.

stimulus-seeking, high extraversion, and a dramatic style of communication. The disorder was renamed "histrionic" to emphasize the dramatic flair believed to characterize these patients, most of whom are female. But it is fair to say that with almost no research support, this category can easily be dropped from the DSM.

Other Variables Influencing Treatment

Assessment and Diagnosis

The most important thing to know about PDs is that they are often missed in clinical evaluations. Diagnosis is strongly influenced by what mental health professionals have in their treatment armamentarium. A failure to acknowledge PDs has been well documented (Paris, 2020). The main reason is the focus of both pharmacologically oriented physicians and cognitively oriented psychologists on targeting symptoms. Another is that many patients with PDs need therapies that are expensive and often poorly insured.

Comorbidity

Comorbidity is a misleading term because it seems to imply that patients have more than one disorder. In fact, the diagnostic system tends to favor multiple diagnoses that overlap with each other. By and large, successful treatment of PDs can be effective in managing a wide range of symptoms.

Demographics

In clinical settings the vast majority of patients with PDs are female (Zimmerman et al., 2008). However, research in community samples shows that there is a large number of males who have the same disorders but do not seek help (Trull et al., 2010). There is very little research on ethnicity or race in PDs, though a report based on a large sample in the UK suggested that Black people have a lower prevalence than do White people (McGilloway et al., 2010). It may be relevant that Black people also have a much lower rate of suicide than do White people (Ramchand et al., 2021).

Medication

Even as specific therapies for borderline personality disorder have been developed and researched, patients may still receive mainly pharmacological treatment. Since the symptoms of borderline personality disorder overlap with mood or anxiety disorders, a PD diagnosis may not even be made. Yet research shows that patients with PD diagnoses, even when depressed or anxious, do not consistently benefit from pharmacotherapy (Newton-Jones et al., 2006). Ironically, when patients fail to respond to these agents, they can receive more aggressive pharmacotherapy leading to polypharmacy. When a nonpsychotic patient is taking five or more medications, it is worth considering whether they may have a PD that does not respond to any of these agents.

Conclusion

Research on PDs, especially borderline personality disorder, has made great progress in the last few decades. We now know that many (if not most) patients with borderline personality disorder do well in the long run. Psychotherapy specifically designed for this population can speed up this recovery process. However, we do not yet know whether these findings can be applied to other categories.

These findings support a more optimistic view of treatment for borderline personality disorder. For many years, this condition has been underdiagnosed or misdiagnosed. This is much less true now, as clinicians have become aware that therapy tends to be effective. But borderline personality disorder is a diagnosis that affects at least 1% of the general population (Trull et al., 2010) and is much more common in clinical populations (Zimmerman et al., 2005).

Other PDs need more research, and we lack well-validated methods of treating them. We will lack the resources needed to manage any of these patients unless we can find a way to shorten therapy and apply the principles of stepped care (Paris, 2015, 2017). One of the unfortunate aspects of the domain of psychotherapy is the existence of several competing methods, most with a three-letter acronym, with results over-interpreted by therapists with allegiance to one or another approach. The most parsimonious conclusion could be that all well-structured methods are superior to TAU, but that none is clearly superior (Choi-Kain, 2020). There should be only one kind of psychotherapy for PD – the one that works best. An integrated approach should use the best ideas from all sources, and put them together into one package (Paris, 2020). But, given the strong evidence for DBT, its ideas are likely to be a crucial element in any plan for psychotherapy integration. We now have a good beginning for identifying effective approaches, but we have a long way to go to make them accessible.

Useful Resources

- Choi-Kain, L., Sharp, C. (2021). *Handbook of good psychiatric management for adolescents with borderline personality disorder*. American Psychiatric Publishing. (up-to-date book on adolescent PD)
- Linehan, M. M. (2014). *DBT skills training manual* (2nd ed.). Guilford. (an essential guide to DBT)

- Paris, J. (2020). *Treatment of borderline personality disorder* (2nd ed.). Guilford. (up to date summary of the research literature)
- Porr, V. (2010). *Overcoming borderline personality disorder: A family guide for healing and change*. Oxford University Press. (best book for families and patients)

References

American Psychiatric Association (APA) (2022). *Diagnostic and statistical manual of mental disorders* (5th ed., text revision). American Psychiatric Publishing.

Bateman, A., & Fonagy, P. (1999). Effectiveness of partial hospitalization in the treatment of borderline personality disorder: A randomized controlled trial. *American Journal of Psychiatry*, 156, 1563–1569.

Bateman, A., & Fonagy, P. (2006). *Mentalization-based treatment: A practical guide*. John Wiley.

Bateman, A., & Fonagy, P. (2008). 8-year follow-up of patients treated for borderline personality disorder: Mentalization-based treatment versus treatment as usual. *American Journal of Psychiatry*, 165(5), 631–638

Bateman, A., & Fonagy, P. (2009). Randomized controlled trial of out-patient mentalization-based treatment versus structured clinical management for borderline personality disorder. *American Journal of Psychiatry*, 166, 1355–1364

Bateman, A., Constantinou, M. P., Fonagy, P., & Holzer, S. (2021). Eight-year prospective follow-up of mentalization-based treatment versus structured clinical management for people with borderline personality disorder. *Personal Disorders*, 12, 291–299

Biskin, R., Paris J., Zelkowitz, P., et al. (2021). Non-suicidal self-injury in early adolescence as a predictor of borderline personality disorder features in early adulthood. *Journal of Personality Disorders*, 35, 764–775.

Black, D. W. (2022). *Bad boys, bad men: Confronting antisocial personality disorder (sociopathy)*, 3rd ed. Oxford University Press,

Blum, N., & Black, D. W. (2020). Systems Training for Emotional Predictability and Problem Solving (STEPPS) for the treatment of BPD. In *Borderline Personality Disorder* (pp. 171–186). Routledge.

Blum, N., St John, D., Pfohl, B., & Black, D. W. (2008). Systems Training for Emotional Predictability and Problem Solving (STEPPS) for outpatients with borderline personality disorder: A randomized controlled trial and 1-year follow-up. *American Journal of Psychiatry*, 165, 468–478

Bornstein, R. F. (1992). The dependent personality: Developmental, social, and clinical perspectives. *Psychological Bulletin*, 112, 3–23.

Bos, E., van der Wel, E., Appelo, M., & Verbraak, M. (2010): A randomized controlled trial of a Dutch version of Systems Training for Emotional Predictability and Problem Solving for Borderline Personality Disorder. *Journal of Nervous and Mental Disease*, 198, 299–304.

Cain, N. M., Ansell, E. B., Simpson, H. B., & Pinto, A. (2015). Interpersonal functioning in obsessive-compulsive personality disorder. *Journal of Personality Assessment*, 97, 90–99.

Campbell, E. W. K., & Miller, J. D. (2011). *The handbook of narcissism and narcissistic personality disorder: Theoretical approaches, empirical findings, and treatments*. Wiley.

Chanen A. M, & McCutcheon, L. (2013): Prevention and early intervention for borderline personality disorder: Current status and recent evidence. *British Journal of Psychiatry*, 202, S24, 29.

Choi-Kain, L. W. (2020). Debranding treatment for borderline personality disorder: A call to balance access to care with therapeutic purity. *Harvard Review Psychiatry*, 28, 143–145.

Clarkin, J. F., Levy, K. N., Lenzenweger, M. F., & Kernberg, O. F. (2007): Evaluating three treatments for borderline personality disorder: A multiwave study. *American Journal of Psychiatry*, 164, 1–8.

Crowell, S. E., Beauchaine, T. P., & Linehan, M. M. (2009). A biosocial developmental model of borderline personality: Elaborating and extending Linehan's theory. *Psychological Bulletin*, 135, 495–510.

Doering S., Hörz S., Rentrop M., et al. (2010). Transference-focused psychotherapy vs. treatment by community psychotherapists for borderline personality disorder: Randomised controlled trial. *British Journal of Psychiatry*, 196, 389–395.

Engel G. (1980). The clinical application of the biopsychosocial model. *American Journal of Psychiatry*, 137, 535–544.

Esterberg, M. L., Goulding, S. M., & Walker, E. F. (2010). Cluster A personality disorders: Schizotypal, schizoid and paranoid personality disorders in childhood and adolescence. *Journal of Psychopathology Behavioral Assessment*, 32, 515–528.

Finch E. F., Iliakis, E. A., Masland, S. R., & Choi-Kain, L. W. (2019). A meta-analysis of treatment as usual for borderline personality disorder. *Personality Disorders*, 10, 491–499.

Giesen-Bloo, J., van Dyck, R., Spinhoven, P., et al. (2006). Outpatient psychotherapy for borderline personality disorder: Randomized trial of schema-focused therapy vs transference-focused psychotherapy. *Archives of General Psychiatry*, 63, 649–658.

Glenn, C. R., Esposito, E. C., Porter, A. C., & Robinson, D. J. (2019). Evidence base update of psychosocial treatments for self-injurious thoughts and behaviors in youth. *Journal of Clinical Child & Adolescent Psychology*, 48(3), 357–392.

Gunderson, J. G., Stout, R. L., McGlashan, T. H., et al. (2011). Ten-year course of borderline personality disorder: Psychopathology and function from the collaborative longitudinal personality disorders study. *Archives of General Psychiatry*, 68, 827–837.

Hopwood, C. J. Mulay, A. L., & Waugh, M., eds. (2019). *The DSM-5 alternative model for personality disorders*. Routledge.

Jørgensen C. R., Freund C., Bøye, R., et al. (2013). Outcome of mentalization-based and supportive psychotherapy in patients with borderline personality disorder: A randomized trial. *Acta Psychiatrica Scandinavica*, 127, 305–317.

Koenigsberg, H. W. (2010). Affective instability: toward an integration of neuroscience and psychological perspectives. *Journal of Personality Disorders*, 24, 60–82.

Kramer, U., Kolly, S., Charbon, P., Ilagan, G. S., & Choi-Kain, L. W. (2021). Brief psychiatric treatment for borderline personality disorder as a first step of care: Adapting general psychiatric management to a 10-session intervention. *Personality Disorders*, 13(5), 516–526. https://doi.org/10.1037/per0000511.

Lambert, M. J. (2013). Outcome in psychotherapy: The past and important advances. *Psychotherapy*, 50, 42–45

Lambert, M., & Bergin, A. (2021). *Handbook of psychotherapy and behavior change*. Wiley

Laporte, L., Paris, J., Zelkowitz, P., & Cardin, J. F. (2018): Clinical outcomes of stepped care for the treatment of borderline personality disorder. *Personality Mental Health*, 12, 49–58.

Levy, K. N., McMain, S., Bateman, A., & Clouthier, T. (2018). Treatment of borderline personality disorder. *Psychiatric Clinics of North America*, 41, 711–728.

Linehan M. M., Heard, H. L., & Armstrong, H. E. (1993). Naturalistic follow-up of a behavioral treatment for chronically parasuicidal borderline patients. *Archives of General Psychiatry*, 50, 971–974.

Linehan, M. M. (1993). *Cognitive behavior therapy for borderline personality disorder.* Guilford.

Linehan, M. M., Comtois, K. A., Murray, A. M., et al. (2006). Two-year randomized controlled trial and follow-up of dialectical behavior therapy vs therapy by experts for suicidal behaviors and borderline personality disorder. *Archives of General Psychiatry*, 63, 757–766.

Lynch, T. (2018). *Radically open dialectical behavior therapy: Theory and practice for treating disorders of overcontrol.* New Harbinger Publications.

Markham, M., Lutz, W., Castonguay, L. G., eds. (2021). *Bergin and Garfield's handbook of psychotherapy and behavior change*, 7th ed. Wiley

McGilloway A., Hall R. E., Lee T., & Bhui, K. S. (2010). A systematic review of personality disorder, race and ethnicity: Prevalence, aetiology and treatment. *BMC Psychiatry.* May 11;10:33. https://doi.org/10.1186/1471-244x-10-33. PMID: 20459788; PMCID: PMC2882360.

McMain, S. F., Chapman, A. L., Kuo, J. R., et al. (2022). The effectiveness of 6 versus 12 months of dialectical behavior therapy for borderline personality disorder: A noninferiority randomized clinical trial. *Psychotherapy and psychosomatics*, 91(6), 382–397.

McMain, S. F., Chapman, A. L., Kuo, J. R., et al. (2018). The effectiveness of 6 versus 12-months of dialectical behaviour therapy for borderline personality disorder: The feasibility of a shorter treatment and evaluating responses (FASTER) trial protocol. *BMC Psychiatry*, 18, 230–237.

McMain, S. F., Guimond, T., Streiner, D., & Links, P. S. (2012). Dialectical behavior therapy compared with general psychiatric management for borderline personality disorder: Clinical outcomes and functioning over a 2-year follow-up. *American Journal of Psychiatry*, 169, 650–661.

McMain, S. F., Links, P., Gnam, W. H., et al. (2009). A randomized trial of dialectical behavior therapy versus general psychiatric management for borderline personality disorder. *American Journal of Psychiatry*, 166, 1365–1374

Newton-Howes, G., Tyrer, P., & Johnson, T. (2006). Personality disorder and the outcome of depression: Meta-analysis of published studies. *British Journal of Psychiatry*, 188, 13–20.

Nock, M. K. (2009). Why do people hurt themselves? New insights into the nature and functions of self-injury. *Current Directions in Psychological Science*, 18(2), 78–83. https://doi.org/10.1111/j.1467-8721.2009.01613.x.

Novais, F., Araujo, A., & Godinho, P. (2015). Historical roots of histrionic personality disorder. *Frontiers in Psychology*, 6, 1463–1470. https://doi.org/10.3389/fpsyg.2015.01463.

Ogrodiczuk, J. S. (2013). *Understanding and treating pathological narcissism. American Psychological Association.*

Ogrodniczuk, J. S. (Ed.). (2013). *Understanding and treating pathological narcissism.* American Psychological Association.

Oldham, J. M., Gabbard, G. O., Goin, M. K., et al. (2001). Practice guideline for the treatment of borderline personality disorder. *American Journal of Psychiatry*, 158, Supp 1–52.

Paris, J. (2015). Making psychotherapy for borderline personality disorder accessible. *Annals of Clinical Psychiatry*, 27, 297–301.

Paris, J. (2017). *Stepped care for borderline personality disorder*. Academic Press.

Paris, J. (2019). *Treatment of borderline personality disorder: A guide to evidence-based practice*. Guilford Publications.

Paris, J. (2020). *Treatment of borderline personality disorder*, 2nd ed. Guilford.

Ramchand R., Gordon, J. A., & Pearson, J. L. (2021). Trends in suicide rates by race and ethnicity in the United States. *JAMA Network Open*, 4(5), e2111563. https://doi.org/10.1001%2Fjamanetworkopen.2021.11563.

Sanislow, C. A., Cruz, K. Gianoli, M., & Reagan, E. (2012). Avoidant personality disorder, traits, and type. In T. A. Widiger (Ed.), *The Oxford handbook of personality disorders* (pp. 549–565). Oxford University Press.

Sharp, C., & Tackett, J. (Eds.) (2014). *Handbook of borderline personality disorder in children and adolescents*. Springer.

Skodol, A. E., Buckley, P., & Charles, E. (1983). Is there a characteristic pattern in the treatment history of clinic outpatients with borderline personality? *Journal of Nervous and Mental Disease*, 171, 405–410.

Society for Clinical Psychology (SCP) (n.d.a.). Borderline personality disorder. https://div12.org/diagnosis/borderline-personality-disorder/ (accessed March 3, 2023).

Society for Clinical Psychology (SCP) (n.d.b.). Radically open dialectical behavior therapy for disorder of overcontrol. https://div12.org/treatment/radically-open-dialectical-behavior-therapy-for-disorders-of-overcontrol/ (accessed March 3, 2023).

Stanley, B., Brodsky, B., Nelson, J., & Dulit, R. (2007). Brief dialectical behavior therapy for suicidality and self-injurious behaviors. *Archives of Suicide Research*, 11, 337–341.

Storebø O. J., Stoffers-Winterling, J. M., Völlm, B. A., et al. (2020). Psychological therapies for people with borderline personality disorder. *Cochrane Database of Systematic Reviews* 2020(5). Art. No.: CD012955. https://doi.org/10.1002/14651858.cd012955.pub2.

Storebø, O. J., Stoffers-Winterling, J. M., Völlm, B. A., et al. (2018). Psychological therapies for people with borderline personality disorder. *Cochrane Database of Systematic Reviews*, Issue 2. Art. No.: CD012955. https://doi.org/10.1002/14651858.cd012955.pub2.

Trull, T. J., Jahng, S., & Tomko, R. L. (2010). Revised NESARC personality disorder diagnosis: Gender, prevalence, and comorbidity with substance dependence disorders. *Journal of Personality Disorders*, 24, 412–426.

Verheul, R., Bartak, A., & Widiger, T. (2007). Prevalence and construct validity of Personality Disorder Not Otherwise Specified (PDNOS). *Journal of Personality Disorders*, 21, 359–370.

Wampold, B. E., & Imel, Z. E. (2015): *The great psychotherapy debate: The evidence for what makes psychotherapy work* (2nd ed.). Routledge.

Widiger, T., & Costa, P. (Eds.). (2013). *Personality disorders and the five-factor model of personality* (3rd ed.). American Psychological Association.

World Health Organization. (2018). *International classification of diseases* (11th rev.). Geneva, Switzerland.

Young, J. E. (1999). *Cognitive therapy for personality disorders: A schema-focused approach* (3rd ed.). Professional Resource Press.

Yuan, Y., Lee, H., Eack, S., & Newhlle, C. E. (2023). A systematic review of the association between early childhood trauma and borderline personality disorder. *Journal of Personality Disorders*, 37. https://doi.org/10.1521/pedi.2023.37.1.16.

Zanarini, M. C. (2009). Psychotherapy of borderline personality disorder. *Acta Psychiatrica Scandinavica*, 120, 373–377.

Zanarini, M. C. (2019). *In the fullness of time: Recovery from borderline personality disorder.* Oxford University Press.

Zimmerman, M., Chelminski, I., & Young, D. (2008). The frequency of personality disorders in psychiatric patients. *Psychiatric Clinics of North America*, 31(3), 405–420.

Zimmerman, M., Rothschild, L., & Chelminski, I. (2005). The prevalence of DSM-IV personality disorders in psychiatric outpatients. *American Journal of Psychiatry*, 162, 1911–1918.

16

Psychosis and Schizophrenia

Elizabeth Thompson, Katherine Visser, Madeline Ward,
and Brandon A. Gaudiano

Psychosis is a broad category of mental health symptoms defined by distorted thoughts and experiences that cause some level of disconnection from reality. Recent estimates indicate that approximately 1 in 150 individuals worldwide will develop a psychotic disorder during their lifetime (Moreno-Küstner et al., 2018). On an individual level, psychosis impairs functional capacity, social engagement, and quality of life. On a global level, meta-analytic data from 24 countries demonstrate yearly healthcare costs ranging between $94 million and $102 billion US dollars for individuals with schizophrenia, one specific and severe form of psychotic disorder (Chong et al., 2016). In recent years these costs have increased substantially, as 2019 estimates indicate that the economic burden of schizophrenia in the US has reached $343.2 billion, with the majority of costs attributed to caregiving (33%), premature mortality (23%), direct health care (18%), and unemployment (16%; Kadakia et al., 2022).

"Positive" symptoms of psychosis, named as such because they are additional experiences that are not typically present for most individuals, include hallucinations (i.e., perceptual experiences in the absence of stimuli), delusions (i.e., belief in ideas that are extreme or not grounded in reality), and disorganized thoughts or behavior (i.e., confused or bizarre thoughts, speech, or behavior). In contrast, "negative" symptoms of psychosis indicate a deficit in typical experiences, such as low levels of motivation, emotional expression, and social engagement. The presence of positive and negative symptoms, accompanied by distress and functional interference, are among the criteria for diagnosing a psychotic disorder (American Psychiatric Association [APA], 2022). Schizophrenia is one severe form of psychotic disorder that is often chronic in nature (at least six months) and accompanied by emotional distress and significant interference in cognitive, social, and role-related functioning (e.g., school or work). Another persistent form of psychosis is schizoaffective disorder, a chronic condition accompanied by major mood episodes (e.g., depression or mania) for the majority of the illness duration. Other psychosis spectrum disorders differ in the duration and scope of illness, such as major depression with psychotic features or bipolar disorders with psychotic features (psychosis occurring only in the context of the mood episode), brief psychotic disorder (marked by short duration symptoms), delusional disorder (defined by delusions only), temporary psychosis caused by a substance (e.g., recreational drugs or medications) or medical condition, catatonia (marked by immobility and abnormal or slowed movements), or other psychotic symptoms that cause some level of distress and interference (e.g., attenuated psychosis, or hallucinations without other psychotic features).

Etiology and Theoretical Underpinnings of Treatment

The diathesis-stress model provides an etiological explanation for the emergence of psychosis and presents a theoretical framework for multiple empirically supported treatments. This model suggests that an underlying biological vulnerability, oftentimes genetic predisposition (e.g., having a close biological relative with a psychotic disorder), may interact with an individual's capacity to manage daily stressors and/or exposure to traumatic life events, which subsequently contributes to either the onset or exacerbation of psychotic symptoms (DeVylder et al., 2013; Walker & Diforio, 1997). Stress reactivity is also known to increase following the onset of a psychotic disorder (Malla et al., 1990), suggesting a decreased capacity to cope with stress overall. This can lead to increased distress and poorer functioning (Corcoran et al., 2003). Accordingly, many treatments for psychosis include elements of stress reduction and emotion regulation skills, to help individuals manage their stress response (and, thus, help reduce the total symptom burden).

Throughout much of the history of mental health care, the medical model has focused squarely on a goal of symptom elimination (Resnick et al., 2005). This cure-focused approach is problematic for many individuals who, despite treatment, continue to experience symptoms, which can lead to demoralization and overemphasis on disability and impairment. In contrast, the recovery model takes a person-centered and strengths-based approach that emphasizes knowledge, empowerment, hope, and satisfaction with life (Resnick et al., 2004). This model focuses on incorporating multifaceted, research-backed interventions designed to foster optimism, enhance collaboration across treatment providers, and incorporate peer support and stigma reduction while promoting re-engagement with work and valued activities (Warner, 2009). Many of the psychosocial interventions that will be detailed herein rely upon these tenets.

Brief Overview of Treatments

For decades, randomized controlled trials (RCTs) have demonstrated that certain psychosocial interventions significantly improve outcomes compared to medication treatment alone for patients with schizophrenia and related psychotic disorders

(Mueser et al., 2013), and, therefore, clinical practice guidelines have recommended their use (Dixon et al., 2010). However, only a minority of patients are being offered such interventions to this day (Drake et al., 2009; Kopelovich et al., 2022). Factors related to the poor uptake of psychosocial interventions for psychosis include the historically low rates of reimbursement and funding to deliver these types of interventions relative to medications, the dearth of clinicians who specialize in treating psychosis, and the lack of systematic training and support for implementing these empirically supported psychosocial interventions in the community (Kopelovich et al., 2019).

Antipsychotic medication is considered the front-line treatment for psychosis, at least during acute episodes (Keepers et al., 2020). Although medications are effective in targeting positive symptoms of psychosis (i.e., hallucinations and delusions) for many individuals, they often fail to adequately address negative symptoms, functioning, and quality of life (Leucht et al., 2017). Therefore, it is critical that the public and professionals become more educated about the various empirically supported psychosocial treatments (Solmi et al., 2023) currently available for patients suffering from psychosis so that they can help to expand the use of these interventions and ultimately increase their reach and uptake. The psychosocial interventions for psychosis with the most consistent empirical support to date are briefly summarized next.

Cognitive-Behavioral Therapies

Cognitive-behavioral therapy for psychosis (CBTp) is an adaptation of traditional CBT, which is one of the best-validated therapies for treating common psychiatric conditions, including depressive and anxiety disorders (Hofmann et al., 2012). CBTp posits that psychotic symptoms are, at least in part, due to and maintained by common cognitive information processing biases, such as "jumping to conclusions" and other attributional biases that cause distorted perceptions and reasoning (Garety et al., 2005). CBTp aims to address these underlying cognitive biases and related behavioral manifestations to decrease distress, improve functioning, and help patients better cope with their psychotic experiences. There is no one specific CBTp treatment program, but rather many variations around this theme (Morrison & Barratt, 2010); all such approaches are structured, emphasize a collaboration between patient and therapist to work on present-focused goals, include in-session skills training, and involve between-session practice (i.e., homework; Morrison et al., 2004). Common cognitive and behavioral techniques are first applied to nonpsychotic symptoms, such as depression and anxiety (Kingdon & Turkington, 2005). Such strategies include Socratic questioning aimed at identifying and correcting distorted thinking patterns, with the use of corresponding behavioral experiments to test out faulty assumptions. As therapy continues and trust is established, the therapist slowly applies Socratic questioning and behavioral experiments to hallucinations and delusions in a nonargumentative and collaborative fashion based on the patient's comfort and motivation levels. Additional strategies are employed for negative symptoms, such as behavioral activation and social skills training, as appropriate.

The current National Institute for Health and Care Excellence (NICE, 2014) guidelines for psychosis and schizophrenia recommend that individual therapy with CBTp be provided to patients in all phases of illness (early, acute, and chronic) and that it be delivered in hospital and outpatient settings. These recommendations are based on evidence from multiple RCTs and more than 20 meta-analyses that have found CBTp to be helpful for improving symptoms and functioning in schizophrenia (Kingdon & Turkington, 2019). For example, one meta-analysis of RCTs demonstrated that CBTp produces significant improvements compared to supportive therapy on overall symptoms (g = 0.42) and positive symptoms (g = 0.23) (Turner et al., 2014).

Assertive Community Treatment

Assertive community treatment (Stein & Test, 1980) was developed in the 1970s in the United States to address the problem of frequent rehospitalizations for patients with severe mental illness (SMI), including schizophrenia, which resulted from the deinstitutionalization movement of the 1950s (Dixon, 2000). Assertive community treatment is a model of care rather than a specific treatment, and over the years it has been adapted and implemented successfully in many countries around the world (Rochefort, 2019). The program is multidisciplinary, multicomponent, and holistic in that it includes a range of services such as psychotherapy, family support, and medication, as well as housing, finance, and education/work support (Bond & Drake, 2015). Furthermore, the team provides services directly to patients and there is a low client-to-staff ratio given the intensity of treatment. Because patients leaving the hospital often have poor rates of engagement with community treatments (Kreyenbuhl et al., 2009), an assertive outreach approach is used to support patients remaining in treatment on a long-term basis.

Based on more than 45 years of efficacy and effectiveness research, assertive community treatment is recommended as a gold-standard intervention in treatment guidelines for schizophrenia (Thorning & Dixon et al., 2017), and meta-analyses have shown that the program reduces days hospitalized (mean reduction = –0.86 days) and improves treatment retention (relative risk = 0.70) (Dieterich et al., 2017). Evidence has been less consistently found for its ability to improve housing, symptom management, and quality of life, as these outcomes have varied based on the particular study. Recent work has focused more on addressing implementation challenges and determining how best to integrate assertive community treatment into modern and ever-changing healthcare systems (Thorning & Dixon, 2020).

Family Therapy

Family therapy is based on the premise that it is not just the affected individual who needs to understand their symptoms and diagnoses; family members should also be included as collaborators, provided with psychoeducation, and taught skills to support their loved one in treatment and at home (Mueser et al., 2015). Family programs are designed to educate families on the signs and symptoms of psychosis and biomedical aspects of psychopathology, while also helping family members to build skills in communication, problem solving, and assisting the client in setting and working toward treatment goals (Mueser et al., 2015). A primary goal of this family work is to reduce family conflict and stress while bolstering empathy and familial support, thereby minimizing vulnerability for relapse and comorbid mental health concerns (e.g., mood and anxiety symptoms, substance use, trauma).

Family therapy has been indicated as one of the first-line treatments for psychotic disorders, along with antipsychotic medication, with a specific emphasis on psycho-education early on in treatment (NICE, 2014). There is a strong evidence base for family therapy and psychoeducation (Rodolico et al., 2022; Solmi et al., 2023), and family therapy is central to several empirically supported interventions, including family-aided assertive community treatment (FACT; McFarlane at al., 1992), family-focused therapy (FFT; Miklowitz et al., 2014), and the Navigate Family Education Program (Glynn & Gingerich, 2020; Mueser et al., 2015). Additionally, family therapy is routinely included at the start of other individual therapies, including CBTp (Steel & Smith, 2013).

Social Learning/Token Economy Programs

Social cognition deficits are considered a significant problem in schizophrenia (Green et al., 2015). Social skills training (SST) refers to several similar interventions developed to ameliorate social cognition deficits in schizophrenia by providing structured instruction on core social skills (e.g., how to begin or leave a conversation, how to say "no"). Skills are taught in a stepwise, scaffolded fashion that incorporates role-play, feedback, and coaching, frequently in a group format (Wallace et al., 1980). SST is recommended by the American Psychiatric Association as part of their guidelines for the treatment of schizophrenia (Lehman et al., 2004). Research indicates that SST is helpful in learning social skills, decreasing negative symptoms of schizophrenia above and beyond the impact of medication, and improving functioning in the community (Kurtz & Mueser, 2008; Turner et al., 2018). Meta-analytic research indicates significant improvements in negative symptoms (e.g., blunted affect, social withdrawal, rapport) in particular, as well as general symptoms (e.g., anxiety, depression, attention) in comparison to control samples (e.g., treatment-as-usual, waitlist controls), but effects were not found for positive symptoms (Turner et al., 2018). Importantly, there are some concerns as to the generalizability of skills into daily life (NICE, 2014), and more research is needed to assess sustained effects across time (Turner et al., 2018).

SST began to be implemented around the same time as another intervention purported to assist with reinforcing appropriate social engagement: token economies (Dickerson et al., 2008; Hersen, 1976; Kazdin, 1977). Based on the principles of operant conditioning (Skinner, 1953) and initially implemented in psychiatric hospitals, token economies involve providing patients with "tokens" to attempt to reinforce desired behavior. The type and purpose of the token varies and is unique to each setting implementing such a program. Research indicates that providing behavioral reinforcement in this manner is effective in institutional settings, primarily for addressing problematic behaviors (Dickerson et al., 2008; Lecomte et al., 2014).

Supported Employment

Individuals with psychotic disorders often have ongoing difficulties in "role functioning" (i.e., engaging in and fulfilling school and/or work responsibilities), and role functioning has been linked to positive, negative, disorganized, and cognitive symptoms, as well as social dysfunction (Dickinson et al., 2007; Fulford et al., 2013; McGurk & Mueser, 2004). Given marked difficulties in vocational functioning among adults with psychosis, supported employment interventions were designed to provide vocational placement and skills development, aiming to improve employment outcomes for participants (Mellen & Danley, 1987). Specifically, supported employment interventions assess the strengths and abilities of clients, help them to obtain competitive work that aligns with their preferences in community settings, navigate disclosure of mental health difficulties to employers, plan for job supports, and offer training in skills necessary for gaining and maintaining employment (McGurk & Mueser, 2004).

Meta-analytic studies (Modini et al., 2016) and nontrial routine programs (Richter & Hoffmann, 2019) indicate that individuals who engage in supported employment interventions such as individual placement and support (IPS) have been shown to be more than twice as likely to gain competitive employment when compared to traditional vocational rehabilitation programs (i.e. a tiered training approach that begins with sheltered job placement in low-paying, segregated settings for individuals with mental illness; Lutfiyya et al., 1988). Supported employment outcomes are sustained over the course of multiyear follow-ups, and international evidence indicates that outcomes associated with IPS were not impacted by geographic location or unemployment rates, suggesting the effectiveness of these interventions across different settings and economic circumstances (Modini et al., 2016). Furthermore, participation in supported employment programs may weaken the negative influence of symptoms (e.g., cognitive, negative, and positive symptoms) on work functioning by bolstering compensatory skills (McGurk & Mueser, 2004), and participation in work has been linked to greater social functioning, fewer symptoms, and sustained periods of remission (Burns et al., 2009).

Cognitive Remediation

Cognitive impairments are a well-studied symptom of schizophrenia (Schaefer et al., 2013). Cognitive remediation is an umbrella term referring to skills-building interventions created to improve cognitive functioning across multiple domains (including processing speed, attention, working memory, visual learning, verbal learning, problem solving, and social cognition; Wykes et al., 2011). These interventions, which are also often used to assist individuals who have developed a traumatic brain injury, may include use of a specialized computer program (Fisher et al., 2009) or involve a trained therapist providing instruction in compensatory skills.

Cognitive remediation is well studied in schizophrenia and consistently shows improvements across phases of the disorder (Revell et al., 2015) and multiple domains of cognitive functioning (McGurk et al., 2007). Meta-analytic research also indicates that cognitive remediation not only improves cognitive function but is also linked to improvements in psychosocial functioning as well as symptom improvement (McGurk et al., 2007), particularly when combined with psychiatric rehabilitation (Fitapelli & Lindenmayer, 2022). While, similarly to SST, there have been questions about the generalizability of cognitive remediation interventions, research does indicate that there are small generalized effects on cognitive functioning dimensions excluded from instruction (e.g., social cognition and global function), particularly when provided in psychiatric rehabilitation settings (Vita et al., 2021).

Peer Support

Peer support for psychosis consists of services and support from individuals who have lived experience (i.e. experienced psychosis themselves; Davidson et al., 2006). Peer-support programs are not based on psychiatric models and may not be theory driven; however, service users, researchers, and professionals have advocated for these programs as they align with the recovery model. Specifically, peer-support services include information about psychosis, effective use of medication, identification and management of symptoms, access to services, coping with stress, crisis planning, building social support, preventing relapse, and setting personal recovery goals (Lloyd-Evans et al., 2014).

A systematic review and meta-analysis of 18 trials consisting of mutual support, peer support, and peer-delivered service programs found considerable variation across program content (Lloyd-Evans et al., 2014). While there was evidence for gains in measures of hope, recovery, and empowerment that were maintained beyond the end of peer-support programs, heavy risk of bias was noted in these studies, and lack of consistency between programs led to inconsistent findings. Current guidelines (Dixon et al., 2010; NICE, 2014) suggest peer support should be delivered by a trained individual who has recovered or is stable in their illness. Further, peer-support specialists should be embedded within a care team and receive support and mentorship from other experienced peer workers (DuBrul et al., 2017).

Credible Components of Treatments

Although the previous section illustrates the various specific empirically supported treatments that have been found to be effective for treating psychosis, each of these treatment packages contains a number of different elements and components, many of which are shared across interventions. Rosen and Davison (2003) argued that it is crucial to understand and promote *empirically supported principles of change* that may underlie effective therapies, rather than just the specific treatment packages themselves. In the remainder of the chapter, we describe the most credible treatment components that can be distilled from what we currently know about effective approaches to treating psychosis.

Psychoeducation

Because psychosis can be characterized by a lack of insight (McCormack et al., 2014), psychoeducational approaches are important to increase both knowledge and insight about one's illness and treatment options in order to improve coping skills. Psychoeducation is also a useful tool to normalize experiences and reduce stigma,

---

Box 16.1 Support and Empathy

Chapter 21 highlights the importance of therapy relationship variables, but they warrant a brief mention in this chapter as well. The so-called "nonspecific" or "common" factors of psychotherapy (e.g., alliance, empathy, genuineness, etc.) play a significant role in treatment outcomes regardless of therapy modality (Wampold, 2015). Empathy – the process by which therapists communicate compassionate understanding of a client's experience – is considered a primary common factor (Wampold, 2015) and significantly influences therapy outcomes (Elliott et al., 2011). Furthermore, research indicates that when therapists are perceived as genuine and empathic by their clients with schizophrenia, alliance is likely to improve (Shattock et al., 2018). As individuals with schizophrenia are known to experience social cognition difficulties (Green et al., 2015) that may impact the extent to which they can develop supportive relationships (Hooley, 2010), and individuals with paranoid delusions in particular may have difficulty establishing trust, a warm, empathic, supportive relationship with a therapist may be an important and primary source of connection and recovery.

particularly internalized stigma, which can improve treatment adherence and bolster hope (Xia et al., 2011). Incorporating psychoeducation into psychosocial treatment for psychosis has been shown to reduce relapse and readmission and to encourage medication adherence, thus demonstrating both clinical and economic benefits, and its benefits extend to both the patient and their caregivers (Xia et al., 2011; Maheshwari et al., 2020). Psychoeducation is best provided within the framework of the recovery model and in the context of a broader intervention such as CBTp or family therapy, rather than in isolation.

Skill Acquisition

CBTp, family psychoeducation, SST, and other therapies for psychosis all teach patients effective coping skills and strategies for managing illness and promoting recovery. Such strategies include goal setting, symptom identification and monitoring, functional analysis to understand the antecedents and consequences of behaviors, examination of interfering/avoidance behaviors, problem solving, treatment adherence promotion, social and communication skills, stress management, behavioral activation, exposure exercises, cognitive change techniques (e.g., Socratic questioning), use of worksheets and between-session homework assignments, safety planning, and relapse prevention work (Morrison & Barratt, 2010; Mueser et al., 2013). Thus, empirically supported psychotherapies for psychosis tend to incorporate a wide range of techniques and strategies based on their particular theoretical frameworks to help patients actively cope with their symptoms and improve their ability to function (Dickerson & Lehman, 2011).

Emotion Regulation

Emotion regulation is defined as the use of strategies to decrease the frequency, intensity, and/or duration of emotional responses (Gross, 1998). Such strategies are frequently taught in cognitive-behavioral interventions such as CBTp. For example, identifying and shifting thought distortions can be thought of as a form of the cognitive reappraisal emotion regulation strategy; cognitive reappraisal is considered an important mechanism of change for CBTp patients (Morrison et al., 2017). Research has indicated that individuals with schizophrenia try to regulate their emotions but may utilize less contextually appropriate strategies and implement them less effectively than healthy individuals (Visser et al., 2018). This has important treatment implications, as individuals with psychotic symptoms are shown to be increasingly sensitized to stress, which is linked to worsening symptoms (Myin-Germeys et al., 2005). Furthermore, meta-analytic findings indicate that individuals with psychotic disorders may use more maladaptive emotion regulation strategies, which are associated with positive symptoms (Ludwig et al., 2019). Accordingly, including supportive instruction in coping skills that are designed to effectively regulate emotion (e.g., cognitive reappraisal, emotion regulation-focused components of dialectical behavior therapy [Linehan, 1987]) can be a powerful component of interventions delivered to individuals with psychosis and aid with the management of negative emotions in particular (Ludwig et al., 2020; Opoka et al., 2021). Such interventions may aid in increasing belief in the ability to manage negative emotions (Khoury et al., 2015, Ryan et al., 2021; Lawlor et al., 2022), improve symptoms of anxiety and depression (Khoury et al., 2015), foster confidence and hope, increase motivation toward goals (Ryan et al., 2021), and improve self care (Khoury et al., 2015). However, generalization of research-taught skills into daily life is unclear (Lawlor et al., 2022). Research in this area is ongoing.

Interpersonal Support

Family-focused intervention strategies aim to reduce family stress, as research suggests that family conflict may influence the course of psychotic illness over time (O'Driscoll et al., 2019). High levels of "expressed emotion," characterized by family members' emotional overinvolvement and critical or hostile attitudes toward the individual with schizophrenia, are consistently associated with negative outcomes (e.g., relapse, rehospitalization; Amaresha & Venkatasubramanian, 2012; Butzlaff & Hooley, 1998). The negative impact of expressed emotion may be particularly harmful for those in the early phases of illness who are more likely to reside with parents and family caregivers (Miklowitz et al., 2014). Family therapy focused on psychoeducation, problem solving, and healthy communication skills may bolster perceived caregiver support, as well as decrease stress and increase family functioning (Glynn & Gingerich, 2020; McFarlane, 2016; Miklowitz et al., 2014).

Interpersonal relationships outside of the family are also important to consider in the context of treatment. Given that diminished social functioning and skills deficits are common among individuals with psychotic disorders, interventions targeting social skills and building social connectedness are an integral part of the recovery process. Social impairments seem to emerge prior to illness onset, are linked to increased risk for future psychosis among individuals at clinical high risk (Addington et al., 2019), and are often persistent, impacting long-term quality of life. Smaller networks of social support among people with psychosis have been linked to negative outcomes including hospitalization, poorer functioning, and worse symptoms (Mazzi et al., 2018). In addition to previously reviewed SST and peer-support interventions, enhancing social integration through involvement in social activities and building meaningful interpersonal relationships (with peers and romantic partners) may be important to expand an individual's support network beyond family, enhance feelings of belongingness and self-confidence, and reduce internalized stigma, loneliness, and isolation (Mazzi et al., 2018).

Care Coordination

A core feature of empirically supported treatment for schizophrenia and psychosis is care coordination, which can include case management and involves the organization and integration of client-care activities in the community (Edwards et al., 1999). Information-sharing, service linkage, and treatment planning across a team of multi-disciplinary providers promotes more consistent, safer, and effective care for each client. Case coordination within mental health services (e.g., psychiatry, psychosocial therapy, and other skills-based interventions such as vocational, cognitive, and social skills supports) and across physical health services is emphasized within the NICE guidelines (2014) and is integral to the assertive community treatment model described earlier. Given the complex needs of many individuals with psychosis, including the high rates of comorbid mental (e.g. depression, suicidality, trauma, substance use) and physical (e.g., metabolic, cardiovascular, sleep, and nutrition) concerns, coordination of services is particularly important to ensure that clients are receiving the wraparound care they need in a timely and effective manner.

Approaches for Youth

Early-onset schizophrenia, defined as onset prior to the age of 18, is rare, with incidence estimated to be less than 0.04% of the population, and childhood-onset schizophrenia (prior to age 13) affects less than 1 in 10,000 children (Stevens et al., 2014). Despite the rarity of full-threshold schizophrenia among children, research indicates that early signs of psychosis often develop during later adolescence, as up to 20% of adults report onset of symptoms prior to the age of 18 (Maloney et al., 2012; Stevens et al., 2014). Thus, recent research has highlighted that schizophrenia and other psychotic disorders can be considered from a developmental framework, as subthreshold symptoms often appear in advance of a diagnosable disorder and may appear early in childhood. Given the young age and ongoing neural development of young individuals, certain special considerations need to be highlighted when treating children and adolescents, and treatments should be tailored to individual presentations and needs. If a young person is showing signs and symptoms of psychosis but has not yet developed a fully diagnosable disorder as indicated by thorough assessment, psychosocial treatments should be considered the first-line approach, as opposed to antipsychotic medications that may impact the developing brain and are known to have increased metabolic impacts on pediatric populations (Conroy et al., 2018). On the other hand, antipsychotics have demonstrated efficacy for younger individuals who have a full-threshold disorder, and as younger age does often equate to increased severity and poorer prognosis (Eggers & Bunk, 1997), antipsychotics are typically recommended despite the concerns related to high-potency antipsychotic medications (McClellan & Stock, 2013).

Similar to adult intervention, the NICE guidelines for treatment of child and adolescent psychosis include FFT, with an emphasis on psychoeducation and adaptive skills to enhance problem solving and crisis management while incorporating the family's preferences (NICE, 2013). Family-focused intervention is particularly important for children given their reliance on and cohabitation with caregivers. In addition, the team-based coordinated specialty care (CSC) service model is a recovery-oriented treatment program for people with first-episode psychosis, including adolescents (Dixon et al., 2018). CSC teams take a multidisciplinary team approach to care in order to enhance supports through wraparound care. Services for these youth emphasize coordinated support services for the school setting, age-appropriate peer groups focused on normalization, social skills acquisition, emotion regulation, and interventions targeting identity-related and transition-age issues. Evidence-based individual therapy for this age group includes CBT, with a focus on psychosis and/or comorbid difficulties (e.g., depression, anxiety, trauma) as indicated.

Other Variables Influencing Treatment

Assessment and Diagnosis

Prior to the initiation of treatment, thorough assessment is necessary to determine an individual's specific diagnosis, as the presentation and type of psychotic disorder will drive treatment planning. There are several well-validated clinician-administered interviews that systematically assess diagnostic criteria for various mental health disorders and include specific modules for psychosis spectrum disorders. Examples of comprehensive gold-standard interviews include the Structured Clinical Interview for DSM-5, Clinician Version (SCID-5-CV; First et al., 2016) which is specific to adults. There are also several psychosis-specific interviews that assess the full spectrum of experiences (e.g., attenuated and psychotic intensity symptoms) and are specifically designed to probe subtle characteristics that distinguish psychosis-risk syndromes from various presentations of full-threshold psychosis (e.g., the Structured Interview for Psychosis-risk Syndromes or SIPS; McGlashan et al., 2001). These structured interviews and other clinician-rated symptom checklists (e.g., Positive and Negative Syndrome Scale or PANSS; Kay et al., 1987) can also be used to track symptom changes (e.g., persistence, progression, or remission of symptoms) over time and with treatment. In addition to thorough diagnostic evaluation, neuropsychological and cognitive assessment, measurement of social and role functioning, and medical workups are recommended to inform conceptualization, rule out nonpsychiatric factors that may better explain or contribute to symptoms, and guide treatment goals.

The particular type of psychotic disorder for which the patient meets diagnostic criteria can impact prognosis and treatment response. For example, patients with mood disorders (depressive or bipolar) with psychotic features will no longer exhibit psychotic symptoms when their mood episode remits (Rothschild, 2013). Furthermore, patients with schizoaffective disorder (i.e., who meet full criteria for schizophrenia along with having repeated mood episodes) tend to have better outcomes compared with those with schizophrenia, and patients with psychotic mood disorders have better outcomes than do patients with either schizophrenia or schizoaffective disorder (Harrow et al., 2000). Additionally, some patients with schizophrenia develop chronic symptoms and treatment resistance, whereas others demonstrate symptom remission with treatment, although full functional recovery (i.e., return to pre-illness functioning) is difficult to attain and maintain for the majority of patients with schizophrenia (Haro et al., 2018).

Comorbidity

Comorbid medical or psychiatric conditions are common in individuals with schizophrenia, impacting at least half of those diagnosed (Carney et al., 2006; Green et al., 2003). Accordingly, assessing and treating comorbid conditions (e.g., depression, anxiety, substance use, PTSD) along with the primary psychotic disorder may be essential in providing the most impactful and effective care. Of particular note, individuals with schizophrenia are at high risk for suicide, particularly in the year following a first episode (Carlborg et al., 2010). Medical comorbidities are also a concern as they can impact quality of life and increase the likelihood of comorbid depression (Carney et al., 2006). Unfortunately, individuals with schizophrenia are more likely to experience more disease across a variety of domains (including cardiovascular, pulmonary, neurological, and endocrine conditions) as compared to the general population, and they are more likely to die prematurely (Olfson et al., 2015).

Demographics

Psychotic disorders most frequently onset between late teens and early 30s, with men typically being diagnosed from late teens to early 20s, and women from early 20s to early 30s, with an additional peak in postmenopausal women, possibly due to the protective effects of estrogen diminishing with age (Falkenburg & Tracy, 2014; McGrath et al., 2008). The five years following onset are often considered a critical period in treatment in terms of psychoeducation and future treatment engagement, as well as reducing risk of relapse. Men and women also tend to show differences in symptom presentation, with men showing more negative symptoms and the content of positive symptoms differing across genders (Falkenburg & Tracy, 2014). Psychosis diagnoses may also be more common in transgender individuals compared to cisgender peers, although more research is needed in this area (Barr et al., 2021). These demographic differences among patients with psychosis have implications for both psychopharmaceutical and psychosocial treatments. There may be risk for overdiagnosis/misdiagnosis due to bias, and gender affirmation and tailored care may be more important in treatment for these individuals. Finally, an array of health disparities exist in racial/ethnic minority patients with serious mental illness, including diagnostic biases, reduced quality of services, poorer outcomes, increased stigma, and lower levels of treatment engagement (Maura & Weisman de Mamani, 2017). Thus, clinicians may need to place greater emphasis on facilitating trust in the healthcare system, inquiring about religious and spiritual beliefs, acknowledging cultural differences, seeking consultation to aid in culturally adapted care, reducing stigma of mental health treatment, and involving family in care.

Medication

Psychological interventions should be administered in conjunction with antipsychotic medication for maximum benefit, at least during acute phases of illness. However, benefits and side effects of medication should be considered when choosing an antipsychotic, such as metabolic, extrapyramidal, cardiovascular, hormonal, and other concerns (NICE, 2014). Due to factors such as poor treatment response, intolerable side effects, and comorbid substance misuse, medication nonadherence in schizophrenia has been estimated at a rate of almost 50% (Lacro et al., 2002). Further, treatment-resistance to antipsychotic medication is a considerable problem (Howes et al., 2017), in which case psychosocial interventions such as CBT and family intervention are recommended (NICE, 2014).

Conclusion

Schizophrenia and related psychotic disorders are impairing and challenging conditions to treat. They negatively impact patients, their families, and the larger society. Fortunately, science offers various empirically supported treatment options to help those with psychosis that have been shown to decrease symptoms and impairment. In this chapter, we described several psychological therapies that have been demonstrated to improve outcomes for individuals with psychosis beyond medications alone. We also detailed credible and efficacious treatment components found across these interventions. Unfortunately, many individuals are not given the opportunity to receive empirically supported psychosocial treatment for psychosis. It will take a concerted effort on the part of mental health and medical professionals, policy makers, and the public to improve the dissemination and implementation of science-backed treatments for psychosis so that individuals with psychosis are given the best chances of achieving the long-term recovery that they deserve. We hope that this chapter will contribute to that aspirational goal.

Useful Resources

Treatment Manuals

- Assertive Community Treatment (ACT): Evidence-Based Practices (EBP) KIT: https:// store.samhsa.gov/product/Assertive-Community-Treatment-ACT-Evidence-Based- Practices-EBP-KIT/SMA08-4344
- Landa, Y. (2017). *Cognitive behavioral therapy for psychosis (CBTp): An introductory manual for clinicians*. Mental Illness Research, Education & Clinical Center. www.mirecc .va.gov/visn2/docs/CBTp_Manual_VA_Yulia_Landa_2017.pdf

Journals

- *Psychosis: Psychological, Social and Integrative Approaches*: www.tandfonline.com/journals/ rpsy20
- *Schizophrenia Bulletin*: https://academic.oup.com/schizophreniabulletin

Organizations

- Hearing Voices Network: www.hearing-voices.org/
- Schizophrenia International Research Society: https://schizophreniaresearchsociety.org/

Clinical Practice Guidelines

- Addington, J., Addington, D., Abidi, S., Raedler, T., & Remington, G. (2017). Canadian treatment guidelines for individuals at clinical high risk of psychosis. *Canadian Journal of Psychiatry*, 62, 656–661. https://doi.org/10.1177/0706743717719895
- Keepers, G. A., Fochtmann, L. J., Anzia, J. M., et al. (2020). The American Psychiatric Association practice guideline for the treatment of patients with schizophrenia. *American Journal of Psychiatry*, 177, 868–872. https://doi.org/10.1176/appi.ajp.2020.177901

References

Addington, J., Farris, M., Stowkowy, J., et al. (2019). Predictors of transition to psychosis in individuals at clinical high risk. *Current Psychiatry Reports*, 21(6), 1–10.

Amaresha, A. C., & Venkatasubramanian, G. (2012). Expressed emotion in schizophrenia: an overview. *Indian Journal of Psychological Medicine*, 34(1), 12–20.

American Psychiatric Association. (2022). *Diagnostic and statistical manual of mental disorders* (5th ed., text revision). https://doi.org/10.1176/appi.books.9780890425596

Barr, S. M., Roberts, D., & Thakkar, K. N. (2021). Psychosis in transgender and gender non-conforming individuals: A review of the literature and a call for more research. *Psychiatry Research*, 306, Article e114272.

Bond, G. R., & Drake, R. E. (2015). The critical ingredients of assertive community treatment. *World Psychiatry: Official Journal of the World Psychiatric Association (WPA)*, 14(2), 240–242. https://doi.org/10.1002/wps.20234

Burns, T., Catty, J., White, S., et al. (2009). The impact of supported employment and working on clinical and social functioning: results of an international study of individual placement and support. *Schizophrenia Bulletin*, 35(5), 949–958.

Butzlaff, R. L., & Hooley, J. M. (1998). Expressed emotion and psychiatric relapse: A meta-analysis. *Archives of General Psychiatry*, 55(6), 547–552.

Carlborg, A., Winnerbäck, K., Jönsson, E. G., Jokinen, J., & Nordström, P. (2010). Suicide in schizophrenia. *Expert Review of Neurotherapeutics*, 10(7), 1153–1164.

Carney, C. P., Jones, L., & Woolson, R. F. (2006). Medical comorbidity in women and men with schizophrenia. *Journal of General Internal Medicine*, 21(11), 1133–1137.

Chong, H. Y., Teoh, S. L., Wu, D. B. C., et al. (2016). Global economic burden of schizophrenia: A systematic review. *Neuropsychiatric Disease and Treatment*, 12, 357–373.

Conroy, S. K., Francis, M. M., & Hulvershorn, L. A. (2018). Identifying and treating the prodromal phases of bipolar disorder and schizophrenia. *Current Treatment Options in Psychiatry*, 5(1), 113–128.

Corcoran, C., Walker, E., Huot, R., et al. (2003). The stress cascade and schizophrenia: Etiology and onset. *Schizophrenia Bulletin*, 29(4), 671–692.

Davidson, L., Chinman, M., Sells, D., & Rowe, M. (2006). Peer support among adults with serious mental illness: A report from the field. *Schizophrenia Bulletin*, 32(3), 443–450. https://doi.org/10.1093/schbul/sbj043

DeVylder, J. E., Ben-David, S., Schobel, S. A., et al. (2013). Temporal association of stress sensitivity and symptoms in individuals at clinical high risk for psychosis. *Psychological Medicine*, 43(2), 259–268.

Dickerson, F. B. (2008). Schizophrenia: Advances in psychotherapy, evidence-based practice. *The Journal of Nervous and Mental Disease*, 196(5), 435–436.

Dickerson, F. B., & Lehman, A. F. (2011). Evidence-based psychotherapy for schizophrenia: 2011 update. *The Journal of Nervous and Mental Disease*, 199(8), 520–526.

Dickinson, D., Bellack, A. S., & Gold, J. M. (2007). Social/communication skills, cognition, and vocational functioning in schizophrenia. *Schizophrenia Bulletin*, 33(5), 1213–1220.

Dieterich, M., Irving, C. B., Bergman, H., et al. (2017). Intensive case management for severe mental illness. *The Cochrane Database of Systematic Reviews*, (1), CD007906. https://doi.org/10.1002/14651858.CD007906.pub2

Dixon, L. (2000). Assertive community treatment: twenty-five years of gold. *Psychiatric Services*, 51(6), 759–765.

Dixon, L. B., Dickerson, F., Bellack, A. S., et al. (2010). Schizophrenia Patient Outcomes Research Team (PORT). The 2009 schizophrenia PORT psychosocial treatment recommendations and summary statements. *Schizophrenia Bulletin*, 36(1), 48–70. https://doi.org/ 10.1093/schbul/sbp115. Epub 2009 Dec 2. PMID: 19955389; PMCID: PMC2800143.

Dixon, L. B., Goldman, H. H., Srihari, V. H., & Kane, J. M. (2018). Transforming the treatment of schizophrenia in the United States: The RAISE initiative. *Annual Review of Clinical Psychology*, 14, 237–258.

Drake, R. E., Bond, G. R., & Essock, S. M. (2009). Implementing evidence-based practices for people with schizophrenia. *Schizophrenia Bulletin*, 35(4), 704–713.

DuBrul, S.A., Deegan, D., Bello, I., et al. (2017). *Peer specialist manual. OnTrack New York. Center for Practice Innovations Columbia Psychiatry*, New York State Psychiatric Institute.

www.ontrackny.org/portals/1/Files/Resources/Peer%20Specialist%20Manual%20Final%
202_17.17.pdf?ver=2017-04-04-063602–080.

Edwards, J., Cooks, J., & Bott, J. (1999). Preventive case management in first-episode psychosis. In P. D. McGorry & H. J. Jackson (Eds.), *The recognition and management of early psychosis: A preventive approach* (pp. 308–375). Cambridge University Press.

Eggers, C., & Bunk, D. (1997). The long-term course of childhood-onset schizophrenia: A 42-year followup. *Schizophrenia Bulletin*, 23(1), 105–117.

Elliott, R., Bohart, A. C., Watson, J. C., & Greenberg, L. S. (2011). Empathy. In J. Norcross (ed.), *Psychotherapy relationships that work* (2nd ed.) (pp. 132–152). Oxford University Press.

Falkenburg, J. & Tracy, D. K. (2014). Sex and schizophrenia: A review of gender differences, *Psychosis*, 6:1, 61–69, https://doi.org/10.1080/17522439.2012.733405.

First, M. B., Williams, J. B. W., Karg, R. S., & Spitzer, R. L. (2016). *User's guide for the SCID-5-CV Structured Clinical Interview for DSM-5® disorders: Clinical version.* American Psychiatric Publishing, Inc.

Fisher, M., Holland, C., Merzenich, M. M., & Vinogradov, S. (2009). Using neuroplasticity-based auditory training to improve verbal memory in schizophrenia. *American Journal of Psychiatry*, 166(7), 805–811.

Fitapelli, B., & Lindenmayer, J. P. (2022). Advances in cognitive remediation training in schizophrenia: A review. *Brain Sciences*, 12(2), 129.

Fulford, D., Niendam, T. A., Floyd, E. G., et al. (2013). Symptom dimensions and functional impairment in early psychosis: More to the story than just negative symptoms. *Schizophrenia Research*, 147(1), 125–131.

Garety, P. A., Freeman, D., Jolley, S., et al. (2005). Reasoning, emotions, and delusional conviction in psychosis. *Journal of Abnormal Psychology*, 114(3), 373.

Glynn, S.M., & Gingerich, S. (2020). NAVIGATE Family Education Program. Navigate Consultants.

Green, A. I., Canuso, C. M., Brenner, M. J., & Wojcik, J. D. (2003). Detection and management of comorbidity in patients with schizophrenia. *Psychiatric Clinics*, 26(1), 115–139.

Green, M. F., Horan, W. P., & Lee, J. (2015). Social cognition in schizophrenia. Nature *Reviews Neuroscience*, 16(10), 620–631.

Gross J. J. (1998). The emerging field of emotion regulation: An integrative review. *Review of General Psychology*, 2, 271–299.

Haro, J. M., Altamura, C., Corral, R., et al. (2018). Understanding the course of persistent symptoms in schizophrenia: Longitudinal findings from the pattern study. *Psychiatry Research*, 267, 56–62.

Harrow, M., Grossman, L. S., Herbener, E. S., & Davies, E. W. (2000). Ten-year outcome: patients with schizoaffective disorders, schizophrenia, affective disorders and mood-incongruent psychotic symptoms. *The British Journal of Psychiatry*, 177(5), 421–426.

Hersen, M. (1976). Token economies in institutional settings: Historical, political, deprivation, ethical, and generalization issues. *The Journal of Nervous and Mental Disease*, 162(3), 206–211.

Hofmann, S. G., Asnaani, A., Vonk, I. J., Sawyer, A. T., & Fang, A. (2012). The efficacy of cognitive behavioral therapy: A review of meta-analyses. *Cognitive Therapy and Research*, 36(5), 427–440.

Hooley, J. M. (2010). Social factors in schizophrenia. *Current Directions in Psychological Science*, 19(4), 238–242.

Howes, O. D., McCutcheon, R., Agid, O., et al. (2017). Treatment-resistant schizophrenia: Treatment Response and Resistance in Psychosis (TRRIP) working group consensus guidelines on diagnosis and terminology. *American Journal of Psychiatry*, 174(3), 216–229. https://doi.org/10.1176/appi.ajp.2016.16050503

Kadakia, A., Catillon, M., Fan, Q., et al. (2022). The economic burden of schizophrenia in the United States. *The Journal of Clinical Psychiatry*, 83(6), 43278.

Kay, S. R., Fiszbein, A., & Opler, L. A. (1987). The positive and negative syndrome scale (PANSS) for schizophrenia. *Schizophrenia Bulletin*, 13(2), 261–276.

Kazdin, A. E. (1977). The influence of behavior preceding a reinforced response on behavior change in the classroom. *Journal of Applied Behavior Analysis*, 10(2), 299–310.

Keepers, G. A., Fochtmann, L. J., Anzia, J. M., et al. (2020). The American Psychiatric Association practice guideline for the treatment of patients with schizophrenia. *The American Journal of Psychiatry*, 177(9), 868–872. https://doi.org/10.1176/appi.ajp.2020.177901.

Khoury, B., Lecomte, T., Comtois, G., & Nicole, L. (2015). Third-wave strategies for emotion regulation in early psychosis: A pilot study. *Early Intervention in Psychiatry*, 9(1), 76–83.

Kingdon, D. G., & Turkington, D. (2005). *Cognitive therapy of schizophrenia*. Guilford Press.

Kingdon, D., & Turkington, D. (2019). Cognitive therapy of psychosis: Research and implementation. *Schizophrenia Research*, 203, 62–65.

Kopelovich, S. L., Hughes, M., Monroe-DeVita, M. B., et al. (2019). Statewide implementation of cognitive behavioral therapy for psychosis through a learning collaborative model. *Cognitive and Behavioral Practice*, 26(3), 439–452.

Kopelovich, S. L., Nutting, E., Blank, J., Buckland, H. T., & Spigner, C. (2022). Preliminary point prevalence of Cognitive Behavioral Therapy for psychosis (CBTp) training in the US and Canada. *Psychosis*, 14(4), 344–354.

Kreyenbuhl, J., Nossel, I. R., & Dixon, L. B. (2009). Disengagement from mental health treatment among individuals with schizophrenia and strategies for facilitating connections to care: a review of the literature. *Schizophrenia Bulletin*, 35(4), 696–703.

Kurtz, M. M., & Mueser, K. T. (2008). A meta-analysis of controlled research on social skills training for schizophrenia. *Journal of Consulting and Clinical Psychology*, 76(3), 491.

Lacro, J. P., Dunn, L. B., Dolder, C. R., Leckband, S. G., & Jeste, D. V. (2002). Prevalence of and risk factors for medication nonadherence in patients with schizophrenia: A comprehensive review of recent literature. *The Journal of Clinical Psychiatry*, 63(10), 892–909. https://doi.org/10.4088/jcp.v63n1007.

Lawlor, C., Vitoratou, S., Duffy, J., et al. (2022). Managing emotions in psychosis: Evaluation of a brief DBT-informed skills group for individuals with psychosis in routine community services. *British Journal of Clinical Psychology*, 61(3), 735–756.

Lecomte, T., Corbière, M., Simard, S., & Leclerc, C. (2014). Merging evidence-based psychosocial interventions in schizophrenia. *Behavioral Sciences*, 4(4), 437–447.

Lehman, A. F., Lieberman, J. A., Dixon, L. B et al. (2004). American Psychiatric Association; Steering Committee on Practice Guidelines. Practice guideline for the treatment of patients with schizophrenia, second edition. *American Journal Psychiatry*, 161, 1–56.

Leucht, S., Leucht, C., Huhn, M., et al. (2017). Sixty years of placebo-controlled antipsychotic drug trials in acute schizophrenia: Systematic review, Bayesian meta-analysis, and meta-regression of efficacy predictors. *American Journal of Psychiatry*, 174(10), 927–942.

Linehan, M. M. (1987). Dialectical behavior therapy for borderline personality disorder: Theory and method. *Bulletin of the Menninger Clinic*, 51(3), 261.

Lloyd-Evans, B., Mayo-Wilson, E., Harrison, B., et al. (2014). A systematic review and meta-analysis of randomized controlled trials of peer support for people with severe mental illness. *BMC Psychiatry* 14, 39. https://doi.org/10.1186/1471-244X-14-39.

Ludwig, L., Mehl, S., Krkovic, K., & Lincoln, T. M. (2020). Effectiveness of emotion regulation in daily life in individuals with psychosis and nonclinical controls – An experience-sampling study. *Journal of Abnormal Psychology*, 129(4), 408–421. https://doi.org/10.1037/abn0000505

Ludwig, L., Werner, D., & Lincoln, T. M. (2019). The relevance of cognitive emotion regulation to psychotic symptoms – A systematic review and meta-analysis. *Clinical Psychology Review*, 72, 101746.

Lutfiyya, Z. M., Rogan, P., & Shoultz, B. (1988). *Supported employment: A Conceptual overview*. Center on Human Policy Research and Training Center on Community Integration. Syracuse University. Syracuse, NY. https://thechp.syr.edu/chp-archives-supported-employment-a-conceptual-overview.

Maheshwari, S., Manohar, S., Chandran, S., & Rao, T. S. S. (2020). Psycho-education in schizophrenia. In A. Shrivastava & A. De Sousa (eds.), *Schizophrenia treatment outcomes.* Springer. https://doi.org/10.1007/978-3-030-19847-3_2410.1002/14651858.CD002831.pub2. PMID: 21678337; PMCID: PMC4170907.

Malla, A., Cortese, L., Shaw, T. S., & Ginsberg, B. (1990). Life events and relapse in schizophrenia. *Social Psychiatry and Psychiatric Epidemiology*, 25(4), 221–224.

Maloney, A. E., Yakutis, L. J., & Frazier, J. A. (2012). Empirical evidence for psychopharmacologic treatment in early-onset psychosis and schizophrenia. *Child and Adolescent Psychiatric Clinics*, 21(4), 885–909.

Maura, J., & Weisman de Mamani, A. (2017). Mental health disparities, treatment engagement, and attrition among racial/ethnic minorities with severe mental illness: A review. *Journal of Clinical Psychology in Medical Settings*, 24(3), 187–210.

Mazzi, F., Baccari, F., Mungai, F., et al. (2018). Effectiveness of a social inclusion program in people with non-affective psychosis. *BMC Psychiatry*, 18(1), 1–9.

McClellan, J., & Stock, S. (2013). Practice parameter for the assessment and treatment of children and adolescents with schizophrenia. *Journal of the American Academy of Child & Adolescent Psychiatry*, 52(9), 976–990.

McCormack, M., Tierney, K., Brennan, D., Lawlor, E., & Clarke, M. (2014). Lack of insight in psychosis: Theoretical concepts and clinical aspects. *Behavioural and Cognitive Psychotherapy*, 42(3), 327–338. https://doi.org/10.1017/S1352465813000155.

McFarlane, W. R. (2016). Family interventions for schizophrenia and the psychoses: A review. *Family Process*, 55(3), 460–482.

McFarlane, W. R., Stastny, P., & Deakins, S. (1992). Family-aided assertive community treatment: A comprehensive rehabilitation and intensive case management approach for persons with schizophrenic disorders. *New Directions for Mental Health Services*, 1992(53), 43–54.

McGlashan, T. H., Walsh, B. C., Woods, S. W., et al. (2001). *Structured interview for psychosis-risk syndromes*. Yale School of Medicine.

McGrath, J., Saha, S., Chant, D., & Welham, J. (2008). Schizophrenia: A concise overview of incidence, prevalence, and mortality. *Epidemiologic Reviews*, 30, 67–76. https://doi.org/10.1093/epirev/mxn001.

McGurk, S. R., & Mueser, K. T. (2004). Cognitive functioning, symptoms, and work in supported employment: A review and heuristic model. *Schizophrenia Research*, 70(2-3), 147-173.

McGurk, S. R., Twamley, E. W., Sitzer, D. I., McHugo, G. J., & Mueser, K. T. (2007). A meta-analysis of cognitive remediation in schizophrenia. *American Journal of Psychiatry*, 164(12), 1791–1802.

Mellen, V., & Danley, K. (1987). Supported employment for persons with severe mental illness. *Psychosocial Rehabilitation Journal*, 11(2), 3–4.

Miklowitz, D. J., O'Brien, M. P., Schlosser, D. A., et al. (2014). Family-focused treatment for adolescents and young adults at high risk for psychosis: Results of a randomized trial. *Journal of the American Academy of Child & Adolescent Psychiatry*, 53(8), 848–858.

Modini, M., Tan, L., Brinchmann, B., et al. (2016). Supported employment for people with severe mental illness: Systematic review and meta-analysis of the international evidence. *The British Journal of Psychiatry*, 209(1), 14–22.

Moreno-Küstner, B., Martin, C., & Pastor, L. (2018). Prevalence of psychotic disorders and its association with methodological issues. A systematic review and meta-analyses. *PloS One*, 13(4), e0195687.

Morrison, A. P. (2017). A manualised treatment protocol to guide delivery of evidence-based cognitive therapy for people with distressing psychosis: learning from clinical trials. *Psychosis*, 9(3), 271–281.

Morrison, A. P., & Barratt, S. (2010). What are the components of CBT for psychosis? A Delphi study. *Schizophrenia Bulletin*, 36(1), 136–142.

Morrison, A. P., Renton, J. C., Dunn, H., Williams, S., & Bentall, R. P. (2004). *Cognitive therapy for psychosis: A formulation-based approach.* Brunner-Routledge.

Mueser, K. T., Deavers, F., Penn, D. L., & Cassisi, J. E. (2013). Psychosocial treatments for schizophrenia. *Annual Review of Clinical Psychology*, 9, 465–497.

Mueser, K. T., Penn, D. L., Addington, J., et al. (2015). The NAVIGATE program for first-episode psychosis: rationale, overview, and description of psychosocial components. *Psychiatric Services*, 66(7), 680–690.

Myin-Germeys, I., Delespaul, P. H., & Van Os, J. (2005). Behavioural sensitization to daily life stress in psychosis. *Psychological Medicine*, 35(5), 733–741.

National Institute for Health and Care Excellence (NICE) (2013). Psychosis and schizophrenia in children and young people: Recognition and management (NICE Clinical Guidelines, No. 155). NICE. www.nice.org.uk/guidance/cg178.

National Institute for Health and Care Excellence (NICE) (2014). Psychosis and schizophrenia in adults: Prevention and management (NICE Clinical Guidelines, No. 178). NICE. www.nice.org.uk/guidance/cg178.

O'Driscoll, C., Sener, S. B., Angmark, A., & Shaikh, M. (2019). Caregiving processes and expressed emotion in psychosis, a cross-cultural, meta-analytic review. *Schizophrenia Research*, 208, 8–15.

Olfson, M., Gerhard, T., Huang, C., Crystal, S., & Stroup, T. S. (2015). Premature mortality among adults with schizophrenia in the United States. *JAMA Psychiatry*, 72(12), 1172–1181.

Opoka, S. M., Sundag, J., Riehle, M., & Lincoln, T. M. (2021). Emotion-regulation in psychosis: Patients with psychotic disorders apply reappraisal successfully. *Cognitive Therapy and Research*, 45, 31–45.

Resnick, S. G., Fontana, A., Lehman, A. F., & Rosenheck, R. A. (2005). An empirical conceptualization of the recovery orientation. *Schizophrenia Research*, 75(1), 119–128.

Resnick, S. G., Rosenheck, R. A., & Lehman, A. F. (2004). An exploratory analysis of correlates of recovery. *Psychiatric Services*, 55(5), 540–547.

Revell, E. R., Neill, J. C., Harte, M., Khan, Z., & Drake, R. J. (2015). A systematic review and meta-analysis of cognitive remediation in early schizophrenia. *Schizophrenia Research*, 168(1–2), 213–222.

Richter, D., & Hoffmann, H. (2019). Effectiveness of supported employment in non-trial routine implementation: Systematic review and meta-analysis. *Social Psychiatry and Psychiatric Epidemiology*, 54(5), 525–531.

Rochefort, D. A. (2019). Innovation and its discontents: Pathways and barriers in the diffusion of assertive community treatment. *The Milbank Quarterly*, 97(4), 1151–1199.

Rodolico, A., Bighelli, I., Avanzato, C., et al. (2022). Family interventions for relapse prevention in schizophrenia: A systematic review and network meta-analysis. *The Lancet Psychiatry*, 9(3), 211–221.

Rosen, G. M., & Davison, G. C. (2003). Psychology should list empirically supported principles of change (ESPs) and not credential trademarked therapies or other treatment packages. *Behavior Modification*, 27(3), 300–312. https://doi.org/10.1177/0145445503027003003.

Rothschild, A. J. (2013). Challenges in the treatment of major depressive disorder with psychotic features. *Schizophrenia Bulletin*, 39(4), 787–796.

Ryan, A., Crehan, E., Khondoker, M., et al. (2021). An emotional regulation approach to psychosis recovery: The Living Through Psychosis group programme. *Journal of Behavior Therapy and Experimental Psychiatry*, 72, 101651.

Schaefer, J., Giangrande, E., Weinberger, D. R., & Dickinson, D. (2013). The global cognitive impairment in schizophrenia: Consistent over decades and around the world. *Schizophrenia Research*, 150(1), 42–50.

Shattock, L., Berry, K., Degnan, A., & Edge, D. (2018). Therapeutic alliance in psychological therapy for people with schizophrenia and related psychoses: A systematic review. *Clinical Psychology & Psychotherapy*, 25(1), e60–e85.

Skinner, B. F. (1953). *Science and human behavior*. The Free Press.

Solmi, M., Croatto, G., Piva, G., et al. (2023). Efficacy and acceptability of psychosocial interventions in schizophrenia: Systematic overview and quality appraisal of the meta-analytic evidence. *Molecular Psychiatry*, 28(1), 354–368.

Steel, C., & Smith, B. (2013). CBT for psychosis: An introduction. In C. Steel (Ed.), *CBT for schizophrenia: Evidence-based interventions and future directions* (pp. 1–12). John Wiley & Sons.

Stein, L. I., & Test, M. A. (1980). Alternative to mental hospital treatment. I. Conceptual model, treatment program, and clinical evaluation. *Archives of General Psychiatry*, 37(4), 392–397. https://doi.org/10.1001/archpsyc.1980.01780170034003.

Stevens, J. R., Prince, J. B., Prager, L. M., & Stern, T. A. (2014). Psychotic disorders in children and adolescents: A primer on contemporary evaluation and management. *The Primary Care Companion for CNS Disorders*, 16(2), 27187.

Thorning, H., & Dixon, L. (2020). Forty-five years later: The challenge of optimizing assertive community treatment. *Current Opinion in Psychiatry*, 33(4), 397–406.

Turner, D. T., McGlanaghy, E., Cuijpers, P., et al. (2018). A meta-analysis of social skills training and related interventions for psychosis. *Schizophrenia Bulletin*, 44(3), 475–491. https://doi.org/10.1093/schbul/sbx146.

Turner, D. T., van der Gaag, M., Karyotaki, E., & Cuijpers, P. (2014). Psychological interventions for psychosis: A meta-analysis of comparative outcome studies. *American Journal of Psychiatry*, 171(5), 523–538.

Visser, K. F., Esfahlani, F. Z., Sayama, H., & Strauss, G. P. (2018). An ecological momentary assessment evaluation of emotion regulation abnormalities in schizophrenia. *Psychological Medicine*, 48(14), 2337–2345.

Vita, A., Barlati, S., Ceraso, A., et al. (2021). Effectiveness, core elements, and moderators of response of cognitive remediation for schizophrenia: A systematic review and meta-analysis of randomized clinical trials. *JAMA Psychiatry*, 78(8), 848–858.

Walker, E. F., & Diforio, D. (1997). Schizophrenia: A neural diathesis-stress model. *Psychological Review*, 104(4), 667–685.

Wallace, C. J., Nelson, C. J., Liberman, R. P., et al. (1980). A review and critique of social skills training with schizophrenic patients. *Schizophrenia Bulletin*, 6(1), 42–63. https://doi.org/10.1093/schbul/6.1.42.

Wampold, B. E. (2015). How important are the common factors in psychotherapy? An update. *World Psychiatry*, 14(3), 270–277.

Warner, R. (2009). Recovery from schizophrenia and the recovery model. *Current Opinion in Psychiatry*, 22(4), 374–380.

Wykes, T., Huddy, V., Cellard, C., McGurk, S. R., & Czobor, P. (2011). A meta-analysis of cognitive remediation for schizophrenia: methodology and effect sizes. *American Journal of Psychiatry*, 168(5), 472–485.

Xia, J., Merinder, L. B., & Belgamwar, M. R. (2011). Psychoeducation for schizophrenia. *The Cochrane Database of Systematic Reviews*, 2011(6), CD002831. https://doi.org/10.1002/14651858.CD002831.pub2.

17

Autism Spectrum and Intellectual Developmental Disorder

Frank R. Cicero

Autism spectrum disorder (ASD) is a neurodevelopmental disorder characterized by issues with social communication and idiosyncratic behavior. Formal diagnosis in the United States is made through diagnostic criteria as per the *Diagnostic and Statistical Manual of Mental Disorders: Fifth Edition* (DSM-5-TR; American Psychological Association [APA], 2022). In order to receive a diagnosis, individuals must display a range of deficits affecting the ability to socialize with others. This includes both verbal and nonverbal behaviors used to communicate with others in a social setting (APA, 2022). Individuals must also engage in a range of restricted and repetitive behaviors across multiple settings. This can include behaviors such as maintaining routines, sensory stimulation, motor movements, verbal perseveration, and fixed interests (APA, 2022). In order to formally give a diagnosis, these characteristics of autism must be noted in the early developmental period.

ASD has formally been considered a spectrum disorder since the publication of the DSM-5 in 2013. As a spectrum, a range of affectedness is noted across persons when it comes to behavior severity, communication deficits, and cognitive ability (Steinbrenner et al., 2020). Although usually diagnosed in childhood, autism will affect an individual across the lifespan. Epidemiological data indicate global prevalence rates for ASD ranging from 0.7% to 2.6% of the childhood population (Lyall et al., 2017), with the current estimate in the United States standing at 2.3% of eight-year-olds (Maenner et al., 2021). Studies investigating the population rates for ASD in adulthood are limited. The most current studies indicate prevalence estimates ranging from 1.1% of the adult population in England (Brugha et al., 2016) to 2.2% of the adult population in the United States (Dietz et al., 2020). Although we do not have definitive epidemiological data, research indicates that the number of adults with ASD is increasing over the years (Laugeson et al., 2015).

Intellectual developmental disorder (IDD) is a condition most characterized by clinically significant deficits in cognitive abilities and adaptive functioning. As with ASD, a formal diagnosis of IDD in the United States is made through diagnostic criteria as per the DSM-5-TR. According to the criteria, individuals must display significant deficits in cognitive functioning as measured through a standardized assessment of intellectual abilities. Typically, derived scores must fall approximately two standard deviations below the population mean (APA, 2022). Individuals must also display significant limitations in adaptive behavior as compared to culturally appropriate standards. Adaptive deficits must be displayed across various areas including communication skills, social skills, personal independence, and/or school/ work functioning. Symptoms of IDD must manifest in the developmental period and will show lifelong effects on skills and behavior (McKenzie et al., 2016). The global prevalence rate of IDD is reported to be approximately 1% of the population; however, estimates vary widely due to methodological differences across studies (McKenzie et al., 2016). Prevalence rates are also difficult to determine due to comorbidity with other developmental conditions (i.e., ASD) and the presence of diagnostic overlap leading to misdiagnosis (Pedersen et al., 2017). Within the diagnosis of IDD, the DSM-5-TR indicates levels of severity as mild, moderate, severe, and profound. Classifications of level are made based on the severity of cognitive and adaptive skill deficits displayed by an individual. Prevalence of severe IDD in the general population falls at approximately 0.6%, or 6 out of 1,000 persons (Saad & ElAdl, 2019).

Etiology and Theoretical Underpinnings of Treatment

ASD is a complex condition with differing forms of behavioral and cognitive expression. Therefore, it is likely that various causes contribute to its development. At the present time, there are no definitive risk factors, simple etiological explanations, or genetic markers for a diagnosis of ASD (Yoon et al., 2020). The current theory is that the condition is a result of a combination of genetic, prenatal environmental, and epigenic factors (Yoon et al., 2020) with genetic factors likely exerting more influence than environmental factors (Bailey et al., 1995). With regard to IDD, etiology of the condition varies according to the specific diagnosis. Causal factors are never discovered for at least 50% of cases of mild IDD, whereas definitive biological causes are noted for at least 75% of cases of severe IDD (Patel et al., 2018). Results of a recent systematic review implicated ten prenatal factors correlated with IDD, including variables such as maternal age, maternal alcohol use, maternal tobacco use, and maternal health issues such as hypertension and epilepsy. Preterm birth and low birth weight were also found to be correlates (Huang et al., 2016).

Interventions for ASD are generally separated into two categories: comprehensive and focused treatment models (Steinbrenner et al., 2020). In a comprehensive treatment model, the goal of intervention is to have a broad positive impact on the core deficits of ASD through the use of a structured set of practices following one conceptual philosophy of therapy (Wong et al., 2015). Two examples of comprehensive treatments are the Early Intensive Behavioral Intervention (EIBI) program of

Lovaas and colleagues (e.g., Lovaas, 1987; Smith & Lovaas, 1998) and the TEACCH program by Schopler and colleagues (1995). Focused treatments, on the other hand, are designed to treat only a single skill or behavior rather than being considered a global treatment for ASD (Steinbrenner et al., 2020). They are often considered the discrete interventions that, when put together, make up comprehensive treatments (Wong et al., 2015). Interventions for adults with IDD can break down in a similar fashion.

When it comes to establishing evidence-based practice for either comprehensive or focused interventions for adults, the problem is that the majority of treatment research has been conducted only with children. In their review of 150 autism intervention studies, Seaman and Cannella-Malone (2016) found that 63% were conducted with participants aged eight years of age or less, and only 2% with participants aged 20 or older. Recent task forces investigating evidence-based practices for ASD treatment in children have indicated 28 practices that meet criteria (Hume et al., 2021). The definitions and procedures for establishing evidence-based practice vary by discipline and by evaluator. Some procedures, such as those outlined by Schalock and colleagues, which were described for use with treatments for IDD, are relatively broad. According to the authors, evidence-based practice is defined as "practices for which there is a demonstrated relation between specific practices and measured outcomes" (Schalock et al., 2017, p. 115). Operational definitions are provided for the terms "evidence," "practices," and "demonstrated relation." A more quantitative and objective method of establishing evidence-based practice for treatments of ASD was explained by Reichow (2011). In his method, Reichow establishes three formulas/rubrics for evaluating evidence-based practice: one for evaluating research report rigor, one for determining research report strength, and finally a quantitative formula used for evaluating if a treatment has enough research to be considered evidence-based. In their task force report, Hume et al. (2021) relied on several evidence-based practice procedures, including a method outlined by Horner and colleagues (2005) which was specifically designed to identify evidence-based practice through single-subject design research. Similar to Reichow (2011), Horner and colleagues' method uses a rubric of quality indicators and a formula across studies to determine if a specific treatment can be considered evidence-based.

The majority of evidence-based practices for ASD treatment follow applied behavior analytic methodology and philosophy (Steinbrenner et al., 2020). In fact, one of the most effective comprehensive treatments for children with ASD has been found to be the EIBI program (Wong et al., 2015). Although we have considerable data supporting evidence-based practice with children, we cannot be sure that those same practices would be effective with adults with ASD. High-quality treatment research of psychosocial interventions with adults with ASD is lacking and those studies that are published tend not to focus on the core symptoms of ASD or use outcome measures designed for different populations or purposes (Brugha et al., 2015; Eack et al., 2018).

Unfortunately, many studies with adults with ASD do not provide outcome evidence of globally significant change, such as measures of overall mental health and quality of life (Lorenc et al., 2018).

There are also issues with establishing evidence-based practice in the treatment of behaviors and characteristics associated with IDD. Treatment studies in IDD often have inadequate numbers of participants, rely on poor research designs, lack control groups, and report different outcome measures between studies (Bhaumik et al., 2011). Because of this, treatments for IDD populations are often based on research conducted with neurotypical populations with mental health issues (Bhaumik et al., 2011). This generalization, however, may not be appropriate.

Brief Overview of Treatments

Recent task force data indicate that, at this time, 28 intervention practices have met criteria to be considered evidence-based practice for use with children with ASD (Hume et al., 2021; Steinbrenner et al., 2020). Unfortunately, research with adults with ASD remains weak and therefore specific evidence-based practices to use with adults with ASD have not yet been established (Howlin & Moss, 2012). The majority of the intervention strategies commonly employed with adults with ASD and IDD broadly fall into the category of applied behavior analytic interventions (Steinbrenner et al., 2020).

In its most general definition, applied behavior analysis (ABA) is the science of learning. It employs the principles of learning theory, including such concepts as reinforcement, shaping, chaining, punishment, and motivation, to increase socially significant behavior in clients (Cooper et al., 2020). In this way, the principles and procedures of ABA form the foundation for behavior therapy, an evidence-based practice. For a much more comprehensive and detailed review of ABA, the reader is referred to comprehensive texts such as Cooper et al. (2020) and Vargas (2020). Roth et al. (2014) conducted a meta-analysis of the literature on behavioral interventions used with adults with ASD. Out of 43 qualifying studies, strong positive effects were obtained for behavioral interventions used to increase academic skills (nonoverlap of all pairs [NAP] effect sizes ranging from 83.24 to 100), decrease phobic avoidance behaviors (NAP score of 100), and increase vocational skills (NAP scores ranging from 85.09 to 100). Medium effect sizes were noted for interventions addressing adaptive living skills (NAP scores ranging from 65.7 to 100), problem behavior (NAP scores ranging from 76.9 to 95), and social skills (NAP scores ranging from 59.9 to 100). True efficacy was difficult to determine, however, because 77% of the reviewed studies lacked a treatment integrity measure. This means it could not be determined whether the behavioral interventions were implemented as described. The specific behavioral interventions that showed efficacy included behavioral skills training, task

Box 17.1 Co-occurring Mental Health Conditions

Research indicates that adults with ASD and/or IDD are at an elevated risk of being diagnosed with co-occurring mental health conditions (Evans & Randle-Phillips, 2020; Hollocks et al., 2019; Lai et al., 2019). Prevalence estimates are difficult to determine and vary across studies (Levy & Perry, 2011); however it has been found that up to 70% of adults with ASD have a comorbid mental health diagnosis and over 40% have multiple comorbid mental health diagnoses (Lai et al., 2019). The prevalence of co-occurring mental health issues in IDD is estimated to be at 10–40% (Evans & Randle-Phillips, 2020). Co-occurring mental health issues are typically diagnosed early in adulthood, with the majority of mental health issues in adults with ASD diagnosed before age 30 (Levy & Perry, 2011). It is difficult to estimate the prevalence of co-occurring conditions because reports of behavioral changes are usually made by third parties instead of the person (Levy & Perry, 2011) and ASD characteristics can overshadow symptoms of other mental health conditions (Hollocks et al., 2019; Lai et al., 2019).

Out of all co-occurring mental health conditions, anxiety conditions, depression, and attention deficits show the highest rates of comorbidity with ASD in adults. In their systematic review, Hollocks et al. (2019) found that adults with ASD in their selected studies showed high comorbidities with anxiety disorders (27% current prevalence, 42% lifetime prevalence), depression (23% current prevalence, 37% lifetime), social anxiety (29% current prevalence, 20% lifetime), and obsessive-compulsive disorder (24% current prevalence, 22% lifetime). As a comparison, prevalence rates for anxiety conditions in the general population range from 1–12%, and for depression rates are reported to be approximately 7% of the general population (Hollocks et al., 2019). Attention-deficit /hyperactivity disorder has been found to the be most frequently occurring co-diagnosis in adults with ASD (Lugo-Marin et al., 2019). Elevations have also been seen with co-occurring Tourette's syndrome, epilepsy, bipolar disorder, and schizophrenia (Levy & Perry, 2011; Lai et al., 2019). Given the effects of diagnostic overshadowing and issues with third-party reporting of thoughts, feelings, and behaviors it is possible that these reported comorbidity prevalence rates are lower than the actual rates.

It is highly important to recognize and treat co-occurring mental health issues in adults with ASD and IDD. Higher than typical rates of co-occurring diagnoses may be the result of genetic vulnerabilities resulting from or correlating with their developmental disabilities, increased frequency of negative life events, increased exposure to abuse, awareness of their disability and how it affects their quality of life and social relationships, increased frequency of bullying in childhood, rejection from peers, and social communication deficits (Evans & Randle-Phillips, 2020; Lugo-Marin et al., 2019; Wigham et al., 2017). Left untreated, co-occurring mental health conditions lead to worsened long-term outcomes for adults with ASD. Co-occurring attention-deficit/hyperactivity disorder has been linked to increased impairments in adaptive living skills; co-occurring anxiety has been correlated with an exacerbation of ASD symptoms; and co-occurring depression has been associated with the presence of aggressive behavior, self injury, and oppositional behavior in adults with ASD (Lai et al., 2019). Activities of daily living such as eating, sleeping, and socialization can also be affected (Lugo-Marin et al., 2019). Frequent screening for mental health issues in adults with ASD and IDD as part of ongoing treatment is indicated.

analyses, prompting, video modeling, differential reinforcement, and role playing. NAP effect sizes ranged from 91.35 to 93.37, supporting efficacy (Roth et al., 2014).

Research has shown that adults with developmental disabilities, including IDD and ASD, display decreases in problem behavior and increases in reported quality of life when treated with behavioral interventions that are often incorporated into ABA (Gregori et al., 2020). As described in the next section, these interventions include behavioral skills training, video modeling, role playing, task analysis, prompting, differential reinforcing, and functional communication training. Other evidence-based practices, also described in the next section, include cognitive-behavioral therapy, social skills interventions, employment-based interventions, educational practices, and other psychosocial techniques (i.e., mindfulness therapies).

Credible Components of Treatments

Applied Behavior Analysis

Behavioral Skills Training

Behavioral skills training (BST) is an evidence-based behavioral teaching procedure consisting of four components: instructions, modeling, rehearsal, and feedback (Nuernberger et al., 2013). Training sessions start off by providing learners with clear instructions on the target behavior that they are expected to perform in a given situation. Instructions can be written, verbal, visual, or a combination of modalities. Instructors then provide a model of what is expected. This is followed by having the learners practice what was modeled while feedback is given by instructors. This is repeated until the skill is mastered under training conditions and then generalized to naturally occurring conditions. Nuernberger et al. (2013) demonstrated the effectiveness of BST by teaching three young adults with ASD to improve their social conversation skills. BST sessions were conducted for 10 minutes each session, 1–5 times per day over a 4-week period. Gains in conversation skills were still maintained 8 weeks post-training with BST. In a systematic review of BST literature related to skill acquisition in autistic children, Lucchesi (2022) found 24 studies that met her predetermined inclusion criteria. Using procedures from Reichow (2011), results indicated that BST reached the level of evidence-based practice for use with autistic children to teach skills including abduction prevention, gun safety, poison safety, street crossing, seeking help when lost, conversation skills, sports skills, daily living skills, and academics.

Video Modeling

Video modeling is an instructional procedure whereby learners are required to watch a video demonstrating a model engaging in a target behavior in a given situation. After video exposure, the learner is asked to perform the target skill under a simulated or real-life condition. Feedback on performance is given by the instructor and the entire procedure can be repeated as needed until the skill is mastered. Videos can depict the learner themselves engaging in the target behavior (self as model) or others engaging in the target behavior (other as model) (Park et al., 2019). Video modeling procedures have been used to teach a wide variety of target behaviors to children and adults with ASD and/or IDD. Bross et al. (2021) conducted a meta-analysis of video modeling with regard to interventions to improve job-related skills in autistic adults. In their review, 11 single-subject research studies met their inclusion criteria and were determined to be methodologically sound. To analyze effectiveness, 66 effect sizes were calculated from the data of 33 participants. Tau-U analyses were used to assess effect size. Across all 11 studies, an omnibus Tau-U of 0.91 (range 0.84–0.97) was obtained, indicating a very large magnitude of change across targets. Job-related targets included a variety of skills including, but not limited to, clerical activities, gardening, and food preparation. One relevant finding with regard to moderating variables is that effect sizes were found to be higher for ASD participants who did not have a comorbid diagnosis of IDD (Bross et al., 2021).

Role Playing

Role playing is a procedure whereby a learner is asked to perform a target skill, according to a pre-introduced script, within a simulated setting including actors playing the roles of persons within those settings. Feedback is provided by instructors either during or after the role play, and role plays continue until the skill is mastered in the simulated setting. The target behavior is then generalized to naturally occurring conditions. Role playing is often used as one of the components of BST. For example, through role playing within a BST intervention, Fisher et al. (2013) successfully taught five young adults with IDD to avoid lures from strangers by engaging in appropriate verbal and physical responses when approached. In their meta-analysis of safety skills interventions for children and adults with ASD, Wiseman et al. (2017) compared effect sizes across studies utilizing four different interventions: video modeling with or without rehearsal, live modeling with or without rehearsal, role play, and single error corrections procedure. The highest average Tau-U scores (all indicating large effect sizes) were obtained for studies utilizing role play as compared to other interventions.

Task Analysis

Task analysis is a breakdown of a complex task into its component parts. Component parts are taught individually and then linked together by behavioral chaining proced-ures so that the learner eventually masters the entire complex task (Cooper et al., 2020). In treatment, task analyses are often used in combination with other teaching techniques, such as video modeling, video prompting, differential reinforcement, and chaining. Task analyses have been shown to be an efficacious component of effective interventions in the teaching of a wide variety of skills in adults with ASD and/or IDD, including vocational skills, leisure skills, and activities of daily living (Roth et al., 2014). In their 2014 meta-analysis, Roth et al. reviewed outcome data for nine studies that included a task analysis as a treatment component. Eight of the nine studies had a level of research rigor to be considered "conclusive certainty of evidence" and had NAP effect size scores ranging from 86.4 to 100. Task analysis was also determined to be an evidence-based practice for children and adults with ASD according to a systematic review conducted by Hume et al. (2021). In their review, the authors found 13 single-subject design studies that met predetermined inclusion criteria, published between 1990 and 2017, that supported the use of interventions including task analysis as a component. Although rising to the level of evidence-based practice as per Hume et al. (2021) and Roth et al. (2014), it is important to note that task analysis is not a treatment by itself, but rather an efficacious component of treatment packages consisting of additional teaching techniques (i.e., video modeling, chaining, prompting, etc.)

Prompting

Prompting refers to the use of physical, gestural, verbal, or other forms of cues to guide a learner to engage in a correct response. As with task analyses, prompting is often used in combination with other behavioral teaching techniques and can be implemented in a least-to-most or most-to-least format with regard to intrusiveness level (Cooper et al., 2020). For example, a skill may be taught through gradually increasing the prompt level as needed from unintrusive verbal prompts (telling an individual how to do something) and modeling prompts (showing an individual how to do something) to more intrusive prompts such as full physical prompts (guiding an individual through a task using hand-over-hand physical manipulation). However, to best foster independence in a skill, an instructor may choose to gradually reduce the intrusiveness of the prompt level, starting off by ensuring a correct response with the most intrusive prompting level (i.e., full physical prompt), then reducing to a less intrusive prompt (i.e., gestural prompt), and ultimately fading the need for all prompts (independence).

Prompting has been used across a wide range of skill areas with both autistic adults and adults with intellectual deficits. Nepo et al. (2021) used a most-to-least prompt hierarchy to promote independent leisure engagement with an iPad in six adults with IDD and ASD between 34 and 45 years of age. Treatment consisted of prompting starting with full physical prompts, fading to gestural prompts, then to verbal prompts, and finally to independence without prompts. Verbal praise and tangible reinforcement were delivered contingent on independent completion of a skill. The research was conducted using a multiple-probe across participants, single-subject experimental design. Results showed attainment of skill independence for all participants as well as an increase in duration of leisure engagement (Nepo et al., 2021). In another example of the use of prompting, Vedora and Conant (2015) used both echoic prompts (verbal imitation) and textual prompts (written words) in the teaching of social question answering to three autistic young adults. Prompting was used along with verbal praise and edible reinforcement for correct responding. Results of an alternating treatments single-subject design indicated that both forms of prompting (echoic and textual) were successful in promoting independent question answering; however, the form that was most effective was individualized between participants (Vedora & Conant, 2015).

Differential Reinforcement

Differential reinforcement refers to a broad range of interventions in which reinforcement is provided for some behaviors, often within the same response class, while reinforcement is withheld for other behaviors (Cooper et al., 2020). Differential reinforcement procedures can be used to systematically increase or decrease target behaviors depending on which behaviors receive reinforcement (Cooper et al., 2020). For example, May and Catrone (2021) successfully taught three adults with Down Syndrome to reduce their pace of eating by using a differential reinforcement of low rate behavior reinforcement schedule. Participants were presented with a meal and a timer was used to identify inter-response times that would result in reinforcement. If a bite of food was taken after a predetermined interval, that response resulted in verbal praise. Tokens to be exchanged for preferred reinforcers were also provided contingent on successful inter-response times. Tokens were not provided when bites were taken before target inter-response times. Data, collected within a combination changing criterion and reversal design, showed improvement for all three participants. Differential reinforcement procedures can be implemented in isolation or can be included within part of a more comprehensive behavior intervention program. In their systematic review of differential reinforcement procedures, implemented without extinction, in the treatment of problem behavior in autistic adults, MacNaul and Neely (2018) reviewed 10 studies that met predetermined inclusion criteria. Out of the 10 studies, 9 were determined to show conclusive evidence as assessed by quality of research rigor and Tau-U effect sizes ranging from large (seven analyses), to medium (five analyses), to small (four analyses).

Functional Communication Training

Functional Communication Training (FCT) is another behavioral strategy that has shown to be an effective intervention for adults with autism and/or IDD. In an FCT intervention, a target challenging behavior is decreased through an assessment of the behavior's function followed by the introduction of a communication response that the learner can use in place of the target challenging behavior in order to get their wants and needs met. The new communicative response, which can be verbal, visual through pictures, electronically spoken, manually signed, and so forth, is taught through a differential reinforcement procedure (Cooper et al., 2020). In their systematic review of FCT intervention studies used with adults with ASD, Gregori et al. (2020) found that all reviewed studies demonstrated moderate or strong evidence of effectiveness. Decreases in targets were noted across a diverse group of participants and for a wide range of challenging behaviors.

Cognitive-Behavioral Therapy

In broad terms, cognitive-behavioral therapy is a short term, goal-oriented psychotherapy used to encourage change in the thought patterns and behaviors of individuals (Spain et al., 2015). The primary goal of CBT is to have a client understand the interrelation of their thoughts, behaviors, and emotions so that they can develop new ways of thinking about, coping with, and responding to challenging situations that they encounter (Spain et al., 2015). Falling into the realm of a talk therapy (Spain et al., 2015), effectively employing CBT techniques with individuals with challenges in communication and introspection (i.e., adults with ASD and/or IDD) can be problematic. Research indicates, however, that CBT may be appropriately used with adults with ASD if what is emphasized during therapy sessions is the development of behavioral coping and social strategies (Kiep et al., 2015). CBT has been shown to be effective in the treatment of obsessive-compulsive disorder comorbid with ASD in adults in both the short term and at 12-month follow up (Russell et al., 2013). In their systematic review of CBT and adults with ASD, Spain et al. (2015) found decreases in comorbid mental health symptoms in all reviewed studies. Six studies met the authors' predetermined inclusion criteria. Of these studies, two were randomized control trials, one was a quasi-experimental study, one was a group-based case series intervention, and the remaining two were case studies. All six studies passed a quality review before data were extracted for analysis. Interventions included in the studies consisted of various forms of CBT, such as exposure-based therapy, relaxation techniques, distraction techniques, restructuring of thoughts and beliefs, and psycho education. It is important, however, to note that some modifications to standard procedures were reported in order to effectively implement CBT procedures with autistic participants.

Due to communication deficits, introspection difficulties, theory of mind deficits, issues with cognitive flexibility, and weak central coherence, Spain et al. (2015) outlined modifications to traditional CBT procedures that may increase its effectiveness for adults with ASD. Suggested modifications include (1) using written and picture cues to enhance discussion and recall, (2) individualizing descriptions of emotions, (3) individualizing outcome measures, (4) teaching emotional literacy prior to initiating CBT, (5) emphasizing behavior change and skill development, and (6) relying less on a "talk therapy" style of sessions (Spain et al., 2015). These adaptations may also be useful when using CBT or other forms of talk therapy with individuals with IDD without ASD. There are also often difficulties with applying what is learned in therapy sessions to everyday situations, completing homework assignments, and in maintaining change over time (Evans & Randle-Phillips, 2020). Including family members and/or support workers in psychotherapy sessions may prove beneficial for these reasons.

Mindfulness-Based Therapy

Mindfulness interventions have been shown to improve mental health and wellness in adults both with and without ASD (Hartley et al., 2019). Effects have been displayed across a variety of physical and psychological conditions (Sizoo & Kuiper, 2017). In 2005, Kabat-Zinn defined mindfulness as the conscious awareness of oneself that arises by focusing thoughts and attention only on environmental stimuli that are present in the moment without judgment (Sizoo & Kuiper, 2017). The ability to engage in mindful thought is gained by working with a therapist on attention exercises within MBT sessions and practicing mindfulness outside of sessions through homework assignments (Sizoo & Kuiper, 2017). There are various forms of MBT that are seen in the literature with ASD; two examples are mindfulness-based stress reduction (MBSR) and mindfulness-based cognitive therapy (MBCT). In MBSR, symptoms of stress and anxiety are treated through procedures such as breathing exercises, meditation, identifying physical reactions to stress, listening exercises, dealing with persistent negative thoughts, and so forth. Therapists assist clients in implementing these procedures through structured therapy sessions, often scheduled once per week, in addition to homework assignments for practice outside of sessions. MBCT includes both the procedures used in MBSR along with the theories, procedures, and goals of traditional CBT (Hartley et al., 2019; Sizoo & Kuiper, 2017).

In their review of 10 independent studies in which MBT was used with children and adults with ASD, Hartley et al. (2019) found preliminary evidence to support its use with this population. Both short- and long-term improvements in measures of subjective well-being were obtained in the studies; however, effects on specific symptoms of ASD or mental health were not reported. Similar conclusions were reported by Cachia et al. (2016) in their systematic review of MBT in children and adults with ASD with and without IDD. Data from 161 participants across six studies that met inclusion criteria and quality review were analyzed. Of those 161 participants, 91 were adults. Results of the systematic review indicated that MBT is a potentially effective intervention that promotes psychological well-being in adults with ASD, including decreases in symptoms of anxiety, depression, and rumination along with increases in positive affect (Cachia et al., 2016). Kiep et al. (2015) employed MBT with 50 adults with ASD without IDD with the goal of treating symptoms of depression, anxiety, and rumination. A modified MBT protocol was utilized in order to increase the effectiveness of MBT procedures with an ASD population. Specifically, a focus on one's own thoughts was eliminated, metaphors and ambiguous terms were avoided, the length of treatment was extended by one week, and breathing exercises were extended from 3 to 5 minutes. The study consisted of 9 weekly sessions, of 2.5 hours each plus 40–60 minutes of at-home practice 6 days a week. Results indicated improvements in symptoms of anxiety, depression, agoraphobia, somatization, sleeping problems, rumination, positive affect, and measures of general physical and psychological well-being (Kiep et al., 2015). Future research on MBT should investigate the effects of MBT on specific mental health symptoms as well as on the core deficits of ASD through objective observation of behavior. The effectiveness of procedures when used with individuals with and without IDD should be explored so that modified protocols can be standardized as needed. Studies need to be designed and implemented with stronger research rigor so that the evidence-base of the effects of MBT with adults with ASD and/or IDD can be properly investigated.

Social Skills Interventions

Despite improvements in many areas over the course of development and education, adults with ASD often continue to struggle with social relationships and social competence. Social competence is a complex construct that refers to the ability to use social behaviors to successfully form relationships and achieve desired social goals while ensuring that behaviors are appropriate given ever-changing contexts (Ke et al., 2018). Interventions targeting social skills may improve outcomes for adults with ASD related to social-communication behaviors and increase engagement in social activities (Lorenc et al., 2018). Unfortunately, there are not many packaged social skills interventions that have reached the status of evidence-based practice for use with adults with ASD (Laugeson et al., 2015). Social skills training is typically conducted in group settings and relies on behavioral strategies based on social learning theory to shape new social behaviors in learners (Dubreucq et al., 2022). Specific treatment strategies often include goal setting, role modeling, behavioral rehearsal, positive reinforcement, corrective feedback, and homework assignments to promote generalization (Dubreucq et al., 2022). In their meta-analysis of 18 studies in which social skills training was implemented with adults with ASD without IDD, Dubreucq and colleagues (2022) found that individuals who received social skills training improved more on measures of social responsiveness than individuals who did not receive training. Of the 18 studies, four employed modified PEERS (Program for the Education and Enrichment of Relational Skills) interventions, two focused on social skills in vocational settings, and the remainder were individualized interventions using a variety of techniques and targets. The results of the meta-analysis reflected the treatment data of 145 adult participants with ASD. A positive effect size of 0.93 was obtained using a forest plot analysis of parent-reported social responsiveness after treatment. One caveat to note, however, is that the majority of included studies were found to be below accepted standards of research rigor. Studies were found to have small sample sizes, issues with randomization, missing comparison groups, and group allocation masking. The authors further suggested that the effects of social skills training may be enhanced if the training is conducted in contexts that facilitate practice: for example, directly in an office setting with coworkers if the treatment was designed to shape social skills in vocational settings, or in a park if the treatment was designed to shape social skills in a less structured setting. Although it is unlikely that any one social skills intervention strategy will show effectiveness with all adults with ASD (Ke et al., 2018), the PEERS program is showing some positive results (Laugeson et al., 2015). Originally developed for children aged 11–16 on the ASD spectrum, PEERS® is a small-group social skills intervention utilizing a combination of didactic lessons, role plays, behavioral rehearsal, coaching, parent facilitators, and homework assignments (McVey et al., 2016). Since 2009, research has shown the program to be efficacious with children with ASD (Gantman et al., 2012). The program focuses on the improvement of social skills associated with the making and maintenance of friendships. Specific skills taught in the PEERS® program include conversation, peer entry and exit, developing friendship networks, teasing, bullying, arguments, good sportsmanship, host behavior, and changing a bad reputation (McVey et al., 2016). The program has since been adapted for a young adult population. In their adaptation, Gantman and colleagues (2012) maintained the majority of the original PEERS® content and methods; however, some topics that were deemed not necessary for adult learners were removed, and other topics that were not in the children's version were added. Modules that were added included lessons on dating etiquette and handling peer pressure. Self-derived goals were used to increase motivation and treatment compliance. The PEERS® for Young Adults program, which has now been manualized, has shown efficacy with improving overall social skills in young adults, including increases in social responsiveness, increases in the frequency of social get-togethers, increases in social skills knowledge, and reported decreases in loneliness, restricted interests, and repetitive behaviors. These effects were demonstrated through independent randomized controlled trials (Gantman et al., 2012; Laugeson et al., 2015; McVey et al., 2016). Due to some limitations in the studies (e.g., lack of ASD-specific standardized outcome measures, lack of third-party raters, reliance on self-report measures, and small sample sizes), further research is required before the PEERS® for Young Adults can be considered an evidence-based practice; however, treatment results so far seem promising.

Employment-Related Interventions

Successfully maintained full- or part-time employment is often a primary goal of education and therapy. Unfortunately, data indicate that employment rates for adults with ASD and/or IDD are significantly less than for neurotypical adults and for adults with other developmental diagnoses (Almalky, 2020). Higher rates of unemployment in ASD, as compared to adults in other disability groups, have been found in the United States, the United Kingdom, Australia, and Canada (Hedley et al., 2017). Employment rates for adults with ASD vary between 10–50% (Nicholas et al., 2015) with between 50–70% of adults with ASD being unemployed (Jacob et al., 2015). Research data indicate that only 39% of adults with IDD are competitively employed eight years after high school graduation (Almalky, 2020). When employed, adults with ASD and/or IDD often work for significantly less pay and work fewer hours than do other adults (Nicholas et al., 2015; Almalky, 2020). Jobs are often held in occupations such as food preparation, cleaning, and maintenance, regardless of cognitive level (Seaman & Cannella-Malone, 2016). Including "underemployment," it is estimated that 90% of adults with ASD are not fully employed to their potential (Walsh et al., 2017).

These statistics are particularly alarming given the benefits to psychological and emotional well-being that being employed provides. Competitive employment allows an individual to be less dependent on others, increases friendships, boosts self-esteem, and improves overall quality of life (Nicholas et al., 2015). Employment has been found to correlate with an increased sense of purpose, meaning, independence, and identity for individuals with ASD (Jacob et al., 2015). Adults with IDD have reported that being gainfully employed reduces negative feelings associated with being disabled (Almalky, 2020).

Comprehensive employment training programs for adults with ASD and/or IDD are often separated into three general categories; sheltered workshop employment, supported employment, and customized employment. In a sheltered workshop model, individuals are placed in a segregated setting, often with a large number of individuals all working on similar tasks and all with similar developmental diagnoses. There are two types of sheltered workshop models. In a transitional sheltered workshop, employees of the workshop are expected to be there for only the length of time it takes to master skills needed for competitive employment in the community. Extended sheltered workshops, on the other hand, are more long-term employment placements (Almalky, 2020). In a supported employment model, a trained job coach is used to maintain an individual within a community-based job setting (Nicholas et al., 2015). Customized employment is a form of supported employment designed for adults who require additional individualization tailored to a person's strengths, interests, and preferences (Wehman et al., 2018). Both forms of integrated employment models – supported employment and customized employment – consist of four phases: (1) becoming familiar with the client, (2) matching the client to an appropriate job, (3) providing on-the-job training and support, and (4) job retention services (Wehman et al., 2018).

Although research studies are often limited by small participant numbers and vague outcome measures (Nicholas et al., 2015), there is evidence that indicates better outcomes for supported employment models over sheltered workshop models. With supported employment, adults with ASD were more likely to secure a job, to get a job with a higher salary, and to be able to choose from a wider variety of jobs than were adults who did not enroll in a supported employment program (Nicholas et al., 2015; Hedley et al., 2017). Although one purported purpose of the transitional sheltered workshop model is the ability to teach people skills needed to transition into community-based job settings, data indicate that there is no difference in employment outcome based on whether or not a person was first instructed in a sheltered workshop (Almalky, 2020). Customized employment has been found to result in employment positions with 30% more work hours per week and three times the amount of pay as compared to sheltered workshop outcomes (Almalky, 2020). Although supported employment programs are efficacious, there are, unfortunately, three times as many adults with ASD in sheltered workshops than in supported employment programs (Hedley et al., 2017).

One issue with the integrated employment models is the amount of training and expertise that is required. Agencies and staff must know how to assess learner choice, arrange for funding, identify potential jobs in the community, interact with parents, approach potential employers, help secure Social Security income benefit determinations, arrange transportation to and from job sites, and effectively train learners on all necessary job skills (Wehman et al., 2018). The success of supported employment programs relies on the skills of job coaches at both finding/ securing job placement and in providing one-on-one evidence-based training on the jobsite (Nicholas et al., 2015). With their focus on individualization, customized employment models require even higher levels of competence and flexibility on the part of the employment specialists and job coaches (Wehman et al., 2018). Unfortunately, these hurdles have resulted in segregated work settings (i.e., sheltered workshops) and nonwork day programs being used at an ever-increasing frequency as compared to more effective, integrated, and competitive employment programs (Wehman et al., 2018).

With any employment training program, successful employment outcome relies on the effectiveness of the teaching practices being used. Literature reviews have shown that there are various intervention strategies that are effective when teaching both vocational skills and "soft skills" to adults with ASD and/or IDD. Vocational skills are those skills that are necessary to hold a specific job, whereas soft skills are general social skills that are necessary for any job (organizational skills, conversation skills, time management, etc.). As with other skills, research has found that employment-related skills can be effectively learned through behavioral teaching techniques (Hedley et al., 2017) and that the effectiveness of job coaching can be enhanced with the use of media and technology (Nicholas et al., 2015). As outlined by Seaman and Cannella-Malone (2016), use of technology in employment training has several advantages. First, teaching sessions can be repeated for practice in the absence of the job coach if audio or video recordings were used for instruction. Second, the use of audio coaching through earphones allows a job coach to provide unintrusive and unnoticeable prompts to a learner in natural settings. Third, modern forms of technology are often cost effective and time efficient, and, fourth, using technology in employment training allows intervention to be conducted easily in natural employment settings. Through avoiding the need for simulated settings, this increases independence and generalization of learned skills.

Technological interventions that have been used successfully to enhance behavioral instruction include video modeling, audio cuing, video prompting, various mobile apps, and virtual reality (Walsh et al., 2017). In their review of the literature, Walsh and colleagues concluded that there is enough evidence for the overall use of technology-aided interventions to be considered probable evidence-based practice for teaching employment-related skills to adults with ASD; however, there is not yet enough research evidence to consider any one single intervention (video modeling, audio cuing, virtual reality, etc.) evidence-based for this purpose and population. Studies demonstrated the efficacy of technology-aided interventions across a wide variety of target skills, including specific vocational skills such as clerical skills, cleaning skills, and clothes folding, as well as soft skills such as time management, appropriate conversation skills, hygiene behaviors, reasoning skills, and decision-making (Walsh et al., 2017).

Approaches for Youth

Many of the interventions already discussed are also considered practices for use with children and adolescents with ASD and/or IDD. In fact, the majority of treatment research for people with ASD and/or IDD has been conducted with children. In their review of the literature on evidence-based practice for children with ASD five years of age and younger, Smith and Iadarola (2015) reviewed the effects of interventions based on the two predominant theories of autism intervention: applied behavior analysis (ABA) and developmental social-pragmatic (DSP) models. As discussed earlier in this chapter, ABA interventions are primarily based on the principles of operant conditioning, which postulates that behaviors that result in reinforcement will increase in future circumstances and behaviors that are not reinforced will decrease (Cooper et al., 2020). ABA interventions can be employed with children in both educational and therapeutic settings regardless of diagnosis. DSP interventions are based on the theory that communication, social, and behavioral issues in autistic children are the result of an impaired ability to engage jointly with other people from infancy (Smith & Iadarola, 2015). Interventions based on this theoretical model aim to treat autistic symptoms through initiating semistructured interactions that foster adult–child joint engagement. Data from their review indicate that both ABA and DSP interventions are showing some level of evidence, with individual comprehensive ABA (EIBI) and teacher-implemented ABA with DSP interventions being identified as "well-established" interventions (Smith & Iadarola, 2015). For listings of specific interventions that have been determined to be evidence-based practice for autistic youth, the reader is referred to Hume et al. (2021) and Steinbrenner et al. (2020).

Similar to treatment with children with ASD, interventions for children and adolescents with IDD typically focus on increasing adaptive and academic skills and decreasing problem behavior in order to allow for greater independence and improved overall quality of life. Educational and therapeutic interventions based on the principles of ABA are most frequently employed. Antecedent-based strategies (e.g., behavioral momentum, providing choices, using visual or auditory cues, etc.) as well as consequence-based strategies (e.g., differential reinforcement of appropriate responding, token economy systems, time out from reinforcement, etc.) have been found to have empirical support. Treatments should be based on objective assessments of need, generalized across settings, and parent involvement fostered (Scherr et al., 2018).

Other Variables Influencing Treatment

Assessment and Diagnosis

Both ASD and IDD are diagnosed through diagnostic criteria in the DSM-5-TR (APA, 2022). Although they are separate diagnoses, they can be codiagnosed by using the specifier "with accompanying intellectual impairment" under the ASD category. Standardized screening tools and diagnostic measures have been developed to assist diagnosticians in conducting diagnostics assessment for ASD. These instruments consist of interviews and direct observation measures that investigate the presence or absence of core ASD symptoms including social communicative deficits and restricted and repetitive patterns of behavior (Maye et al., 2017). Examples of ASD screening and diagnostic instruments include the Autism Diagnostic Interview-Revised (ADI-R; Lord et al., 1994), Autism Diagnostic Observation Schedule – Second Edition (ADOS-2; Lord et al., 2012), Childhood Autism Rating Scale – Second Edition (CARS2; Schopler et al., 2010), and the Modified Checklist for Autism in Toddlers, Revised with Follow up (M-CHAT-R/F; Robins & Fein, 2018). For a diagnosis of IDD, deficits in intellectual functions (i.e., reasoning, problem solving, abstract thinking, etc.) must be displayed through the results of a standardized test of intelligence in addition to deficits displayed in one or more activities of daily life across multiple contexts (APA, 2022).

Once a diagnosis is made, it is important to determine goals to be worked on within education and therapy. Goals are often developed through a multidisciplinary team approach, including parents/guardians where appropriate. Professionals on the team frequently consist of special education teachers, behavior analysts, speech therapists, residential service providers, nurses, psychologists, occupational therapists, physical therapists, social workers, vocational specialists, and nutritionists. Psychiatrists, primary care physicians, and medical specialists are often part of the team as needed.

Once treatment goals have been determined, it is important to conduct several other assessments to help guide treatment. When treating problem behavior, it is important to first conduct a functional behavior assessment to determine why the person is exhibiting the problem behavior. This is done by collecting and analyzing data on the antecedents (what happens before the behavior) and consequences (what happens after the behavior) in natural settings. Treatment plans are then tailored to the function of the problem behavior (Hanley & Slaton, 2019). Preference and reinforcer assessments are other forms of data-based assessment procedures that are used to guide instruction and treatment. Through these assessments, a person's likes and dislikes are determined through systematic presentations of various tangible items and activities. This is done so that items can be selected to be used as reinforcers (rewards) for behaviors that are targeted for increase in treatment (Cannella-Malone, 2020). It is also important to more broadly assess variables such as learning style, treatment history, environmental supports, and comorbid conditions when designing and implementing treatments for persons with ASD and IDD.

When treating people with ASD and IDD with comorbid mental health conditions, it is important to first diagnose the specific mental health conditions of concern and assess the severity levels of the conditions as well as assess progress over the course of treatment. Unfortunately, many assessment instruments used for treatment with an adult ASD population have been designed for different purposes than they are being used for or were validated only on a non-ASD population (Brugha et al., 2015). Therefore, there is a need for research into the development of mental health assessment instruments geared to this population (Lai et al., 2019).

Comorbidity

At the present time, there are no interventions that have been demonstrated to directly cure ASD or IDD in affected individuals. This relates to both children and adults. The majority of evidence-based interventions are designed to treat behavioral issues and skill deficits resulting from ASD and/or IDD or to treat emotional/behavioral issues associated with comorbid mental health conditions. It is therefore highly important to assess the presence of comorbid conditions, behavioral symptoms, and skill deficits when developing intervention strategies and choosing evidence-based treatments.

Medication

This lack of evidence-based psychotherapy practices with adults with ASD, as well as with IDD, may account for the high rate of pharmacological interventions used to treat behavioral issues in these populations (Howlin & Moss, 2012; Sheehan et al., 2015). It has been found that pharmacological interventions, especially anti-psychotic medications, are often prescribed to individuals with IDD in place of psychosocial interventions and in the absence of a diagnosed comorbid mental health condition (Sheehan et al., 2015). At the present time, there are no medications that have been found to directly cure ASD or IDD, although some medications (e.g., risperidone) have been found effective in reducing specific problem behavior associated with ASD/IDD such as aggression, self injury, and stereotypy. Although there are empirically supported pharmacological interventions for the treatment of mental health conditions in neurotypical adults (e.g., antidepressants, anti-anxiety medications), more research is needed on the use of pharmacological interventions for mental health conditions when comorbid with ASD and IDD. Medications are also frequently used to treat comorbid health conditions in adults with ASD and IDD (e.g., epilepsy, sleep disorders, gastrointestinal issues, etc.). Again, however, more research is needed on how pharmacological treatments for health-related conditions are affected by ASD/IDD.

Conclusion

Adults with ASD and/or IDD have a wide range of skills that can be taught and behaviors that can be treated with interventions that are showing promising levels of empirical support in the research literature. As with children with ASD and/or IDD, many of these interventions are consistent with applied behavior analytic philosophy and practice. Comorbid mental health concerns, which are frequent in this population, have been successfully treated with various cognitive-behavioral therapies, including the relatively recent introduction of mindfulness-based interventions. Unfortunately, the mental health needs of adults with ASD continue to go unmet due to a lack of therapist knowledge and expertise on ASD treatment, as well as a lack of knowledge on how to tailor evidence-based mental health practices to this population (Lipinski et al., 2022). Long-term outcomes have been improved through the use of comprehensive social skills interventions as well as employment training programs. Although much has been done, there is still much to do. More high-quality research is required to establish a range of evidence-based comprehensive and focused treatments to improve the quality of life of adults with ASD and/or IDD.

Useful Resources

Books

- Pennington R. C. (2019). *Applied behavior analysis for everyone: Principles and practices explained by applied researchers who use them.* AAPC Publishing.
- Cooper, J., Heron, T., & Heward, W. (2020). *Applied Behavior Analysis* (3rd ed.). Pearson/ Merrill-Prentice-Hall.
- Vargas J. S. (2020). *Behavior analysis for effective teaching.* Routledge.
- Volkmar, F. R., Rogers, S. J., Paul, R., & Pelphrey, K. A. (2014). *Handbook of autism and pervasive developmental disorders* (4th ed.) John Wiley & Sons.

Websites

- American Association on Intellectual and Developmental Disabilities: www.aaidd.org/home
- Association for Behavior Analysis International: www.abainternational.org
- Association for Behavioral and Cognitive Therapies: www.abct.org/
- Association for Professional Behavior Analysts: www.apbahome.net/
- Association for Science in Autism Treatment: https://asatonline.org/
- Autism Speaks: www.autismspeaks.org/
- Behavior Analyst Leadership Council: https://balcllc.org/
- Cambridge Center for Behavioral Studies: https://behavior.org/
- Different Roads: https://difflearn.com/
- Diverse-City Press: https://diverse-city.com/
- Organization for Autism Research: https://researchautism.org/

References

Almalky, H. A. (2020). Employment outcomes for individuals with intellectual and developmental disabilities: A literature review. *Children and Youth Services Review*, 109, 1–10. https://doi.org/10.1016/j.childyouth.2019.104656.

American Psychiatric Association. (2022). *Diagnostic and statistical manual of mental disorders* (5th ed., text revision). https://doi.org/10.1176/appi.books.9780890425596.

Bailey, A., Le Couteur, A., Gottesman, I., et al. (1995). Autism as a strongly genetic disorder: evidence from a British twin study. *Psychological Medicine*, 25(1), 63–78.

Bhaumik, S., Gangadharan, S., Hiremath, A., & Russell, P. S. S. (2011). Psychological treatments in intellectual disability: The challenges of building a good evidence base. *The British Journal of Psychiatry*, 198(6), 428–430.

Bross, L. A., Travers, J. C., Huffman, J. M., Davis, J. L., & Mason, R. A. (2021). A meta-analysis of video modeling interventions to enhance job skills of autistic adolescents and adults. *Autism in Adulthood : Challenges and Management*, 3(4), 356–369. https://doi.org/10.1089/ aut.2020.0038.

Brugha, T. S., Doos, L., Tempier, A., Einfeld, S., & Howlin, P. (2015). Outcome measures in intervention trials for adults with autism spectrum disorders: A systematic review of assessments of core autism features and associated emotional and behavioural problems. *International Journal of Methods in Psychiatric Research*, 24(2), 99–115. https://doi.org/10.1002/mpr.1466.

Brugha, T. S., Spiers, N., Bankart, J., et al. (2016). Epidemiology of autism in adults across age groups and ability levels. *The British Journal of Psychiatry: The Journal of Mental Science*, 209(6), 498–503. https://doi.org/10.1192/bjp.bp.115.174649.

Cachia, R., Anderson, A., & Moore, D. (2016). Mindfulness in individuals with autism spectrum disorder: A systematic review and narrative analysis. *Review Journal of Autism and Developmental Disorders*, 3(2), 165–178. https://doi.org/10.1007/s40489-016-0074-0.

Canella-Malone, H. (2019). Assessing preferences. In R. C. Pennington (Ed.), *Applied behavior for everyone* (pp. 98–107). AAPC Publishing.

Cannella-Malone, H. I., & Sabielny, L. M. (2020). Preference assessments, choice, and quality of life for people with significant disabilities. *Choice, preference, and disability: Promoting self-determination across the lifespan*, 195–206.

Cooper, J. O., Heron, T. E., & Heward, W. L. (2020). *Applied behavior analysis* (3rd ed.). Pearson Education, Inc.

Dietz, P. M., Rose, C. E., McArthur, D., & Maenner, M. (2020). National and state estimates of adults with autism spectrum disorder. *Journal of Autism & Developmental Disorders*, 50(12), 4258–4266. https://doi.org/10.1007/s10803-020-04494-4.

Dubreucq, J., Haesebaert, F., Plasse, J., Dubreucq, M., & Franck, N. (2022). A Systematic review and meta-analysis of social skills training for adults with autism spectrum disorder. *Journal of Autism and Developmental Disorders*, 52(4), 1598–1609. https://doi.org/10.1007/s10803-021-05058-w.

Eack, S. M., Hogarty, S. S., Greenwald, D. P., et al. (2018). Cognitive enhancement therapy for adult autism spectrum disorder: Results of an 18-month randomized clinical trial. *Autism Research*, 11(3), 519–530. https://doi.org/10.1002/aur.1913.

Evans, L., & Randle-Phillips, C. (2020). People with intellectual disabilities' experiences of psychological therapy: A systematic review and meta-ethnography. *Journal of Intellectual Disabilities*, 24(2), 233–252.

Fisher, M. H., Burke, M. M., & Griffin, M. M. (2013). Teaching young adults with disabilities to respond appropriately to lures from strangers. *Journal of Applied Behavior Analysis*, 46(2), 528–533. https://doi.org/10.1002/jaba.32.

Gantman, A., Kapp, S. K., Orenski, K., & Laugeson, E. A. (2012). Social skills training for young adults with high-functioning autism spectrum disorders: A randomized controlled pilot study. *Journal of Autism and Developmental Disorders*, 42(6), 1094–1103. https://doi.org/10.1007/SI0803-011-1350-6.

Gregori, E., Wendt, O., Gerow, S., et al. (2020). Functional communication training for adults with autism spectrum disorder: A systematic review and quality appraisal. *Journal of Behavioral Education*, 29(1), 42–63. https://doi.org/10.1007/s10864-019-09339-4.

Hanley, G. M. & Slaton, J. (2019). Practical functional assessment of problem behavior. In R. C. Pennington (Ed.), *Applied behavior analysis for everyone* (pp. 75–97). AAPC Publishing.

Hartley, M., Dorstyn, D., & Due, C. (2019). Mindfulness for children and adults with autism spectrum disorder and their caregivers: A meta-analysis. *Journal of Autism and Developmental Disorders*, 49(10), 4306–4319. https://doi.org/10.1007/s10803-019-04145-3.

Hedley, D., Uljarević, M., Cameron, L., et al. (2017). Employment programmes and interventions targeting adults with autism spectrum disorder: A systematic review of the literature. *Autism: The International Journal of Research and Practice*, 21(8), 929–941. https://doi.org/10.1177/1362361316661855.

Hollocks, M. J., Lerh, J. W., Magiati, I., Meiser-Stedman, R., & Brugha, T. S. (2019). Anxiety and depression in adults with autism spectrum disorder: A systematic review and meta-analysis. *Psychological Medicine*, 49(4), 559–572. https://doi.org/10.1017/S0033291718002283.

Horner, R. H., Carr, E. G., Halle, J., et al. (2005). The use of single-subject research to identify evidence-based practice in special education. *Exceptional Children*, 71(2), 165–179. https://doi.org/10.1177/001440290507100203.

Howlin, P., & Moss, P. (2012). Adults with autism spectrum disorders. Canadian Journal of Psychiatry. *Revue Canadienne de Psychiatrie*, 57(5), 275–283. https://doi.org/10.1177/070674371205700502.

Huang, J., Zhu, T., Qu, Y., & Mu, D. (2016). Prenatal, perinatal and neonatal risk factors for intellectual disability: A systemic review and meta-analysis. *PloS One*, 11(4), 1–12. https://doi.org/10.1371/journal.pone.0153655.

Hume, K., Steinbrenner, J. R., Odom, S. L., et al. (2021). Evidence-based practices for children, youth, and young adults with autism: Third generation review. *Journal of Autism and Developmental Disorders*, 51(11), 4013–4032. doi:10.1007/s10803-020-04844-2.

Jacob, A., Scott, M., Falkmer, M., & Falkmer, T. (2015). The costs and benefits of employing an adult with autism spectrum disorder: A systematic review. *PLoS ONE*, 10(10), 1–15. https://doi.org/10.1371/journal.pone.0139896.

Kabat-Zinn, J. (2005). *Coming to our senses: Healing ourselves and the world through mindfulness*. Hachette UK.

Ke, F., Whalon, K., & Yun, J. (2018). Social skill interventions for youth and adults with autism spectrum disorder: A systematic review. *Review of Educational Research*, 88(1), 3–42.

Kiep, M., Spek, A. A., & Hoeben, L. (2015). Mindfulness-based therapy in adults with an autism spectrum disorder: Do treatment effects last? *Mindfulness*, 6(3), 637–644. https://doi.org/10.1007/s12671-014-0299-x.

Lai, M.-C., Kassee, C., Besney, R., et al. (2019). Prevalence of co-occurring mental health diagnoses in the autism population: a systematic review and meta-analysis. *The Lancet Psychiatry*, 6(10), 819–829. https://doi.org/10.1016/S2215-0366(19)30289-5.

Laugeson, E., Gantman, A., Kapp, S., Orenski, K., & Ellingsen, R. (2015). A randomized controlled trial to improve social skills in young adults with autism spectrum disorder: The UCLA PEERS Program. *Journal of Autism & Developmental Disorders*, 45(12), 3978–3989. https://doi.org/10.1007/s10803-015-2504-8.

Levy, A., & Perry, A. (2011). Outcomes in adolescents and adults with autism: A review of the literature. *Research in Autism Spectrum Disorders*, 5(4), 1271–1282. https://doi.org/10.1016/j.rasd.2011.01.023.

Lipinski, S., Boegl, K., Blanke, E. S., Suenkel, U., & Dziobek, I. (2022). A blind spot in mental healthcare? Psychotherapists lack education and expertise for the support of adults on the autism spectrum. *Autism: The International Journal of Research and Practice*, 26(6), 1509–1521. https://doi.org/10.1177/13623613211057973.

Lord, C., Rutter, M., & Le Couteur, A. (1994). Autism Diagnostic Interview-Revised: A revised version of a diagnostic interview for caregivers of individuals with possible pervasive developmental disorders. *Journal of Autism and Developmental Disorders*, 24(5), 659–685. https://doi.org/10.1007/bf02172145.

Lord., C., Rutter, M., DiLavore, P. C., et al. (2012). *Autism Diagnostic Observation Schedule: ADOS-2*. Western Psychological Services.

Lorenc, T., Rodgers, M., Marshall, D., et al. (2018). Support for adults with autism spectrum disorder without intellectual impairment: Systematic review. *Autism: The International Journal of Research and Practice*, 22(6), 654–668.

Lovaas, O. I. (1987). Behavioral treatment and normal educational and intellectual functioning in young autistic children. *Journal of Consulting and Clinical Psychology*, 55(1), 3.

Lucchesi, K. E. (2022). The effects of behavioral skills training on skill acquisition in autistic children: A systematic review. eRepository @ Seton Hall, Master's thesis. https://scholarship.shu.edu/cgi/viewcontent.cgi?article=4117&context=dissertations.

Lugo-Marín, J., Magán-Maganto, M., Rivero-Santana, A., et al. (2019). Prevalence of psychiatric disorders in adults with autism spectrum disorder: A systematic review and meta-analysis. *Research in Autism Spectrum Disorders*, 59, 22–33. https://doi.org/10.1016/j.rasd.2018.12.004.

Lyall, K., Croen, L., Daniels, J., et al. (2017). The changing epidemiology of autism spectrum disorders. *Annual Review of Public Health*, 38, 81–102. https://doi.org/10.1146/annurev-publhealth-031816-044318.

MacNaul, H. L. & Neely, L. C. (2018). Systematic review of differential reinforcement of alternative behavior without extinction for individuals with autism. *Behavior Modification*, 42(3), 398–421. https://doi.org/10.1177/0145445517740321.

Maenner, M. J., Shaw, K. A., Bakian, A. V., et al. (2021). Prevalence and characteristics of autism spectrum disorder among children aged 8 years – Autism and developmental disabilities monitoring network, 11 Sites, United States, 2018. *Morbidity and Mortality Weekly Report. Surveillance Summaries (Washington, D.C.: 2002)*, 70(11), 1–16. https://doi.org/10.15585/mmwr.ss7011a1.

May, B. K., & Catrone, R. (2021). Reducing rapid eating in adults with Down syndrome: Using token reinforcement to increase interresponse time between bites. *Behavior Analysis: Research and Practice*, 21(3), 273–281. https://doi.org/10.1037/bar0000213

Maye, M. P., Kiss, I. G., & Carter, A. S. (2017). Definitions and classification of autism spectrum disorders. In D. Zager, D. F. Cihak, & A. Stone-MacDonald (Eds.), *Autism spectrum disorders: Identification, education, and treatment.*, 4th ed. (pp. 1–22). Routledge/Taylor & Francis Group.

McKenzie, K., Milton, M., Smith, G., & Ouellette-Kuntz, H. (2016). Systematic review of the prevalence and incidence of intellectual disabilities: Current trends and issues. *Current Developmental Disorders Reports*, 3(2), 104–115.

McVey, A., Dolan, B., Willar, K., et al. (2016). A replication and extension of the PEERS® for Young Adults Social Skills Intervention: Examining effects on social skills and social anxiety in young adults with autism spectrum disorder. *Journal of Autism & Developmental Disorders*, 46(12), 3739–3754. https://doi.org/10.1007/s10803-016-2911-5.

Nepo, K., Tincani, M., & Axelrod, S. (2021). Teaching mobile device-based leisure to adults with autism spectrum disorder and intellectual disability. *Focus on Autism & Other Developmental Disabilities*, 36(2), 83–94. https://doi.org/10.1177/1088357620943500.

Nicholas, D. B., Attridge, M., Zwaigenbaum, L., & Clarke, M. (2015). Vocational support approaches in autism spectrum disorder: A synthesis review of the literature. *Autism: The International Journal of Research and Practice*, 19(2), 235–245.

Nuernberger, J. E., Ringdahl, J. E., Vargo, K. K., Crumpecker, A. C., & Gunnarsson, K. F. (2013). Using a behavioral skills training package to teach conversation skills to young adults with autism spectrum disorders. *Research in Autism Spectrum Disorders*, 7(2), 411–417. https://doi.org/10.1016/j.rasd.2012.09.004.

Park, J., Bouck, E., & Duenas, A. (2019). The Effect of video modeling and video prompting interventions on individuals with intellectual disability: A systematic literature review. *Journal of Special Education Technology*, 34(1), 3–16.

Patel, D. R., Apple, R., Kanungo, S., & Akkal, A. (2018). Intellectual disability: Definitions, evaluation and principles of treatment. *Pediatric Medicine*, 1, 11.

Pedersen, A. L., Pettygrove, S., Lu, Z., et al. (2017). DSM criteria that best differentiate intellectual disability from autism spectrum disorder. *Child Psychiatry and Human Development*, 48(4), 537. https://doi.org/10.1007/s10578-016-0681-0.

Reichow, B. (2011). Development, procedures, and application of the evaluative method for determining evidence-based practices in autism. In B. Reichow, P. Doehring, D. V. Cicchetti & F. R. Volkmar (Eds.), *Evidence-based practices and treatments for children with autism* (pp. 25–39). Springer Science + Business Media. https://doi.org/10.1007/978-1-4419-6975-0_2.

Robins, D. L., & Fein, D. (2018). *Modified checklist for autism in toddlers, revised, with follow-up (M-CHAT-R/ F), also M-CHAT*. Springer International Publishing. https://doi.org/10.1007/978-3-319-57111-9_1569.

Roth, M. E., Gillis, J. M., & DiGennaro Reed, F. D. (2014). A meta-analysis of behavioral interventions for adolescents and adults with autism spectrum disorders. *Journal of Behavioral Education*, 23(2), 258–286. https://doi.org/10.1007/s10864-013-9189-x.

Russell, A. J., Jassi, A., Fullana, M. A., et al. (2013). Cognitive behavior therapy for comorbid obsessive-compulsive disorder in high-functioning autism spectrum disorders: A randomized controlled trial. *Depression and Anxiety*, 30(8), 697–708. https://doi.org/10.1002/da.22053.

Saad, M. A. E., & ElAdl, A. M. (2019). Defining and determining intellectual disability (intellectual developmental disorder): Insights from DSM-5. *International Journal of Psych-Educational Sciences*, 8(1), 51–54.

Schalock, R. L., Gomez, L. E., Verdugo, M. A., & Claes, C. (2017). Evidence and evidence-based practices: Are we there yet? *Intellectual and Developmental Disabilities*, 55(2), 112–119. https://doi.org/10.1352/1934-9556-55.2.112.

Scherr, J. F., Kryszak, E. M., & Mulick, J. A. (2018). Intellectual and adaptive functioning. In S. Hupp (Ed.), *Child and adolescent psychotherapy: Components of evidence-based treatments for youth and their parents.* (pp. 12–29). Cambridge University Press.

Schopler, E., Mesibov, G. B., & Hearsey, K. (1995). Structured teaching in the TEACCH system. *Learning and Cognition in Autism*, 243–268.

Schopler, E., Van Bourgondien, M., Wellman, J., & Love, S. (2010). *Childhood autism rating scale – Second Edition (CARS2): Manual*. Western Psychological Services.

Seaman, R. L., & Cannella-Malone, H. I. (2016). Vocational skills interventions for adults with autism spectrum disorder: A review of the literature. *Journal of Developmental and Physical Disabilities*, 28(3), 479–494. https://doi.org/10.1007/s10882-016-9479-z.

Sheehan, R., Hassiotis, A., Walters, K., et al. (2015). Mental illness, challenging behaviour, and psychotropic drug prescribing in people with intellectual disability: UK population based cohort study. *British Medical Journal*, 351, 1–9. https://doi.org/10.1136/bmj.h4326.

Sizoo, B. B., & Kuiper, E. (2017). Cognitive behavioural therapy and mindfulness based stress reduction may be equally effective in reducing anxiety and depression in adults with autism spectrum disorders. *Research in Developmental Disabilities*, 64, 47–55. https://doi.org/10.1016/j.ridd.2017.03.004.

Smith, T., & Iadarola, S. (2015). Evidence base update for autism spectrum disorder. *Journal of Clinical Child and Adolescent Psychology*, 44(6), 897–922. https://doi.org/10.1080/15374416.2015.1077448.

Smith, T., & Lovaas, I. O. (1998). Intensive and early behavioral intervention with autism: The UCLA young autism project. *Infants & Young Children*, 10(3), 67–78.

Spain, D., Sin, J., Chalder, T., Murphy, D., & Happé, F. (2015). Cognitive behaviour therapy for adults with autism spectrum disorders and psychiatric co-morbidity: A review. *Research in Autism Spectrum Disorders*, 9, 151–162. https://doi.org/10.1016/j.rasd.2014.10.019.

Steinbrenner, J. R., Hume, K., Odom, S. L., et al. (2020). Evidence-based practices for children, youth, and young adults with autism. Report. The University of North Carolina at Chapel Hill, Frank Porter Graham Child Development Institute, National Clearinghouse on Autism Evidence and Practice Review Team. https://fpg.unc.edu/publications/evidence-based-practices-children-youth-and-young-adults-autism-spectrum-disorder-1.

Vargas, J. (2020). *Behavior analysis for effective teaching* (3rd ed.). Routledge.

Vedora, J., & Conant, E. (2015). A comparison of prompting tactics for teaching intraverbals to young adults with autism. *The Analysis of Verbal Behavior*, 31(2), 267–276. https://doi.org/10.1007/s40616-015-0030-6.

Vereenooghe, L., & Langdon, P. E. (2013). Psychological therapies for people with intellectual disabilities: A systematic review and meta-analysis. *Research in Developmental Disabilities*, 34(11), 4085–4102. https://doi.org/10.1016/j.ridd.2013.08.030.

Walsh, E., Holloway, J., McCoy, A., & Lydon, H. (2017). Technology-aided interventions for employment skills in adults with autism spectrum disorder: A systematic review. *Review Journal of Autism and Developmental Disorders*, 4(1), 12–25. https://doi.org/10.1007/s40489-016-0093-x

Wehman, P., Taylor, J., Brooke, V., et al. (2018). Toward competitive employment for persons with intellectual and developmental disabilities: What progress have we made and where do we need to go? *Research & Practice for Persons with Severe Disabilities*, 43(3), 131–144. https://doi.org/10.1177/1540796918777730.

Wigham, S., Barton, S., Parr, J. R., & Rodgers, J. (2017). A systematic review of the rates of depression in children and adults with high-functioning autism spectrum disorder. *Journal of Mental Health Research in Intellectual Disabilities*, 10(4), 267–287.

Wiseman, K. V., McArdell, L. E., Bottini, S. B., & Gillis, J. M. (2017). A meta-analysis of safety skill interventions for children, adolescents, and young adults with autism spectrum disorder. *Review Journal of Autism and Developmental Disorders*, 4(1), 39–49. https://doi.org/10.1007/s40489-016-0096-7.

Wong, C., Odom, S. L., Hume, K. A., et al. (2015). Evidence-based practices for children, youth, and young adults with autism spectrum disorder: A comprehensive review. *Journal of Autism and Developmental Disorders*, 45(7), 1951–1966. https://doi.org/10.1007/s10803-014-2351-z.

Yoon, S. H., Choi, J., Lee, W. J., & Do, J. T. (2020). Genetic and epigenetic etiology underlying autism spectrum disorder. *Journal of Clinical Medicine*, 9(4), 966–993. https://doi.org/10.3390/jcm9040966.

18

Attention-Deficit/Hyperactivity Disorder

Mary V. Solanto

Attention-deficit/hyperactivity disorder (ADHD) is a neurodevelopmental disorder which is usually first apparent in childhood, and, as described in the DSM-5-TR, is characterized by high levels of inattention, hyperactivity-impulsivity, or both (American Psychiatric Association, 2022). Once thought to be limited to childhood, longitudinal outcome studies confirmed that impairing symptoms persist to adulthood in approximately 60% of childhood cases (Faraone et al., 2015), although more recent research has identified variable patterns of remission in adulthood (Sibley et al., 2021). Longitudinal and cross-sectional studies have documented significant impairment in virtually every domain of functioning – academic, occupational, social and emotional – for adults with ADHD (Barkley et al., 2006), as well as high rates of comorbid mood, anxiety, and substance abuse disorders (Kessler et al., 2006).

Etiology and Theoretical Underpinnings of Treatment

Although the etiology of ADHD is not fully understood, the primary cause appears to be genetic, as evidenced by markedly higher rates of concordance for ADHD in monozygotic versus dizygotic twin pairs (Fitzallen et al., 2023), and identification of genetic variants that increase risk for ADHD (Agnew-Blais et al., 2021; Demontis et al., 2019). The neuro-pathophysiology appears to predominantly reside in attentional networks and involves under-activation of the dorsolateral prefrontal cortex, which is important for executive function, as well as under-activation of subcortical reward centers important for sustained motivation, as revealed by fMRI studies (Faraone et al., 2015).

Executive dysfunction is a primary mediator of impairment in ADHD across functional domains and age groups (Barkley, 2012). Given its substantial correlation with educational and occupational impairment (Barkley & Fischer, 2011), executive dysfunction has been the primary target of cognitive-behavioral intervention for adult ADHD (Young et al., 2016). The goal of CBT for ADHD is to help the individual to develop behavioral and cognitive strategies to counteract or compensate for deficits in executive self-management in specific contexts, and with respect to specific goals, problems, and tasks. A positive synergy evolves such that improvements in cognitive self-instruction generate improvements in behavioral self-management, which in turn generate more adaptive and self-enhancing cognitions,

Other interventions, such as dialectical behavior therapy (DBT) and mindfulness-based CBT, have targeted a broad array of other ADHD-related difficulties, including emotional dysregulation, impulsivity, comorbid internalizing symptoms, and social function, as well as the core difficulties related to inattention.

Brief Overview of Treatments

Cognitive-Behavioral Therapy

CBT programs that target executive dysfunction in ADHD aim to impart both behavioral and cognitive skills and strategies to facilitate time management, organization, and planning. Behavioral aids and corresponding habits include consistent use of a planner (agenda), systems to organize digital and paper files, a flow-chart to aid in planning, and removal of distractors (e.g., cell phones) from the workspace. Cognitive strategies are conveyed and rehearsed in the form of self-instructional "rules" to guide daily scheduling, prioritizing, and self-activation These programs typically also incorporate cognitive reframing to target negative automatic beliefs that generate demoralization, anxiety, and perfectionism (Beck, 1995). Generalization and maintenance of treatment gains are facilitated through intensive practice within the sessions and at home via the at-home exercises, as well as through positive reinforcement and support from the therapist and group members.

Following upon successful open trials of CBT to enhance executive function, Safren et al. (2010) and Solanto et al. (2010) each conducted randomized controlled trials to test the efficacy of individual and group-based CBT interventions, respectively. These studies employed an active control ("psychological placebo") for the nonspecific effects of CBT (relaxation therapy and a support group, respectively). The sample size for each study was ample at 86 and 88 patients, respectively, who were randomized to CBT or to the active control group. Results showed that the effect sizes for the active treatment, as assessed by independent evaluators on structured interviews of ADHD symptoms, were moderate at 0.52 and 0.58, respectively (standardized mean difference). Responder rates to CBT were, depending on the outcome measure, 53–67% (Safren et al., 2010) and 42–53% (Solanto et al., 2010).

The importance of an active control condition in clinical trials of therapies for ADHD was underscored by the results of a meta-analysis by Young and colleagues (2016) that reported that the effect size for five studies that lacked an adequate control for CBT was substantially larger (0.76) than for four studies that included an appropriate active control condition (0.43).

On the basis of findings such as those described here, CBT for ADHD has been designated a *well-established* intervention by Division 12 (Clinical Psychology) of the American Psychological Association (https://div12.org/treatment/cognitive-behavioral-therapy-for-adult-adhd/).

Dialectical Behavior Therapy

There are commonalities between ADHD and borderline personality disorder (Ditrich et al., 2021) with respect to impulsive behavior, emotional dysregulation (Beheshti et al., 2020), relationship problems (Wymbs et al., 2021), and low self-esteem (Harpin et al., 2016). DBT, originally designed to treat borderline personality disorder, aims to increase emotional and cognitive self-regulation by increasing awareness of the triggers that lead to reactive states, and by facilitating the application of coping skills to avoid undesired reactions. In addition to emotion regulation, DBT includes skills to increase tolerance of distress, increase mindfulness to counteract inattention, and improve interpersonal relations.

DBT has been adapted to address the specific needs of adults with ADHD. Following upon the positive pre- to posttreatment results of an open trial of DBT in 72 participants (Philipsen et al., 2007), Philipsen and colleagues (2015) randomized 419 adults with ADHD to 1 of 4 12-week treatment alternatives: adapted group DBT, combined with either methylphenidate or placebo, or clinical management (CM) which included supportive counseling and was also combined with either methylphenidate or placebo. The design thus included active controls in the form of a placebo for methylphenidate and CM for DBT. Treatment was comprised of psychoeducation, behavioral analysis, emotional regulation, and mindfulness. The range of topics, each of which was addressed during one of the 13 weekly 2-hour sessions, was broad and included the neurobiology of ADHD, disorganization, emotional regulation, depression, impulse control, stress, addictive behaviors, and relationships. Results revealed no differences between DBT and CM on the Conners' Adult ADHD Rating Scales (CAARS) self-report measure of ADHD symptoms, either at three months or at one-year follow-up. By contrast, participants who received methylphenidate experienced reduced ADHD symptoms compared to those receiving placebo, regardless of whether they also received DBT or CM.

A more recent RCT of 121 adults reported that DBT group treatment was more effective than treatment-as-usual in improving executive function on the Behavior Rating Inventory of Executive Function – Adult Form (BRIEF-A) (Halmoy et al., 2022). However, there was no active control for DBT, and change in ADHD symptoms was not measured. It may be the case that although DBT is well-conceptualized as a potential intervention for ADHD, the very multiplicity of topics addressed in the context of only 13 weekly sessions militates against the efficacy of any one target of the intervention, necessitating a longer period of intervention.

Box 18.1 Effects on Co-occurring Conditions

An important question for clinicians is whether CBT affects co-occurring conditions, especially anxiety and depression, which, as described, are common comorbidities in adults with ADHD (Kessler et al., 2006). The results of a recent meta-analysis (Lopez-Pinar et al., 2020) have been enlightening in this regard. This meta-analysis included 20 randomized controlled trials of CBT, of which 5 had active controls and 12 had uncontrolled pre-test/post-test comparisons. CBT significantly improved anxiety and depression symptoms, as well as quality of life and emotional dysregulation. Furthermore, these changes were predicted by the reduction in ADHD symptoms, suggesting a cause–effect relationship. However, treatment was significantly less effective for depression and anxiety outcomes when compared with active controls, suggesting that remediation of internalizing symptoms is a nonspecific result of therapy.

Credible Components of Treatments

Tolin and colleagues (2015) observed that while recent intervention research has adduced empirical clinical support for the efficacy of treatment "packages" with manualized protocols, there has been little investigation of the active principles of change that underlie these treatments, and little testing of the efficacy of the individual components (i.e., dismantling studies). Although the efficacy of the individual components of CBT for ADHD have not been determined, it is possible to delineate these components and to generate hypotheses regarding their mechanisms of action. Illustrations of specific strategies are taken from the published CBT treatment protocol for therapists, developed by Solanto (2011).

The Centrality of Learning Theory

Like other cognitive and behavioral interventions, CBT is grounded in learning theory, particularly operant conditioning: namely, that behaviors that are rewarded/reinforced will increase in frequency (Beck, 1995). In cognitive-behavioral interventions, that reinforcement comes initially from the therapist who describes to the patient the rewards which will be available contingent upon shifting to a more effective behavior. As the patients begin to test out an adaptive behavior, and they experience the positive results, the new behaviors become self-reinforcing and ultimately autonomous. Group therapy adds therapeutic elements – specifically, the opportunity for positive modeling and vicarious reinforcement of successful strategies. Support and encouragement from other group members provide additional opportunities for positive reinforcement of adaptive behavior changes. In some programs (Solanto, 2011), self-reinforcement (i.e., planned access to discrete preferred activities) upon completion of aversive, boring, or unpleasant tasks is explicitly guided and encouraged via a home exercise as an early strategy in the program.

Time Estimation

Multiple studies have shown that adults with ADHD have deficits in time perception, including time estimation and time awareness, which may represent a fundamental substrate of dysfunction in ADHD, and may be mediated by anomalies in the cerebellum (Barkley et al., 2001). Difficulty estimating how long things take, and poor awareness of the passage of time, will obviously impair planning and will inhibit efforts to adjust one's pace according to situational demands. An exercise in the CBT group protocol is intended to increase time awareness and improve time estimation by having participants estimate how long they believe certain routine tasks and activities at home or at the office require (e.g., getting ready to leave the house in the morning, cleaning up after dinner, producing a given type of report at work) and then actually timing those activities to assess the accuracy of estimation. It is conjectured that repeated exercises of this type will improve time perception, but there is virtually no research literature on the effectiveness of this or any intervention to improve time perception in adults with ADHD.

Temporal Discounting

A major problem for most people with ADHD is the tendency to avoid or delay the initiation or completion of tasks that are perceived as effortful, difficult, and/or lacking in stimulation or gratification. So, for example, a college student with ADHD may succumb to the desire to go out partying with friends on a given night rather than stay home to study for an upcoming test. This tendency, which may be conceptualized as the preference for smaller sooner over larger delayed rewards, is otherwise known as "temporal discounting," and has been demonstrated in both children and adults with ADHD (Jackson & MacKillop, 2016) when they make choices between smaller and larger rewards at different time delays on computerized laboratory measures. Repeated over thousands of iterations across the lifespan and exhibited in the workplace as well as in school, this tendency may account for the lessened success of many individuals with ADHD both academically and occupationally, as documented in the longitudinal outcome studies. A strategy to counteract this tendency is to increase the salience of the distant reward in order to motivate the individual to pursue that larger/more important reward (e.g., a better grade on the test or in the course) in preference to immediately available rewards.

In the group CBT program (Solanto, 2011), this goal is pursued by having the participant actively "fast-forward" and envision, as vividly as possible, the tangible and intangible rewards that will accompany the distant goal. In the laboratory, an analogous process, termed "Episodic Future Thinking" (EFT), in which the individual is instructed to imagine the rewards associated with achievement of the larger delayed reward, has been shown to reduce temporal discounting (Scholten et al., 2019) and would appear to be a good candidate for evaluation of "real-world" clinical effectiveness in ADHD. Early in the CBT program this approach is applied to the goal of helping participants cease engrossing late-night activities (the "immediate" reinforcers) and get to bed early enough to get adequate sleep, thereby avoiding fatigue, grogginess, and lateness to school or work the next day, which are chronic difficulties for many with ADHD.

Prioritizing and Planning

Awareness of and attention to important future events is also facilitated by the use of several aids incorporated into the program. These include plotting tasks and activities on a 2×2 (i.e., urgency × importance) matrix, in which "urgent" items are those which are time-sensitive, with no implications for their importance. Regular use of the matrix, included in the session on prioritization, is intended to help the individual weigh the benefits of future "important" gains (e.g., a possible promotion at the office for working overtime on a project) against the appeal of more immediate ("urgent") gratifications (e.g., watching TV all evening instead).

Use of a flow-chart is incorporated into the module on planning as a visual aid to planning a complex task or project. Completion of the chart facilitates identification of all the steps that must be executed to complete the project, their sequence, and the anticipated time which must be allocated for each in order to complete the entire project by a given deadline.

Self-Instruction via "Mantras"

Throughout treatment, patients are helped to develop self-instructive cognitions which cue the application of adaptive strategies. Some of these are crystallized as aphorisms or "mantras" which are repeated strategically throughout treatment in the hope that they will be internalized as automatic guides to behavior and thereby serve to facilitate generalization and maintenance of adaptive strategies. One of these is "If it's not in the planner, it doesn't exist," meaning that unless appointments and (especially) tasks are entered into the planner, they are unlikely to be accomplished. Another mantra is, "If I am having trouble getting started (i.e., procrastinating), then the first step is too big," which is the cue to chunk a difficult or aversive task/activity into more manageable parts. This mantra also takes advantage of "if–then" thinking which cues both the problem situation and an appropriate solution. Research has demonstrated that administration of methylphenidate and the use of if–then planning equivalently improved inhibition of an unwanted response on a "Go/NoGo" task, and increased the P300 attending response on EEG (Paul-Jordanov et al., 2010). The strategy of chunking itself, and the verbally encoded aids to facilitate it, represent good targets for future dismantling research.

Cognitive Reframing

As also included in the programs developed by Ramsay and Rostain (2014), the programs by Safren et al. (2005) and Solanto (2011) included sessions on identifying and debunking or reframing automatic negative thoughts such as those reflecting "overgeneralization," "disqualifying the positive," "all-or-none thinking," "personalization," and "catastrophizing." Such thoughts generate anxiety and depression, and serve to inhibit positive changes in behavior. It would be of interest to test the incremental efficacy of this approach when included with the behavioral strategies described earlier.

Mindfulness

Mindfulness, which is described as purposeful, nonjudgmental attention to the present moment, is developed through meditation and other practices. In the teaching of mindfulness, an individual is guided to become aware of incoming thoughts, feelings, and sensations, to observe and accept them without judgment, and then to disengage from them (Kabat-Zinn, 1996). Originally inspired by teachings from the East, training in mindfulness has been applied to relieve patient stress, anxiety, pain, and other problems. Mindfulness-based cognitive therapy (MBCT) combines the clinical application of mindfulness training with elements of cognitive-behavioral intervention, such as cognitive reframing, and showed early promise as an intervention to improve focus for people with ADHD (Househam & Solanto, 2016). Zylowska and colleagues (2008) reported the results of an open trial of an 8-week program of mindfulness meditation with 24 adults and 8 adolescents, which showed improvement on self-report ratings of ADHD symptoms, depression, and anxiety, as well as increased performance on cognitive tests of attention and impulse control. The results of more recent research, however, have been mixed. Positive findings have been reported in comparison with treatment-as-usual (Janssen et al., 2019; Mitchell et al., 2017) but not when compared with an active control condition (Bachmann et al., 2018; Hoxhaj et al., 2018).

Approaches for Youth

The most effective form of psychosocial therapy for children with ADHD is behavior therapy, which focuses upon the child's overt behaviors rather than their thoughts/cognitions. Behavior therapy is grounded in learning theory, principally operant conditioning. The well-established types of behavior therapy for youth with

ADHD include behavioral classroom management, behavior parent training, and behavioral peer interventions (Evans et al., 2014). Organizational training is also well established (Abikoff et al., 2013). These approaches involve the systematic manipulation, primarily by parents and teachers, of the antecedents and consequences of targeted behaviors, with positive reinforcement for desired behaviors and time-out, loss of privileges, or penalties for negative behaviors.

Over the 50 years since its introduction, an extensive literature has documented the effectiveness of behavior therapy (Fabiano et al., 2009). The landmark NIMH-sponsored MTA study (Multi-modal Treatment of ADHD) found that although behavior therapy was less effective than stimulant medication (MTA Cooperative Group, 1999), it added to the benefit of medication for some outcomes (Swanson et al., 2001), notably parent–child conflict, academic difficulties, and anxiety. More recently, Sonuga-Barke and colleagues (2013) conducted a meta-analysis of 14 randomized controlled trials of behavior therapy and reported that inclusion of studies involving both "probably blinded" and "unblinded" raters yielded a significant effect size of 0.40–0.64 (moderate) for core symptoms of ADHD, whereas limiting the analysis to those trials (k=7) which were "probably blinded" reduced the effect of the treatment to insignificance. However, a follow-up meta-analysis of the same set of studies (Daley et al., 2014) found that effects were significant for other outcomes (parenting quality, conduct problems, academic performance, and social skills) in studies involving probably blinded and unblinded raters, whether considered separately or together.

Other Variables Influencing Treatment

Assessment and Diagnosis

Moderating effects of clinical variables on response to psychotherapy for adult ADHD have generally not been investigated. Solanto et al. (2010) found no moderating effect on response to treatment on the basis of ADHD subtype or concurrent medication for ADHD. In that study, however, severity of self-rated (but not clinician-rated) inattentive ADHD symptoms at baseline predicted a better response to treatment on self-reported (but not clinician-rated) ADHD symptoms. That study also reported that within the CBT group, the number of completed Home Exercises was a significant positive predictor of reduction in posttreatment clinician-rated inattentive symptoms.

Comorbidity

No studies have reported that presence of comorbid anxiety or depression was a predictor of response to CBT. Rather, as referenced earlier, there is evidence indicating that CBT has a salutary effect on comorbid anxiety or depression.

Demographics

Patient demographic variables have been insufficiently examined as potential moderators of treatment outcome. Solanto et al. (2010) found no effect of gender, race, education, household income, marital status, employment status, or IQ on outcome of treatment. Age had no moderating effect when examined as a continuous variable. However, in a subsequent study (Solanto et al., 2018) in which the same sample was dichotomized into subgroups of individuals 50 years of age or older and those less than 50, it was found that the older group responded as well to CBT as did the younger patients. Interestingly, they responded to support as well as they did to CBT, demonstrating a better response to support than did the younger group of patients.

Medication

Consistent with the conceptualization of ADHD as a brain-based condition, stimulant medication has been shown to be highly effective and is considered the drug class of choice for treatment of the core attentional and impulsive symptoms of ADHD. However, response rates in adults are lower than they are in children (Cortese, 2020), and it is apparent that additional, nonpharmacological interventions are needed to address the executive dysfunction, emotional dysregulation, impulsivity, relationship problems, comorbid anxiety and depression, and low self-esteem which persist among adults with ADHD, even after stimulant medication is optimally titrated.

An important issue for clinicians, therefore, is whether CBT augments the benefit of medication to treat ADHD, and, conversely, whether medication augments the benefit of CBT. In the absence of a fully crossed 2 × 2 design, in which adults with ADHD are randomly assigned to receive either CBT or an active control therapy, combined with either medication or placebo, we must rely on studies that have conducted these comparisons separately.

Does CBT add to the benefit of medication? Five studies have assessed the benefits of adding CBT to medication, with four studies reporting positive results (Emilsson et al., 2011; Pan et al., 2022; Wettstein et al., 2021; Young et al., 2015) and one study reporting negative results (Corbisiero et al., 2018). None of these five studies included an active control for CBT, however, so these results must be viewed as tentative, and more research is needed.

Medication clearly added to the benefit of CBT in one controlled, adequately powered study (Cherkasova et al., 2020) in which adults with ADHD were randomized to receive CBT + stimulant medication (n=42) or CBT + placebo (n=46). Medication was individually titrated and optimized. Results were superior for the CBT + medication group with respect to ADHD symptoms, organizational skills, and self-esteem. An earlier study (Weiss et al., 2012) had reported that medication did *not* add to the benefits of CBT – that is, the effects of CBT alone and CBT + medication were not significantly different. Yet another result, reported by Pan et al. (2019) was that CBT + medication (n=57) was not superior to CBT alone (n=67) in improving ADHD symptoms, emotional symptoms, or social functional outcomes, but was more effective with respect to executive function. However, this study was not a randomized trial. Patients in the CBT + medication group had been titrated and stabilized on medication in the clinic before the study began, and were then asked to participate in a study of CBT. Thus, poor or nonresponders to medication may have self-selected to receive additional treatment with CBT. In the study by Cherkasova and colleagues (2020), by contrast, patients were randomly assigned to treatment conditions and titration was initiated within the study proper. Insufficiently explored is whether CBT and medication each target different clinical outcomes, which might be predicted given their differing mechanisms of action.

Conclusion

Although stimulant medication is broadly effective in reducing core symptoms of ADHD, other therapies are needed to address commonly co-occurring conditions in adults, including executive dysfunction, emotional dysregulation, comorbid internalizing disorders, and social difficulties. CBT primarily targets executive dysfunction, and appears to fully meet criteria as a well-established intervention by the APA Division 12. By contrast, a large-scale well-designed study of DBT (Philipsen et al., 2015) which addressed a broad array of accompanying conditions, including emotional dysregulation, impulse control, stress, addictive behaviors, and social relationships, performed no better than "clinical management," suggesting that over-inclusion of treatment targets militates against the successful treatment of any one dysfunction. Positive results have been reported for mindfulness when compared to treatment-as-usual, but not when compared to an active control condition.

CBT for ADHD has yet to be fully evaluated against the criteria delineated by Tolin et al. (2015) for an empirically supported treatment (EST). Treatment and patient variables yet to be fully addressed include: the long-term maintenance of treatment gains, effectiveness in "real-world" contexts with demographically and clinically diverse samples, and dismantling to identify the efficacy and mechanisms of action of individual treatment components. All in all, however, with continued research and refinement, CBT has the potential to substantially improve the functioning of adults with ADHD in multiple domains.

Useful Resources

Books For Therapists

- Ramsay, J. R., & Rostain, A. L. (Eds.). (2014). *Cognitive-Behavioral Therapy for Adult ADHD: An Integrative Psychosocial and Medical Approach* (2nd ed.). Routledge.
- Safren, S. A., Sprich, S., Perlman, C., & Otto, M. (2005). *Mastering Your Adult ADHD: A Cognitive-Behavioral Treatment Program (Therapist Workbook).* Oxford University Press.
- Solanto, M. V. (2011). *Cognitive-Behavioral Therapy for Adult ADHD: Targeting Executive Dysfunction.* Guilford Press.

For Patients

- Safren, S. A., Sprich, S., Perlman, C., & Otto, M. (2005). *Mastering Your Adult ADHD: A Cognitive-Behavioral Treatment Program (Client Workbook).* Oxford University Press.
- Surman, C., Bilkley, T., & Weintraub, K. (2014). *Fast Minds: How to Thrive If You Have ADHD (Or Think You Might).* Penguin Publishing Group.
- Tuckman, A. (2009). *More Attention, Less Deficit: Success Strategies for Adults with ADHD.* Specialty Press/ADD Warehouse.
- Zylowska, L. (2012). *The Mindfulness Prescription for Adult ADHD: An 8-Step Program for Strengthening Attention, Managing Emotions, and Achieving Your Goals*: Shambhala Press.

References

Abikoff, H., Gallagher, R., Wells, K. C., et al. (2013). Remediating organizational functioning in children with ADHD: Immediate and long-term effects from a randomized controlled trial. *Journal of Consulting and Clinical Psychology*, 81(1), 113–128.

Agnew-Blais, J. C., Belsky, D. W., Caspi, A., et al. (2021). Polygenic risk and the course of attention-deficit/hyperactivity disorder from childhood to young adulthood: Findings from a nationally-representative cohort. *Journal of Clinical Child & Adolescent Psychology*, 60(9), P1147–56. https://doi.org/10.1016/j.jaac.2020.12.033.

American Psychiatric Association. (2013). *Diagnostic and statistical manual of mental disorders* (5th ed.). American Psychiatric Publishing.

Bachmann, K., Lam, A. P., Soros, P., et al. (2018). Effects of mindfulness and psychoeducation on working memory in adult ADHD: A randomised, controlled fMRI study. *Behaviour Research and Therapy*, 106, 47–56. https://doi.org/10.1016/j.brat.2018.05.002.

Barkley, R. A. (2012). *Executive functions: What they are, how they work, and why they evolved.* Guilford.

Barkley, R. A., & Fischer, M. (2011). Predicting impairment in major life activities and occupational functioning in hyperactive children as adults: Self-reported executive function (EF) deficits vs. EF tests. *Developmental Neuropsychology*, 36(2), 137–161.

Barkley, R. A., Fischer, M., Smallish, L., & Fletcher, K. (2006). Young adult outcome of hyperactive children: Adaptive functioning in major life areas. *Journal of the American Academy of Child and Adolescent Psychiatry*, 45, 192–202.

Barkley, R. A., Murphy, K. R., & Bush, T. (2001). Time perception and reproduction in young adults with attention deficit hyperactivity disorder. *Neuropsychology*, 15, 351–360.

Beck, J. S. (1995). *Cognitive therapy: Basics and beyond*. Guilford Press.

Beheshti, A., Chavanon, M. L., & Christiansen, H. (2020). Emotion dysregulation in adults with attention deficit hyperactivity disorder: a meta-analysis. *BMC Psychiatry*, 20(1), 120. https://doi.org/10.1186/s12888-020-2442-7.

Cherkasova, M. V., French, L. R., Syer, C. A., et al. (2020). Efficacy of cognitive behavioral therapy with and without medication for adults with ADHD: A randomized clinical trial. *Jornal of Attention Disorders*, 24(6), 889–903. https://doi.org/10.1177/1087054716671197.

Corbisiero, S., Bitto, H., Newark, P., et al. (2018). A comparison of cognitive-behavioral therapy and pharmacotherapy vs. pharmacotherapy alone in adults with attention-deficit/hyperactivity disorder (ADHD): A randomized controlled trial. *Frontiers in Psychiatry*, 9, 571. https://doi.org/10.3389/fpsyt.2018.00571.

Cortese, S. (2020). Pharmacologic treatment of attention deficit-hyperactivity disorder. *New England Journal of Medicine*, 383(11), 1050–1056. https://doi.org/10.1056/NEJMra1917069.

Daley, D., van der Oord, S., Ferrin, M., et al. (2014). Behavioral interventions in attention-deficit/ hyperactivity disorder: A meta-analysis of randomized controlled trials across multiple outcome domains. *Journal of the American Academy of Child & Adolescent Psychiatry*, 53(8), 835–847, 847.e831–835. https://doi.org/10.1016/j.jaac.2014.05.013.

Demontis, D., Walters, R. K., Martin, J., et al. (2019). Discovery of the first genome-wide significant risk loci for attention deficit/hyperactivity disorder. *Nature Genetics*, 51(1), 63–75. https://doi.org/10.1038/s41588-018-0269-7.

Ditrich, I., Philipsen, A., & Matthies, S. (2021). Borderline personality disorder (BPD) and attention deficit hyperactivity disorder (ADHD) revisited: A review-update on common grounds and subtle distinctions. *Borderline Personal Disorder and Emotion Dysregulation*, 8(1), 22. https://doi.org/10.1186/s40479-021-00162-w.

Emilsson, B., Gudjonsson, G., Sigurdsson, J. F., et al. (2011). Cognitive behaviour therapy in medication-treated adults with ADHD and persistent symptoms: A randomized controlled trial. *BMC Psychiatry*, 11, 116. https://doi.org/10.1186/1471-244x-11-116.

Evans, S. W., Owens, J. S., & Bunford, N. (2014). Evidence-based psychosocial treatments for children and adolescents with attention-deficit/hyperactivity disorder. *Journal of Clinical Child and Adolescent Psychology*, 43(4), 527–551. https://doi.org/10.1080/15374416.2013.850700.

Fabiano, G. A., Pelham, W. E., Jr., Coles, E. K., et al. (2009). A meta-analysis of behavioral treatments for attention-deficit/hyperactivity disorder. *Clinical Psychology Review*, 29(2), 129–140. https://doi.org/10.1016/j.cpr.2008.11.001.

Faraone, S. V., Asherson, P., Banaschewski, T., et al. (2015). Attention-deficit/hyperactivity disorder. *Nature Reviews Disease Primers*, 1, 15020. https://doi.org/10.1038/nrdp.2015.20.

Fitzallen, G. C., Taylor, H. G., Liley, H. G., & Bora, S. (2023). Within- and between-twin comparisons of risk for childhood behavioral difficulties after preterm birth. *European Society for Paediatric Research*. https://doi.org/10.1038/s41390-023-02579-1.

Halmoy, A., Ring, A. E., Gjestad, R., et al. (2022). Dialectical behavioral therapy-based group treatment versus treatment as usual for adults with attention-deficit hyperactivity disorder: A multicenter randomized controlled trial. *BMC Psychiatry*, 22(1), 738. https://doi.org/10.1186/s12888-022-04356-6.

Harpin, V., Mazzone, L., Raynaud, J. P., Kahle, J., & Hodgkins, P. (2016). Long-term outcomes of ADHD: A systematic review of self-esteem and social function. *Journal of Attention Disorders*, 20(4), 295–305. https://doi.org/10.1177/1087054713486516.

Househam, A., & Solanto, M. (2016). Mindfulness as an intervention for ADHD. *The ADHD Report*, 24, 1–9.

Hoxhaj, E., Sadohara, C., Borel, P., et al. (2018). Mindfulness vs psychoeducation in adult ADHD: A randomized controlled trial. *European Archives of Psychiatry and Clinical Neuroscience*, 268(4), 321–335. https://doi.org/10.1007/s00406-018-0868-4.

Jackson, J. N., & MacKillop, J. (2016). Attention-Deficit/Hyperactivity Disorder and Monetary Delay Discounting: A Meta-Analysis of Case-Control Studies. *Yonsei Medical Journal*, 1(4), 316–325. https://doi.org/10.1016/j.bpsc.2016.01.007.

Janssen, L., Kan, C. C., Carpentier, P. J., et al. (2019). Mindfulness-based cognitive therapy v. treatment as usual in adults with ADHD: A multicentre, single-blind, randomised controlled trial. *Psychological Medicine*, 49(1), 55–65. https://doi.org/10.1017/s0033291718000429.

Kabat-Zinn, J. (1996). *Full catastrophe living: How to cope with stress, pain and illness using mindfulness meditation*. Piatkus.

Kessler, R. C., Adler, L. A., Barkley, R. A., et al. (2006). The prevalence and correlates of adult ADHD in the United States: Results from the national comorbidity survey replication. *American Journal of Psychiatry*, 163(4), 716–723.

Lopez-Pinar, C., Martinez-Sanchis, S., Carbonell-Vaya, E., Sanchez-Meca, J., & Fenollar-Cortes, J. (2020). Efficacy of nonpharmacological treatments on comorbid internalizing symptoms of adults with attention-deficit/hyperactivity disorder: A meta-analytic review. *Journal of Attention Disorders*, 24(3), 456–478. https://doi.org/10.1177/1087054719855685.

Mitchell, J. T., McIntyre, E. M., English, J. S., et al. (2017). A pilot trial of mindfulness meditation training for ADHD in adulthood: Impact on core symptoms, executive functioning, and emotion dysregulation. *Journal of Attention Disorders*, 21(13), 1105–1120. https://doi.org/10.1177/1087054713513328.

MTA Cooperative Group. (1999). A 14-month randomized clinical trial of treatment strategies for Attention-Deficit/Hyperactivity Disorder. *Archives of General Psychiatry*, 56, 1073–1086.

Pan, M. R., Huang, F., Zhao, M. J., et al. (2019). A comparison of efficacy between cognitive behavioral therapy (CBT) and CBT combined with medication in adults with attention-deficit/hyperactivity disorder (ADHD). *Psychiatry Research*, 279, 23–33. https://doi.org/10.1016/j.psychres.2019.06.040.

Pan, M. R., Zhang, S. Y., Qiu, et al. (2022). Efficacy of cognitive behavioural therapy in medicated adults with attention-deficit/hyperactivity disorder in multiple dimensions: A randomised controlled trial. *European Archives of Psychiatry and Clinical Neuroscience*, 272(2), 235–255. https://doi.org/10.1007/s00406-021-01236-0.

Paul-Jordanov, I., Bechtold, M., & Gawrilow, C. (2010). Methylphenidate and if-then plans are comparable in modulating the P300 and increasing response inhibition in children with ADHD. *Attention Deficit Hyperactivity Disorder*, 2(3), 115–126. https://doi.org/10.1007/s12402-010-0028-9.

Philipsen, A., Jans, T., Graf, E., et al. (2015). Effects of group psychotherapy, individual counseling, methylphenidate, and placebo in the treatment of adult attention-deficit/hyperactivity disorder: A randomized clinical trial. *JAMA Psychiatry*, 72(12), 1199–1210. https://doi.org/10.1001/jamapsychiatry.2015.2146.

Philipsen, A., Richter, H., Peters, J., et al. (2007). Structured group psychotherapy in adults with attention deficit hyperactivity disorder: Results of an open multicentre study. *Journal of Nervous and Mental Disease*, 195(12), 1013–1019.

Ramsay, J. R., & Rostain, A. L. (Eds.). (2014). *Cognitive-behavioral therapy for adult ADHD: An integrative psychosocial and medical approach* (2nd ed.). Routledge.

Safren, S. A., Sprich, S., Mimiaga, M. J., et al. (2010). Cognitive behavioral therapy vs. relaxation with educational support for medication-treated adults with ADHD and persistent symptoms: A randomized controlled trial. *Journal of the American Medical Association*, 304(8), 875–880.

Safren, S. A., Sprich, S., Perlman, C., & Otto, M. (2005). *Mastering your adult ADHD: A cognitive-behavioral treatment program (TherapistWorkbook)*. Oxford University Press.

Scholten, H., Scheres, A., de Water, E., Graf, U., Granic, I., & Luijten, M. (2019). Behavioral trainings and manipulations to reduce delay discounting: A systematic review. *Psychon Bull Rev*, 26(6), 1803–1849. https://doi.org/10.3758/s13423-019-01629-2.

Sibley, M. H., Arnold, L. E., Swanson, J. M., et al. (2021). Variable patterns of remission from ADHD in the multimodal treatment study of ADHD. *American Journal of Psychiatry*. https://doi.org/10.1176/appi.ajp.2021.21010032.

Solanto, M. V. (2011). *Cognitive-Behavioral Therapy for Adult ADHD: Targeting Executive Dysfunction*. Guilford Press.

Solanto, M. V., Marks, D. J., Wasserstein, J., et al. (2010). Efficacy of meta-cognitive therapy for adult ADHD. *American Journal of Psychiatry*, 167(8), 958–968. https://doi.org/10.1176/appi.ajp.2009.09081123.

Solanto, M. V., Surman, C. B., & Alvir, J. M. J. (2018). The efficacy of cognitive-behavioral therapy for older adults with ADHD: A randomized controlled trial. *Attention Deficit Hyperactivity Disorder*, 10(3), 223–235. https://doi.org/10.1007/s12402-018-0253-1.

Sonuga-Barke, E. J., Brandeis, D., Cortese, S., et al. (2013). Nonpharmacological interventions for ADHD: Systematic review and meta-analyses of randomized controlled trials of dietary and psychological treatments. *American Journal of Psychiatry*, 170(3), 275–289. https://doi.org/10.1176/appi.ajp.2012.12070991.

Swanson, J. M., Kraemer, H. C., Hinshaw, S. P., et al. (2001). Clinical relevance of the primary findings of the MTA: Success rates based on severity of ADHD and ODD symptoms at the end of treatment. *Journal of the American Academy of Child & Adolescent Psychiatry*, 40(2), 168–79.

Tolin, D. F., McKay, K. E., Evan, E. M., Klonsky, E. D., & Thomba, B. D. (2015). Empirically supported treatment: Recommendations for a new model. *Clinical Psychology: Science and Practice*, 22, 317–38.

Weiss, M., Murray, C., Wasdell, M., et al. (2012). A randomized controlled trial of CBT therapy for adults with ADHD with and without medication. *BMC Psychiatry*, 12, 30. https://doi.org/10.1186/1471-244X-12-30.

Wettstein, R., Klabbers, Y., Romijn, E., et al. (2021). Cognitieve gedragstherapie bij medica-menteuze behandeling van ADHD bij volwassenen [Cognitive behavioral therapy in combination with pharmacotherapy for adults with ADHD]. *Tijdschrift voor psychiatrie*, 63(7), 550–556. www.ncbi.nlm.nih.gov/pubmed/34523707.

Wymbs, B. T., Canu, W. B., Sacchetti, G. M., & Ranson, L. (2021). Adult ADHD and romantic relationships: What we know and what we can do to help. *Journal of Marital and Family Therapy*, 47(3), 664–681. https://doi.org/10.1111/jmft.12475.

Young, S., Khondoker, M., Emilsson, B., et al. (2015). Cognitive-behavioural therapy in medication-treated adults with attention-deficit/hyperactivity disorder and co-morbid psychopathology: A randomized controlled trial using multi-level analysis. *Psychological Medicine*, 45(13), 2793–2804. https://doi.org/10.1017/S0033291715000756.

Young, Z., Moghaddam, N., & Tickle, A. (2016). The efficacy of cognitive behavioral therapy for adults with ADHD: A systematic review and meta-analysis of randomized controlled trials. *Journal of Attention Disorders*. https://doi.org/10.1177/1087054716664413.

Zylowska, L., Ackerman, D. L., Yang, M. H., et al. (2008). Mindfulness meditation training in adults and adolescents with ADHD: A feasibility study. *Journal of Attention Disorders*, 11(6), 737–746.

19

Tic Disorders

Kirsten Bootes, Emily Braley, and Michael B. Himle

Tics are sudden, rapid, recurrent, nonrhythmic movements and/or vocalizations (i.e., motor and vocal tics; APA, 2022) that fall along a continuum of complexity ranging from simple to complex. Simple tics are brief, purposeless movements involving a small number of discrete muscle groups (e.g., blinking, head-jerking) or the production of brief, meaningless sounds (e.g., sniffing, snorting, chirping). Complex tics have a more purposeful and sustained appearance and involve orchestrated patterns of movement or elaborate vocalizations that mimic goal-directed actions or speech (e.g., patterned touching and tapping, shouting of words or phrases, echo- and coprophenomena). Diagnostically, there are three primary, hierarchically arranged, tic disorder (TD) diagnoses that are differentiated by the types of tics present (i.e., motor, vocal, or both) and the duration of symptoms since initial onset (APA, 2022). Tourette's disorder involves multiple motor and at least one vocal tic that have been present for at least one year. Persistent motor or vocal tic disorder involves single or multiple motor or vocal tics (but not both) that have been present for at least one year. Finally, provisional tic disorder involves single or multiple motor and/or vocal tics that have been present for less than one year. In all three cases, diagnosis requires that tics begin prior to 18 years of age and that they are not attributable to the physiological effects of a substance or another medical condition. Subjectively, most individuals with TDs report that their tics are preceded by unpleasant somatic sensations, referred to as premonitory urges, that are typically described as an uncomfortable feeling localized to the area of the tic or a vague sense that something is "just not right" in the body. Most individuals report that their premonitory urges worsen when they attempt to suppress their tics and that they are temporarily alleviated when the tic is performed (Kwak et al., 2003).

The clinical course of TDs is highly variable; however, tics typically first emerge in early childhood, take a notable waxing and waning course, spontaneously change in appearance over time, and reach peak severity in early adolescence. In approximately 50–75% of cases, tics significantly improve by early adulthood (Bloch & Leckman, 2009). For those for whom tics persist into adulthood, they can be a source of significant distress, discrimination, impairment, and reduced quality of life (Conelea et al., 2013). Adult-onset tics are relatively rare, and in most cases are secondary to substance exposure, an identifiable medical condition, or adult re-emergence of childhood tics (Jankovic et al., 2010). Epidemiological studies have shown that TDs affect 1–3% of school-aged children (Hornsey et al., 2001; Robertson, 2008); however, precise prevalence estimates in adults have been difficult to determine, due in part to the removal of the distress and impairment criteria from recent editions of the DSM and uncertainty regarding how longitudinal course should be considered when conferring a diagnosis.

Etiology and Theoretical Underpinnings of Treatment

Current empirically supported treatments for tics are based on a biobehavioral model that incorporates what is known about the underlying pathophysiology of tics with principles of learning theory to explain how internal and external contextual stimuli and tic-contingent consequences exacerbate and maintain tics (Woods et al., 2008). While the exact etiology of TDs remains unclear, there is converging evidence that tics are the result of structural and functional abnormalities within cortico-striatal-thalamic-cortical (CSTC) circuitry that subserve a host of important integrative motor and sensorimotor functions, including the selection and execution of goal-directed and habitual actions, inhibition, habit formation, and reward processing, among others (Ganos et al., 2013). Tic disorders are also highly heritable. Recent genome-wide association studies suggest the inheritance patterns responsible for TDs are complex and polygenetic, but the specific genes and risk factors involved remain unknown (Lin et al., 2022).

The behavioral component of the biobehavioral model centers around two primary tenets. First, studies have shown that tics can be influenced by internal and external contextual factors (i.e., antecedents; Conelea & Woods, 2008). For example, most individuals report that their tics fluctuate in specific settings, when engaged in certain activities, and in response to their emotional state (Himle et al., 2014). Likewise, studies have shown that tics can be exacerbated or attenuated by tic-contingent consequences such as attention and/or avoidance of nonpreferred tasks (Himle et al., 2014). Importantly, the impact of specific antecedents and consequences on tics is highly idiosyncratic and believed to be based on an individualized learning history. The second primary tenet of the behavioral model is that tics function to temporarily remove or reduce aversive premonitory urges, and thus tics are hypothesized to be strengthened through automatic negative reinforcement (Evers & van de Wetering, 1994). Furthermore, because tics are executed regularly across contexts and are immediately reinforced by a reduction in the premonitory urge, they become overlearned (i.e., habitual) behaviors that occur outside of immediate awareness (Singer, 2016). Based on these two tenets, the primary goals of behavioral approaches

to tic management are to systematically identify and modify tic-exacerbating antecedents and consequences, to increase the individual's awareness of tics and associated urges, and to teach patients to interrupt or suppress tics, especially when in the
presence of tic-eliciting stimuli. Doing so is thought to disrupt the reinforcement
processes maintaining tics and facilitate habituation to premonitory urges (Himle
et al., 2006; Verdellen et al., 2008).

Brief Overview of Treatments

Habit Reversal Training

Habit reversal training (HRT) is a collection of behavior modification techniques that
was originally developed to treat a broad range of problematic repetitive behaviors,
including motor and vocal tics (Azrin & Nunn, 1973). The rationale for HRT is based
on the assumptions that tics occur outside of the patient's immediate awareness and
are reinforced through both automatic and socially mediated reinforcement contingencies. The goal of HRT is to extinguish the reinforcement contingencies maintaining tics by increasing the patient's awareness of when a tic is about to occur (or has
occurred) and then teaching and reinforcing tic suppression strategies to interrupt or
prevent tic occurrence. The original HRT treatment package consisted of a set of
sequentially delivered therapeutic techniques that included self-monitoring, awareness training, competing response training, social support, and several additional
therapeutic procedures to enhance motivation and generalization (Azrin & Nunn,
1973). Subsequent dismantling studies have shown that a simplified version of HRT
that involves only awareness training, competing response training, and social support
may be sufficient (Miltenberger & Fuqua, 1985). Each component of HRT is applied
sequentially to each tic in the patient's repertoire, typically with one tic targeted per
week, and the patient is assigned to practice using competing responses between
sessions in settings and contexts in which the tic is likely to occur.

Comprehensive Behavioral Intervention for Tics

Comprehensive Behavioral Intervention for Tics (CBIT) is a multicomponent treatment package that combines several behavioral tic management strategies into
a single comprehensive treatment package. The primary components of CBIT include
psychoeducation, simplified HRT (i.e., awareness training, competing response training, and social support), a function-based assessment and intervention (FBAI) protocol designed to systematically identify and modify or eliminate tic-exacerbating
antecedents and consequences, relaxation training, and motivational techniques to
increase treatment compliance and the use of tic management strategies outside of
sessions (Woods et al., 2008). The CBIT treatment protocol is designed to be flexibly

administered across eight weekly sessions, delivered over the course of 10–12 weeks, with a different tic targeted in treatment each week (Woods et al., 2008; Piacentini et al., 2010; Wilhelm et al., 2012).

Exposure and Response Prevention

Like HRT, the rationale for applying exposure and response prevention (ERP) to treat tics assumes that tics are strengthened through automatic negative reinforcement (i.e., function to reduce aversive premonitory urges). As such, the ERP approach hypothesizes that if a patient suppresses their tics for a prolonged period of time (i.e., response prevention) they will be repeatedly "exposed" to their premonitory sensations, which will result in habituation to the urge and a decrease in the overall frequency and severity of tics (Verdellen et al., 2004). Within the ERP protocol, patients are encouraged to suppress all tics for increasingly longer durations of time while also periodically reporting the strength of their premonitory urges in order to reinforce the notion that premonitory urges will eventually decrease if tics are suppressed. Treatment typically consists of 12 2-hour sessions, and patients are encouraged to practice tic suppression while engaged in tic-exacerbating activities (Hoogduin et al., 1997).

Overall Level of Research Support

The Society of Clinical Psychology does not identify any empirically supported treatments for TDs at this time. Several small-N and uncontrolled group design studies and small randomized controlled trials provided early support for the efficacy of HRT; however, these studies had methodological shortcomings that limited confidence in their findings (see Himle et al., 2006 for a review). More recently, the efficacy of behavior therapy for TDs was demonstrated in two large multisite randomized controlled trials (parallel adult and child trials) comparing CBIT to psychoeducation plus supportive therapy (PST). In the child trial (n=126 children with TD), 53% of children who received CBIT were classified as treatment responders, compared to 19% of children who received PST (Piacentini et al., 2010). CBIT also resulted in a significantly greater decrease in overall tic severity compared to PST, and treatment gains were durable, with 87% of CBIT responders maintaining their gains 6-months posttreatment. In the adult trial (122 patients, ages 16–69 years), 38% of patients who received CBIT were rated as treatment responders versus 6% of those who received PST, and 80% of CBIT responders maintained their gains at 6-month follow-up (Wilhelm et al., 2012). Those who received CBIT also showed a significantly greater reduction in overall tic severity. The efficacy of HRT/CBIT is further supported by several meta-analytic studies showing medium-to-large treatment effect sizes across randomized control trials (McGuire et al., 2014; Wile &

Pringsheim, 2013; Yu et al., 2020). Based on the current state of evidence supporting CBIT, it is now recommended within several practice guidelines as a first-line intervention for treating tics in both children and adults whose tics are bothersome (Pringsheim et al., 2019). ERP has been less extensively studied but has been shown to be effective in several small studies and three randomized controlled trials (Andren et al., 2019; Hollis et al., 2021; Hoogduin et al., 1997; Verdellen et al., 2004; Wetterneck & Woods, 2006; Woods et al., 2000). A recent meta-analysis found a small-to-medium effect size for ERP for TDs; however, this study included only three studies in their analysis, two of which examined a therapist-supported online delivery format (Yan et al., 2022).

Credible Components of Treatments

Although the treatment packages described herein differ with respect to the specific therapeutic procedures they employ, each is based on a similar biobehavioral model and shares several specific, theoretically driven treatment components designed to alter internal and external learning processes hypothesized to strengthen and maintain tics. The primary credible treatment components shared across HRT, CBIT, and ERP are described in the following sections.

Increasing Awareness of Tics

Most individuals with TDs are largely unaware of their tics and associated urges on a moment-to-moment basis (Müller-Vahl et al., 2014; Singer, 2016). Because awareness of tics and associated premonitory urges is thought to facilitate and enhance tic suppression, awareness training strategies are a central component of behavioral interventions for TDs. Within the HRT protocol, awareness training is an explicit multistep process. It begins with response description, which involves asking the patient to describe the progression of body parts, movements, sensations, and premonitory urges involved in the target tic. The second step of awareness training involves teaching the patient to recognize and acknowledge discrete occurrences of the target tic as early in the tic chain as possible, ideally before it occurs, by detecting the associated premonitory urge. In-session awareness training procedures are supplemented with between-session practice and self-monitoring. In contrast to HRT, the ERP protocol does not contain specific instructions or activities for increasing awareness prior to teaching tic suppression. Rather, strategies to increase awareness are embedded into the ERP suppression protocol.

Although awareness training is considered a theoretically important component of behavioral treatment packages for TDs (especially for HRT), additional research is needed to better understand whether awareness training is an essential component of the HRT/CBIT treatment package, as well as the level of awareness that is necessary and/or sufficient for optimal treatment outcomes. Furthermore, whether embedded (i.e., ERP) or explicit (i.e., HRT) procedures are differentially effective for increasing awareness of tics and associated premonitory urges is unknown. Finally, although awareness training alone has been shown to decrease tics in a few uncontrolled case studies (Wiskow & Klatt, 2013; Wright & Miltenberger, 1987), there have been no systematic investigations examining awareness training as a stand-alone treatment for TDs.

Tic Suppression

Therapeutic strategies aimed at teaching and/or encouraging patients to suppress their tics are also a core component of treatment. Tic suppression is believed to disrupt the negative reinforcement cycle, facilitate habituation to the premonitory urge, and weaken urge-tic associations (Himle et al., 2006). Within HRT (and CBIT), tic suppression is accomplished through competing response training, which involves teaching the patient to engage in a behavior that is physically incompatible with the tic (i.e., a competing response) whenever a tic occurs or is about to occur. As a general rule, an effective competing response is a behavior that: (1) is physically incompatible with the tic or interferes with performance of the tic to the greatest extent possible, (2) a response that can be maintained without difficulty for several minutes, (3) is less conspicuous than the tic itself, and (4) does not interfere with routine activities (e.g., walking, driving, talking). The patient is instructed to engage in the selected competing response whenever they recognize that a tic has occurred or begun, or, ideally, whenever they detect a premonitory urge. The patient is also instructed to maintain the competing response for at least one minute or until the urge to tic subsides, whichever is longer. Whenever the patient exhibits a tic, the therapist prompts them to use the competing response, and unprompted use of the competing response is reinforced with praise. The patient is then instructed to practice using the competing response regularly between sessions, particularly when in high-risk settings or engaged in tic-exacerbating activities. In one small component analysis study, competing response training was found to be necessary (above and beyond awareness training, self-monitoring, and social support) for reducing motor tics in two of four children (Woods et al., 1996); however, additional dismantling studies with larger sample sizes are needed to better understand its incremental benefit when delivered as part of the HRT/CBIT treatment package.

ERP also emphasizes tic suppression as a primary component of treatment; however, the patient is not typically taught a specific strategy for suppressing their tics. Rather, patients are asked to suppress their tics for as long as possible and are challenged to do so for increasing durations of time (Verdellen et al., 2011a; Verdellen et al., 2011b). In addition, whereas HRT focuses on treating one tic at a time, in ERP patients are instructed to suppress all of their tics simultaneously.

Finally, unlike in HRT, in which patients are encouraged to practice inhibiting their tics while multitasking (i.e., distracted), in ERP patients are explicitly encouraged to focus on and tolerate premonitory urges until habituation occurs. This later element of ERP is presumably based on the assumption that distraction will interfere with habituation and/or expectancy violation (i.e., providing corrective information to counter the belief that urges will not decrease); however, these assumptions have not been empirically tested.

Social Support

Social support involves recruiting a supportive person, such as a spouse, partner, friend, or family member, to assist the patient in practicing therapeutic techniques between sessions. The social support person's role primarily involves assisting with between-session awareness training exercises (HRT/CBIT), prompting and reinforcing the use of competing responses (HRT/CBIT), assisting with tic suppression practice (ERP), and providing general encouragement and support. Although a component analysis study of HRT applied to treat adults with body-focused repetitive behaviors suggested that the social support component of HRT did not add incremental benefit (Flessner et al., 2005), there is evidence to support the use of social support when applying HRT/CBIT to treat tics. For example, Woods et al. (1996) sequentially applied the core components of HRT for four children with motor tics and found that social support improved outcomes in three of the four participants. In addition, follow-up analysis of the child and adult CBIT trials found that compliance with between-session homework predicted better treatment response (Essoe et al., 2021). More research is needed, however, to better understand the relative importance of the specific activities assigned to the social support person (e.g., assisting with awareness activities, reinforcing use of the competing response, etc.) and how to tailor social support to individual patients to maximize therapeutic benefit.

Identifying and Modifying Tic-Exacerbating Antecedents and Consequences

A primary component of treatment for tics involves identifying and modifying or eliminating antecedents and tic-contingent consequences associated with tic exacerbations. Within CBIT, this process is referred to as function-based assessment and intervention (FBAI; Woods et al., 2008). The FBAI process begins with a systematic functional assessment, in which patients are queried about specific antecedent stimuli (i.e., tic triggers) and consequences (i.e., tic reactions) that have been shown in the research literature to be commonly associated with tic worsening (Himle et al., 2014). Patients are also assigned to regularly self-monitor their tics between sessions and to record both antecedents and consequences associated with situational tic worsening. Based on the information gleaned from the functional assessment and self-monitoring, a collection of individualized function-based interventions is collaboratively created and implemented with the goal of eliminating or reducing tic-exacerbating contextual factors (i.e., creating a "tic-neutral" environment; Walkup et al., 2012). Function-based environmental modification strategies have been shown to be effective for reducing tics in several small studies (Conelea & Woods, 2008; Roane et al., 2002; Wagaman et al., 1995; Watson & Sterling, 1998); however, additional research is needed to validate the function-based assessment procedures utilized in CBIT and to determine the extent to which FBAI procedures contribute to therapeutic outcomes (and for whom).

When tic-exacerbating antecedents and consequences cannot be feasibly eliminated, the patient is assigned to practice *in vivo* tic suppression strategies within that context or to engage in in-session simulations (Woods et al., 2008; Verdellen et al., 2011a). Although tic-exacerbating functional variables are unique to each patient, most individuals report that stress, anxiety, and muscle tension increase tics (Caurin et al., 2014). As such, within CBIT all patients are taught relaxation techniques such as deep breathing and progressive muscle relaxation (Woods et al., 2008). Although research has shown that relaxation training can situationally reduce tics (Tilling & Cavanna, 2020), results of a comparison study show that relaxation training is less effective than self-monitoring and HRT (32% tic reduction compared to 44% and 55%, respectively; Peterson & Azrin, 1992), and therefore there is insufficient support to recommend relaxation techniques as a stand-alone monotherapy for TDs (Tilling & Cavanna, 2020). Furthermore, acute stress has been shown to undermine tic suppression (Conelea et al., 2011), suggesting that relaxation techniques might enhance suppression-based therapeutic techniques, though further research is needed to test that hypothesis.

Motivational Techniques

Studies have shown that between-session practice of therapeutic activities, especially later in the course of treatment, increases the likelihood that patients will ultimately benefit (Essoe et al., 2021). Strategies to increase motivation are thus interspersed throughout treatment protocols – for example, through frequent encouragement and reinforcement for treatment engagement, self-managed reward programs (e.g., token economies), and regularly tracking and reviewing treatment progress (Woods et al., 2008). Although follow-up analysis of the child and adult CBIT trials found that compliance with between-session homework predicted better treatment response (Essoe et al., 2021), the most effective strategies for motivating treatment engagement and compliance remain unknown.

Generalization, Mastery, and Maintenance Strategies

Embedded within treatments for tics are strategies that support the generalization and mastery of skills taught in treatment. For example, patients are encouraged to self-monitor their tics outside of session and to practice awareness and tic suppression procedures across a wide range of contexts, especially those associated with tic worsening. In addition, even treatment responders are likely to have new tics emerge (Peterson et al., 2016) and/or to encounter novel situations that exacerbate residual tics (e.g., stressful life events). Thus, relapse prevention strategies are included as part of treatment. For example, in CBIT, the final two sessions are dedicated to topics such as monitoring for the onset of new tics and the re-emergence of successfully treated tics, continued monitoring for tic-exacerbating antecedents and consequences, and simulated practice applying CBIT skills to novel tics to ensure that the patient can apply the primary components of treatment to new tics (Woods et al., 2008). Patients are also encouraged to periodically attend booster sessions, as needed, following the acute phase of treatment in order to maintain treatment gains (Woods et al., 2008). Although the effectiveness of booster sessions within CBIT has not been specifically examined, such sessions have been shown to result in larger and longer-lasting treatment gains in studies of other behavioral treatments for youth (Gearing et al., 2013). Long-term follow-up data from a subset of treatment responders from the CBIT trials also provides indirect evidence for the utility of the generalization and mastery approach employed in CBIT. Espil and colleagues (2022) identified and reassessed 80 of the 126 participants from the original trials 11 years posttreatment (on average) and found that CBIT responders were more likely than PST responders to achieve partial or full remission of symptoms (67% versus 0%, respectively), with no differences between groups with respect to the use of adjunctive intervention in the 11-year interim (Espil et al., 2022). While promising, additional research is clearly needed to understand the relative role of the various HRT/CBIT treatment components in the maintenance and durability of treatment gains, especially given the tendency for tics to naturally improve over time for most patients.

Psychoeducation and Other Credible Ancillary Components

Several additional credible components are often incorporated into treatment to enhance therapeutic outcomes or as ancillary techniques to minimize the impact of tics on functioning. For example, psychoeducation is often provided to ensure that patients have an accurate understanding of their TD, to provide a rationale for treatment, to reduce stigma, and to correct common myths and misunderstandings about TDs that could decrease treatment engagement and expectations (Cox et al., 2019). Cognitive restructuring, emotion regulation strategies, collaborative problem solving, and mindfulness-based techniques have also shown promise as ancillary or stand-alone techniques for reducing tic-related impairment, distress, and self-stigma (McGuire et al., 2015; Reese et al., 2015). Mindfulness strategies, in particular, could theoretically serve to increase interoceptive awareness and urge tolerance, which might enhance patients' ability to identify and tolerate premonitory urges (Reese et al., 2015); however, this remains speculative. Although there is insufficient evidence to consider these techniques to be credible components, they have generally been shown to be efficacious behavior change techniques and fit within the biobehavioral conceptual model of TDs, though more research is needed to understand their incremental benefit, if any.

Approaches for Youth

Approaches to treating tics in children largely parallel those used with adults (Woods et al., 2008; Verdellen et al., 2011b). For example, as noted earlier, the standard CBIT protocol has been shown to be efficacious for reducing tics in children ages 8–17 years (Piacentini et al., 2010). The primary difference between adult and child CBIT protocols is the involvement of parents when treating children. In addition, research has shown that compliance with homework activities early in the course of treatment predicts treatment response in youth receiving CBIT (Essoe et al., 2021). As such, the child-focused protocol has an increased emphasis on early homework compliance and motivation. For example, reward programs are typically employed to reinforce attending sessions, active participation during sessions, and completing homework (Woods et al., 2008), though it is unclear whether parental involvement or extrinsic reward programs influence compliance or add incremental benefit. Further, an adapted version of CBIT, referred to as CBIT-Junior, is a developmentally modified protocol for children as young as five. CBIT-Junior contains several developmental modifications to increase understanding and make tic suppression practice easier, and has an increased emphasis on parental involvement in treatment (Bennett et al., 2020). A small open pilot study with 15 youth with TDs found that CBIT-Junior was effective for reducing tics, with response rate, symptom reduction, and maintenance of treatment gains similar to those reported in the larger child CBIT trial (Bennett et al., 2020), though larger randomized controlled efficacy trials are needed. ERP has also been shown to be efficacious in children, with many of the same modifications described for CBIT-Junior (e.g., increased parental involvement and developmentally tailored language; Mateu et al., 2018).

Other Variables Influencing Treatment

Assessment and Diagnosis

The sole features that differentiate the primary TD diagnoses, the types of tics present (motor, vocal, or both) and the duration of symptoms since initial onset (more or less than one year) are important for diagnosis but have little practical relevance for treatment. Both motor and vocal tics have been shown to respond to treatment, and age of tic onset did not moderate or predict treatment response in the CBIT trials (Sukhodolsky et al., 2017). A thorough assessment of TDs and common comorbid conditions is essential for differential diagnosis, treatment planning and prioritization, and outcome monitoring. Identification of comorbid conditions that might interfere with the treatment of tics is particularly important prior to initiating treatment. At a minimum, it is essential to carefully assess for the presence of comorbid attention-deficit/hyperactivity disorder (ADHD), obsessive-compulsive disorder (OCD), and depressive and anxiety disorders, as these are exceptionally common in TDs and can complicate the treatment of tics (see section on "Comorbidity"). Several psychometrically sound structured clinical interviews and symptom measures are available for this purpose. A comprehensive assessment of tics is also strongly recommended to inform the course of treatment and specific intervention components, and to monitor treatment outcomes. For example, information regarding the sequence of complex tics and understanding a patient's degree of awareness of their tics and premonitory urges can be useful for planning HRT. The most widely used assessment measures for TDs are the Yale Global Tic Severity Scale (YGTSS; Leckman et al., 1989) and the Premonitory Urge for Tics Scale (PUTS; Woods et al., 2005). The YGTSS is a semistructured clinician-administered rating scale that contains a checklist of common motor and vocal tics; anchored ratings of the number, frequency, intensity, complexity, and interference caused by motor and vocal tics (rated separately to create a 0–50 Total Tic Score [TTS]); and a global rating of tic-related impairment. The PUTS is a brief self-report measure that asks the patient to rate the presence and strength of premonitory urges. A 25% decrease on the YGTSS-TTS has been shown to predict a clinically meaningful response to treatment (Jeon et al., 2013), and higher premonitory urge ratings have been shown to predict poorer response to CBIT (Sukhodolsky et al., 2017).

Comorbidity

Psychiatric comorbidity is exceptionally common in TDs. Large international clinical samples have shown that that up to 85% of patients report a lifetime history of at least one comorbid condition, with over half experiencing multiple comorbidities (Freeman et al., 2000; Hirschtritt et al., 2015). ADHD (35–60%) and OCD (30–60%) are particularly prevalent; mood, anxiety, and personality disorders are also common

(Hirschtritt et al., 2015; Robertson et al., 2018). The high rate of psychiatric comorbidity in TDs has several implications for treatment. First, prioritizing treatment targets can be challenging, as it is often the case that both tics and comorbid symptoms uniquely contribute to distress and impairment, and the symptoms can interact in complex ways (e.g., anxiety can exacerbate tics, and tics can be a source of anxiety). Second, it can sometimes be difficult to differentiate tics from comorbid symptoms. For example, complex tics can sometimes be difficult to differentiate from compulsions. These factors can make it challenging to decide what treatment to utilize (e.g., HRT versus cognitive and behavioral techniques for OCD). Finally, it is our clinical experience that comorbid symptoms can complicate the delivery of treatments for tics. For example, inattention, distractibility, and impulsivity can interfere with HRT. Likewise, unmanaged depression and/or anxiety can decrease treatment motivation, compliance, and treatment expectations, which have been shown to predict response to CBIT (Essoe et al., 2021; Sukhodolsky et al., 2017). While a secondary analysis of the CBIT trials found that comorbidity status did not moderate treatment response in children or adults, the presence of an anxiety disorder did predict less improvement in tic severity at posttreatment (Sukhodolsky et al., 2017). It is important to note, however, that patients were excluded from those studies if they had unmanaged comorbidity requiring more immediate treatment, raising questions about the generalizability of the findings to patients with more severe comorbid symptoms.

Demographics

To date, few studies have examined the association between demographic or cultural variables and treatment outcomes for tics, and the vast majority of existing treatment studies have been conducted with predominantly White, non-Hispanic samples. Understanding the impact of cultural variables in the treatment of tics and the development and testing of culturally informed protocols is sorely needed, as the limited information that is available suggests there may be important cross-cultural differences in how tics and behavioral approaches to treatment are viewed (Stiede et al., 2021). In addition, factors such as lack of awareness of effective treatment options, misperceptions about behavioral approaches to tic treatment, access to trained providers, and the cost and time associated with treatment are commonly cited barriers to receiving CBIT, suggesting that TD-related health literacy, socioeconomic status, and factors related to healthcare access are worthy of additional research (Woods et al., 2010).

Medication

Several effective medication options are available for treating tics and are often used alongside behavioral therapies, especially for those with severe and/or impairing tics. Typical and atypical neuroleptics have been shown to produce the most robust tic suppression, but their use is often limited by adverse side effects (Weisman et al., 2013). Alpha-2 adrenergic agonists have also shown to be moderately effective for reducing tics, especially for those with comorbid ADHD, and are generally better tolerated (Weisman et al., 2013). Several other novel therapeutic agents are currently under investigation (Quezada & Coffman, 2018). Head-to-head comparisons of medication and behavior therapy (or their combination) have not been conducted with adults. Importantly, secondary analysis of the CBIT trials found that medication status moderated treatment response, with a smaller between-group effect size (CBIT vs. PST) for those on tic-suppressing medications (Sukhodolsky et al., 2017). This effect was largely accounted for by the fact that patients who were on alpha-2 agonists showed a greater response to PST. However, participants not on tic-suppressing medications were more likely to show a positive response to CBIT than those on tic-suppressing medications. Reasons for these findings are unclear. Speculatively, it is possible that these findings are accounted for by group differences in pre-medication tic severity, differences in patient characteristics among those who are and are not prescribed medication, or that some tic-suppressing medications interfere with CBIT (Sukhodolsky et al., 2017).

Conclusion

Behavioral approaches to tic management have been shown to be effective for reducing tics in both adults and children. The intervention packages with the strongest support are HRT, CBIT (which includes HRT as a primary component), and ERP. Although these treatment packages have important procedural differences, they share a set of theoretically driven components designed to reduce tics and associated impairment. The primary credible components of treatments for tics include techniques for increasing tic awareness, teaching and facilitating tic suppression, the identification and modification of environmental factors known to exacerbate tics, strategies to increase motivation and treatment compliance, and techniques to promote generalization and maintenance of treatment gains. Several additional therapeutic elements, including psycho-education, relaxation training, relapse prevention, homework compliance, social support, and behavioral reward programs, are also commonly included as part of treatment. The development and testing of culturally adapted protocols, strategies for enhancing treatment outcomes, and a better understanding of how to effectively and efficiently treat psychiatrically complex cases are important directions for future research.

Box 19.1 Treatment Format

Treatment for tics have primarily been developed and tested as individually delivered, face-to-face protocols with therapeutic sessions dispersed across several weeks. However, alternative delivery modalities and formats have started to emerge. Several studies have shown that CBIT and ERP can be effectively delivered via telehealth technologies, with high rates of patient satisfaction and treatment effect sizes similar to those reported with in-person delivery (Capriotti et al., 2023; also see Woods et al., 2023 for a review). A few small, uncontrolled studies have also examined the feasibility and efficacy of intensively delivered CBIT (delivered over the course of four days to two weeks) and have found treatment response rates and symptom reduction similar to what has been reported in studies utilizing the standard 10-week protocol (Blount et al., 2014; Kennedy et al., 2016). However, to date, there have been no controlled studies directly comparing intensive delivery to the standard CBIT protocol, and studies with longer follow-up periods are needed to understand if treatment gains following intensive delivery are durable. Group-delivered HRT and CBIT protocols have also been tested in several small randomized controlled trials with children. These studies have generally shown that group-delivered CBIT is more effective than education-only control conditions for decreasing motor tics but not vocal tics (Yates et al., 2016; Zimmerman-Brenner et al., 2022). It is not known why vocal tics would be less responsive to group-delivered CBIT. In the only adult study to date, Bekk and colleagues (2023) treated 26 adults with tics using a group-delivered CBIT protocol and found significant reduction in overall tic severity at posttreatment and 1-year follow-up; however, this study lacked a control comparison group. In addition, similar to what has been reported in studies of children, vocal tics showed a less robust response compared to motor tics. Combining group and intensive protocols, Heijerman-Holtgrefe and colleagues (2021) conducted an initial pilot study of a four-day intensive group-delivered ERP protocol for 14 children with tics and found that 23% of patients were rated as treatment responders at posttreatment and 54% were rated as responders at 2-month follow-up; however, symptom reduction was lower than has generally been reported in studies utilizing the standard ERP protocol, and this study lacked a control comparison condition. Finally, online self-help and hybrid online + therapist-support versions of CBIT and ERP have also shown promise in initial studies, with response rates and degree of tic reduction similar to those observed in the traditional in-person, therapist-delivered protocols (Hollis et al., 2021; Rachamim et al., 2022). Although these alternative delivery formats are potentially promising avenues for addressing known dissemination and utilization barriers for treatment for tics (e.g., lack of access to trained therapists; Woods et al., 2010), additional studies examining their efficacy, acceptability, and durability of treatment gains are needed, especially in adults.

Useful Resources

Books

- McGuire, J. F., Murphy, T. K., Piacentini, J., & Storch, E. A. (2018). *The clinician's guide to treatment and management of youth with Tourette syndrome and tic disorders*. Elsevier.
- Verdellen, C. W. J., van de Griendt, J. M. T. M., Kriens, S., & van Oostrum, I. (2011). *Tics: Therapist manual*. Boom Publishers.
- Woods, D. W., Piacentini, J. C., Chang, S. W., et al. (2008). *Managing Tourette syndrome: A behavioral intervention for children and adults*. Oxford University Press.

Websites

- European Society for the Study of Tourette Syndrome: www.essts.org
- Tourette Association of America: www.tourette.org
- Tourettes Action: www.tourettes-action.org.uk

References

American Psychiatric Association [APA] (2022). *Diagnostic and statistical manual of mental disorders* (5th ed., text rev.). American Psychiatric Association. https://doi.org/10.1176/appi.books.9780890425787.

Andren, P., Aspvall, K., Fernandez de la Cruz, L., et al. (2019). Therapist-guided and parent-guided internet-delivered behaviour therapy for paediatric Tourette's disorder: A pilot randomized controlled trial with long-term follow-up. *BMJ Open*, 9, e024685. https://doi.org/10.1136/bmjopen-2018-024685.

Azrin, N. H., & Nunn, R. G. (1973). Habit-reversal: A method of eliminating nervous habits and tics. *Behavior Research and Therapy*, 11, 619–628. https://doi.org/10.1016/0005-7967(73)90119-8.

Bekk, M., Meland, K. J., Moen, E., et al. (2023). Group-based comprehensive behavioral intervention for tics (CBIT) for adults with Tourette syndrome or chronic tic disorders: A pilot study. *Scandinavian Journal of Psychology*, 64, 784–793. https://doi.org/10.1111/sjop.12942.

Bennett, S. M., Capriotti, M., Bauer, C., et al. (2020). Development and open trial of a psychosocial intervention for young children with chronic tics: The CBIT-JR study. *Behavior Therapy*, 51, 659–669. https://doi.org/10.1016/j.beth.2019.10.114.

Bloch, M. H., & Leckman, J. F. (2009). Clinical course of Tourette syndrome. *Journal of Psychosomatic Research* 67, 497–501. https://doi.org/10.1016/j.jpsychores.2009.09.002.

Blount, T. H., Lockhart, A. T., Garcia, R. V., Raj, J. J., & Peterson, A. L. (2014). Intensive outpatient comprehensive behavioral intervention for tics: A case series. *World Journal of Clinical Cases*, 2, 569–577. https://doi.org/10.12998/wjcc.v2.i10.569.

Capriotti, M. R., Wellen, B. C. M., Young, B. N., et al. (2023). Evaluating the feasibility, acceptability, and preliminary effectiveness of tele-comprehensive behavior therapy for tics (teleCBIT) for Tourette syndrome in youth and adults. *Journal of Telemedicine and Telecare.* https://journals.sagepub.com/doi/10.1177/1357633X231189305.

Caurin, B., Serrano, M., Fernandez-Alvarez, E., Campistol, J., & Perez-Duenas, B. (2014). Environmental circumstances influencing tic expression in children. *European Journal of Paediatric Neurology* 18, 157–162. https://doi.org/10.1016/j.ejpn.2013.10.002.

Conelea, C. A., & Woods, D. W. (2008). The influence of contextual factors on tic expression in Tourette's syndrome: A review. *Journal of Psychosomatic Research*, 65, 487–496. https://doi.org/10.1016/j.jpsychores.2008.04.010.

Conelea, C. A., Woods, D. W., & Brandt, B. C. (2011). The impact of a stress induction task on tic frequencies in youth with Tourette syndrome. *Behaviour Research and Therapy*, 49, 492–497. https://doi.org/10.1016/j.brat.2011.05.006.

Conelea, C. A., Woods, D. W., Zinner, S. H., et al. (2011). Exploring the impact of chronic tic disorders on youth: Results from the Tourette syndrome impact survey. *Child Psychiatry & Human Development*,42, 219–242. https://doi.org/10.1007/s10578-010-0211-4.

Conelea, C. A., Woods, D. W., Zinner, S. H., et al. (2013). The impact of Tourette syndrome in adults: Results from the Tourette syndrome impact survey. *Community Mental Health Journal*, 49, 110–120. https://doi.org/10.1007/s10597-011-9465-y.

Cox, J. H., Nahar, A., Termine, C., et al. (2019). Social stigma and self-perception in adolescents with Tourette syndrome. *Adolescent Health, Medicine, and Therapeutics* 10, 75–82. https://doi.org/10.2147/AHMT.S175765.

Espil, F. M., Woods, D. W., Specht, M. W., et al. (2022). Long-term outcomes of behavior therapy for youth with Tourette disorder. *Journal of the American Academy of Child and Adolescent Psychiatry*, 61, 764–771. https://doi.org/10.1016/j.jaac.2021.08.022.

Essoe, J. K., Ricketts, E. J., Ramsey, K. A., et al. (2021). Homework adherence predicts therapeutic improvement from behavior therapy in Tourette's disorder. *Behaviour Research and Therapy* 140, 103844. https://doi.org/10.1016/j.brat.2021.103844.

Evers, R. A. F., & van de Wetering, B. J. M. (1994). A treatment model for motor tics based on a specific tension-reduction technique. *Journal of Beahvior Therapy and Experimental Psychiatry*, 25(3), 255–260. https://doi.org/10.1016/0005-7916(94)90026-4.

Flessner, C. A., Miltenberger, R. G., Egemo, K., et al. (2005). An evaluation of the social support component of simplified habit reversal. *Behavior Therapy*, 36, 35–42. https://doi.org/10.1016/S0005-7894(05)80052-8.

Freeman, R. D., Fast, D. K., Burd, L., et al. (2000). An international perspective on Tourette syndrome: Selected findings from 3,500 individuals in 22 countries. *Developmental Medicine and Child Neurology*, 42, 436–447. https://doi.org/10.1017/s0012162200000839.

Ganos, C., Roessner, V., & Münchau, A. (2013). The functional anatomy of Gilles de la Tourette syndrome. *Neuroscience & Biobehavioral Reviews*, 37(6), 1050–1062.

Gearing, R. E., Schwalbe, C. S., & Hoagwood, K. E. (2013). The effectiveness of booster sessions in CBT treatment for child and adolescent mood and anxiety disorders. *Depression and Anxiety*, 30, 800–808. https://doi.org/10.1002/da.22118.

Heijerman-Holtgrefe, A. P., Verdellen, C. W. J., van de Griendt, J. M. T. M., et al. (2021). Tackle your tics: Pilot findings of a brief, intensive group-based exposure therapy program for children with tic disorders. *European Journal of Child and Adolescent Psychiatry*, 30, 461–473. https://doi.org/10.1007/s00787-020-01532-5.

Himle, M. B., Capriotti, M. R., Hayes, L. P., et al. (2014). Variables associated with tic exacerbation in children with chronic tic disorders. *Behavior Modification* 38, 168–183. https://doi.org/10.1177/0145445514531016.

Himle, M. B., Woods, D. W., Piacentini, J. C., & Walkup, J. T. (2006). Brief review of habit reversal training for Tourette syndrome. *Journal of Child Neurology*, 21, 719–725. https://doi.org/10.1177/08830738060210080101.

Hirschtritt, M. E., Lee, P. C., Pauls, D. L., et al. (2015). Lifetime prevalence, age of risk, and genetic relationships of comorbid psychiatric disorders in Tourette syndrome. *JAMA Psychiatry*, 72, 325–333. https://doi.org/10.1001/jamapsychiatry.2014.2650.

Hollis, C., Hall, C.L., Jones, R., et al. (2021). Therapist-supported online remote behavioural intervention for tics in children and adolescents in England (ORBIT): A multicentre, parallel group, single-blind, randomized controlled trial. *Lancet Psychiatry*, 8, 871–882. https://doi.org/10.1016/S2215-0366(21)00235-2.

Hoogduin, K., Verdellen, C., & Cath, D. (1997). Exposure and response prevention in the treatment of Gilles de la Tourette's syndrome: Four case studies. *Clinical Psychology and Psychotherapy*, 4, 125–137.

Hornsey, H., Banerjee, S., Zeitlin, H., & Robertson, M. (2001). The prevalence of Tourette syndrome in 13-14-year-olds in mainstream schools. *Journal of Child Psychology and Psychiatry, and Allied Disciplines*, 42, 1035–1039. https://doi.org/10.1111/1469-7610.00802.

Jankovic, J., Gelineau-Kattner, R., & Davidson, A. (2010). Tourette's syndrome in adults. *Movement Disorders*, 25, 2171–2175. https://doi.org/10.1002/mds.23199.

Jeon, S., Walkup, J. T., Woods, D. W., et al. (2013). Detecting a clinically meaningful change in tic severity in Tourette syndrome: A comparison of three methods. *Contemporary Clinical Trials*, 36, 414–420. https://doi.org/10.1016/j.cct.2013.08.012.

Kennedy, T. M., Morris, A. T., Walkup, J. T., et al. (2016). Rapid-response behavioral triage for tics (RRBTT): A 2-week clinical case series. *Clinical Practice in Pediatric Psychology*, 4, 373–382. https://doi.org/10.1037/cpp000151.

Kwak, C., Dat Vuong, K., & Jankovic, J. (2003). Premonitory sensory phenomenon in Tourette's syndrome. *Movement Disorders*, 18, 1530–1533. https://doi.org/10.1002/mds.10618.

Leckman, J. F., Riddle, M. A., Hardin, M. T., et al. (1989). The Yale Global Tic Severity Scale: Initial testing of a clinician-rated scale of tic severity. *Journal of the American Academy of Child and Adolescent Psychiatry*, 28, 566–573. https://doi.org/10.1097/00004583-198907000-00015.

Lin, W. D., Tsai, F. J., & Chou, I. C. (2022). Current understanding of the genetics of Tourette syndrome. *Biomedical Journal*, 45, 271–279. https://doi.org/10.1016/j.bj.2022.01.008.

Mateu, A., McFarlane, F., & Heyman, I. (2018). Exposure with response prevention for Tourette's syndrome: A case study of a 6 year-old. *Archives of Disease in Childhood*, 103, A065. https://doi.org/10.1136/goshabs.65.

McGuire, J. F., Piacentini, J., Brennan, E. A., et al. (2014). A meta-analysis of behavior therapy for Tourette syndrome. *Journal of Psychiatric Research*, 50, 106–112. https://doi.org/10.1016/j.jpsychires.2013.12.009.

McGuire, J. F., Ricketts, E. J., Piacentini, J., et al. (2015). Behavior therapy for tic disorders: An evidenced-based review and new directions for treatment research. *Current Developmental Disorders Reports*, 2, 309–317. https://doi.org/10.1007/s40474-015-0063-5.

Miltenberger, R. G., & Fuqua, R. W. (1985). A comparison of contingent vs non-contingent competing response practice in the treatment of nervous habits. *Journal of Behavior Therapy and Experimental Psychiatry* 16, 195–200. https://doi.org/10.1016/0005-7916(85)90063-1.

Müller-Vahl, K. R., Riemann, L., & Bokemeyer, S. (2014). Tourette patients' misbelief of a tic rebound is due to overall difficulties in reliable tic rating. *Journal of Psychosomatic Research*, 76, 472–476. https://doi.org/10.1016/j.jpsychores.2014.03.003.

Peterson, A. L., & Azrin, N. H. (1992). An evaluation of behavioral treatments for Tourette syndrome. *Behaviour Research and Therapy*, 30, 167–174. https://doi.org/10.1016/0005-7967(92)90140-c.

Peterson, A. L., McGuire, J. F., Wilhelm, S., et al. (2016). An empirical examination of symptom substitution associated with behavior therapy for Tourette's disorder. *Behavior Therapy*, 47, 29–41. https://doi.org/10.1016/j.beth.2015.09.001.

Piacentini, J., Woods, D. W., Scahill, L., et al. (2010). Behavior therapy for children with Tourette Disorder. *Journal of American Medical Association*, 303, 1929. https://doi.org/10.1001/jama.2010.607.

Pringsheim, T., Okun, M. S., Müller-Vahl, K., et al. (2019). Practice guideline recommendations summary: Treatment of tics in people with Tourette syndrome and chronic tic disorders. *Neurology* 92, 896–906. https://doi.org/10.1212/WNL.0000000000007466.

Quezada, J., & Coffman, K. A. (2018). Current approaches and new developments in the pharmacological management of Tourette syndrome. *CNS Drugs* 32, 33–45. https://doi.org/10.1007/s40263-017-0486-0.

Rachamim, L., Zimmerman-Brenner, S., Rachamim, O., et al. (2022). Internet-based guided self-help comprehensive behavioral intervention for tics (ICBIT) for youth with tic disorders: A feasibility and effectiveness study with 6 month-follow-up. *European Child & Adolescent Psychiatry*, 31, 275–287. https://doi.org/10.1007/s00787-020-01686-2.

Reese, H. E., Vallejo, Z., Rasmussen, J., et al. (2015). Mindfulness-based stress reduction for Tourette Syndrome and Chronic Tic Disorder: A pilot study. *Journal of Psychosomatic Research*, 78, 293–298. https://doi.org/10.1016/j.jpsychores.2014.08.001.

Roane, H. S., Piazza, C. C., Cercone, J. J., & Grados, M. (2002). Assessment and treatment of vocal tics associated with Tourette's syndrome. *Behavior Modification*, 26, 482–498. https://doi.org/10.1177/0145445502026004003.

Robertson, M. M. (2008). The prevalence and epidemiology of Gilles de la Tourette syndrome. Part 1: The epidemiological and prevalence studies. *Journal of Psychosomatic Research*, 65(5): 461–472. https://doi.org/10.1016/j.jpsychores.2008.03.006.

Robertson, M. M., Banerjee, S., Fox-Hiley, P. J., & Tannock, C. (2018). Personality disorder and psychopathology in Tourette's syndrome: A controlled study. *The British Journal of Psychiatry*, 171(3), 283–286. https://doi.org/10.1192/bjp.171.3.283.

Singer, H. S. (2016). Habitual and goal-directed behaviours and Tourette syndrome. *Brain*, 139, 312–316. https://doi.org/10.1093/brain/awv378.

Stiede, J. T., Woods, D. W., Anderson, S., et al. (2021). Cultural differences in reactions to tics and tic severity. *Child and Family Behavior Therapy*, 43, 161–180. https://doi.org/10.1080/07317107.2021.1940586.

Sukhodolsky, D. G., Woods, D. W., Piacentini, J., et al. (2017). Moderators and predictors of response to behavior therapy for tics in Tourette syndrome. *Neurology*, 88, 1029–1036. https://doi.org/10.1212/WNL.0000000000003710.

Tilling, F., & Cavanna, A. E. (2020). Relaxation therapy as a treatment for tics in patients with Tourette syndrome: A systematic literature review. *Neurological Sciences*, 41, 1011–1017. https://doi.org/10.1007/s10072-019-04207-5.

Verdellen, C. W. J., Hoogduin, C. A. L., Kato, B. S., et al. (2008). Habituation of premonitory sensations during exposure and response prevention treatment in Tourette's syndrome. *Behavior Modification*, 32(2), 215–227. https://doi.org/10.1177/0145445507309020.

Verdellen, C. W. J., Keijsers, G. P., Cath, D. C., & Hoogduin, C. A. (2004). Exposure with response prevention versus habit reversal in Tourette's syndrome: A controlled study. *Behaviour Research and Therapy* 42, 501–511. https://doi.org/10.1016/S0005-7967(03)00154-2.

Verdellen, C. W. J., van de Griendt, J. M. T. M., Kriens, S., & van Oostrum, I. (2011a). *Tics: Therapist manual*. Boom Publishers.

Verdellen, C. W. J., van de Griendt, J. M. T. M., Kriens, S., & van Oostrum, I. (2011b). *Tics: Therapist manual and workbook for children*. Boom Publishers.

Wagaman, J. R., Miltenberger, R. G., & Williams, D. E. (1995). Treatment of a vocal tic by differential reinforcement. *Journal of Behavior Therapy and Experimental Psychiatry*, 26, 35–39. https://doi.org/10.1016/0005-7916(94)00068-w.

Walkup, J. T., Mink, J. W., & McNaught, K. (2012). *A family's guide to Tourette syndrome*. iUniverse, Inc.

Watson, T. S., & Sterling, H. E. (1998). Brief functional analysis and treatment of a vocal tic. *Journal of Applied Behavior Analysis*, 31, 471–474. https://doi.org/10.1901/jaba.1998.31-471.

Weisman, H., Qureshi, I. A., Leckman, J. F., Scahill, L., & Bloch, M. H. (2013). Systematic review: Pharmacological treatment of tic disorders- efficacy of antipsychotic and alpha-2 adrenergic agonist agents. *Neuroscience and Biobehavioral Reviews*, 37, 1162–1171. https://doi.org/10.1016/j.neubiorev.2012.09.008.

Wetterneck, C. T., & Woods, D. W. (2006). An evaluation of the effectiveness of exposure and response prevention on repetitive behaviors associated with Tourette's syndrome. *Journal of Applied Behavior Analysis*, 39, 441–444. https://doi.org/10.1901/jaba.2006.149-03.

Wile, D. J., & Pringsheim, T. M. (2013). Behavior therapy for Tourette syndrome: A systematic review and meta-analysis. *Current Treatment Options in Neurology*, 15, 385–395. https://doi.org/10.1007/s11940-013-0238-5.

Wilhelm, S., Peterson, A. L., Piacentini, J., et al. (2012). Randomized trial of behavior therapy for adults with Tourette syndrome. *Archives of General Psychiatry*, 69, 795. https://doi.org/10.1001/archgenpsychiatry.2011.1528.

Wiskow, K. M., & Klatt, K. P. (2013). The effects of awareness training on tics in a young boy with Tourette syndrome, Asperger syndrome, and attention deficit hyperactivity disorder. *Journal of Applied Behavior Analysis* 46, 695–698. https://doi.org/10.1002/jaba.59.

Woods, D. W., Conelea, C. A., & Himle, M. B. (2010). Behavior therapy for Tourette's disorder: Utilization in a community sample and an emerging area of practice for psychologists. *Professional Psychology: Research and Practice*, 41, 518–525. https://doi.org/10.1037/a0021709.

Woods, D. W., Himle, M. B., Stiede, J. T., & Pitts, B. X. (2023). Behavioral interventions for children and adults with tic disorders. *Annual Review of Clinical Psychology*, 19, 207–232. https://doi.org/10.1146/annurev-clinpsy-080921-074307.

Woods, D. W., Hook, S. S., Spellman, D. F., & Friman, P. C. (2000). Case study: Exposure and response prevention for an adolescent with Tourette's syndrome and OCD. *Journal of the American Academy of Child and Adolescent Psychiatry*, 39, 904–907. https://doi.org/10.1097/00004583-200007000-00020.

Woods, D. W., Miltenberger, R. G., & Lumley, V. A. (1996). Sequential application of major habit reversal components to treat motor tics in children. *Journal of Applied Behavior Analysis* 29, 483–493. https://doi.org/10.1901/jaba.1996.29-483.

Woods, D. W., Piacentini, J. C., Chang, S. W., et al. (2008). *Managing Tourette syndrome: A behavioral intervention for children and adults*. Oxford University Press.

Woods, D., Piacentini, J., Himle, M. B., & Chang, S. (2005). Premonitory urge for tics scale (PUTS). *Journal of Developmental & Behavioral Pediatrics*, 26, 397–403. https://doi.org/10.1097/00004703-200512000-00001.

Wright, K. M., & Miltenberger, R. G. (1987). Awareness training in the treatment of head and facial tics. *Journal of Behavior Therapy and Experimental Psychiatry*, 18, 269–274. https://doi.org/10.1016/0005-7916(87)90010-3.

Yan, J., Cui, L., Wang, M., Cui, Y., & Li, Y. (2022). The efficacy and neural correlates of ERP-based therapy for OCD and TS: A systematic review and meta-analysis. *Journal of Integrative Neuroscience*, 21, 97. https://doi.org/10.31083/j.jin2103097.

Yates, R., Edwards, K., King, J., et al. (2016). Habit reversal training and educational group treatments for children with Tourette syndrome: A preliminary randomized controlled trial. *Behaviour Research and Therapy*, 80, 43–50. https://doi.org/10.1016/j.brat.2016.03.003.

Yu, L., Li, Y., Zhang, J., et al. (2020). The therapeutic effect of habit reversal training for Tourette syndrome: A meta-analysis of randomized control trials. *Expert Review of Neurotherapeutics*, 20, 1189–1196. https://doiorg/10.1080/14737175.2020.1826933.

Zimmerman-Brenner, S., Pilowsky-Peleg, T., Rachamim, L., et al. (2022). Group behavioral interventions for tics and comorbid symptoms in children with chronic tic disorders. *European Child and Adolescent Psychiatry*, 31, 637–648. https://doi.org/10.1007/s00787-020-01702-5.

20

Couples Discord

Matthew D. Johnson and Erin F. Reto

Unlike most of the chapters that precede this one, the goal of couple therapy usually is not the treatment of a disorder found in the *Diagnostic and Statistical Manual of Mental Disorders* (DSM-5-TR; American Psychiatric Association, 2022). Rather, the target of couple therapy is the improvement of a couple's intimate relationship. By "intimate relationship" we mean a close relationship that, at minimum, has the potential for sex – relationships such as those experienced by couples who are dating, living together, or married. We are not referring to other close relationships, such as between other family members, friends, or business partners. While there is some evidence that couple therapy approaches can be used with other types of close relationships and couple therapy has demonstrated efficacy in treating problems beyond the relationship (e.g., psychopathology, physical ailments, and parenting), the vast majority of the research – and our focus in this chapter – is on employing couple therapy to improve intimate relationships.

Couple therapy tends to have two conceptual goals: (1) the prevention or treatment of relationship distress and (2) the prevention of relationship dissolution. Relationship distress is usually operationalized with self-report measures of relationship satisfaction, relationship quality, or relationship adjustment (and is included in the DSM-5-TR under Other Conditions that May be a Focus of Clinical Attention). Psychometrically, these are essentially the same underlying concept, with distress being the opposite of satisfaction (Balderrama-Durbin et al., 2015; Mattson et al., 2013; Norton, 1983); therefore, for the purposes of this chapter, we will use the terms "relationship distress" and "relationship satisfaction." Relationship dissolution simply means a divorce for married couples and a break-up for unmarried couples.

Etiology and Theoretical Underpinnings of Treatment

There are several broad theories from which couple therapies have been derived (Paolino & McCrady, 1978). All of the approaches that have been subjected to research feature the ongoing exchange of behavior within the couple. In this sense, one can make the case – as we do – that social learning theory is at least part of, if not central to, all of the couple therapies that have any empirical support. In social learning theory (Bandura, 1977), basic operant learning principles guide social behaviors among people. In other words, social learning theory is based on the idea that people modify each other's behavior specifically through the rewards and punishments that follow those behaviors (Bandura, 1969). In couples, the theory posits that relationship partners routinely and mutually reward and punish each other's behaviors. Dysfunction develops when problematic behaviors are rewarded and desirable behaviors are punished. All forms of couple therapy to one degree or another attempt to alter maladaptive learning that has taken place between partners. In other words, in various ways, couple therapies try to reinforce adaptive interpersonal behaviors while ignoring or punishing maladaptive interpersonal behaviors (Stuart, 1969).

These theoretical principles became the foundation for couple therapies designed to prevent (Markman, 1979) and treat (Jacobson & Margolin, 1979; Stuart, 1980) relationship distress. Not only were social learning theory and behavioral principles eagerly adapted for couple therapy, they are widely accepted by many people in WEIRD (Western, Educated, Industrialized, Rich, and Democratic; Henrich et al., 2010) societies. The most shared article in *The New York Times* is one in which a reporter covering animal trainers used the same operant learning techniques the trainers were using on animals on her husband. In the article, she described how she stopped inadvertently reinforcing her husband's dysfunctional behaviors (Sutherland, 2006). Of course, most couples do not describe their problems as dysfunctional learning problems, they describe them as "communication" problems. What is communication if not the ongoing exchange of behavior within the couple, which rests at the heart of social learning theory? It is understandable that couples and their therapists find social learning theory appealing because the ongoing exchange of behaviors is the most proximal and parsimonious means of connecting to a partner and assessing the strength of that connection. Each of the couple therapies described herein relies to one degree or another on this theoretical principle.

Brief Overview of Treatments

There are many approaches to couple therapy that have empirical support and have been subjected to randomized controlled trials (RCTs); for a full review of these, see Lebow and Snyder (2022), and for a meta-analysis, see Roddy and colleagues (2020). For the purposes of this chapter, we focus on behavioral couple therapy and therapies that developed out of it (i.e., what some have termed "third-wave" therapies).

As noted previously, in first-wave behavioral couple therapy the goal was to alter the dysfunctional learning that has taken place between partners and to relearn more functional behavioral patterns (Jacobson & Margolin, 1979; Stuart, 1980). RCTs of behavioral couple therapy demonstrated improvement in partners' relationship satisfaction. A meta-analysis found that it was more effective ($d = 0.59$) than no-treatment control groups (Shadish & Baldwin, 2005). However, fewer than half of couples treated with behavioral couple therapy had improved to the point that they were no longer different from couples who were not seeking treatment (Jacobson et al., 1984) and thus considered successful. Of the couples successfully treated, only about 70% maintained the improvement for two years (Jacobson et al., 1987); 15% of successfully treated couples dissolved their relationship within two years (Christensen et al., 2006) and 30% dissolved their relationship within five years (Christensen et al., 2010).

After publicly declaring that behavioral couple therapy was ineffective, Neil Jacobson – one of the original developers of the intervention – collaborated with Andrew Christensen to develop integrated behavioral couple therapy (IBCT; Jacobson & Christensen, 1996). This approach, like other third-wave therapies, combined elements of the behavioral approach with acceptance of some aspects of their relationship and partner. Jacobson and Christensen then conducted a rigorous two-site RCT comparing IBCT to behavioral couple therapy. After five years, recovery rates were similar for both groups, as were the rates of couples who deteriorated and divorced (Christensen et al., 2010). Thus, ICBT does not appear to be more efficacious than behavioral couple therapy.

Another couple therapy approach that was gaining attention at the same time was emotionally focused therapy (EFT; Johnson & Greenberg, 1995), which is described by its developers as an attachment-based, experiential-humanistic, systemic intervention (Greenman & Johnson, 2013). Nevertheless, the first stage in the EFT approach involves "cycle de-escalation," followed by a restructuring of couples' interactions. These are the core components of a behavioral approach. EFT leads to 39% of couples being indistinguishable from nontreatment-seeking couples, 7% to improvement but still below the satisfaction of nontreatment-seeking couples, 21% who experienced no change, and 32% who experienced deterioration or dissolution (Beasley & Ager, 2019; Wiebe et al., 2017). In other words, the outcome research on EFT did not differ substantially from that of behavioral couple therapy and IBCT.

Although there are other couple therapy approaches that have empirical support, behavioral couple therapy, IBCT, and EFT are the three with a substantial body of RCTs behind them. Other approaches that have been carefully researched, including with outcome research, are as follows:

- Cognitive-behavioral couple therapy is very similar conceptually to behavioral couple therapy, but with more of a focus on dysfunctional thoughts (i.e., second-wave). The outcome data on this approach is similar to other behavioral approaches (Baucom et al., 2022).
- Insight-oriented couple therapy is based on the couple understanding the origin of their problems. It yielded similar results to behavioral couple therapy initially and at six months

Box 20.1 Preventative Interventions

Preventative interventions for couples, often called couple relationship education (CRE), were developed contemporaneously with behavioral couple therapy, with the same fundamental principles (e.g., Gottman et al., 1976; Markman & Floyd, 1980). The most widely studied of the CREs is the Prevention and Relationship Enhancement Program (PREP). Developed by Howard Markman, PREP was designed to teach couples how to communicate more effectively, especially while discussing topics on which there is disagreement (Markman et al., 1994). Others have developed programs that include acceptance, commitment, empathy, stress management, and relationship maintenance (e.g., Bodenmann & Shantinath, 2004; Halford, 2011; Ragan et al., 2009; Rogge et al., 2013). Nevertheless, all of these CREs have the goal of preventing declines in satisfaction by teaching couples better ways to communicate and handle the inevitable stresses on their relationships.

Meta-analyses of RCTs indicate that prevention programs have a small to medium effect on communication ($d = 0.44$) and relationship quality ($d = 0.36$) immediately after the program (Hawkins et al., 2008). The problem is that there are some indications that CRE programs can have negative impacts on couples, such as leading some to feel less safe in the relationship (e.g., Bir et al., 2012; Wood et al., 2014). The effects of CREs on relationships in the subsequent few years are null (Johnson, 2012, 2013; Johnson & Bradbury, 2015). A meta-analysis of CREs showed that effectiveness was predicted neither by the type of skill being taught nor the rigor of the program (Hawkins et al., 2012). In the end, couples not receiving CREs and states not pushing CREs fare no worse than do couples participating in CRE programs or states with more CRE funding in terms of divorce rates (Johnson, 2014). In conclusion, the prevention of relationship problems through CREs lacks the effectiveness to be considered empirically supported.

following treatment (Snyder & Wills, 1989). In one study, it also had a substantially lower divorce rate (3% compared with 38%; Snyder et al., 1991).

Despite the assortment of approaches to choose from, at this time IBCT and EFT are the couple therapies with the most evaluation research behind them; however, there is no reason to think that cognitive-behavioral couple therapy and insight-oriented couple therapy would fare any differently (for efficacy reviews, see Bradbury & Bodenmann, 2020; Roddy et al., 2020).

Credible Components of Treatments

As noted previously, meta-analyses of couple therapy support a large effect ($d \geq 0.80$) immediately following termination of treatment, with 60–72% of couples having noticeably better relationship satisfaction. As for whether these improvements last, here are five-year posttreatment data from a rigorous study: 31–33% of couples have recovered; 13–19% have improved but are still distressed; 50–54% have not changed, deteriorated, or dissolved their relationship (Christensen et al., 2010). Returning to the meta-analytic findings, caution should be used in interpreting the efficacy studies of couple therapy overall because of the heterogeneity in the study designs, sample sizes, and characteristics, and the involvement of the developers of the treatments in the evaluation studies. As with all evaluation studies, the degree to which placebo effects inflate treatment effects is not known without an active control group. Most of these studies only used a passive no-treatment group. With those qualifications and all things being equal (which they never are), one could argue that distressed couples seeking treatment with a competent therapist have a one-in-three chance of experiencing improvement that lasts for at least five years.

None of the therapeutic approaches have been declared the clear winner, therefore the field is considering which components of couple therapy increase its impact. Although these lines of research are ongoing, Bradbury and Bodenmann (2020) identified the following components of couple therapy as having promising results.

Early Assessment of Goals and Commitment

Couple therapy is a bitter pill. By the time they call a therapist, many couples find themselves in relationships that are very near the point of dissolution. As many as half are already actively considering separation and feel hopeless about whether the relationship can be salvaged (Doss et al., 2004). Assessing couples' goals for treatment in the initial appointments is essential to understanding the prognosis of therapy. The IBCT model (Christensen et al., 2020) suggests meeting with couples conjointly in the first session and splitting the second session into two individual sessions. This allows therapists to assess the couples' and individuals' goals for treatment; commitment to the relationship, including whether there are any ultimatums on the table (e.g., a secession to extramarital relationships); optimism/hopelessness for treatment; and willingness to work on improving the relationship. This assessment (via interview and self-report measures) provides important prognostic information because the rate of relationship dissolution within six months of therapy is 10% for couples in which both partners have the goal of improving the relationship, 45% if only one partner seeks improvement, and 56% if both partners have the goal of determining whether the relationship can be saved (Owen et al., 2012; see Baucom et al., 2015, for similar five-year data). If one or both partners seem to be questioning the viability of the relationship or have the goal of an amicable dissolution, there are other models of intervention available, such as discernment counseling (Doherty et al., 2016) and planning for divorce in couple therapy (Lebow, 2022). In the end, a careful assessment at the onset of treatment is likely to enable either triaging couples poorly suited for couple therapy or improved efficacy of couple therapy (for a more thorough review of couple assessment, see Snyder & Balderrama-Durbin, 2022).

Measurement-Based Care

Assessment should not end at the onset of treatment; rather, ongoing assessment with psychometrically validated instruments should continue through treatment. The powerful force of confirmation bias makes it difficult for therapists to gauge progress using their own observations of the couple. In individual psychotherapy, research shows that session-by-session monitoring and feedback of symptoms improves treatment outcomes (Lambert et al., 2018). In couple therapy, measurement-based approaches allow for more precise prediction of couples who are not benefiting from couple therapy (e.g., Pepping et al., 2015). In two studies in which couples were randomly assigned to either session-by-session monitoring of treatment progress and alliance versus treatment as usual, the couples in the measurement-based treatment had twice the rate of recovery or reliable improvement at the end of treatment compared with the control group (Anker et al., 2009; Reese et al., 2010). In summary, session-by-session data appears to improve couple therapy outcomes, at least by the end of therapy. It is likely that the mechanism for this is providing the therapist insights not easily gained from observation alone that allow for course-correction during treatment (for more discussion of this, see Halford et al., 2016).

Focusing on Positive Exchanges Between Partners

The two couple therapy approaches with long-term efficacy studies – IBCT and EFT – show the same pattern: treatment effects fade over time (Christensen et al., 2010; Wiebe et al., 2017). Christensen and colleagues found that, of the couples who reliably improved or fully recovered by termination, half reverted to pretreatment levels of relationship satisfaction or deteriorated even further. So, what distinguishes the couples with lasting beneficial effects from those who deteriorate? It appears that couples who maintain their relationship gains for five years posttreatment have greater levels of problem-solving ability, display more positive behavior toward their partner, reciprocate more positive behavior from their partner, and display more empathy during conflict. In reviewing the list of five-year outcome predictors in the previous sentence, note that these are all positive behaviors, whereas changes in negative behaviors/skills and withdrawal/avoidance (either during treatment or measured following treatment) did not predict five-year outcomes (Baucom et al., 2015; Baucom et al., 2011). These findings, which are consistent with basic longitudinal marital research (Johnson et al., 2005), offer hope that more of a focus on positive skills and behaviors may allow couples to sustain the benefits of treatment for the long-term. This is particularly challenging for therapists given couples' reasonable focus on addressing the negative interactions that brought them to therapy initially, but it is likely worth rising to this challenge. Even if this challenge is met, understanding how to focus on positive exchanges is fraught with the potential for partners to dismiss positive acts because their partner is just doing what the therapist told them to do; therefore, we explore some of the techniques from EFT and IBCT with promising findings.

In both EFT and IBCT, improvements in relationship satisfaction appear linked to in-session emotional responses, intimate disclosures and responsive affiliative statements, and discussion of attachment issues. While the exact procedures are beyond the scope of this chapter, therapists work to soften the emotion of an aggrieved partner. As part of this, the therapist attempts to elicit the aggrieved partner's expression of a desire for closeness that in turn may lower the defenses of the other partner and bring that person back into the conversation (Wiebe et al., 2017). In different studies, this process has covaried concurrently with session-by-session increases in relationship satisfaction and in attachment security (Johnson & Whiffen, 1999; McKinnon & Greenberg, 2017; Moser et al., 2018). In these tactics, therapists are explicitly attempting to change expressions of affect from anger, contempt, and fear to affect that is vulnerable, warm, and affiliative (Christensen et al., 2020; Schade et al., 2015; Zuccarini et al., 2013).

Other Variables Influencing Treatment

Assessment of Intimate Partner Violence

Initial and ongoing rigorous assessment has been demonstrated to enhance immediate and long-term efficacy. In this section, we focus on the assessment of intimate partner violence (IPV) as essential to determining whether couple therapy is indicated. The common belief among therapists is that IPV is not a homogeneous phenomenon, but rather that it falls into distinct categorical groups. The belief in an IPV typology, such as those proposed by Michael Johnson (1995) and Amy Holtzworth-Munroe (Holtzworth-Munroe & Stuart, 1994) is widely accepted. However, there is scant evidence to support these theories (Alexander & Johnson, 2023; Alexander & Johnson, under review) and no validated assessment instrument that distinguishes them (Alexander et al., 2021). Our recommendation is to ask about violence with both partners present, then conduct a brief interview with each partner individually and administer the HITS: a validated four-item measure that stands for Hurt, Insulted, Threatened, and Screamed (Sherin et al., 1998). If there is a low level of violence (e.g., pushing or slapping), it is worth administering a validated couple-based IPV intervention (Heyman & Schlee, 2003); however, if the violence is serious with a high potential for lethality, it is recommended that the victim(s) become unavailable to the perpetrator (de Becker, 1997).

Comorbidity

Relationship satisfaction is so strongly correlated with mental health that all but one of the 11 most common mental illnesses tend to be comorbid with relationship distress (Whisman, 2007), a finding consistent across racial and ethnic groups (McShall & Johnson, 2015). Therefore, it is no surprise that, although the goal of couple therapy is typically to improve relationship quality, it can be effectively used to reduce symptoms of comorbid illnesses (Meis et al., 2013). As the efficacy of couple-based approaches to treating psychopathology has become better known, the acceptance of it as a treatment has grown.

The mental illness for which couple therapy has been studied the most is depression. The efficacy of couple therapy approaches to depression has been described and reviewed with meta-analyses (e.g., Barbato & D'Avanzo, 2020). Importantly, there appears to be no clear differences between couple therapy and various efficacious individual psychotherapies for depression, but couple therapy has the added benefit of being more efficacious than individual therapy at treating relationship distress. This is particularly notable because a systematic review of the research evidence on the comorbidity of depression and relationship distress led to the conclusion that "summating across the evidence obtained from research using correlational, genetically informed, and intervention methods, we conclude that relationship distress is a causal risk factor for depression" (Whisman et al., 2021, p. 250).

More and more diagnoses are demonstrating improved or as-good-as efficacy by employing couple-based therapies instead of individual treatment. For example, alcohol and drug problems are also a frequent target for couple-based interventions. A meta-analysis of RCTs of alcohol abuse treatments found that couple-based interventions were more efficacious than individual-based treatment (and again increased relationship satisfaction; Powers et al., 2008). As the role of relationships in the etiology and treatment of various forms of psychopathology becomes more evident, we expect to see couple therapy used more widely with more mental health disorders.

Demographics

There are some couple-based interventions that have been adapted for different developmental stages and couples experiencing distinctive stressors. Most of the adaptations that have had some outcome data collected tend to be primary or secondary interventions. For example, a cognitive-behavioral secondary intervention was designed for low-income African American couples with children. In this in-home intervention, couples received instruction on how to work together to address stressors likely to impact them (e.g., racism). An RCT of the project revealed that the vast majority of the couples completed all six sessions, with treated

Box 20.2 Self-Directed and Brief Programs

With the onset of the pandemic, telemedicine and video therapy have become the norm and widely accepted. Much has been written about the ways in which this will enable more people to access these services. There were some couple-based interventions that preceded the pandemic that have rigorous data. Initial work suggests that self-directed programs have comparable effects with in-person programs (e.g., Braithwaite & Fincham, 2014; Zemp et al., 2017). For example, OurRelationship is an interactive web-based program marketed as a "relationship counseling alternative." It has many of the components of in-person couple therapy, including a self-assessment stage, a goal-setting stage, a problem-identification stage, an understand-the-problem stage, and, finally, a resolution stage that employs acceptance and problem solving. Couples also participate in four coaching sessions in which they can ask questions, review progress, and tweak the program (Doss et al., 2013). In an RCT of OurRelationship with 300 couples who were initially distressed, treated couples reported greater satisfaction at termination compared with a waitlist control condition ($d = 0.69$), and 57% improved their relationship satisfaction, 36% had no change, and 7% deteriorated (Doss et al., 2016). These effects were maintained a year following treatment and appear to be beneficial for parenting as well (Doss et al., 2020; Doss et al., 2019; Roddy et al., 2021). It is also worth noting that a brief two-session in-person couple therapy program also led to demonstrable reductions in marital distress (Córdova et al., 2014). Based on these data, it appears that online or minimal interventions may be as effective as traditional in-person couple therapy while also greatly expanding access to care.

couples reporting better satisfaction, communication, and parenting relationships at 17- and 25-month follow ups compared with the couples who received a workbook on relationship communication (Barton et al., 2017; Barton et al., 2018; Lavner et al., 2019, 2020). The success of this intervention points to the benefits of taking stressors associated with distinct demographic characteristics into account in couple therapy.

The transition to parenthood is a particularly challenging time for couples (Doss & Rhoades, 2017; Johnson, 2016). Unfortunately, a meta-analysis of specialized interventions for couples transitioning to parenthood revealed negligible effects on relationship satisfaction ($d = 0.12$) and small effects on communication ($d = 0.29$) over one year (Pinquart & Teubert, 2010). However, there is evidence that couples with several known risk factors for divorce benefit from couples-based interventions as they transition to parenthood (Petch et al., 2012), and these benefits last more than two years later (Heyman et al., 2019). Thus, there is still much to learn about tailoring interventions for couples at particular life stages, particularly with regard to secondary interventions.

Conclusion

Relationship problems are not only common but important. Overall life satisfaction is most closely aligned with relationship satisfaction (Diener et al., 2000; Diener et al., 1999), and it is associated with nearly everything we care about, including physical health (e.g., Langhinrichsen-Rohling et al., 2011), mental health (Whisman, 2007), and job performance (e.g., Forthofer et al., 1996; Leigh & Lust, 1988). Notably, many of these associations appear to be causal, with relationship problems leading to other problems (e.g., Whisman et al., 2021). So, what do we know about preventing and treating relationship distress? We know that many couples will remain mostly happy and that relationship education programs for these couples is probably unnecessary. Many other couples have the deck stacked against them and will struggle to make their relationships work because of their circumstances. We know that alleviating the stress in their lives is more likely than therapy or relationship education programs to prevent relationship dissolution (Johnson, 2013). Finally, we know that many other couples will become distressed and fall into patterns of conflict or malaise in their relationship. The approaches to couple therapy that have been empirically tested using rigorous methods offer some hope for these couples. IBCT and EFT, with their focus on emotional connection and acceptance, perform reasonably well in RCTs, and research on the efficacious mechanisms of change suggest that there are some common factors and principles at work across couple therapeutic approaches. Common factors, such as the quality of the alliance between patient and therapist, reliably predict outcomes in therapy (Cuijpers et al., 2019) and this is true in couple therapy as well (Davis, 2022). Beyond these common factors there are credible components of a science-based approach to couple therapy outlined by Bradbury and Bodenmann (2020) as well as Christensen (2010). Some have proposed a unified protocol for couple therapy with five common principles: "(a) altering the couple's view of the presenting problem to be more objective, contextualized, and dyadic; (b) decreasing emotion-driven, dysfunctional behavior; (c) eliciting emotion-based, avoided, private behavior; (d) increasing constructive communication patterns; and (e) emphasizing strengths and reinforcing gains" (Benson et al., 2012, p. 25). To varying degrees, science-based approaches to couple therapy incorporate all five principles of the unified protocol. Based on the current empirical literature, couple therapists would do well to heed these principles no matter the model they prefer to employ.

Useful Resources

- An approach to treating relationship distress by watching movies: www.rochester.edu/news/divorce-rate-cut-in-half-for-couples-who-discussed-relationship-movies/
- An efficacious online self-directed couple therapy: www.ourrelationship.com/
- EFT, another efficacious couple therapy: http://iceeft.com/
- IBCT, an efficacious couple therapy: https://ibct.psych.ucla.edu/

References

Alexander, E. F., Backes, B. L., & Johnson, M. D. (2021). Evaluating measures of intimate partner violence using consensus-based standards of validity. *Trauma, Violence, & Abuse*, 15248380211013413. https://doi.org/10.1177/15248380211013413

Alexander, E. F., & Johnson, M. D. (under review). *Comparing typologies of intimate partner violence using finite mixture modeling.*

Alexander, E. F., & Johnson, M. D. (2023). On categorizing intimate partner violence: A systematic review of exploratory clustering and classification studies. *Journal of Family Psychology*, 37(5), 743–752. https://doi.org/10.1037/fam0001075

American Psychiatric Association. (2022). *Diagnostic and statistical manual of mental disorders* (5th ed., Text Revision). American Psychiatric Publishing.

Anker, M. G., Duncan, B. L., & Sparks, J. A. (2009). Using client feedback to improve couple therapy outcomes: A randomized clinical trial in a naturalistic setting. *Journal of Consulting and Clinical Psychology*, 77(4), 693–704. https://doi.org/10.1037/a0016062.

Balderrama-Durbin, C., Snyder, D. K., & Balsis, S. (2015). Tailoring assessment of relationship distress using the Marital Satisfaction Inventory – Brief Form. *Couple and Family Psychology: Research and Practice*, 4(3), 127–135. https://doi.org/10.1037/cfp0000042.

Bandura, A. (1969). *Principles of behavior modification*. Holt, Rinehart and Winston.

Bandura, A. (1977). *Social learning theory*. Prentice-Hall.

Barbato, A., & D'Avanzo, B. (2020). The findings of a Cochrane meta-analysis of couple therapy in adult depression: Implications for research and clinical practice. *Family Process*, 59(2), 361–375.. https://doi.org/10.1111/famp.12540.

Barton, A. W., Beach, S. R. H., Lavner, J. A., et al. (2017). Is communication a mechanism of relationship education effects among rural African Americans? *Journal of Marriage and Family*, 79(5), 1450–1461. https://doi.org/10.1111/jomf.12416.

Barton, A. W., Beach, S. R. H., Wells, A. C., et al. (2018). The protecting strong African American families program: A randomized controlled trial with rural African American couples. *Prevention Science*, 19(7), 904–913. https://doi.org/10.1007/s11121-018-0895-4.

Baucom, B. R., Atkins, D. C., Rowe, L. S., Doss, B. D., & Christensen, A. (2015). Prediction of treatment response at 5-year follow-up in a randomized clinical trial of behaviorally based couple therapies. *Journal of Consulting and Clinical Psychology*, 83(1), 103–114. https://doi.org/10.1037/a0038005.

Baucom, D. H., Epstein, N., Fischer, M. S., Kirby, J. S., & LaTaillade, J. J. (2022). Cognitive aspects of cognitive-behavioral marital therapy. In J. Lebow & D. K. Snyder (Eds.), *Clinical handbook of couple therapy* (6th ed., pp. 53–78). Guilford.

Baucom, K. J. W., Sevier, M., Eldridge, K. A., Doss, B. D., & Christensen, A. (2011). Observed communication in couples two years after integrative and traditional behavioral couple therapy: Outcome and link with five-year follow-up. *Journal of Consulting and Clinical Psychology*, 79(5), 565–576. https://doi.org/10.1037/a0025121.

Beasley, C. C., & Ager, R. (2019). Emotionally Focused Couples Therapy: A systematic review of its effectiveness over the past 19 years. *Journal of Evidence-Based Social Work*, 16(2), 144-159. https://doi.org/10.1080/23761407.2018.1563013.

Benson, L. A., McGinn, M. M., & Christensen, A. (2012). Common principles of couple therapy. *Behavior Therapy*, 43(1), 25-35. https://doi.org/10.1016/j.beth.2010.12.009.

Bir, A., Corwin, E., MacIlvain, B., et al. (2012). The community healthy marriage initiative evaluation: Impacts of a community approach to strengthening families, OPRE Report #2012-34A.

Bodenmann, G., & Shantinath, S. D. (2004). The Couples Coping Enhancement Training (CCET): A new approach to prevention of marital distress based upon stress and coping. *Family Relations: An Interdisciplinary Journal of Applied Family Studies*, 53(5), 477–484. https://doi.org/10.1111/j.0197-6664.2004.00056.x.

Bradbury, T. N., & Bodenmann, G. (2020). Interventions for couples. *Annual Review of Clinical Psychology*, 16(1), 99–123. https://doi.org/10.1146/annurev-clinpsy-071519-020546.

Braithwaite, S. R., & Fincham, F. D. (2014). Computer-based prevention of intimate partner violence in marriage. *Behaviour Research and Therapy*, 54, 12–21. https://doi.org/10.1016/j.brat.2013.12.006.

Christensen, A. (2010). A unified protocol for couple therapy. In K. Hahlweg, M. Grawe-Gerber, & D. H. Baucom (Eds.), *Enhancing couples: The shape of couple therapy to come* (pp. 33–46). Hogrefe.

Christensen, A., Atkins, D. C., Baucom, B., & Yi, J. (2010). Marital status and satisfaction five years following a randomized clinical trial comparing traditional versus integrative behavioral couple therapy. *Journal of Consulting and Clinical Psychology*, 78(2), 225–235. https://doi.org/10.1037/a0018132.

Christensen, A., Atkins, D. C., Yi, J., George, W. H., & Baucom, D. H. (2006). Couple and individual adjustment for 2 years following a randomized clinical trial comparing traditional versus integrative behavioral couple therapy. *Journal of Consulting and Clinical Psychology*, 74(6), 1180–1191. https://doi.org/10.1037/0022-006X.74.6.1180.

Christensen, A., Doss, B. D., & Jacobson, N. S. (2020). *Integrative behavioral couple therapy: A therapist's guide to creating acceptance and change* (2nd ed.). Norton.

Córdova, J. V., Fleming, C. J. E., Morrill, M. I., et al. (2014). The Marriage Checkup: A randomized controlled trial of annual relationship health checkups. *Journal of Consulting and Clinical Psychology*, 82(4), 592–604. https://doi.org/10.1037/a0037097

Cuijpers, P., Reijnders, M., & Huibers, M. J. H. (2019). The role of common factors in psychotherapy outcomes. *Annual Review of Clinical Psychology*, 15, 207–231. https://doi.org/10.1146/annurev-clinpsy-050718-095424.

Davis, S. (2022). Common factors in couple therapy. In J. Lebow & D. K. Snyder (Eds.), *Clinical handbook of couple therapy* (6th ed., pp. 295–317). Guilford.

de Becker, G. (1997). *The gift of fear: Survival signals that protect us from violence*. Little, Brown and Company.

Diener, E., Gohm, C. L., Suh, E., & Oishi, S. (2000). Similarity of the relations between marital status and subjective well-being across cultures. *Journal of Cross-Cultural Psychology*, 31(4), 419–436. https://doi.org/10.1177/0022022100031004001.

Diener, E., Suh, E. M., Lucas, R. E., & Smith, H. L. (1999). Subjective well-being: Three decades of progress. *Psychological Bulletin*, 125(2), 276–302. https://doi.org/10.1037/0033-2909.125.2.276.

Doherty, W. J., Harris, S. M., & Wilde, J. L. (2016). Discernment counseling for "mixed-agenda" couples. *Journal of Marital and Family Therapy*, 42(2), 246–255. https://doi.org/10.1111/jmft.12132.

Doss, B. D., & Rhoades, G. K. (2017). The transition to parenthood: Impact on couples' romantic relationships. *Current Opinion in Psychology*, 13, 25–28. https://doi.org/10.1016/j.copsyc.2016.04.003.

Doss, B. D., Benson, L. A., Georgia, E. J., & Christensen, A. (2013). Translation of integrative behavioral couple therapy to a web-based intervention. *Family Process*, 52(1), 139–153. https://doi.org/10.1111/famp.12020.

Doss, B. D., Cicila, L. N., Georgia, E. J., et al. (2016). A randomized controlled trial of the web-based OurRelationship program: Effects on relationship and individual functioning. *Journal of Consulting and Clinical Psychology*, 84(4), 285–296. https://doi.org/10.1037/ccp0000063.

Doss, B. D., Roddy, M. K., Llabre, M. M., Georgia Salivar, E., & Jensen-Doss, A. (2020). Improvements in coparenting conflict and child adjustment following an online program for relationship distress. *Journal of Family Psychology*, 34(1), 68–78. https://doi.org/10.1037/fam0000582.

Doss, B. D., Roddy, M. K., Nowlan, K. M., Rothman, K., & Christensen, A. (2019). Maintenance of gains in relationship and individual functioning following the online OurRelationship program. *Behavior Therapy*, 50(1), 73–86. https://doi.org/10.1016/j.beth.2018.03.011.

Doss, B. D., Simpson, L. E., & Christensen, A. (2004). Why do couples seek marital therapy? *Professional Psychology: Research and Practice*, 35(6), 608–614. https://doi.org/10.1037/0735-7028.35.6.608.

Forthofer, M. S., Markman, H. J., Cox, M., Stanley, S., & Kessler, R. C. (1996). Associations between marital distress and work loss in a national sample. *Journal of Marriage and The Family*, 58(3), 597–605. https://doi.org/10.2307/353720.

Gottman, J. M., Notarius, C. I., Gonzo, J., & Markman, H. J. (1976). *A couple's guide to communication*. Research Press.

Greenman, P. S., & Johnson, S. M. (2013). Process research on Emotionally Focused Therapy (EFT) for couples: Linking theory to practice. *Family Process*, 52(1), 46–61. https://doi.org/10.1111/famp.12015.

Halford, W. K. (2011). *Marriage and relationship education: What works and how to provide it*. Guilford.

Halford, W. K., Pepping, C. A., & Petch, J. (2016). The gap between couple therapy research efficacy and practice effectiveness. *Journal of Marital and Family Therapy*, 42(1), 32-44. https://doi.org/10.1111/jmft.12120.

Hawkins, A. J., Blanchard, V. L., Baldwin, S. A., & Fawcett, E. B. (2008). Does marriage and relationship education work? A meta-analytic study. *Journal of Consulting and Clinical Psychology*, 76(5), 723–734. https://doi.org/10.1037/a0012584.

Hawkins, A. J., Stanley, S. M., Blanchard, V. L., & Albright, M. (2012). Exploring programmatic moderators of the effectiveness of marriage and relationship education programs: A meta-analytic study. *Behavior Therapy*, 43(1), 77–87. https://doi.org/10.1016/j.beth.2010.12.006.

Henrich, J., Heine, S. J., & Norenzayan, A. (2010). The weirdest people in the world? *The Behavioral and Brain Sciences*, 33(2–3), 45–67. https://doi.org/10.1017/S0140525X0999152X.

Heyman, R. E., & Schlee, K. (2003). Stopping wife abuse via physical aggression couples treatment. *Journal of Aggression, Maltreatment & Trauma*, 7(1-2), 135–157. https://doi.org/10.1300/J146v07n01_07.

Heyman, R. E., Slep, A. M. S., Lorber, M. F., et al. (2019). A randomized, controlled trial of the impact of the Couple CARE for Parents of Newborns program on the prevention of intimate partner violence and relationship problems. *Prevention Science*, 20(5), 620–631. https://doi.org/10.1007/s11121-018-0961-y.

Holtzworth-Munroe, A., & Stuart, G. L. (1994). Typologies of male batterers: Three subtypes and the differences among them. *Psychological Bulletin*, 116(3), 476–497. https://doi.org/10.1037/0033-2909.116.3.476.

Jacobson, N. S., & Christensen, A. (1996). *Integrative couple therapy: Promoting acceptance and change*. Norton.

Jacobson, N. S., & Margolin, G. (1979). *Marital therapy: Strategies based on social learning and behavior exchange principles*. Brunner/Mazel.

Jacobson, N. S., Follette, W. C., Revenstorf, D., et al. (1984). Variability in outcome and clinical significance of behavioral marital therapy: A reanalysis of outcome data. *Journal of Consulting and Clinical Psychology*, 52, 497–504. https://doi.org/10.1037/0022-006X.52.4.497.

Jacobson, N. S., Schmaling, K. B., & Holtzworth-Munroe, A. (1987). Component analysis of behavioral marital therapy: 2-year follow-up and prediction of relapse. *Journal of Marital and Family Therapy*, 13, 187–195. https://doi.org/10.1111/j.1752-0606.1987.tb00696.x.

Johnson, M. D. (2012). Healthy marriage initiatives: On the need for empiricism in policy implementation. *American Psychologist*, 67(4), 296–308. https://doi.org/10.1037/a0027743.

Johnson, M. D. (2013). Optimistic or quixotic? More data on marriage and relationship education programs for lower income couples. *American Psychologist*, 68(2), 111–112. https://doi.org/10.1037/a0031793.

Johnson, M. D. (2014). Government-supported healthy marriage initiatives are not associated with changes in family demographics: A comment on Hawkins, Amato, and Kinghorn (2013). *Family Relations*, 63(2), 300–304. https://doi.org/10.1111/fare.12060.

Johnson, M. D. (2016). Have children? Here's how kids ruin your romantic relationship. *TheConversation.com*. https://theconversation.com/have-children-heres-how-kids-ruin-your-romantic-relationship-57944.

Johnson, M. D., & Bradbury, T. N. (2015). Contributions of social learning theory to the promotion of healthy relationships: Asset or liability? *Journal of Family Theory & Review*, 7, 13–27. https://doi.org/10.1111/jftr.12057.

Johnson, M. D., Cohan, C. L., Davila, J., et al. (2005). Problem-solving skills and affective expressions as predictors of change in marital satisfaction. *Journal of Consulting and Clinical Psychology*, 73(1), 15–27. https://doi.org/10.1037/0022-006x.73.1.15.

Johnson, M. P. (1995). Patriarchal terrorism and common couple violence: Two forms of violence against women. *Journal of Marriage & the Family*, 57(2), 283–294. https://doi.org/10.2307/353683.

Johnson, S. M., & Greenberg, L. S. (1995). The emotionally focused approach to problems in adult attachment. In N. S. Jacobson & A. S. Gurman (Eds.), *Clinical handbook of couple therapy* (pp. 121–141). Guilford.

Johnson, S. M., & Whiffen, V. E. (1999). Made to measure: Adapting emotionally focused couple therapy to partners' attachment styles. *Clinical Psychology: Science and Practice*, 6(4), 366–381. https://doi.org/10.1093/clipsy.6.4.366.

Lambert, M. J., Whipple, J. L., & Kleinstäuber, M. (2018). Collecting and delivering progress feedback: A meta-analysis of routine outcome monitoring. *Psychotherapy*, 55(4), 520–537. https://doi.org/10.1037/pst0000167.

Langhinrichsen-Rohling, J., Snarr, J. D., Slep, A. M. S., Heyman, R. E., & Foran, H. M. (2011). Risk for suicidal ideation in the US Air Force: An ecological perspective. *Journal of Consulting and Clinical Psychology*, 79(5), 600–612. https://doi.org/10.1037/a0024631.

Lavner, J. A., Barton, A. W., & Beach, S. R. H. (2019). Improving couples' relationship functioning leads to improved coparenting: A randomized controlled trial with rural African American couples. *Behavior Therapy*, 50(6), 1016–1029. https://doi.org/10.1016/j.beth.2018.12.006.

Lavner, J. A., Barton, A. W., & Beach, S. R. H. (2020). Direct and indirect effects of a couple-focused preventive intervention on children's outcomes: A randomized controlled trial with African American families. *Journal of Consulting and Clinical Psychology*, 88(8), 696–707. https://doi.org/10.1037/ccp0000589.

Lebow, J. (2022). Divorce issues in couple therapy. In J. Lebow & D. K. Snyder (Eds.), *Clinical handbook of couple therapy* (6th ed., pp. 472–491). Guilford.

Lebow, J., & Snyder, D. K. (Eds.). (2022). *Clinical handbook of couple therapy* (6th ed.). Guilford.

Leigh, J. P., & Lust, J. (1988). Determinants of employee tardiness. *Work & Occupations*, 15(1), 78–95.

Markman, H. J. (1979). Application of a behavioral model of marriage in predicting relationship satisfaction of couples planning marriage. *Journal of Consulting and Clinical Psychology*, 47, 743–749. https://doi.org/10.1037/0022-006X.47.4.743.

Markman, H. J., & Floyd, F. (1980). Possibilities for the prevention of marital discord: A behavioral perspective. *American Journal of Family Therapy*, 8(2), 29–48. https://doi.org/10.1080/01926188008250355.

Markman, H. J., Stanley, S., & Blumberg, S. L. (1994). *Fighting for your marriage*. Jossey-Bass.

Mattson, R. E., Rogge, R. D., Johnson, M. D., Davidson, E. K. B., & Fincham, F. D. (2013). The positive and negative semantic dimensions of relationship satisfaction. *Personal Relationships*, 20, 328–355. https://doi.org/10.1111/j.1475-6811.2012.01412.x.

McKinnon, J. M., & Greenberg, L. S. (2017). Vulnerable emotional expression in emotion focused couples therapy: Relating interactional processes to outcome. *Journal of Marital and Family Therapy*, 43(2), 198–212. https://doi.org/10.1111/jmft.12229.

McShall, J. R., & Johnson, M. D. (2015). The association between relationship distress and psychopathology is consistent across racial and ethnic groups. *Journal of Abnormal Psychology*, 124(1), 226–231. https://doi.org/10.1037/a0038267.

Meis, L. A., Griffin, J. M., Greer, N., et al. (2013). Couple and family involvement in adult mental health treatment: A systematic review. *Clinical Psychology Review*, 33(2), 275–286. https://doi.org/10.1016/j.cpr.2012.12.003.

Moser, M. B., Johnson, S. M., Dalgleish, T. L., Wiebe, S. A., & Tasca, G. A. (2018). The impact of blamer-softening on romantic attachment in Emotionally Focused Couples Therapy. *Journal of Marital and Family Therapy*, 44(4), 640–654. https://doi.org/10.1111/jmft.12284.

Norton, R. (1983). Measuring marital quality: A critical look at the dependent variable. *Journal of Marriage and The Family*, 45(1), 141–151. https://doi.org/10.2307/351302.

Owen, J., Duncan, B., Anker, M., & Sparks, J. (2012). Initial relationship goal and couple therapy outcomes at post and six-month follow-up. *Journal of Family Psychology*, 26(2), 179–186. https://doi.org/10.1037/a0026998.

Paolino, T. J., & McCrady, B. S. (1978). *Marriage and marital therapy: Psychoanalytic, behavioral and systems theory perspectives*. Brunner/Mazel.

Pepping, C. A., Halford, W. K., & Doss, B. D. (2015). Can we predict failure in couple therapy early enough to enhance outcome? *Behaviour Research and Therapy*, 65, 60–66. https://doi.org/10.1016/j.brat.2014.12.015.

Petch, J. F., Halford, W. K., Creedy, D. K., & Gamble, J. (2012). A randomized controlled trial of a couple relationship and coparenting program (Couple CARE for Parents) for high- and low-risk new parents. *Journal of Consulting and Clinical Psychology*, 80(4), 662–673. https://doi.org/10.1037/a0028781.

Pinquart, M., & Teubert, D. (2010). A meta-analytic study of couple interventions during the transition to parenthood. *Family Relations: An Interdisciplinary Journal of Applied Family Studies*, 59(3), 221–231. https://doi.org/10.1111/j.1741-3729.2010.00597.x.

Powers, M. B., Vedel, E., & Emmelkamp, P. M. G. (2008). Behavioral couples therapy (BCT) for alcohol and drug use disorders: A meta-analysis. *Clinical Psychology Review*, 28(6), 952–962. https://doi.org/10.1016/j.cpr.2008.02.002.

Ragan, E. P., Einhorn, L. A., Rhoades, G. K., Markman, H. F., & Stanley, S. M. (2009). Relationship education programs: Current trends and future directions. In J. H. Bray & M. Stanton (Eds.), *The Wiley-Blackwell handbook of family psychology* (pp. 450–462). Wiley-Blackwell.

Reese, R. J., Toland, M. D., Slone, N. C., & Norsworthy, L. A. (2010). Effect of client feedback on couple psychotherapy outcomes. *Psychotherapy: Theory, Research, Practice, Training*, 47(4), 616–630. https://doi.org/10.1037/a0021182.

Roddy, M. K., Knopp, K., Georgia Salivar, E., & Doss, B. D. (2021). Maintenance of relationship and individual functioning gains following online relationship programs for low-income couples. *Family Process*, 60(1), 102–118. https://doi.org/10.1111/famp.12541.

Roddy, M. K., Walsh, L. M., Rothman, K., Hatch, S. G., & Doss, B. D. (2020). Meta-analysis of couple therapy: Effects across outcomes, designs, timeframes, and other moderators. *Journal of Consulting and Clinical Psychology*, 88(7), 583–596. https://doi.org/10.1037/ccp000051410.1037/ccp0000514.

Rogge, R. D., Cobb, R. J., Lawrence, E., Johnson, M. D., & Bradbury, T. N. (2013). Is skills training necessary for the primary prevention of marital distress and dissolution? A 3-year experimental study of three interventions. *Journal of Consulting and Clinical Psychology*, 81(6), 949–961. https://doi.org/10.1037/a0034209.

Schade, L. C., Sandberg, J. G., Bradford, A., et al. (2015). A longitudinal view of the association between therapist warmth and couples' in-session process: An observational pilot study of emotionally focused couples therapy. *Journal of Marital and Family Therapy*, 41(3), 292–307. https://doi.org/10.1111/jmft.12076.

Shadish, W. R., & Baldwin, S. A. (2005). Effects of behavioral marital therapy: A meta-analysis of randomized controlled trials. *Journal of Consulting and Clinical Psychology*, 73(1), 6–14. https://doi.org/10.1037/0022-006x.73.1.6.

Sherin, K. M., Sinacore, J. M., Li, X. Q., Zitter, R. E., & Shakil, A. (1998). HITS: A short domestic violence screening tool for use in a family practice setting. *Family Medicine*, 30(7), 508–512.

Snyder, D. K., & Balderrama-Durbin, C. (2022). Couple assessment. In J. Lebow & D. K. Snyder (Eds.), *Clinical handbook of couple therapy* (6th ed., pp. 22–51). Guilford.

Snyder, D. K., & Wills, R. M. (1989). Behavioral versus insight-oriented marital therapy: Effects on individual and interspousal functioning. *Journal of Consulting and Clinical Psychology*, 57, 39–46. https://doi.org/10.1037/0022-006X.57.1.39.

Snyder, D. K., Wills, R. M., & Grady-Fletcher, A. (1991). Long-term effectiveness of behavioral versus insight-oriented marital therapy: A 4-year follow-up study. *Journal of Consulting and Clinical Psychology*, 59(1), 138–131. https://doi.org/10.1037/0022-006X.59.1.138.

Stuart, R. B. (1969). Operant-interpersonal treatment for marital discord. *Journal of Consulting and Clinical Psychology*, 33, 675–682. https://doi.org/10.1037/h0028475.

Stuart, R. B. (1980). *Helping couples change: A social learning approach to marital therapy.* Guilford.

Sutherland, A. (2006). What Shamu taught me about a happy marriage. *The New York Times*, June 25. www.nytimes.com/2006/06/25/fashion/what-shamu-taught-me-about-a-happy-marriage.html.

Whisman, M. A. (2007). Marital distress and DSM-IV psychiatric disorders in a population-based national survey. *Journal of Abnormal Psychology*, 116(3), 638–643. https://doi.org/10.1037/0021-843X.116.3.638.

Whisman, M. A., Sbarra, D. A., & Beach, S. R. H. (2021). Intimate relationships and depression: Searching for causation in the sea of association. *Annual Review of Clinical Psychology*, 17(1), 233–258. https://doi.org/10.1146/annurev-clinpsy-081219-103323.

Wiebe, S. A., Johnson, S. M., Burgess Moser, M., Dalgleish, T. L., & Tasca, G. A. (2017). Predicting follow-up outcomes in emotionally focused couple therapy: The role of change in trust, relationship-specific attachment, and emotional engagement. *Journal of Marital and Family Therapy*, 43(2), 213–226. https://doi.org/10.1111/jmft.12199.

Wood, R. G., Moore, Q., Clarkwest, A., & Killewald, A. (2014). The long-term effects of Building Strong Families: A program for unmarried parents. *Journal of Marriage and Family*, 76(2), 446–463. https://doi.org/10.1111/jomf.12094.

Zemp, M., Merz, C. A., Nussbeck, F. W., et al. (2017). Couple relationship education: A randomized controlled trial of professional contact and self-directed tools. *Journal of Family Psychology*, 31(3), 347–357. https://doi.org/10.1037/fam0000257.

Zuccarini, D., Johnson, S. M., Dalgleish, T. L., & Makinen, J. A. (2013). Forgiveness and reconciliation in emotionally focused therapy for couples: The client change process and therapist interventions. *Journal of Marital and Family Therapy*, 39(2), 148–162. https://doi.org/10.1111/j.1752-0606.2012.00287.x.

21

Psychotherapy Relationships

John C. Norcross and Christie P. Karpiak

The patient–practitioner relationship constitutes the heart and soul of psychotherapy, healing in and of itself. Second only to the client's contribution, the therapy relationship is the most powerful predictor of, and contributor to, successful outcomes. Even when offered as a manualized intervention and delivered via electronic means, therapy is invariably rooted in and dependent on that complex connection between the client and therapist. As such, it warrants substantial attention in any scientific compilation of evidence-based (or science-based) list of psychotherapy components.

The effectiveness of the multiple relationship factors cuts across theoretical orientations (transtheoretical) and largely across client problems (transdiagnostic). The research evidence on the relationship does not favor any single orientation; the probability of a positive client–clinician relationship or a failure in that relationship is not any more characteristic of one psychotherapy system than another. The relationship elements or components considered in this chapter have all been shown, in dozens of individual studies and in rigorous meta-analyses, to associate, predict, and contribute to success. Failure to provide these elements also predicts and contributes to poor treatment outcomes, however measured (e.g., dropout, deterioration).

In this chapter, we review evidence-based psychotherapy relationships, primarily with adults in individual treatment. We begin by defining our terms and diving into effective relationship behaviors or components (what works). That is followed by a few words on ineffective or discredited relationship behaviors (what does not work). We then advance therapeutic and training practices based on this research evidence. The chapter finishes with multiple caveats, concluding thoughts, and useful resources.

Definitions

Many spirited and unproductive debates on psychotherapy fail to operationally define their terms. Antagonists wind up speaking past one another, literally not on the same page. Cases in point are the *psychotherapy relationship* and *evidence-based practice*.

We will not commit the errors of undefined terms and unidentified contexts in this chapter.

An operational definition of the *therapeutic relationship* is the feelings and attitudes that therapist and client have toward one another, and the manner in which these are expressed (Gelso & Carter, 1985, 1994). While this definition is quite general, it is mercifully concise, theoretically neutral, and sufficiently precise.

The *therapeutic alliance* represents a part of the relationship, but only a part. In fact, a pernicious error in the psychotherapy literature equates the totality of the relationship with the therapeutic alliance. In part, this mistake occurs inadvertently because the alliance is the most frequently measured and researched relationship factor in the psychotherapy literature (Horvath et al., 2016). In part, too, this mistake probably occurs intentionally to misrepresent and diminish the cumulative power of the relationship (Norcross & Karpiak, 2023). Ironically, the alliance's association with psychotherapy success is not even the largest of the relationship factors, as discussed shortly. Conflating the entirety of the therapy relationship with only the alliance weakens the power of the therapeutic relationship empirically and clinically.

The short past of *evidence-based practice* (EBP) in behavioral/mental health traces back to the 1980s, originally in Great Britain and then gathering steam in Canada, the United States, and now around the globe (Norcross et al., 2017). The early stirrings of the movement trace back to the United Kingdom and Archie Cochrane's (1979) article calling on medicine to assemble critical summaries of science-based treatments that had proven effective according to randomized clinical trials. Cochrane and others contrasted EBP with expert- or *authority-based practice*, the latter lacking in solid research support and typically resulting in less effective health care.

A consensual and concrete definition of EBP has emerged from the research literature and professional organizations. Adapting a definition from Sackett and colleagues, the Institute of Medicine (2001, p. 147) defined *evidence-based medicine* (EBM) as "the integration of best research evidence with clinical expertise and patient values." The American Psychological Association (APA) Task Force on Evidence-Based Practice (2006, p. 273), beginning with this foundation and expanding it to mental health, defined EBP as "the integration of the best available research with clinical expertise in the context of patient characteristics, culture, and preferences." We use the latter as our operational definition throughout.

Several core features of EBPs become manifest in this definition. First and foremost, EBPs rest on three pillars: available research; clinician expertise; and patient characteristics, culture, and preferences. By definition, the wholesale imposition of research without attending to the clinician or patient is *not* EBP; conversely, the indiscriminate disregard of available research is *not* EBP. Second, the definition requires integrating these three evidentiary sources. The integration flows seamlessly and uncontested when the three evidentiary sources agree; it becomes complicated and contested when the three sources disagree. Third, not all three pillars stand equal: Research assumes priority in EBP. Clinicians begin with research and then integrate with their expertise and patients. Fourth and final, compared to EBM, the patient assumes a more active, prominent position in EBPs in behavioral health and addictions. "Patient values" in EBM rise to the status of "patient characteristics, culture, and preferences" in behavioral health EBPs.

Evidence-Based Therapy Relationships

The centrality of the therapy relationship has been highlighted since the origins of modern psychotherapy. Sigmund Freud described the operation of transference and countertransference, and psychoanalytic scholars developed a rich literature on the relationship. Among the foundational constructs are the establishment of a positive working or therapeutic alliance (Bordin, 1979; Luborsky, 1976) and the management of negative countertransference (Singer & Luborsky, 1977). The real relationship, characterized by realism and genuineness, was emphasized later by psychodynamic therapists (Greenson, 1967; Gelso et al., 2019). All three of these elements have subsequently proven effective in psychotherapy according to the research evidence (Table 21.1; Norcross & Lambert, 2019).

Carl Rogers's legacy includes the three relational *facilitative conditions* for therapeutic change: empathy, positive regard, and genuineness/congruence (Rogers, 1957). Two of Rogers's facilitative conditions are demonstrably effective and the third probably effective based on the meta-analyses (Table 21.1; Norcross & Lambert, 2019). A dedicated scientist, Rogers established psychotherapy process–outcome research, modeling how to scientifically examine the association between specific therapist behaviors and client responses to understand not just whether psychotherapy works but how it works.

Early cognitive-behavioral formulations of the therapy relationship emphasized it as a precondition of change, the soil that enables treatment methods to work, as opposed to a healing process in and of itself. Therapist and patient were to work together, akin to a student–teacher relationship, establishing rapport, cultivating positive expectations, and jointly determining treatment goals (Beck et al., 1979). Recent meta-analyses support the salubrious link between collaboration, goal consensus, and positive expectations and successful psychotherapy (Table 21.1; Norcross & Lambert, 2019).

Subsequent generations of practice and research on the therapy relationship have emphasized transtheoretical conceptualizations (as opposed to theory specific) and research evidence (as opposed to clinical lore or authority). In this context, three American Psychological Association (APA) Interdivisional Task Forces were convened to identify, compile, and disseminate therapy relationships that were evidence based (Norcross, 2002; Norcross, 2011; Norcross & Lambert, 2019). The Task Force

John C. Norcross and Christie P. Karpiak

Table 21.1 *Summary of meta-analytic associations between relationship components and distal psychotherapy outcomes (adapted from Norcross & Lambert, 2019; © Norcross & Lambert)*

Relationship element	# of studies (k)	# of patients (N)	Effect size r	d or g	Consensus on evidentiary strength
Alliance in individual adult psychotherapy	306	30,000+	0.28	0.57	Demonstrably effective
Alliance in child and adolescent therapy	43	3,447	0.20	0.40	Demonstrably effective
Alliances in couple and family therapy	40	4,113	0.30	0.62	Demonstrably effective
Collaboration	53	5,286	0.29	0.61	Demonstrably effective
Goal consensus	54	7,278	0.24	0.49	Demonstrably effective
Cohesion in group therapy	55	6,055	0.26	0.56	Demonstrably effective
Empathy	82	6,138	0.28	0.58	Demonstrably effective
Positive regard and affirmation	64	3,528	0.28		Demonstrably effective
Collecting and delivering client feedback	24	10,921		0.14–0.49	Demonstrably effective
Congruence/ genuineness	21	1,192	0.23	0.46	Probably effective
Real relationship	17	1,502	0.37	0.80	Probably effective
Emotional expression	42	925	0.40	0.85	Probably effective
Cultivating positive expectation	81	12,722	0.18	0.36	Probably effective
Promoting treatment credibility	24	1,504	0.12	0.24	Probably effective
Managing countertransference	9	392*	0.39	0.84	Probably effective
Repairing alliance ruptures	11	1,318	0.30	0.62	Probably effective

* Refers to the number of psychotherapists, not patients.
Note. In the behavioral sciences, an effect size (*d* or *g*) of 0.20 is generally considered a small effect, 0.50 a medium effect, and 0.80 a large effect (Cohen, 2013).

aimed, in addition, to heal some of the damage of the culture wars in psychotherapy that unproductively pit treatment methods against therapeutic relationships.

In its third and most recent iteration, *Psychotherapy Relationships that Work* (Norcross & Lambert, 2019; Norcross & Wampold, 2019) contains two volumes of 30 meta-analyses of therapist and patient contributions to therapy effectiveness. The strength of the scientific evidence is undeniable, and the field has (mostly) matured past polarized positions (relationship vs. method) to consider how all elements optimally operate and interact. Table 21.1 presents, from those volumes, a summary of the meta-analytic associations between relationship elements and distal (end of treatment) psychotherapy outcomes. In the following section, we concentrate on those elements that have proven effective in individual psychotherapy with adults.

What Works

Alliance

The term *alliance* is not easily differentiated from several other relational concepts; in the literature, the words "working," "helping," or "therapeutic" often appear in conjunction with it (Fluckiger et al., 2019). An early tripartite definition by Bordin (1979) emphasized (1) a warm emotional bond, (2) agreement on respective tasks, and (3) consensus on treatment goals. A more recent definition includes mutual collaboration between client and therapist on goals and tasks of psychotherapy, along with the therapeutic bond between the dyad (Del Re et al., 2021). Alliance is interpersonal – therapist and client both contribute to it – but the ability to form an alliance with an array of clients is a therapist characteristic that can be learned (Ackerman & Hilsenroth, 2003; Muran & Eubanks, 2020).

A meta-analysis of more than 30,000 clients found a moderate, but extremely robust, association between the alliance and outcome in adult individual psychotherapy ($d = 0.57$; Fluckiger et al., 2019). The alliance relates to, predicts, and contributes to psychotherapy success. To a lesser extent, success in therapy also strengthens the relationship.

Likewise, with a few wrinkles, the alliance in youth psychotherapy works. Across 43 studies of child and adolescent therapy (3,447 clients and parents), there was a moderate effect size between alliance and treatment outcome ($d = 0.40$; Karver et al., 2019). Importantly, the strength of the alliance–outcome relation did not vary with the type of treatment. Further, the effect size, or clinical impact, of dual alliances – therapist with youth, therapist with parent – was identical. Both the therapist–youth and therapist–caregiver alliance matter mightily.

The average effect size for the alliance in couples/family therapy is in the same range (0.62), based on 40 studies (Friedlander et al., 2019), as is the impact of the alliance in psychopharmacological treatment, based on 8 studies (Totura et al., 2018).

The alliance emerges in the ongoing relationship between therapist and client, and accurate measurement of the alliance at any point during the course of therapy probably requires collecting information from both (or all) participants. Most studies indicate that the client rating is the better predictor of treatment outcome than therapist or observer ratings, but all information proves valuable. Alliance measures completed by the client can be used by a therapist or supervisor to track the development of this vital competency and predictor of therapy outcome.

Goal Consensus and Collaboration

These two relational components are present across theoretical orientations and are sometimes considered part of the therapeutic alliance. Indeed, both are commonly assessed for research purposes via measures of the alliance, completed separately by clinician and client. Goal consensus refers to the agreement between the therapist and the client about the targets of their work together and how to achieve them. A large body of research documents the vital role this factor plays in treatment outcome ($d = 0.49$; Tryon et al., 2019). Collaboration is the active mutual engagement of the therapist and client around the work of therapy. Research also shows that collaboration is substantially associated with treatment outcome, with an effect size (d) of 0.61 (Tryon et al., 2019).

Empathy

The term *empathy* is widely used in the common vernacular to refer to a strong emotional response to the situation of another, and in popular use is often conflated with sympathy or compassion. For clarity, we use Rogers's (1980, p. 85) definition as "the therapist's sensitive ability and willingness to understand the client's thoughts, feelings and struggles from the client's point of view." Empathy can be assessed, according to Barrett-Lennard (1981), as "(a) the therapist's empathic resonance with the client, (b) the observer's perception of the therapist's expressed empathy, and (c) the client's experience of received therapist empathy" (Elliott et al., 2019, p. 248).

Empathic responding is one of the strongest and best-supported contributors to outcome (Elliott et al., 2019). Starting with the groundbreaking research of Carl Rogers, decades of evidence now attest to its value, with meta-analytic effect sizes ranging between moderate to large ($d = 0.58$), from 82 high-quality studies. Even better, the skills and basic stance of empathic understanding can be practiced in everyday relationships outside of a real or simulated therapy situation (see Miller, 2018), as long as others in these relationships are willing and able to provide feedback.

Affirmation and Validation

Therapist positive regard for the client (and expression of that regard, including through affirmation) is another relationship factor originally investigated by Carl Rogers. As with empathy, positive regard has been the subject of much research, with its effect on psychotherapy outcome falling in the moderate range ($d = 0.57$), based on 64 studies of quality appropriate for inclusion in a meta-analysis (Farber et al., 2019).

Like empathy, the terms *positive regard* and *affirmation* are easily misunderstood – mistaken for simple compliments, shallow praise, or other concrete tactics (e.g., preceding requests for compliance). In fact, positive regard is the therapist's genuine nonpossessive liking and expressed appreciation for the client as a unique person. This strengthens the client's sense of agency and self. To contribute to outcome, this regard must be made evident to the client through words and nonverbals. Therapists can express on a regular basis that they value, care about, and believe in the client, ideally over the course of treatment. However, it does *not* need to be (and probably could not be) experienced by the therapist at every moment across treatment with any given client (Farber et al., 2019).

Congruence/Genuineness and Real Relationship

This pair of relational factors includes the last of the three Rogerian core conditions (empathy, unconditional positive regard, and congruence/genuineness) and a concept from the psychodynamic literature: the real relationship. Both have accumulated sufficient evidence to be classified as effective.

Congruence/genuineness has both intrapersonal and interpersonal features, meaning it is both a personal characteristic of the therapist as well as a quality of the therapeutic interaction. When congruent, therapists' actions and behaviors not only fit their words but also who they are as a person – their values and identity – exuding groundedness, thoughtfulness, and genuineness. In short, they are real, not phony, distracted, or playing a role. Studies of this relational component show a moderate association with treatment outcome, making it a reliable contributor to therapeutic success ($d = 0.46$; Kolden et al., 2019).

The real relationship is composed of both genuineness and realism. It's "the personal relationship between therapist and patient marked by the extent to which each is genuine with the other and perceives/experiences the other in ways that befit the other" (Gelso, 2014, p. 119). In contrast to the alliance, it refers to a subset of therapist–client interactions not directly focused on the tasks. These interactions are taken at face value in the here and now. A meta-analysis based on 17 studies and 1,502 patients revealed a large effect between the real relationship and client success ($d = 0.80$; Gelso et al., 2019).

Emotional Expression

Although emotion is obviously core to psychotherapy, organized research on the subject is quite recent. That evidence shows that the facilitation, experience, and expression of client emotion in session are strongly correlated with treatment outcome ($d = 0.85$; Peluso & Freund, 2019). Contributions to this research base come from a wider range of theoretical orientations than do the components reviewed thus far. Because of this variability, the definition of emotional expression is less precise and has failed to achieve consensus in the field. One essential and simple clarification: what is not being referenced here is the "expressed emotion" from family process and relapse prevention research with serious mental illnesses, where reducing expressed emotion is the goal.

Of all the relational elements, emotional expression is possibly the one that can most easily go astray in the absence of a clear plan. Treatment model and case formulation help determine which emotions to address, where a particular emotional expression fits into the therapeutic endeavor, and what to do with it – in other words, how to attend to and make therapeutic use of emotion versus allowing the session to deteriorate into an unfocused rant, wallow, or self-attack.

Repair of Alliance Ruptures

Ruptures are problems or strains in the collaborative relationship between client and therapist related to treatment goals, agreement on the tasks of therapy, or the emotional bond (Eubanks et al., 2019). Two main types occur in session: (1) withdrawal, in which the client moves away from the therapist and the work; and (2) confrontation, in which the client moves against the therapist by expressing anger or dissatisfaction. Although the term *rupture* may connote a dramatic breakdown, many studies point to subtle tensions and minor misalignments as markers.

Therapist efforts to repair alliance ruptures can be overt or indirect. Either way, research shows attending to them improves treatment outcomes. A meta-analysis of 11 studies, involving 1,318 clients, revealed that repair of alliance ruptures in individual therapy is moderately to strongly associated with outcome ($d = 0.62$). That is, addressing ruptures works; ignoring them does not.

Repairing ruptures proves valuable for all psychotherapists, but especially for therapists with less experience and training in negotiating the therapeutic alliance (Eubanks et al., 2019). Moderator analyses revealed that rupture resolutions training is more effective for cognitive-behavioral therapists, many of whom have not received explicit training in processing relationship dynamics with their clients.

Collection of Client Feedback

In collecting feedback from patients – or the more recent term *routine outcome monitoring* (ROM) – psychotherapists inquire directly about the patient's progress on a regular basis, compare those data to benchmarks or norms, address the progress (or lack thereof) directly in session, and, in some cases, offer clinical support tools to identify obstacles and adapt future sessions. A dozen or so ROM systems are now available, but most of the controlled research has employed the Outcome Questionnaire and the briefer PCOMS (Partners in Change Outcome Monitoring System) feedback systems. A meta-analysis of 24 controlled trials (on more than 10,000 patients) conducted on those systems (Lambert et al., 2019; Table 21.1) found that feedback or ROM produced variable but salutatory effects (between 0.14 and 0.49) on distal treatment outcomes. A subsequent and larger meta-analysis (de Jong et al., 2021) on 58 studies, encompassing more than 20,000 patients, reported an overall *d* of 0.15.

Collecting feedback or conducting ROM is thus slightly effective for all patients but more effective for patients not on track in treatment or at risk of an unsuccessful outcome. ROM, in fact, reduces the risk of patient dropout by 20–25% (de Jong et al., 2021; Lambert et al., 2019). All these are additive effects to conducting standard therapy.

Overall

The scientific conclusion emerges that there is a robust, consistent association between these core relational elements and client improvement. On average, the correlation (*r*) is about 0.25–0.30. That translates to an effect size (*d*) of about 0.55 and indicates that clients receiving psychotherapy characterized by high degrees of empathy, regard, and the like will experience a decided advantage over clients that receive (or perceive) relatively lower degrees of those relationship attributes.

Although this estimate of treatment effects may seem rather modest, bear in mind the large number of complex variables that contribute to treatment outcomes, especially clients' contributions and life events that exist before and during the therapeutic encounter (Lambert et al., 1992). Also bear in mind that the average effect size (*d*) between psychotherapy and no psychotherapy hovers about 0.85; any single relational behavior in Table 21.1 comes in at an impressive 0.55.

It would probably prove advantageous to both practice and science to sum the individual effect sizes in Table 21.1 to arrive at a total of relationship contribution to treatment outcome, but reality is not so accommodating. Neither the research studies nor the relationship elements contained in the meta-analyses are independent; hence, the amount of variance accounted for by each element cannot be simply added to estimate the overall contribution. For example, the correlations between empathy and therapeutic alliance are as high as 0.70 (Watson & Geller, 2005). The intercorrelations between the person-centered conditions are also high: in an early research review on client-centered conditions empathy correlated 0.53 with positive regard, 0.62 with congruence, and 0.28 with unconditionally (Gurman, 1977). Unfortunately, the degree of overlap between all the measures (and therefore relationship elements) is not available but is bound to be substantial.

Despite the overlap in relational elements, the best scientific estimates of relationship effects are reliable and robust. The therapeutic relationship contributes as much, and probably more, to client outcomes than the particular treatment method. The effect sizes for relationship behaviors (Table 21.1) of 0.39–0.72 are higher than the effect sizes of 0–0.20 attributable to different treatment methods found in bona fide comparisons (Wampold & Imel, 2015). Although we deplore the mindless dichotomy between relationship and method in psychotherapy, we also need to publicly proclaim what decades of research has discovered: The relationship can heal.

What Does *Not* Work

Translational research is both prescriptive and proscriptive; it tells us what works and what does not (Norcross et al., 2017). Here, we highlight those practitioner relational behaviors that are ineffective, perhaps even hurtful, in psychotherapy (Karpiak & Norcross, 2022; Norcross & Karpiak, 2023).

Of course, we could simply reverse the effective behaviors identified in the meta-analyses (Table 21.1) to identify ineffective qualities of the therapeutic relationship. What does not work, for example, are poor alliances, paucity of collaboration, and inadequate efforts at empathy. The ineffective practitioner will not seek nor be receptive to client feedback on progress and relationship, will ignore alliance ruptures, and will not promote their patients' emotional expression. "One doesn't have to operate with great malice to do great harm," warned Charles Blow. "The absence of empathy and understanding are sufficient."

Another means of identifying ineffective qualities of the relationship is to scour the research literature for clinician behaviors frequently associated with negative outcomes and premature discontinuation (e.g., Hardy et al., 2019; Swift & Greenberg, 2012). Here are several relational behaviors that therapists should avoid according to the Task Forces review of that research (Norcross & Lambert, 2019):

♦ *Confrontations.* Controlled research trials, particularly in the addictions field, consistently find that a confrontational style proves ineffective. In one review (Miller et al., 2003), confrontation was ineffective in all 12 identified trials. And yet it persists. By contrast, expressing empathy, rolling with resistance, developing discrepancy, and supporting self-efficacy characteristic of motivational interviewing have demonstrated large effects in a small number of sessions (Lundahl et al., 2013).

♦ *Negative processes.* Client reports and research studies converge in warning therapists to avoid comments or behaviors that are experienced by clients as hostile, pejorative, critical, rejecting, or blaming (Binder & Strupp, 1997). Therapists who attack a client's dysfunctional thoughts or relational patterns need, repeatedly, to distinguish between attacking the person versus their behavior. When negative processes ensue, then repairing alliance ruptures is amongst the most easily applied skills and strongest relationship behaviors documented in psychotherapy (Eubanks et al., 2019; Table 21.1).

♦ *Assumptions.* Psychotherapists who assume or intuit their client's perceptions of relationship satisfaction and treatment success frequently misjudge these aspects. By contrast, therapists who formally measure and respectfully inquire about their client's perceptions, via feedback or ROM, frequently enhance the alliance and prevent premature termination (Lambert et al., 2019).

♦ *Therapist-centricity.* A recurrent lesson from process–outcome research and the associated meta-analyses is that the client's perspective on the therapy relationship best predicts outcome. Psychotherapy that relies on the therapist's observational perspective alone, while valuable, does not predict outcome as accurately. Therefore, privileging and monitoring the patient's experience of the relationship prove central.

♦ *Rigidity.* By inflexibly and excessively structuring treatment, psychotherapists risk empathic failures and inattentiveness to clients' experiences. Such a therapist is likely to overlook a breach in the relationship and mistakenly assume they have not contributed to that breach. Dogmatic reliance on particular relational or therapy methods, incompatible with the client, imperils treatment (Ackerman & Hilsenroth, 2003).

♦ *Cultural arrogance.* Arrogant impositions of therapists' cultural beliefs in terms of gender, race/ethnicity, sexual orientation, and other intersecting dimensions of identity are culturally insensitive and demonstrably less effective (Soto et al., 2019). By contrast, therapists' expressing cultural humility, offering adapted treatments, and emphasizing cultural responsiveness markedly improve client engagement, retention, and eventual treatment outcome.

We can optimize therapy relationships by simultaneously using what works *and* studiously avoiding what does not work.

Cautions and Caveats

In valuing the therapeutic relationship, it becomes deceptively easy to overplay the impact of that relationship in treatment (Norcross & Lambert, 2014). "It's all the relationship" is a frequent (and inaccurate) refrain among many trainees and some practitioners. The Task Force repeatedly urged restraint and balance in disseminating its meta-analytic findings, pointedly concluding that "The therapy relationship acts in concert with treatment methods, patient characteristics, and other practitioner qualities in determining effectiveness; a comprehensive understanding of effective (and ineffective) psychotherapy will consider all of these determinants and how they work together to produce benefit" (Norcross & Lambert, 2019, p. 632).

Historically, the polarized psychotherapy community rarely found the middle ground in valuing the therapy relationship in context; contemporarily, most psychotherapists avoid the unproductive schism of relationship versus method and frame the therapeutic relationship in comprehensive, scientific contexts. Multiple lines of evidence suggest that humans (including patients) hold two major dimensions of social perception, often called *warmth* and *competence* (Eisenbruch & Krasnow, 2022). The relational warmth of the therapist is typically prioritized by patients over therapist competence (e.g., Swift & Callahan, 2010). Fortunately, the choice is not binary or exclusive. The most effective therapists regularly manifest both relational warmth and technical competence (Castonguay & Hill, 2017; Seewald & Rief, 2022).

The research on these relational elements features additional cautions. The meta-analytic results in Table 21.1 probably underestimate the true effect of the relationship due to the responsiveness problem (Kramer & Stiles, 2015; Stiles et al., 1998). It is a problem for researchers but a boon to practitioners, who flexibly adjust the amount and timing of relational behaviors in psychotherapy to fit the unique individual and singular context. Effective psychotherapists responsively provide varying levels of relationship elements in different cases and, within the same case, at different moments. This responsiveness tends to confound attempts to find naturalistically observed linear relations of outcome with therapist behaviors (e.g., empathy, ROM). As a consequence, the reported statistical association between therapy relationship and outcome cannot always be trusted and tends to be lower than it actually is. By being clinically attuned and flexible, psychotherapists ironically make it more difficult in research studies to discern what works (Norcross & Lambert, 2019).

Nor has the research generated a definitive list of what works in the therapy relationship. We have neither completed the search nor exhausted the relationship behaviors associated with therapy success. Insufficient controlled research exists to draw conclusions at this juncture on many other relationship behaviors advocated by practitioners.

As the evidence base of therapist relationship behaviors develop, we will know more about their effectiveness for particular circumstances and conditions. A case in point is the meta-analysis on collecting client feedback or conducting ROM. The evidence is clear that adding formal feedback/ROM helps clinicians effectively treat patients at risk for deterioration and that adding some form of clinical support tools to assist clinicians boosts its effectiveness. But for most of these relational elements, we do not yet know for whom and when they prove effective.

The strength of the therapy relationship also depends in some instances on the client's principal disorder. The moderator analyses occasionally find some relationship elements less efficacious with some disorders, usually substance abuse, severe anxiety, and eating disorders. Most moderator analyses usually find the relationship equally effective across disorders, but that conclusion may be due to the relatively small number of studies for any single disorder and the resulting low statistical power to find actual differences. And, of course, it gets more complicated as patients typically present with multiple, comorbid disorders.

Finally, we emphasize that, with a couple of exceptions (collecting feedback, repairing alliance ruptures), the meta-analyses reported the association and prediction of the relationship element to psychotherapy outcome. These were overwhelmingly correlational designs, showing that more of, say, collaboration, emotional expression,

Box 21.1 Therapy and Training Practices

Review of the research evidence led the APA Interdivisional Task Force (Norcross & Lambert, 2019) to advance several recommendations for clinical practice and training. Practitioners are encouraged to:

♦ make the creation and cultivation of the therapy relationship a primary aim of treatment. This is especially true for relationship elements found to be demonstrably and probably effective.
♦ assess relational behaviors (e.g., alliance, empathy, cohesion) vis-à-vis cut-off scores on popular clinical measures in ways that lead to more positive outcomes.
♦ assess and responsively attune psychotherapy to clients' cultural identities (broadly defined).
♦ monitor patients' satisfaction with the therapy relationship, comfort with responsiveness efforts, and response to treatment. Such monitoring leads to increased opportunities to re-establish collaboration, improve the relationship, modify technical strategies, and investigate factors external to therapy that may be hindering its effects.
♦ use concurrently evidence-based relationships *and* evidence-based treatments adapted to the whole patient as that is likely to generate the best outcomes in psychotherapy.

In turn, training programs are encouraged to:

♦ provide competency-based training in the demonstrably and probably effective elements of the therapy relationship.
♦ train students in assessing and honoring clients' cultural heritages, values, and beliefs in ways that enhance the therapeutic relationship and inform treatment adaptations.
♦ develop criteria for assessing the adequacy of training in evidence-based therapy relationships and responsiveness.

and positive regard were associated with improved patient success. Of the relationship behaviors reviewed in this chapter, only two (client feedback/ROM, alliance ruptures) have addressed disaggregation by means of RCTs and only one (alliance in individual therapy; Del Re et al., 2012) by other statistical means. And it turns out the evidence is strong that it is the therapist that is important: therapists who generally form stronger alliances generally have better outcomes, but not vice versa (Wampold et al., 2012). It is largely the therapist's contribution, not the patient's, that relates to therapy outcome (Baldwin et al., 2007; Wampold & Imel, 2015). Put differently, for most of these relationship elements, we know with certainty that they characterize, positively correlate with, and predict successful psychotherapy. But that does not necessarily mean that they are therapist contributions. Another type of causal linkage is still needed.

Conclusion

How to improve the outcomes of psychological treatments? Follow the scientific evidence; follow what contributes to treatment outcome as reviewed in this chapter. Begin by leveraging the patient's resources and self-healing capacities; create and cultivate a therapy relationship characterized by these effective elements; avoid use of ineffective and discredited relational behaviors; responsively personalize to the patient's characteristics, personality, and worldviews. That's evidence-based therapy relationships.

All treatment, all health care, all methods are embedded within a relational context. Not only is there a deep synergy between a treatment method and a therapeutic relationship, but one does not exist without the other. This point was convincingly made decades ago in Winnicott's observation that there is no such thing as a baby without a mother. Effective psychotherapy cannot, and does not, exist without a relationship.

The future of mental health services portends the integration of science and service, of the instrumental and the interpersonal, of the technical and the relational in the EBP tradition (Norcross et al., 2016). We can imagine few practices in mental health that can confidently boast that they seamlessly integrate "the best available research with clinical expertise in the context of patient characteristics, culture, and preferences" (APA Task Force, 2006, p. 273) as well as cultivating and customizing the powerful therapy relationship. As Carl Rogers (1980) compellingly demonstrated, there is no inherent tension between a relational approach and a scientific one. Science can and should inform us about what works in psychotherapy – be it relational or otherwise.

Useful Resources

- Norcross, J. C., & Lambert, M. J. (Eds.). (2018). Evidence-based psychotherapy relationship III (special issue). *Psychotherapy*, 55(4), 303–537.
- Norcross, J. C., & Lambert, M. J. (Eds.). (2019). *Psychotherapy relationships that work. Volume 1: Evidence-based therapist contributions* (3rd ed.). Oxford University Press.
- Norcross, J. C., & Wampold, B. E. (2019). (Eds.). *Psychotherapy relationships that work. Volume 2: Evidence-based responsiveness* (3rd ed.). Oxford University Press.
- Norcross, J. C., & Karpiak, C. P. (2023). Relationship factors. In S. D. Miller, D. Chow, S. Malins, & M. A. Hubble (Eds.), *Field guide to better results: Individualizing a deliberate practice*. American Psychological Association.
- Society for the Advancement of Psychotherapy (APA Division of Psychotherapy). (2020). *Teaching and learning evidence-based relationships: Interviews with the experts*. society forpsychotherapy.org/teaching-learning-evidence-based-relationships.

References

Ackerman, S. J., & Hilsenroth, M. J. (2003). A review of therapist characteristics and techniques positively impacting the therapeutic alliance. *Clinical Psychology Review*, 23, 1–33.

American Psychological Association Task Force on Evidence-Based Practice. (2006). Evidence-based practice in psychology. *American Psychologist*, 61, 271–285.

Baldwin, S. A., Wampold, B. E., & Imel, Z. E. (2007). Untangling the alliance-outcome correlation: Exploring the relative importance of therapist and patient variability in the alliance. *Journal of Consulting and Clinical Psychology*, 75, 842–852.

Barrett-Lennard, G. T. (1981). The empathy cycle: Refinement of a nuclear concept. *Journal of Counseling Psychology*, 28, 91–100.

Beck, A. T., Rush, A. J., Shaw, B. F., & Emery, G. (Eds.). (1979). *Cognitive therapy of depression*. Guilford Press.

Binder, J. L., & Strupp, H. H. (1997). "Negative process": A recurrently discovered and underestimated facet of therapeutic process and outcome in the individual psychotherapy of adults. *Clinical Psychology: Science and Practice*, 4, 121–139.

Bordin, E. S. (1979). The generalizability of the psychoanalytic concept of the working alliance. *Psychotherapy*, 16, 252–260.

Castonguay, L., & Hill, C. E. (Eds.). (2017). *How and why are some therapists better than others? Understanding therapist effects*. American Psychological Association.

Cochrane, A. (1979). 1931–1971: A critical review with particular reference to the medical profession. In *Medicines for the year 2000* (pp. 1–11). UK Office of Health Economics.

Cohen, J. (2013). *Statistical power analysis for the behavioral sciences*. Academic Press.

de Jong, K., Conijn, J. M., Gallagher, R., et al. (2021). Using progress feedback to improve outcomes and reduce drop-out, treatment duration, and deterioration: A multilevel meta-analysis. *Clinical Psychology Review*, 85, 102002. https://doi.org/10.1016/j.cpr.2021.102002.

Del Re, A. C., Flückiger, C., Horvath, A. O., & Wampold, B. E. (2021). Examining therapist effects in the alliance–outcome relationship: A multilevel meta-analysis. *Journal of Consulting and Clinical Psychology*, 89, 371–378.

Del Re, A. C., Flückiger, C., Horvath, A. O., Symonds, D., & Wampold, B.E. (2012). Therapist effects in the therapeutic alliance-outcome relationship: A restricted-maximum likelihood meta-analysis. *Clinical Psychology Review*, 32, 642–649.

Eisenbruch, A. B., & Krasnow, M. M. (2022). Why warmth matters more than competence: A new evolutionary approach. *Perspectives on Psychological Science*, 17(6), 1604–1623.

Elliott, R., Bohart, A. C., Watson, J. C., & Murphy, D. (2019). Empathy. In J. C. Norcross & M. J. Lambert (Eds.), *Psychotherapy relationships that work, Volume 1* (3rd ed.). Oxford University Press.

Eubanks, C. F., Muran, J. C., & Safran, J. D. (2019). Repairing alliance ruptures. In J. C. Norcross & M. J. Lambert (Eds.), *Psychotherapy relationships that work, Vol. 1* (3rd ed.). Oxford University Press.

Farber, B. A., Suzuki, J. Y., & Lynch, D. (2019). Positive regard and affirmation. In J. C. Norcross & M. J. Lambert (Eds.), *Psychotherapy relationships that work, Volume 1* (3rd ed.). Oxford University Press.

Flückiger, C., Del Re, A. C., Wampold, B. E., Symonds, D., & Horvath, A.O. (2019). Alliance in adult psychotherapy. In J. C. Norcross & M. J. Lambert (Eds.), *Psychotherapy relationships that work, Volume 1* (3rd ed.). Oxford University Press.

Friedlander, M. L., Escudero, V., Welmers-van de Poll, M. J., & Heatherington, L. (2019). Alliances in couple and family therapy. In J. C. Norcross & M. J. Lambert (Eds.), *Psychotherapy relationships that work, Volume 1* (3rd ed.). Oxford University Press.

Gelso, C. (2014). A tripartite model of the therapeutic relationship: Theory, research, and practice. *Psychotherapy Research*, 24, 117–131.

Gelso, C. J., & Carter, J. A. (1985). The relationship in counseling and psychotherapy: Components, consequences, and theoretical antecedents. *The Counseling Psychologist*, 13, 155–243. https://doi.org/10.1177/0011000085132001.

Gelso, C. J., & Carter, J. A. (1994). Components of the psychotherapy relationship: Their inter-action and unfolding during treatment. *Journal of Counseling Psychology*, 41, 296-306.

Gelso, C. J., Kivlighan, D. M., & Markin, R. D. (2019). The real relationship. In J. C. Norcross & M. J. Lambert (Eds.), *Psychotherapy relationships that work, Vol. 1* (3rd ed.). Oxford University Press.

Greenson, R. R. (1967). *Technique and practice of psychoanalysis*. International University Press.

Gurman, A. S. (1977). Therapist and patient factors influencing the patient's perception of facilitative therapeutic conditions. *Psychiatry*, 40, 218–231.

Hardy, G. E., Bishop-Edwards, L., Chambers, E., et al. (2019). Risk factors for negative experiences during psychotherapy. *Psychotherapy Research*, 29, 403–414.

Horvath, A. O., Symonds, D. B., Fluckiger, C., DelRe, A. C., & Lee, E. (2016, June). *Integration across* professional domains: The helping relationship. Address presented at 32nd conference of Society for the Exploration of Psychotherapy Integration, Dublin, Ireland.

Institute of Medicine. (2001). *Crossing the quality chasm: A new health system for the 21st century*. National Academies Press.

Karpiak, C. P., & Norcross, J. C. (2022). Evidence-based therapy relationships. In G. J. G. Asmundson (Ed.), *Comprehensive clinical psychology, Vol. 2* (2nd ed). Elsevier.

Karver, M. S., De Nadai, A. S., Monahan, M., & Shirk, S. R. (2019). Alliance in child and adolescent psychotherapy. In J. C. Norcross & M. J. Lambert (Eds.), *Psychotherapy relationships that work, Volume 1* (3rd ed.). Oxford University Press.

Kolden, G. G., Wang, C.C., Austin, S. B., Chang, Y., & Klein, M. H. (2019). Congruence / genuineness. In J. C. Norcross & M. J. Lambert (Eds.), *Psychotherapy relationships that work, Volume 1* (3rd ed.). Oxford University Press.

Kramer, U., & Stiles, W. B. (2015). The responsiveness problem in psychotherapy: A review of proposed solutions. *Clinical Psychology: Science and Practice*, 22, 277–295. https://doi.org/10.1111/cpsp.12107.

Lambert, M. J. (2010). *Prevention of treatment failure: The use of measuring, monitoring, & feedback in clinical practice*. American Psychological Association.

Lambert, M. J., Ogles, B. M., & Masters, K. S. (1992). Choosing outcome assessment devices: An organizational and conceptual scheme. *Journal of Counseling & Development*, 70(4), 527–532.

Lambert, M. J., Whipple, J. L., & Kleinstauber, M. (2019). Collecting and delivering client feedback. In J. C. Norcross & M. J. Lambert (Eds.), *Psychotherapy relationships that work, Vol. 1* (3rd ed.). Oxford.

Luborsky, L. (1976). Helping alliances in psychotherapy: The groundwork for a study of their relationship to its outcome. In J. L. Claghorn (Ed.), *Successful psychotherapy*. Brunner/ Mazel.

Lundahl, B., Moleni, T., Burke, B. L., et al. (2013). Motivational interviewing in medical care settings: A systematic review and meta-analysis of randomized controlled trials. *Patient Education and Counseling*, 93, 157–168.

Miller, W. R. (2018). *Listening well: The art of empathic understanding*. Wipf and Stock.

Miller, W. R., Wilbourne, P. L., & Hettema, J. E. (2003). What works? A summary of alcohol treatment outcome research. In R. K. Hester & W. R. Miller (Eds.), *Handbook of alcoholism treatment approaches* (3rd ed., pp. 13–63). Allyn & Bacon.

Muran, J. C. & Eubanks, C. F. (2020). *Therapist performance under pressure: Negotiating emotion, difference, and rupture*. American Psychological Association.

Norcross, J. C. (Ed.). (2002). *Psychotherapy relationships that work*. Oxford University Press.

Norcross, J. C. (Ed.). (2011). *Psychotherapy relationships that work* (2nd ed.). Oxford University Press.

Norcross, J. C., & Karpiak, C. P. (2023). Relationship factors. In S. D. Miller, D. Chow, S. Malins, & M. A. Hubble (Eds.), *Field guide to better results: Individualizing a deliberate practice*. American Psychological Association.

Norcross, J. C., & Lambert, M. J. (Eds.). (2019). *Psychotherapy relationships that work, Volume 1* (3rd ed.). Oxford University Press.

Norcross, J. C., & Lambert, M. J. (2019). What works in the psychotherapy relationship: Results, conclusions, and practices. In J. C. Norcross & M. J. Lambert (Eds.), *Psychotherapy relationships that work, Vol. 1* (3rd ed.). Oxford University Press.

Norcross, J. C., & Lambert, M. J. (2014). Relationship science and practice in psychotherapy: Closing commentary. *Psychotherapy*, 51, 398-403. doi: 10.1037/a0037418

Norcross, J. C., & Wampold, B. E. (Eds.). (2019). *Psychotherapy relationships that work. Volume 2: Evidence-based responsiveness* (3rd ed.). Oxford University Press.

Norcross, J. C., Hogan, T. P., Koocher, G. P., & Maggio, L. A. (2017). *Clinician's guide to evidence-based practices: Behavioral health and addictions* (2nd ed.). Oxford University Press.

Norcross, J. C., VandenBos, G. R., & Freedheim, D. K. (Eds.). (2016). *APA handbook of clinical psychology* (5 volumes). American Psychological Association.

Peluso, P. R., & Freund, R. R. (2019). Emotional expression. In J. C. Norcross & M. J. Lambert, (Eds.), *Psychotherapy relationships that work, Volume 1* (3rd ed.). Oxford University Press.

Rogers, C. R. (1957). The necessary and sufficient conditions of therapeutic personality change. *Journal of Consulting Psychology*, 21, 95–103.

Rogers, C. R. (1980). *A way of being*. Houghton Mifflin.

Seewald, A., & Rief, W. (2022). How to change negative outcome expectations in psycho-therapy? The role of the therapist's warmth and competence. *Clinical Psychological Science*, 11(1), 149–163. https://doi.org/10.1177/21677026221094331.

Singer, B.A., & Luborsky, L. (1977). Countertransference: The status of clinical versus quantitative research. In A. S. Gurman & A. M. Razin (Eds.), *Effective psychotherapy: A handbook of research*. Pergamon.

Soto, A., Smith, T. B., Griner, D., Rodriguez, M. D., & Bernal, G. (2019). Cultural adaptations and multicultural competence In J. C. Norcross & B. E. Wampold (Eds.), *Psychotherapy relationships that work, Vol. 2* (3rd ed.). Oxford University Press.

Stiles, W. B., Honos-Webb, L., & Surko, M. (1998). Responsiveness in psychotherapy. *Clinical Psychology: Science and Practice*, 5, 439–458.

Swift, J. K., & Callahan, J. L. (2010). A comparison of client preferences for intervention empirical support versus common therapy variables. *Journal of Clinical Psychology*, 66 1217–1231.

Swift, J. K., & Greenberg, R. P. (2012). Premature discontinuation in adult psychotherapy: A meta-analysis. *Journal of Consulting and Clinical Psychology*, 80, 547–559.

Totura, C. M. W., Fields, S. A., & Karver, M. S. (2018). The role of the therapeutic relationship in psychopharmacological treatment outcomes: A meta-analytic review. *Psychiatric Services*, 69, 41–47.

Tryon, G. S., Birch, S. E., & Verkuilen, J. (2019). Goal consensus and collaboration. In J. C. Norcross & M. J. Lambert (Eds.), *Psychotherapy relationships that work, Volume 1* (3rd ed.). Oxford University Press.

Wampold, B. E. (2010). The research evidence for the common factor models: A historically situated perspective. In B. L. Duncan, S. D. Miller, B. E. Wampold, & M. A. Hubble (Eds.), *The heart and soul of change: Delivering what works in therapy* (pp. 49–81). American Psychological Association.

Wampold, B. E. (2012). Humanism as a common factor in psychotherapy. *Psychotherapy*, 49(4), 445–449.

Wampold, B. E., & Imel, Z. (2015). *The great psychotherapy debate* (2nd ed.). Erlbaum.

Watson, J. C. & Geller, S. (2005). An examination of the relations among empathy, unconditional acceptance, positive regard and congruence in both cognitive-behavioral and process-experiential psychotherapy. *Psychotherapy Research*, 15, 25–33.

Postscript

Evaluating Treatments with the Science-Based Tolin Criteria: A Call to Action

Cassandra L. Boness, Stephen Hupp, and David F. Tolin

The chapters in this book offer a glimpse of what effective therapies look like, but we are just at the beginning of fully realizing what science-based therapy will become. As described in Chapter 1, the Society of Clinical Psychology (SCP; Division 12 [D12] of the American Psychological Association) provided the first major comprehensive framework for identifying efficacious psychological treatments. Within this framework – sometimes referred to as the "Chambless criteria" – the highest designation that an empirically supported treatment (EST) can be given is to be officially characterized as *well-established* (Chambless & Hollon, 1998; Chambless & Ollendick, 2001) and informally described as having *strong research support* (www.psychologicaltreatments.org). Table 22.1 provides a summary of the psychological treatments for adults that have achieved this highest level of support (for a similar table about treatments for youth, see Hupp & Hupp, 2023).

As can be gleaned from the table, the majority of ESTs fall within the behavioral and cognitive traditions. Moreover, the blended approach of cognitive-behavioral therapy (CBT) – and its many variants – has frequently been identified as being well established. These time-limited behavioral and cognitive therapies have been particularly well suited to being investigated by using randomized controlled trials (RCTs), which many consider to be the "gold standard" for determining treatment efficacy.

However, it's important to recognize that the emphasis on RCTs has been criticized for not being applicable to "real-world" settings (Beutler, 1998; Goldfried & Wolfe, 1996, 1998; Gonzales & Chambers, 2002; Norcross, 1999; Seligman, 1996), and it has been correctly noted that many patients seeking psychological treatment will deviate from the RCT sample in some important ways (Fensterheim & Raw, 1996; Westen et al., 2004b). Whereas RCTs commonly exclude patients for "comorbid" psychiatric conditions (Westen & Morrison, 2001), clinic patients frequently meet criteria for multiple disorders, making it difficult to isolate a single disorder (Goldfried & Eubanks-Carter, 2004; Wachtel, 2010; Westen et al., 2004a). The operationalizing of psychotherapeutic procedures in the form of manualized treatments allowed for greater consistency across therapists, created some minimal

Table 22.1 *Well-established empirically supported treatments: Chambless criteria*

Disorder	Well-established treatments
Attention deficit/ hyperactivity disorder	Cognitive-behavioral therapy
Schizophrenia and other severe mental illnesses	Assertive community treatment Cognitive-behavioral therapy Cognitive remediation Family psychoeducation Social learning/token economy programs Social skills training Supported employment
Bipolar disorder	Psychoeducation (mania) Systemic care (mania) Family-focused therapy (depression)
Depression	Behavioral activation Cognitive therapy Cognitive behavioral analysis system of psychotherapy Cognitive-behavioral therapy (for people with diabetes) Interpersonal psychotherapy Mindfulness-based cognitive therapy Problem-solving therapy Self-management/self-control therapy
Anxiety disorders	Cognitive and behavioral therapies (generalized anxiety disorder) Cognitive-behavioral therapy (panic disorder; social anxiety) Exposure therapies (specific phobias)
Obsessions-compulsive disorder	Cognitive-behavioral therapy Exposure and response prevention
Posttraumatic stress disorder	Cognitive processing therapy Prolonged exposure therapy Seeking safety (with substance use disorders)
Pain	Acceptance and commitment therapy (chronic) Cognitive-behavioral therapy (back; head; irritable bowel) Multicomponent CBT (fibromyalgia; rheumatologic)
Eating disorders	Cognitive-behavioral therapy (bulimia; binge eating disorder) Family-based treatment (anorexia; bulimia) Interpersonal psychotherapy (bulimia; binge eating disorder)
Weight management	Behavioral weight management
Insomnia disorder	Cognitive-behavioral therapy Paradoxical intention Relaxation training Sleep Restriction therapy Stimulus Control therapy

Table 22.1 (*cont.*)

Disorder	Well-established treatments
Substance and alcohol use disorder	Behavioral couples therapy (alcohol)
	MI, MET, and MET+CBT (mixed substances)
	Seeking safety (mixed substance)
Borderline personality	Dialectical behavior therapy
Relationship distress	Emotionally focused couples therapy

Note: A version of this table was originally published in Hupp & Hupp (2023), created in 2023, and influenced by several pages from the website for the Society of Clinical Psychology (SCP) and several systematic reviews. MI = motivational interviewing; MET = motivation enhancement treatment; CBT = cognitive-behavioral therapy.

standards of practice, and allowed practitioners and patients alike to more clearly understand what was to be done. This process, however, raised eyebrows among many (e.g., Fonagy, 1999; Levant, 2004; Norcross, 1999), with some suggesting that these manuals overestimate the degree of homogeneity among patients with a particular diagnosis, forcing a "one-size-fits-all" approach (Wachtel, 2010). Others criticized treatment manuals as a "straightjacket for a talented therapist" (Goldfried & Eubanks-Carter, 2004, p. 670). Aware of these criticisms, some researchers have worked toward including participants with comorbidities, offering treatment manuals that allow for greater flexibility, and prioritizing investigations in real-world settings.

As described in Chapter 1, the updated Division 12 EST guidelines – sometimes referred to as the "Tolin criteria" (Tolin, McKay, et al., 2015) set out to encourage greater emphasis on research in real-word settings. Other priorities of these newer criteria also include a demonstration of meaningful outcome improvement, lasting treatment gains, and other contextual factors such as the identification of active ingredients. Since the publication of these new EST criteria, the evidence base for several psychological treatments has been formally evaluated according to these standards. Psychological treatments that have been evaluated in coordination with the SCP include exposure and response prevention for obsessive-compulsive disorder (Tolin, Melnyk, et al., 2015), CBT for insomnia disorder (Boness et al., 2020), CBT for substance use disorder (Boness et al., 2023), contingency management for drug use (Pfund et al., 2022), and CBT for gambling harm (Pfund et al., 2023). Additional evaluations for psychological treatments are currently in progress. Table 22.2 provides a summary of the results of these reviews, and a current list of completed and in-progress evaluations is maintained by the SCP's Committee on Science and Practice. Treatments evaluated with the "Tolin criteria" are also located on the SCP's website.

Table 22.2 *Empirically supported treatment status: Tolin criteria*

Treatment Target	Treatment	Recommendation
Obsessive-compulsive disorder	Exposure and response prevention	Strong recommendation
Insomnia disorder	Cognitive-behavioral therapy	Strong recommendation
Substance use disorders	Cognitive-behavioral therapy	Strong recommendation
	Contingency management (drug use)	Strong recommendation
Gambling harm	Cognitive-behavioral therapy	Strong recommendation

Note: The possible levels of recommendation are: *very strong recommendation, strong recommendation, and weak recommendation.*

As shown in the table, the treatments evaluated with the Tolin criteria to date have received a *strong recommendation* – but not a *very strong recommendation*. Moreover, very few treatments have been evaluated at all. Thus, the need for rigorous research persists, and the door is open for many more reviews. Our call to action is this: Consider conducting a treatment evaluation using these criteria and submitting that evaluation to Division 12 for consideration as an EST. To do so, a good first step would be to read the brief manual: *The Society of Clinical Psychology's Manual for the Evaluation of Psychological Treatments Using the Tolin Criteria* (Boness et al., 2021), available for free on the SCP website (https://div12.org/psychological-treatments/). The manual describes the next steps, including how to submit a letter of intent to the SCP's Committee on Science and Practice.

Of course, evaluating the empirical support for a treatment with the Tolin criteria is no small undertaking. To aid in the process, there have been attempts to manualize the application of the criteria and offer tools for simplifying the process (Boness et al., 2021). Although there are required elements of evaluating a treatment with the Division 12 Criteria, there is no one "right" way, and specific practices may vary across evaluation teams (e.g., the decision to statistically combine effect sizes or not, which review quality tool to use). The lack of a single "right" way to conduct these evaluations can be a challenge for some teams, particularly in cases where the team lacks sufficient expertise to deviate from the manual.

In our opinion, adequately evaluating the evidence for a particular psychological treatment requires a diverse team with both content and methodological experience. It is valuable to have a team member with expertise in a given treatment for the particular disorder in question (e.g., CBT for insomnia disorder) as well as a team member with expertise in systematic review methodology, including meta-analyses. In ideal circumstances, it can also be helpful to have a team member with expertise in additional or adjacent treatments for the same disorder (e.g., brief behavioral treatment for insomnia disorder), particularly if that person has less allegiance to the treatment being evaluated compared to other team members. Teams might even seek out a member who is critical of the treatment under evaluation as they can bring a healthy level of skepticism to the process.

One of the greatest resources to engage when undertaking a systematic review of any type is a librarian, particularly one with subject matter expertise. Librarians can help formulate comprehensive search strategies and conduct literature searches to ensure all relevant reviews are captured for the evaluation. In some cases, they may also be able to help guide other steps in the evaluation, including the selection of software for screening reviews and extracting data as well as the selection of standardized instruments for evaluating review quality. We strongly advise consulting a librarian early and often in the evaluation process, and even formally including them as a team member. Whether a librarian is included or not, staying organized throughout the evaluation process is critical for transparent reporting and rigorous treatment evaluation.

A final word of advice when conducting these evaluations is to take the consideration of contextual factors seriously. Contextual factors include considering features such as how the current treatment's effect size compares to other well established treatments; whether the current treatment offers an advantage in cost, efficiency, or practicality; evidence that the treatment is effective across diverse individuals, patient populations, and settings; whether the treatment has been studied by a wide array of researchers without strong allegiance to the treatment; and evidence linking the treatment to the purported mechanism of change. These are critical to consider in treatment evaluations because they have the potential to influence the overall treatment rating (i.e., weak, strong, very strong) and can provide insight into what additional work might be needed to strengthen the evidence base for the treatment.

Although evaluating treatments with the Tolin criteria may seem like a massive undertaking, with the right team and robust systems for staying organized, these evaluations are feasible to complete. Evaluation teams are not required to pursue publication of their evaluations, but we strongly encourage them to for the sake of dissemination. As more evaluations are completed, the criteria can also be updated and refined to ensure that the evidence base for psychological treatments is being evaluated with rigor, further supporting the dissemination of effective treatments and the improvement of mental health care for all people.

References

Beutler, L. E. (1998). Identifying empirically supported treatments: What if we didn't? *Journal of Consulting and Clinical Psychology*, 66(1), 113–120. https://doi.org/blatt10.1037/0022-006X.66.1.113.

Boness, C. L., Hershenberg, R., Grasso, D., et al. (2021). *The Society of Clinical Psychology's manual for the evaluation of psychological treatments using the Tolin criteria* [Preprint]. Open Science Framework. https://doi.org/10.31219/osf.io/8hcsz.

Boness, C. L., Hershenberg, R., Kaye, J., et al. (2020). An evaluation of cognitive behavioral therapy for insomnia: A systematic review and application of Tolin's Criteria for empirically supported treatments. *Clinical Psychology: Science and Practice, 27*(4), e12348. https://doi.org/10.1037/h0101780.

Boness, C. L., Votaw, V. R., Schwebel, F. J., et al. (2023). An evaluation of cognitive behavioral therapy for substance use disorders: A systematic review and application of the society of clinical psychology criteria for empirically supported treatments. *Clinical Psychology: Science and Practice*. https://doi.org/10.1037/cps0000131.

Chambless, D. L., & Hollon, S. D. (1998). Defining empirically supported therapies. *Journal of Consulting and Clinical Psychology, 66*(1), 7–18. https://doi.org/10.1037/0022-006X.66.1.7.

Chambless, D. L., & Ollendick, T. H. (2001). Empirically supported psychological interventions: Controversies and evidence. *Annual Review of Psychology, 52*, 685–716. https://doi.org/10.1146/annurev.psych.52.1.685.

Fensterheim, H., & Raw, S. D. (1996). Psychotherapy research is not psychotherapy practice. *Clinical Psychology: Science and Practice, 3*, 168–171. https://doi.org/10.1111/j.1468-2850.1996.tb00067.x.

Fonagy, P. (1999). Achieving evidence-based psychotherapy practice: A psychodynamic perspective on the general acceptance of treatment manuals. *Clinical Psychology: Science and Practice, 6*, 442–444. https://doi.org/10.1093/clipsy.6.4.442.

Goldfried, M. R., & Eubanks-Carter, C. (2004). On the need for a new psychotherapy research paradigm: comment on Westen, Novotny, and Thompson-Brenner (2004). *Psychological Bulletin, 130*(4), 669–673; author reply 677–683. https://doi.org/10.1037/0033-2909.130.4.669.

Goldfried, M. R., & Wolfe, B. E. (1996). Psychotherapy practice and research: Repairing a strained alliance. *American Psychologist, 51*(10), 1007–1016. https://doi.org/10.1037//0003-066X.51.10.1007.

Goldfried, M. R., & Wolfe, B. E. (1998). Toward a more clinically valid approach to therapy research. *Journal of Consulting and Clinical Psychology, 66*(1), 143–150. https://doi.org/10.1037/0022-006X.66.1.143.

Gonzales, J. J., & Chambers, D. A. (2002). The tangled and thorny path of science to practice: Tensions in interpreting and applying "evidence." *Clinical Psychology: Science and Practice, 9*, 204–209. https://doi.org/10.1093/clipsy.9.2.204.

Hupp, S. & Hupp, V. (2023). Science-based clinical psychology. In J. N. Stea & S. Hupp (Eds.), *Investigating Clinical Psychology: Pseudoscience, Fringe Science, and Controversies* (pp. 195–205). Routledge.

Levant, R. F. (2004). The empirically validated treatments movement: A practitioner/educator perspective. *Clinical Psychology: Science and Practice, 11*(2), 219–224. https://doi.org/10.1093/clipsy.bph075.

Norcross, J. C. (1999). Collegially validated limitations of empirically validated treatments. *Clinical Psychology: Science and Practice, 6*, 472–476. https://doi.org/10.1093/clipsy.6.4.472.

Pfund, R. A., Ginley, M. K., Boness, C. L., et al. (2022). Contingency management for drug use disorders: Meta-analysis and application of Tolin's criteria. *Clinical Psychology: Science and Practice* [advance online publication]. https://doi.org/10.1037/cps0000121.

Pfund, R. A., Ginley, M. K., Kim, H. S., et al. (2023). Cognitive-behavioral treatment for gambling harm: Umbrella review and meta-analysis. *Clinical Psychology Review*, 102336.

Seligman, M. E. P. (1996). Science as an ally of practice. *American Psychologist, 51*(10), 1072–1079.

Tolin, D. F., McKay, D., Forman, E. M., Klonsky, E. D., & Thombs, B. D. (2015). Empirically Supported Treatment: Recommendations for a New Model. *Clinical Psychology: Science and Practice, 22*(4), 317–338. https://doi.org/10.1111/cpsp.12122.

Tolin, D. F., Melnyk, T., & Marx, B. (2015). Exposure and response prevention for obsessive-compulsive disorder. www.div12.org/wp-content/uploads/2019/10/Treatment-Review-ERP-for-OCD.pdf.

Wachtel, P. L. (2010). Beyond "ESTs": Problematic assumptions in the pursuit of evidence-based practice. *Psychoanalytic Psychology, 27*(3), 251–272. https://doi.org/10.1037/a0020532.

Westen, D., & Morrison, K. (2001). A multidimensional meta-analysis of treatments for depression, panic, and generalized anxiety disorder: An empirical examination of the status of empirically supported therapies. *Journal of Consulting and Clinical Psychology, 69*(6), 875–899. www.ncbi.nlm.nih.gov/entrez/query.fcgi?cmd=Retrieve&db=PubMed&dopt=Citation&list_uids=11777114.

Westen, D., Novotny, C. M., & Thompson-Brenner, H. (2004a). The empirical status of empirically supported psychotherapies: assumptions, findings, and reporting in controlled clinical trials. *Psychological Bulletin, 130*(4), 631–663. https://doi.org/10.1037/0033-2909.130.4.63.

Westen, D., Novotny, C. M., & Thompson-Brenner, H. (2004b). The next generation of psychotherapy research: Reply to Ablon and Marci (2004), Goldfried and Eubanks-Carter (2004), and Haaga (2004). *Psychological Bulletin, 130*(4), 677–683. www.ncbi.nlm.nih.gov/entrez/query.fcgi?cmd=Retrieve&db=PubMed&dopt=Citation&list_uids=15250817.

Index

www.ingramcontent.com/pod-product-compliance
Ingram Content Group UK Ltd.
Pitfield, Milton Keynes, MK11 3LW, UK
UKHW050238140125
453545UK00010B/38